2014

The Year Book of MEDICINE®

Editors

James A. Barker
Jennifer L. Barton
Kenneth R. DeVault
Renee Garrick
Michael R. Gold
Nancy M. Khardori
Colleen A. Lawton
Derek LeRoith
Randall K. Pearson

ELSEVIER
MOSBY

ELSEVIER
MOSBY

Vice President, Global Medical Reference: Mary E. Gatsch
Developmental Editor: Susan Showalter
Production Supervisor, Electronic Year Books: Donna M. Skelton
Electronic Article Manager: Mike Sheets
Illustrations and Permissions Coordinator: Dawn Vohsen

2014 EDITION

Printed in the United States of America
Composition by TNQ Books and Journals Pvt Ltd, India
Printing/binding by Sheridan Books, Inc.

Editorial Office:
Elsevier
Suite 1800
1600 John F. Kennedy Blvd
Philadelphia, PA 19103-2899

International Standard Serial Number: 0084-3873
International Standard Book Number: 978-0-323-26469-3

Editorial Board

Table of Contents

Journal Represented

Journals represented in this YEAR BOOK are listed below.

Alimentary Pharmacology and Therapeutics
American Journal of Cardiology
American Journal of Gastroenterology
American Journal of Kidney Diseases
American Journal of Medicine
American Journal of Respiratory and Critical Care Medicine
American Journal of Transplantation
Annals of Allergy, Asthma and Immunology
Annals of Internal Medicine
Annals of the American Thoracic Society
Annals of the Rheumatic Diseases
Arthritis & Rheumatology
Arthritis Care & Research
Brachytherapy
British Medical Journal
CA: A Cancer Journal for Clinicians
Canadian Journal of Anaesthesia
Cancer
Chest
Circulation
Clinical Endocrinology
Clinical Infectious Diseases
Clinical Journal of the American Society of Nephrology
Critical Care Medicine
Drugs
European Heart Journal
Fertility and Sterility
Gastroenterology
International Journal of Radiation Oncology *Biology* Physics
Journal of Allergy and Clinical Immunology
Journal of Bone Mineral Research
Journal of Clinical Endocrinology and Metabolism
Journal of Clinical Investigation
Journal of Clinical Microbiology
Journal of Clinical Oncology
Journal of Clinical Sleep Medicine
Journal of Infectious Diseases
Journal of Internal Medicine
Journal of Rheumatology
Journal of the American College of Cardiology
Journal of the American College of Radiology
Journal of the American Medical Association
Journal of the American Medical Association Internal Medicine
Journal of the American Medical Association Pediatrics
Journal of the American Society of Nephrology
Journal of the National Cancer Institute
Journal of Thoracic and Cardiovascular Surgery

Journal of Urology
Kidney International
Lancet
Mayo Clinic Proceedings
Nature
Neurogastroenterology and Motility
New England Journal of Medicine
Oncology (Williston Park, N.Y.)
Osteoporosis International
Pediatrics
Proceedings of the National Academy of Sciences of the United States of America
Radiology
Respiratory Medicine
Rheumatology
Sleep
Spine Journal
Thorax
Transplantation

Standard Abbreviations

The following terms are abbreviated in this edition: acquired immunodeficiency syndrome (AIDS), cardiopulmonary resuscitation (CPR), central nervous system (CNS), cerebrospinal fluid (CSF), computed tomography (CT), deoxyribonucleic acid (DNA), electrocardiography (ECG), health maintenance organization (HMO), human immunodeficiency virus (HIV), intensive care unit (ICU), intramuscular (IM), intravenous (IV), magnetic resonance (MR) imaging (MRI), ribonucleic acid (RNA), and ultrasound (US).

Note

The Year Book of Medicine is a literature survey service providing abstracts of articles published in the professional literature. Every effort is made to assure the accuracy of the information presented in these pages. Neither the editors nor the publisher of the Year Book of Medicine can be responsible for errors in the original materials. The editors' comments are their own opinions. Mention of specific products within this publication does not constitute endorsement.

To facilitate the use of the Year Book of Medicine as a reference tool, all illustrations and tables included in this publication are now identified as they appear in the original article. This change is meant to help the reader recognize that any illustration or table appearing in the Year Book of Medicine may be only one of many in the original article. For this reason, figure and table numbers will often appear to be out of sequence within the Year Book of Medicine.

PART ONE

RHEUMATOLOGY

JENNIFER L. BARTON, MD

1 Osteoarthritis

A Randomized Trial of Epidural Glucocorticoid Injections for Spinal Stenosis

Friedly JL, Comstock BA, Turner JA, et al (Univ of Washington, Seattle; et al)
N Engl J Med 371:11-21, 2014

Background.—Epidural glucocorticoid injections are widely used to treat symptoms of lumbar spinal stenosis, a common cause of pain and disability in older adults. However, rigorous data are lacking regarding the effectiveness and safety of these injections.

Methods.—In a double-blind, multisite trial, we randomly assigned 400 patients who had lumbar central spinal stenosis and moderate-to-severe leg pain and disability to receive epidural injections of glucocorticoids plus lidocaine or lidocaine alone. The patients received one or two injections before the primary outcome evaluation, performed 6 weeks after randomization and the first injection. The primary outcomes were the score on the Roland–Morris Disability Questionnaire (RMDQ, in which scores range from 0 to 24, with higher scores indicating greater physical disability) and the rating of the intensity of leg pain (on a scale from 0 to 10, with 0 indicating no pain and 10 indicating "pain as bad as you can imagine").

Results.—At 6 weeks, there were no significant between-group differences in the RMDQ score (adjusted difference in the average treatment effect between the glucocorticoid–lidocaine group and the lidocaine-alone group, −1.0 points; 95% confidence interval [CI], −2.1 to 0.1; $P = 0.07$) or the intensity of leg pain (adjusted difference in the average treatment effect, −0.2 points; 95% CI, −0.8 to 0.4; $P = 0.48$). A prespecified secondary subgroup analysis with stratification according to type of injection (interlaminar vs. transforaminal) likewise showed no significant differences at 6 weeks.

Conclusions.—In the treatment of lumbar spinal stenosis, epidural injection of glucocorticoids plus lidocaine offered minimal or no short-term benefit as compared with epidural injection of lidocaine alone. (Funded by the Agency for Healthcare Research and Quality; ClinicalTrials.gov number, NCT01238536.)

► Do epidural glucocorticoid injections for lumbar spinal stenosis work to relieve pain? There has been a rapid increase in the number of injections performed in the United States over the past 2 decades. A significant number of injections are received by Medicare patients and those in the VA health care system. Given the devastating cases of fungal meningitis and other infections after the use of contaminated steroids produced at a compounding pharmacy in New England in the fall of 2012 as well as the broad use and expense of the injections, their efficacy as studied in a rigorous, large trial remained unknown until now. Friedly et al conducted a double-blind, multisite, randomized controlled trial of epidural glucocorticoids plus lidocaine vs lidocaine alone in 400 patients with spinal stenosis. The 6-week outcomes of change in pain-related functional disability and leg pain were not statistically significantly different between the 2 groups. It is important to translate these findings into everyday practice.

J. Barton, MD

Milk Consumption and Progression of Medial Tibiofemoral Knee Osteoarthritis: Data From the Osteoarthritis Initiative

Lu B, Driban JB, Duryea J, et al (Brigham and Women's Hosp and Harvard Med School, Boston, MA; Tufts Med Ctr, Boston, MA; et al)

Arthritis Care Res 66:802-809, 2014

Objective.—Milk consumption has long been recognized for its important role in bone health, but its role in the progression of knee osteoarthritis (OA) is unclear. We examined the prospective association of milk consumption with radiographic progression of knee OA.

Methods.—In the Osteoarthritis Initiative, 2,148 participants (3,064 knees) with radiographic knee OA and dietary data at baseline were followed up to 12, 24, 36, and 48 months. Milk consumption was assessed with a Block Brief Food Frequency Questionnaire completed at baseline. To evaluate progression of OA, we used quantitative joint space width (JSW) between the medial femur and tibia of the knee based on plain radiographs. The multivariate linear models for repeated measures were used to test the independent association between milk intake and the decrease in JSW over time, while adjusting for baseline disease severity, body mass index, dietary factors, and other potential confounders.

Results.—We observed a significant dose-response relationship between baseline milk intake and adjusted mean decrease of JSW in women ($P = 0.014$ for trend). With increasing levels of milk intake (none, ≤3, 4–6, and ≥7 glasses/week), the mean decreases of JSW were 0.38 mm, 0.29 mm, 0.29 mm, and 0.26 mm, respectively. In men, we observed no significant association between milk consumption and the decreases of JSW.

Conclusion.—Our results suggest that frequent milk consumption may be associated with reduced OA progression in women. Replication of these novel findings in other prospective studies demonstrating the increase in milk consumption leads to delay in knee OA progression are needed (Table 2).

▶ Celebrities with painted-on white mustaches have decorated the pages of popular magazines with the tag line "Got Milk?" for years. Now, rheumatologists can add to this campaign and ask (primarily older women), "Got OA? Drink milk."

TABLE 2.—Adjusted Mean Decrease (SE) of Joint Space Width (JSW) During Followup by Milk Intake

	Men				Women			
Glasses/Week	N	ΔJSW, mm*	*P*	*P* for Trend	N	ΔJSW, mm*	*P*	*P* for Trend
None	133	0.32 (0.05)	Referent		238	0.38 (0.04)	Referent	
≤3	342	0.35 (0.04)	0.611		473	0.29 (0.03)	0.013	
4–6	173	0.41 (0.04)	0.130		246	0.29 (0.03)	0.025	
≥7	240	0.33 (0.04)	0.820	0.618	303	0.26 (0.03)	0.006	0.014

*Adjusted for age, race, education, marital status, household income, employment, depression, knee injury and knee surgery, smoking, physical activity, body mass index, use of nonsteroidal antiinflammatory drugs, baseline Kellgren/Lawrence grade, weight change, changes of rim distance and beam angle, other dairy products (yogurt, cheese), and intake of other dietary factors (total calories, fat, grain, vegetable and fruit, meat, fish, soft drink, and dietary and supplement vitamin A, C, D, and E).

Reprinted from Lu B, Driban JB, Duryea J, et al. Milk Consumption and Progression of Medial Tibiofemoral Knee Osteoarthritis: Data From the Osteoarthritis Initiative. Arthritis Care Res. 2014;66:802-809.

Researchers in Boston prospectively studied the association of milk consumption with radiographic progression of osteoarthritis (OA) among adults enrolled in the Osteoarthritis Initiative who had moderate radiographic knee OA and dietary information over 48 months. Lu et al noted a significant dose-response relationship between baseline milk consumption, and adjusted mean decrease in joint space width was observed among women (but not seen in men, Table 2). The greatest decrease in joint space width was seen in women who consumed 7 glasses or more of milk per week. Interestingly, the authors did not see the same relationship with cheese consumption and found ≥7 servings per week of cheese compared with no servings in women was associated with worsening OA changes. Information on the type of milk consumed was not available, and it should be noted that high-fat milk may increase risks of obesity or cardiovascular disease. Therefore, frequent consumption of low fat or fat-free milk in women > 50 may help prevent progression of knee OA.

J. Barton, MD

2 Miscellaneous Rheumatic Diseases and Therapies

The global burden of low back pain: estimates from the Global Burden of Disease 2010 study

Hoy D, March L, Brooks P, et al (Univ of Queensland, Herston, Australia; Univ of Sydney Inst of Bone and Joint Res, New South Wales, Australia; Univ of Melbourne, Parkville, Victoria, Australia)

Ann Rheum Dis 73:968-974, 2014

Objective.—To estimate the global burden of low back pain (LBP).

Methods.—LBP was defined as pain in the area on the posterior aspect of the body from the lower margin of the twelfth ribs to the lower glutaeal folds with or without pain referred into one or both lower limbs that lasts for at least one day. Systematic reviews were performed of the prevalence, incidence, remission, duration, and mortality risk of LBP. Four levels of severity were identified for LBP with and without leg pain, each with their own disability weights. The disability weights were applied to prevalence values to derive the overall disability of LBP expressed as years lived with disability (YLDs). As there is no mortality from LBP, YLDs are the same as disability-adjusted life years (DALYs).

Results.—Out of all 291 conditions studied in the Global Burden of Disease 2010 Study, LBP ranked highest in terms of disability (YLDs), and sixth in terms of overall burden (DALYs). The global point prevalence of LBP was 9.4% (95% CI 9.0 to 9.8). DALYs increased from 58.2 million (M) (95% CI 39.9M to 78.1M) in 1990 to 83.0M (95% CI 56.6M to 111.9M) in 2010. Prevalence and burden increased with age.

Conclusions.—LBP causes more global disability than any other condition. With the ageing population, there is an urgent need for further research to better understand LBP across different settings.

▶ The impact of musculoskeletal disease on disability from a global perspective requires careful study of existing literature. As the population grows and resources are not limitless, it is important to focus research on prevalent conditions across the world. The Global Burden of Disease 2010 Study undertook a study of musculoskeletal disease as 1 area of focus. Over 6 years, researchers reviewed the world's literature on low back pain to assess its burden, which they expressed as disability-adjusted life years. The authors found that the number 1 greatest contributor to disability across the globe is indeed low back pain, with an overall prevalence (from age 0 to 100) of 9.4%. Prevalence was higher in men (mean: 10.1%, 95% confidence interval 9.4–10.7) than women (mean 8.7%, 95% confidence interval 8.2–9.3, Fig 2 in the original article). They then broke the prevalence down by region of the world, with the highest prevalence in Western Europe and North Africa/Middle East and the lowest in the Caribbean and central Latin America. Given our aging populations, the burden and disability from low back pain will continue to increase, which underscores the need for intense study to better understand, treat, and prevent this condition.

J. Barton, MD

3 Rheumatoid Arthritis

Does the "Hispanic Paradox" Occur in Rheumatoid Arthritis? Survival Data From a Multiethnic Cohort

Molina E, Haas R, del Rincon I, et al (Univ of Texas Health Science Ctr at San Antonio; et al)

Arthritis Care Res 66:972-979, 2014

Objective.—Despite lower socioeconomic status (SES) and higher disease burden, Hispanics in the US paradoxically display equal or lower mortality on average than non-Hispanic whites. Our objective was to determine if the "Hispanic paradox" occurs among patients with rheumatoid arthritis (RA).

Methods.—In a cohort of 706 RA patients, we compared differences in RA severity and comorbidity between Hispanic and non-Hispanic white ethnic groups at baseline. Cox proportional hazards models were used to estimate and compare mortality risk between Hispanics and non-Hispanic whites.

Results.—We studied 706 patients with RA, of whom 434 were Hispanic and 272 were non-Hispanic white. Hispanics had significantly lower SES, greater inflammation, as well as higher tender and swollen joint counts. Patients were observed for 6,639 patient-years, during which time 229 deaths occurred by the censoring date (rate 3.4 per 100 person-years; 95% confidence interval 3.0, 3.9). Age- and sex-adjusted mortality was not significantly different between the 2 ethnic groups (hazard ratio [HR] 0.96). After adjustment for comorbidities, RA severity, and level of acculturation, mortality among Hispanics was lower (HR 0.56, $P = 0.004$).

Conclusion.—Despite greater severity in most clinical manifestations and lower SES among Hispanics, paradoxically, their mortality was not increased. Further research is needed to understand the mechanisms underlying this survival paradox.

► Over the past several decades, it has been observed that Hispanics with certain medical conditions, such as cancer or heart disease, have lower mortality rates than non-Hispanic whites. This is termed the "Hispanic paradox." Several hypotheses exist for why this may be: the salmon bias (more Hispanics return to their native countries to die), genetic variation, or cultural influences. Molina et al set out to study this question in rheumatoid arthritis (RA). More than 700 RA patients from San Antonio, Texas, were followed from 1996–2000 until May 2010 with a wide range of data collected on clinical disease activity, socioeconomic status (SES), acculturation, social support, and comorbidities. The overall mortality rate was 3.4 per 100 patient years. For Hispanics, the rate was 2.8 per 100 patient years compared with 4.7 for non-Hispanic whites. After adjusting for age, gender, SES, acculturation, disease activity, and comorbidities, the adjusted hazard ratio for Hispanics versus non-Hispanics was 0.56 (95% confidence interval 0.38–0.84). This lower mortality rate was seen despite higher markers of disease activity, higher body mass index, more diabetes, and poorer SES among Hispanics. The authors propose that perhaps genetics plays a role in this variation in mortality, and they could neither refute nor accept the salmon bias hypothesis. This important study points to the need for more study of how and why Hispanics with RA live longer than non-Hispanics.

J. Barton, MD

4 Psoriatic Arthritis

Association between tobacco smoking and response to tumour necrosis factor α inhibitor treatment in psoriatic arthritis: results from the DANBIO registry

Højgaard P, Glintborg B, Hetland ML, et al (Gentofte Hosp, Copenhagen, Denmark; Copenhagen Univ Hosp Glostrup, Denmark; et al)

Ann Rheum Dis 2014 [Epub ahead of print]

Objectives.—To investigate the association between tobacco smoking and disease activity, treatment adherence and treatment responses among patients with psoriatic arthritis (PsA) initiating the first tumour necrosis factor α inhibitor therapy (TNFi) in routine care.

Methods.—Observational cohort study based on the Danish nationwide DANBIO registry. Kaplan–Meier plots, logistic and Cox regression analyses by smoking status (current/previous/never smoker) were calculated for treatment adherence, ACR20/50/70-responses and EULAR-good-response. Additional stratified analyses were performed according to gender and TNFi-subtype (adalimumab/etanercept/infliximab).

Results.—Among 1388 PsA patients included in the study, 1148 (83%) had known smoking status (33% current, 41% never and 26% previous smokers). Median follow-up time was 1.22 years (IQR 0.44–2.96). At baseline, current smokers had lower Body Mass Index (27 kg/m^2 (23–30)/28 kg/m^2 (24–31)) (median (IQR)), shorter disease duration (3 years (1–8)/5 years (2–10)), lower swollen joint count (2 (0–5)/3 (1–6)), higher visualanalogue- scale (VAS) patient global (72 mm (54–87)/68 mm (50–80)), VAS fatigue (72 mm (51–86)/63 mm (40–77)) and Health Assessment Questionnaire (HAQ) score (1.1 (0.7 to 1.5)/1.0 (0.5 to 1.5)) than never smokers (all $p<0.05$). Current smokers had shorter treatment adherence than never smokers (1.56 years (0.97 to 2.15)/ 2.43 years (1.88 to 2.97), (median (95% CI)), log rank $p = 0.02$) and poorer 6 months' EULAR-good-response rates (23%/34%), ACR20 (24%/33%) and ACR50 response rates (17%/24%) (all $p < 0.05$), most pronounced in men. In current smokers, the treatment adherence was poorer for infliximab (HR) 1.62, 95% CI 1.06 to 2.48) and etanercept (HR 1.74, 1.14 to 2.66) compared to never smokers, but not for adalimumab (HR 0.80, 0.52 to 1.23).

Conclusion.—In PsA, smokers had worse baseline patient-reported outcomes, shorter treatment adherence and poorer response to TNFi's compared to non-smokers. This was most pronounced in men and in patients treated with infliximab or etanercept.

▶ It is well known that smoking is associated with poorer outcomes in rheumatoid arthritis and ankylosing spondylitis; however, the impact of smoking on disease activity or adherence in patients with psoriatic arthritis (PsA) initiating tumor necrosis factor (TNF) inhibitors has not been well studied. Investigators using the nationwide Danish registry, DANBIO, examined this question among 1388 PsA patients who had just initiated a TNF inhibitor. One-third of the sample comprised current smokers compared with 41% never and 26% previous smokers. The authors found that current smokers had shorter treatment adherence (over half a year less adherence) and poorer 6-month European League Against Rheumatism (EULAR) good-response rates and American College of Rheumatology score (ACR, 50% improvement—ACR50) response rates compared with never smokers. Fig 1 in the original article depicts Kaplan-Meier drug adherence curves among all patients, highlighting the poorer adherence among smokers compared with never smokers and then by gender with no difference in adherence for women. Fig 2 in the original article reflects the differences in treatment response at 6 months in EULAR good response, ACR20 and ACR50 response for male smokers versus never smokers. These changes were not observed among women. A frank discussion and resources for PsA patients (particularly men) around smoking cessation is needed.

J. Barton, MD

Brodalumab, an Anti-IL17RA Monoclonal Antibody, in Psoriatic Arthritis

Mease PJ, Genovese MC, Greenwald MW, et al (Swedish Med Ctr and Univ of Washington, Seattle; Stanford Univ, Palo Alto; Desert Med Advances, Palm Desert, CA; et al)

N Engl J Med 370:2295-2306, 2014

Background.—We assessed the efficacy and safety of brodalumab, a human monoclonal antibody against interleukin-17 receptor A (IL17RA), in a phase 2, randomized, double-blind, placebo-controlled study involving patients with psoriatic arthritis.

Methods.—We randomly assigned patients with active psoriatic arthritis to receive brodalumab (140 or 280 mg subcutaneously) or placebo on day 1 and at weeks 1, 2, 4, 6, 8, and 10. At week 12, patients who had not discontinued their participation in the study were offered open-label brodalumab (280 mg) every 2 weeks. The primary end point was 20% improvement in American College of Rheumatology response criteria (ACR 20) at week 12.

Results.—Of the 168 patients who underwent randomization (57 in the brodalumab 140-mg group, 56 in the brodalumab 280-mg group, and 55 in the placebo group), 159 completed the double-blind phase and 134 completed 40 weeks of the open-label extension. At week 12, the brodalumab 140-mg and 280-mg groups had higher rates of ACR 20 than the placebo group (37% [$P = 0.03$] and 39% [$P = 0.02$], respectively, vs. 18%);

they also had higher rates of 50% improvement (ACR 50) (14% [$P = 0.05$] and 14% [$P = 0.05$] vs. 4%). Rates of 70% improvement were not significantly higher in the brodalumab groups. Similar degrees of improvement were noted among patients who had received previous biologic therapy and those who had not received such therapy. At week 24, ACR 20 response rates in the brodalumab 140-mg and 280-mg groups were 51% and 64%, respectively, as compared with 44% among patients who switched from placebo to open-label brodalumab; responses were sustained through week 52. At week 12, serious adverse events had occurred in 3% of patients in the brodalumab groups and in 2% of those in the placebo group.

Conclusions.—Brodalumab significantly improved response rates among patients with psoriatic arthritis. Larger studies of longer duration are necessary to assess adverse events. (Funded by Amgen; ClinicalTrials.gov number, NCT01516957.)

▶ New biologic therapies for inflammatory arthritis continue to emerge, and more are on the horizon. One target that has been shown to be involved in the pathogenesis of psoriatic arthritis is interleukin (IL)17, which has been implicated in bone remodeling and inflammation in mouse models of spondyloarthritis. Amgen has produced a fully human monoclonal antibody against IL17 receptor A (IL17RA), brodalumab. Mease et al present the results of a phase II randomized, double-blind, placebo-controlled trial in which 2 doses of brodalumab (140 mg, 280 mg subcutaneous) were compared with placebo with roughly 55 subjects per arm. The primary outcome was the American College of Rheumatology (ACR) score of 20 at 12 weeks. Subjects in the placebo arm at 12 weeks could cross over to brodalumab 280 mg every 2 weeks and were followed in an open label phase for 40 weeks. Of the patients who completed the 12-week study, the majority was female (64%), mean age was 52, and the average duration of psoriatic arthritis was 9 years. Just over half had been on a prior biologic. At 12 weeks, 37% and 39% of the brodalumab arms (140 mg and 280 mg, respectively) achieved the primary endpoint of an ACR20 compared with 18% in the placebo arm (see Fig 1 in the original article). Several other secondary end points showed significant improvement in the treatment arms compared with placebo (change in Clinical Disease Activity Index, Disease Activity Score 28) but no significant difference in dactylitis, enthesitis, Health Assessment Questionnaire, or patient global assessments. Patient-reported outcomes of psoriasis symptoms, the Bath Ankylosing Spondylitis Disease Activity Index, and Short Form (36) Health Survey physical components as well as the physician global did show significant improvements in the brodalumab arms. In terms of safety, there were no deaths, and adverse event rates were similar across all 3 arms, although in the open-label phase, several cancers (breast, metastatic melanoma, lung cancer) and infections (septic arthritis, pyelonephritis) were observed. Biologic therapies targeting IL17 hold great promise for the treatment of psoriatic arthritis and the spondyloarthropathies, and larger trials with longer follow-up are needed.

J. Barton, MD

5 Ankylosing Spondylitis

Higher disease activity leads to more structural damage in the spine in ankylosing spondylitis: 12-year longitudinal data from the OASIS cohort

Ramiro S, van der Heijde D, van Tubergen A, et al (Univ of Amsterdam, The Netherlands; Leiden Univ Med Ctr, The Netherlands; Maastricht Univ Med Ctr, The Netherlands; et al)

Ann Rheum Dis 73:1455-1461, 2014

Objectives.—To analyse the long-term relationship between disease activity and radiographic damage in the spine in patients with ankylosing spondylitis (AS).

Methods.—Patients from the Outcome in AS International Study (OASIS) were followed up for 12 years, with 2-yearly clinical and radiographic assessments. Two readers independently scored the X-rays according to the modified Stoke Ankylosing Spondylitis Spine Score (mSASSS). Disease activity measures include the Bath AS Disease Activity Index (BASDAI), AS Disease Activity Index (ASDAS)-C-reactive protein (CRP), CRP, erythrocyte sedimentation rate (ESR), patient's global assessment and spinal pain. The relationship between disease activity measures and radiographic damage was investigated using longitudinal, autoregressive models with 2-year time lags.

Results.—184 patients were included (70% males, 83% HLA-B27 positive, mean (SD) age 43 (12) years, 20 (12) years symptom duration). Disease activity measures were significantly longitudinally associated with radiographic progression. Neither medication nor the presence of extra-articular manifestations confounded this relationship. The models with ASDAS as disease activity measure fitted the data better than models with BASDAI, CRP or BASDAI +CRP. An increase of one ASDAS unit led to an increase of 0.72 mSASSS units/2 years. A 'very high disease activity state' (ie, ASDAS >3.5) compared with 'inactive disease' (ie, ASDAS <1.3) resulted in an additional 2-year progression of 2.31 mSASSS units. The effect of ASDAS on mSASSS was higher in males versus females (0.98 vs −0.06 mSASSS units per ASDAS unit) and in patients with <18 years vs ≥18 years symptom duration (0.84 vs 0.16 mSASSS units per ASDAS unit).

Conclusions.—This is the first study showing that disease activity contributes longitudinally to radiographic progression in the spine in AS.

This effect is more pronounced in men and in the earlier phases of the disease.

▶ The relationship between disease activity and radiographic progression in rheumatoid arthritis has been well established and has provided a basis for current treatment strategies. To truly determine whether disease activity leads to worsening radiographic changes in another rheumatic disease, ankylosing spondylitis (AS), would require a longitudinal study with multiple time points and reliable measures as well as a relatively large patient population. Rheumatology researchers in Europe report the results of a longitudinal study in which they followed patients with AS over 12 years and collected radiographic and clinical data every 2 years. Of 184 patients who had at least a 2-year interval of radiographic and disease activity scores, 83% were HLA-B27 positive, 70% were male, and 22% had exposure to a tumor necrosis factor inhibitor. The authors consistently demonstrate that disease activity (across multiple measures) is longitudinally associated with radiographic progression in AS (as seen in Fig 1 of the original article) and that this association is stronger in men and in the earlier phases of the disease. Despite this finding, the authors acknowledge that unanswered questions remain as to why there is radiographic progression even in a setting of low or minimal disease activity and what is the true impact of therapies that lower inflammation.

J. Barton, MD

6 Gout and Other Crystal Diseases

Measuring Physician Adherence with Gout Quality Indicators – A Role for Natural Language Processing

Kerr GS, Richards JS, Nunziato CA, et al (Veterans Affairs Med Ctr, Washington, DC; et al)

Arthritis Care Res 2014 [Epub ahead of print]

Objective.—To evaluate physician adherence with gout quality indicators (QI) for medication use and monitoring, and behavioral modification (BM).

Methods.—Gout patients were assessed for the following QI; QI 1: initial allopurinol dose < 300 mg/day for patients with chronic kidney disease (CKD); QI 2: uric acid within 6 months of allopurinol start; QI 3: complete blood count and creatinine phosphokinase within 6 months of colchicine initiation. Natural language processing (NLP) was used to analyze clinical narrative data from electronic medical records (EMR) of overweight (BMI $\geq$ 28 Kg/m^2) gout patients for BM counseling on gout specific dietary restrictions, weight loss and alcohol consumption (QI 4). Additional data included socio-demographics, comorbidities and number of rheumatology and primary care visits. QI compliance versus non-compliance was compared using chi-square analyses and independent-groups t-test.

Results.—In 2,280 gout patients, compliance with QI was as follows: QI 1: 92.1%; QI 2: 44.8%; QI 3: 7.7%. Patients compliant with QI 2 had more rheumatology visits; 3.5 vs. 2.6; ($p < 0.001$), while those compliant with QI 3 had more CKD ($p < 0.01$). Of 1576 eligible patients, BM counseling for weight loss occurred in 1008 patients (64.0%), low purine diet in 390 (24.8%), alcohol abstention in 137 (8.7%) and all three elements in 51 (3.2%). Regular rheumatology clinic visits correlated with frequent advice on weight loss and gout specific diet ($p < 0.0001$).

Conclusions.—Rheumatology clinic attendance was associated with greater QI compliance. NLP proved a valuable tool for measuring BM documented in the clinical narrative of EMR.

▶ The prevalence and incidence of gout in the United States is on the rise, affecting 7.5 million Americans. Choosing the right therapy for patients can be a challenge as chronic kidney disease (CKD) also becomes more prevalent. Quality indicators (QI) for the management of gout have been established and include the following: QI1—initial allopurinol dose <300 mg/day for patients with CKD; QI2—check uric acid level within 6 months of allopurinol start; QI4—behavioral modification counseling on diet, weight, and alcohol consumption among patients with BMI ≥28. How compliant are physicians with these QIs? Kerr et al examined records of more than 2200 veterans with gout at 1 center using data from the VA Decision Support System and a novel technique, natural language processing (NLP), to search for counseling on behavior modification. Table 2 in the original article demonstrates the percentage of eligible patients for each QI and the percent meeting each QI. More than 90% of patients with CKD were started on allopurinol dose <300, yet among those starting allopurinol (572), only 45% had a serum uric acid within 6 months. Of the 1576 patients with a BMI ≥28, 64% had received counseling on weight loss but only 25% on a gout-specific diet, 8.7% on reducing alcohol intake, and 3.2% on all 3 concerns. Gout will continue to be a growing problem in the United States, causing significant pain, disability, and work loss. Behavioral modification and monitoring for efficacy of therapy are essential to ensure high-quality care and better outcomes for our patients.

J. Barton, MD

7 Sjogren's Syndrome

Treatment of Primary Sjögren Syndrome With Rituximab: A Randomized Trial

Devauchelle-Pensec V, Mariette X, Jousse-Joulin S, et al (Centre Hospitalier Universitaire Brest, France; Université Paris-Sud, France; Centre Hospitalier Universitaire Nantes, France; et al)

Ann Intern Med 160:233-242, 2014

Background.—Primary Sjögren syndrome (pSS) is an autoimmune disorder characterized by ocular and oral dryness or systemic manifestations.

Objective.—To evaluate efficacy and harms of rituximab in adults with recent-onset or systemic pSS.

Design.—Randomized, placebo-controlled, parallel-group trial conducted between March 2008 and January 2011. Study personnel (except pharmacists), investigators, and patients were blinded to treatment group. (ClinicalTrials.gov: NCT00740948)

Setting.—14 university hospitals in France.

Patients.—120 patients with scores of 50 mm or greater on at least 2 of 4 visual analogue scales (VASs) (global disease, pain, fatigue, and dryness) and recent-onset (<10 years) biologically active or systemic pSS.

Intervention.—Randomization (1:1 ratio) to rituximab (1 g at weeks 0 and 2) or placebo.

Measurements.—Primary end point was improvement of at least 30 mm in 2 of 4 VASs by week 24.

Results.—No significant difference between groups in the primary end point was found (difference, 1.0% [95% CI, −16.7% to 18.7%]). The proportion of patients with at least 30-mm decreases in at least two of the four VAS scores was higher in the rituximab group at week 6 (22.4% vs. 9.1%; $P = 0.036$). An improvement of at least 30 mm in VAS fatigue score was more common with rituximab at weeks 6 ($P < 0.001$) and 16 ($P = 0.012$), and improvement in fatigue from baseline to week 24 was greater with rituximab. Adverse events were similar between groups except for a higher rate of infusion reactions with rituximab.

Limitation.—Low disease activity at baseline and a primary outcome that may have been insensitive to detect clinically important changes.

Conclusion.—Rituximab did not alleviate symptoms or disease activity in patients with pSS at week 24, although it alleviated some symptoms at earlier time points.

▶ Effective treatment for primary Sjögren syndrome (pSS), a chronic autoimmune disorder manifested largely by dryness of the eyes and mouth, remains elusive. Evidence to support a central role of B cells in the pathogenesis of pSS has emerged in recent years, leading to small trials of B-cell depleting therapy. Given the potential for clinical improvement with B-cell—depleting therapy with rituximab in these small trials, investigators in France conducted a larger, randomized, placebo-controlled, parallel group trial in 120 patients with pSS with a primary end point of at least 30-mm improvement in 2 of 4 visual analogue scales (global disease, pain, fatigue, dryness) at 24 weeks. All patients received a dose of intravenous methylprednisolone 100 mg with each of 2 infusions (active drug or placebo) at week 0 and 2. Disappointingly, there was no significant difference in the primary outcome at 24 weeks between the 2 groups. However, the rituximab group did have a >30-mm reduction in fatigue at weeks 6 and 16, but this did not persist out to 24 weeks. Given the expense and potential for adverse events with the use of rituximab, the authors conclude that this study does not support the use of rituximab for pSS. One challenge for clinicians in interpreting the results of this trial is the lack of a true gold standard measure for improvement in disease activity; however, despite this, there is little evidence to support the use of rituximab in pSS at this time.

J. Barton, MD

8 Systemic Lupus Erythematosus

Prevalence and incidence of systemic lupus erythematosus in a population-based registry of American Indian and Alaska Native people, 2007-2009

Ferucci ED, Johnston JM, Gaddy JR, et al (Alaska Native Tribal Health Consortium, Anchorage)

Arthritis Rheumatol 66:2494-2502, 2014

Objective.—Few studies have investigated the epidemiology of systemic lupus erythematosus (SLE) in American Indian and Alaska Native (AI/AN) populations. The objective of this population-based registry was to determine the prevalence and incidence of SLE in the Indian Health Service (IHS) active clinical population in three regions of the US.

Methods.—For this population-based registry within the IHS, the denominator consisted of individuals: 1) in the IHS active clinical population in 2007, 2008, and/or 2009; and 2) residing in a community in one of three specified regions. Potential SLE cases were identified based on the presence of a diagnostic code for SLE or related disorder in the IHS National Data Warehouse. Detailed medical record abstraction was performed for each potential case. The primary case definition was documentation of four or more of the ACR classification criteria in the medical record. Prevalence was calculated for 2007, and mean annual incidence was calculated from 2007-2009.

Results.—The age-adjusted prevalence and incidence of SLE by the primary definition were 178 per 100,000 (95% CI 157-200) and 7.4 per 100,000 person-years (95% CI 5.1-10.4). In women, the age-adjusted prevalence was 271 (95% CI 238-307) and incidence was 10.4 (95% CI 6.6-14.6). The prevalence was highest in women aged 50-59 and in the Phoenix Area of IHS.

Conclusion.—The first population-based lupus registry in the US AI/AN population has demonstrated that the prevalence and incidence of SLE are high. Our estimates are as high as or higher than the rates reported in US black populations.

► Systemic lupus erythematosus (SLE) is a heterogeneous, complex, and potentially deadly disease that disproportionately affects women. Historically, the severe manifestations of SLE such as renal disease more often occur in racial or ethnic minorities. To capture the impact of SLE, it is important to have accurate estimates of incidence and prevalence across different populations. To date, most studies have focused on differences between whites and blacks, as well as Latinos. Ferucci et al established a population-based registry to examine the prevalence and incidence of SLE among American Indian (AI) and Alaska Native (AN) people, during the years of 2007–2009, through rigorous chart review and the American College of Rheumatology classification criteria (4 or more of the 11 criteria documented) in 3 areas of the Indian Health Service: Alaska, Phoenix, and Oklahoma. The age-adjusted combined prevalence of SLE for these 3 areas was 178 per 100 000, and the age-adjusted mean annual incidence rate was 7.4 per 100 000. The age-adjusted prevalence rates found by Ferucci and colleagues for AI/AN women (271 per 100 000) were higher than those for black women in similar population-based registries based in Georgia and Michigan (196 and 186 per 100 000, respectively). This important study highlights the need for vigilance and heightened awareness of SLE among clinicians caring for patients within the IHS system and for more research to better characterize outcomes in these populations.

J. Barton, MD

Thirty-day Hospital Readmissions in Systemic Lupus Erythematosus: Predictors and Hospital and State-level Variation

Yazdany J, Marafino BJ, Dean ML, et al (Univ of California, San Francisco)

Arthritis Rheumatol 2014 [Epub ahead of print]

Objective.—Systemic lupus erythematosus (SLE) has among the highest hospital readmission rates among chronic conditions. We sought to identify patient-level, hospital-level, and geographic predictors of 30-day hospital readmissions in SLE.

Methods.—Using hospital discharge databases from 5 geographically dispersed states, we performed a study of all-cause SLE readmissions between 2008 and 2009. We evaluated each hospitalization as a possible index event leading up to a readmission, our primary outcome. We accounted for clustering of hospitalizations within patients and within hospitals and adjusted for hospital case-mix. Using multi-level mixed-effects logistic regression, we examined factors associated with 30-day readmissions and calculated risk-standardized hospital-level and state-level readmission rates.

Results.—We examined 55,936 hospitalizations among 31,903 patients with SLE. 9,244 (16.5%) hospitalizations resulted in readmission within 30 days. In adjusted analyses, age was inversely related to risk of readmission. Black and Hispanic patients were more likely to be readmitted compared to white patients, as were those with Medicare or Medicaid insurance (versus private insurance). Several lupus clinical characteristics, including lupus nephritis, serositis and thrombocytopenia were associated with readmission. Readmission rates varied significantly between hospitals after accounting for patient-level clustering and hospital case mix. There

TABLE 2.—Odds of 30-Day Readmission for Adults with Systemic Lupus Erythematosus in California, Florida, New York, Utah, and Washington State in 2008 and 2009

	OR (95% C.I.)	p-value for 95% C.I.
Demographic characteristics		
Age, per year	0.98 (0.98-0.98)	<0.001
Sex		
Female	reference	-
Male	0.93 (0.85-1.03)	0.160
Race		
White	reference	-
Black	1.18 (1.09-1.28)	<0.001
Hispanic	1.12 (1.02-1.22)	0.009
Asian	1.13 (0.97-1.31)	0.110
Other	1.14 (1.01-1.39)	0.042
Income quartile		
Fourth	reference	-
Third	1.08 (0.99-1.18)	0.097
Second	1.01 (0.92-1.11)	0.872
First (lowest)	1.06 (0.97-1.16)	0.230
Primary payer		
Private insurance	reference	-
Medicare	1.57 (1.45-1.69)	<0.001
Medicaid	1.53 (1.40-1.67)	<0.001
Uninsured	1.20 (1.01-1.42)	0.040
Other	1.18 (1.01-1.38)	0.036
Clinical characteristics of hospitalizations		
Clinical conditions		
Nephritis	1.25 (1.16-1.34)	<0.001
Chronic renal failure	1.61 (1.50-1.73)	<0.001
Autoimmune hemolytic anemia	1.06 (0.82-1.37)	0.661
Thrombocytopenia	1.17 (1.04-1.30)	0.006
Pericarditis	1.08 (0.89-1.30)	0.428
Pleuritis	1.13 (0.99-1.27)	0.064
Seizure	1.17 (1.07-1.28)	<0.001
Psychosis	1.11 (1.01-1.23)	0.027
Cancer	1.64 (1.43-1.88)	<0.001
Congestive heart failure	1.40 (1.29-1.52)	<0.001
Myocardial infarction	1.07 (0.90-1.27)	0.439
Cerebrovascular accident	0.78 (0.63-0.96)	0.019
Diabetes	1.10 (1.02-1.18)	0.011
Peripheral vascular disease	1.19 (1.09-1.30)	<0.001
Liver disease	0.96 (0.82-1.12)	0.538
Infection	0.99 (0.92-1.07)	0.847
Length of stay, *per day*	1.01 (1.00-1.01)	<0.001
Community and hospital characteristics at index visit		
Patient geographical location		
Urban	reference	-
Rural	0.86 (0.77-0.95)	0.005
Hospital teaching status		
Non-teaching	reference	-
Teaching	0.94 (0.85-1.03)	0.185
State		
California	reference	-
Florida	1.20 (1.11-1.32)	<0.001
New York	0.77 (0.70-0.85)	<0.001
Utah	0.76 (0.57-1.02)	0.065
Washington	0.91 (0.75-1.12)	0.339

Data presented are adjusted results from a multilevel mixed-effects logistic model in which all of the listed variables were entered.

*Clinical conditions are components of the Charlson-Deyo comorbidity index, Ward lupus mortality index and also validated definitions for infection.

Reprinted from Yazdany J, Marafino BJ, Dean ML, et al. Thirty-day Hospital Readmissions in Systemic Lupus Erythematosus: Predictors and Hospital and State-level Variation. Arthritis Rheumatol. 2014;66(10):2828-36. Copyright 2014, with permission from Arthritis & Rheumatism and John Wiley and Sons, www.interscience.wiley.com.

was also geographic variation, with risk-adjusted readmission rates lower in New York and higher in Florida compared to California.

Conclusions.—We found that about 1 in 6 hospitalized patients with SLE were readmitted within 30 days, with higher rates in historically underserved populations. Significant geographic and hospital-level variation in risk-adjusted readmission rates suggests potential for quality improvement (Table 2).

▶ Almost a quart of all patients with systemic lupus erythematosus (SLE) are admitted to the hospital each year. Readmission to the hospital for many chronic conditions has become a potential marker of quality of care. Yazdany and colleagues examined the important question of 30-day hospital readmission rates among lupus patients across 5 states using hospital discharge data. Of 55 936 hospitalizations for 31 903 lupus patients in New York, Florida, California, Utah, and Washington, there were 9244 readmissions within 30 days (16.5%) during 2008–2009. The authors examined factors associated with readmission rates and found that younger age, black or Hispanic race/ethnicity, and Medicaid or Medicare insurance were all associated with higher odds of readmission within 30 days of discharge, as were more severe SLE disease manifestations, such as nephritis, thrombocytopenia, and serositis (Table 2). In addition, variation among geographic regions was observed with Florida having higher risk-adjusted readmission rates and New York lower rates when compared with California. This important study highlights the need for interventions to improve the quality of care for lupus patients at the time of hospital discharge and immediately after, especially those most vulnerable for poor outcomes.

J. Barton, MD

9 Systemic Sclerosis

Autologous Hematopoietic Stem Cell Transplantation vs Intravenous Pulse Cyclophosphamide in Diffuse Cutaneous Systemic Sclerosis: A Randomized Clinical Trial

van Laar JM, for the EBMT/EULAR Scleroderma Study Group (Newcastle Univ, Newcastle upon Tyne, UK; et al)

JAMA 311:2490-2498, 2014

Importance.—High-dose immunosuppressive therapy and autologous hematopoietic stem cell transplantation (HSCT) have shown efficacy in systemic sclerosis in phase 1 and small phase 2 trials.

Objective.—To compare efficacy and safety of HSCT vs 12 successive monthly intravenous pulses of cyclophosphamide.

Design, Setting, and Participants.—The Autologous Stem Cell Transplantation International Scleroderma (ASTIS) trial, a phase 3, multicenter, randomized (1:1), open-label, parallel-group, clinical trial conducted in 10 countries at 29 centers with access to a European Group for Blood and Marrow Transplantation–registered transplant facility. From March 2001 to October 2009, 156 patients with early diffuse cutaneous systemic sclerosis were recruited and followed up until October 31, 2013.

Interventions.—HSCT vs intravenous pulse cyclophosphamide.

Main Outcomes and Measures.—The primary end point was event-free survival, defined as time from randomization until the occurrence of death or persistent major organ failure.

Results.—A total of 156 patients were randomly assigned to receive HSCT (n = 79) or cyclophosphamide (n = 77). During a median follow-up of 5.8 years, 53 events occurred: 22 in the HSCT group (19 deaths and 3 irreversible organ failures) and 31 in the control group (23 deaths and 8 irreversible organ failures). During the first year, there were more events in the HSCT group (13 events [16.5%], including 8 treatment-related deaths) than in the control group (8 events [10.4%], with no treatment-related deaths). At 2 years, 14 events (17.7%) had occurred cumulatively in the HSCT group vs 14 events (18.2%) in the control group; at 4 years, 15 events (19%) had occurred cumulatively in the HSCT group vs 20 events (26%) in the control group. Time-varying hazard ratios (modeled with treatment × time interaction) for event-free survival were 0.35 (95%CI, 0.16-0.74) at 2 years and 0.34 (95%CI, 0.16-0.74) at 4 years.

Conclusions and Relevance.—Among patients with early diffuse cutaneous systemic sclerosis, HSCT was associated with increased treatment-related mortality in the first year after treatment. However, HCST conferred a significant long-term event-free survival benefit.

Trial Registration.—isrctn.org Identifier: ISRCTN54371254.

▶ Systemic sclerosis with major organ involvement such as lung, heart, or kidney remains a challenging disease to treat effectively and safely. The use of autologous hematopoietic stem cell transplantation (HSCT) to treat scleroderma has been investigated in phase I and small phase II studies dating back to the late 1990s. The Autologous Stem Cell Transplantation International Scleroderma (ASTIS) trial recently published its results describing the efficacy and safety of HSCT in early scleroderma patients (disease duration of <4 years, later reduced to 2 due to recruitment issues) with major organ involvement compared with intravenous (IV) cyclophosphamide. One hundred and fifty-six patients in 10 countries were randomized to either 12 monthly doses of IV cyclophosphamide (control) or HSCT. The primary end point was event-free survival. Over the entire study period, subjects randomized to HSCT had longer event-free survival; however, during the first year, there were more events in the HSCT arm (13 events, which included 8 deaths) than the control (8 events, no deaths). Over the median follow-up of nearly 6 years, the total number of events in the HSCT arm was 22 (19 deaths, 3 organ failures) compared with 31 in the control group (23 deaths, 8 organ failures) as depicted in Fig 2 of the original article. The authors highlight the fact that 7 of 8 treatment-related deaths in the HSCT group were among current or former smokers. It is difficult to look past the 10% mortality rate in the HSCT group when considering therapy for a recently diagnosed patient with systemic sclerosis, and one imagines a future of more personalized medicine that minimizes risk and maximizes efficacy.

J. Barton, MD

Survival and Predictors of Mortality in Systemic Sclerosis–Associated Pulmonary Arterial Hypertension: Outcomes From the Pulmonary Hypertension Assessment and Recognition of Outcomes in Scleroderma Registry

Chung L, Domsic RT, Lingala B, et al (Stanford Univ, CA; Univ of Pittsburgh, PA; et al)

Arthritis Care Res 66:489-495, 2014

Objective.—To assess cumulative survival rates and identify independent predictors of mortality in patients with incident systemic sclerosis (SSc)–associated pulmonary arterial hypertension (PAH) who had undergone routine screening for PAH at SSc centers in the US.

Methods.—The Pulmonary Hypertension Assessment and Recognition of Outcomes in Scleroderma registry is a prospective registry of SSc patients at high risk for PAH or with definite pulmonary hypertension diagnosed by right-sided heart catheterization within 6 months of enrollment. Only patients with World Health Organization group I PAH (mean pulmonary artery pressure ≥25 mm Hg and pulmonary capillary wedge pressure ≤15 mm Hg without significant interstitial lung disease) were included in these analyses.

Results.—In total, 131 SSc patients with incident PAH were followed for a mean ± SD of 2.0 ± 1.4 years. The 1-, 2-, and 3-year cumulative survival rates were 93%, 88%, and 75%, respectively. On multivariate analysis, age >60 years (hazard ratio [HR] 3.0, 95% confidence interval [95% CI] 1.1–8.4), male sex (HR 3.9, 95% CI 1.1–13.9), functional class (FC) IV status (HR 6.5, 95% CI 1.8–22.8), and diffusing capacity for carbon monoxide (DLco) <39% predicted (HR 4.2, 95% CI 1.3–13.8) were significant predictors of mortality.

Conclusion.—This is the largest study describing survival in patients with incident SSc-associated PAH followed up at multiple SSc centers in the US who had undergone routine screening for PAH. The survival rates were better than those reported in other recently described SSc-associated PAH cohorts. Severely reduced DLco and FC IV status at the time of PAH diagnosis portended a poor prognosis in these patients.

▶ Systemic sclerosis (SSc) patients with pulmonary artery hypertension (PAH) have a 3-fold increased risk of death compared with SSc patients without PAH. Research has shown that if PAH is detected and treated early in its course, exercise capacity and survival can improve, and this has led to screening guidelines. Can screening at-risk SSc patients improve health outcomes? Chung et al analyzed data from a prospective registry of scleroderma patients who are at high risk for or who have been diagnosed with PAH by right-sided catheterization. They excluded patients with significant interstitial lung disease. Among 131 SSc patients with PAH followed for a mean of 2 years, their 1- and 3-year survival rates were 93% and 75% (Fig 1 in the original article). These rates are higher than those published previously (72%–86% for 1 year, 39%–67% for 3 year). Factors associated with mortality in this group of patients were age > 60 years, male sex, low predicted diffusing capacity for carbon monoxide, and New York Heart Association functional class IV. Results from this registry promote early screening, detection, and treatment of PAH in scleroderma, which appears to lead to better health outcomes and prolonged survival in this challenging population.

J. Barton, MD

10 Vasculitis

The informational needs of patients with ANCA-associated vasculitis—development of an informational needs questionnaire

Mooney J, Spalding N, Poland F, et al (Univ of East Anglia, Norwich, UK; et al)
Rheumatology 53:1414-1421, 2014

Objective.—The aim of the study was to compare the informational needs of patients with ANCA associated vasculitis (AAV).

Methods.—We developed a Vasculitis Informational Needs Questionnaire that was distributed to members of Vasculitis UK (VUK) by mail and registrants of the Vasculitis Clinical Research Consortium (VCRC) online registry with self-reported AAV. Patients were asked to use a 5-point scale (1 = not important, 5 = extremely important) to rank aspects of information in the following domains: disease, investigations, medication, disease management and psychosocial care. The source and preferred method of educational delivery were recorded.

Results.—There were 314 VUK and 273 VCRC respondents. Respondents rated information on diagnosis, prognosis, investigations, treatment and side effects as extremely important. Information on patient support groups and psychosocial care was less important. There was no difference in the ratings of needs based on group, sex, age, disease duration, disease or method of questionnaire delivery. The most-preferred methods of providing information for both groups were by a doctor (with or without written material) or web based; educational courses and compact disc/digital video disc (CD/DVD) were the least-preferred methods.

Conclusion.—This study demonstrates that people with AAV seek specific information concerning their disease, treatment regimes and side effects and the results of investigations. Individuals preferred to receive this information from a doctor. Patients with AAV should be treated in a similar manner to patients with other chronic illnesses in which patient education is a fundamental part of care.

► Knowledge is power. For patients with chronic disease, of which nearly all rheumatic diseases are, self-management is a critical part of successful treatment, and education and knowledge about one's disease are key. Studies in rheumatoid arthritis have demonstrated that patients want more information about their condition and have a preference to receive information from their physician. Educational needs of patients with rare conditions, such as anti-neutrophil cytoplasmic antibody (ANCA)-associated vasculitis (AAV) are not well known. Mooney and colleagues distributed a survey of information needs that they developed to 2 vasculitis patient groups, 1 in the United Kingdom and 1 largely based in the United States. Not surprisingly, subjects from both geographic areas had high informational needs with an emphasis on disease and treatment domains and less on psychological aspects. Patients preferred to receive information from a doctor and in written form. CD or DVD format was least desirable. When the authors compared the informational needs of the AAV patients to those with cancer, they found striking similarities across domains of information on disease, tests, and treatment. This study is the first of its kind in vasculitis and highlights the unmet needs of AAV patients, who experience significant negative impact on their quality of life and increased anxiety. The creation of literacy-appropriate education materials that describe the disease and treatment and can be reviewed with the rheumatologist are important next steps in the comprehensive treatment of vasculitis patients.

J. Barton, MD

Mutant Adenosine Deaminase 2 in a Polyarteritis Nodosa Vasculopathy

Navon Elkan P, Pierce SB, Segel R, et al (Med Genetics Inst, Jerusalem; Univ of Washington, Seattle; et al)
N Engl J Med 370:921-931, 2014

Background.—Polyarteritis nodosa is a systemic necrotizing vasculitis with a pathogenesis that is poorly understood. We identified six families with multiple cases of systemic and cutaneous polyarteritis nodosa, consistent with autosomal recessive inheritance. In most cases, onset of the disease occurred during childhood.

Methods.—We carried out exome sequencing in persons from multiply affected families of Georgian Jewish or German ancestry. We performed targeted sequencing in additional family members and in unrelated affected persons, 3 of Georgian Jewish ancestry and 14 of Turkish ancestry. Mutations were assessed by testing their effect on enzymatic activity in serum specimens from patients, analysis of protein structure, expression in mammalian cells, and biophysical analysis of purified protein.

Results.—In all the families, vasculitis was caused by recessive mutations in *CECR1*, the gene encoding adenosine deaminase 2 (ADA2). All the Georgian Jewish patients were homozygous for a mutation encoding a Gly47Arg substitution, the German patients were compound heterozygous for Arg169Gln and Pro251Leu mutations, and one Turkish patient was compound heterozygous for Gly47Val and Trp264Ser mutations. In the endogamous Georgian Jewish population, the Gly47Arg carrier frequency was 0.102, which is consistent with the high prevalence of disease. The other mutations either were found in only one family member or patient or were extremely rare. ADA2 activity was significantly reduced in serum specimens from patients. Expression in human embryonic kidney 293T cells revealed low amounts of mutant secreted protein.

Conclusions.—Recessive loss-of-function mutations of ADA2, a growth factor that is the major extracellular adenosine deaminase, can cause polyarteritis nodosa vasculopathy with highly varied clinical expression. (Funded by the Shaare Zedek Medical Center and others.)

▶ The pathogenesis of polyarteritis nodosa (PAN) is not well understood. This necrotizing vasculitis of medium- and small-vessel muscular arteries has a prevalence of 1 to 9 per 100 000 and can affect both adults and children. Elkan et al make the observation that among Israeli Jewish families of Georgian Caucasus ancestry, pediatric PAN occurs repeatedly, and thus they provide a population in which to study the genetic basis of this often severe and life-threatening systemic disease. The authors performed exome sequencing from affected persons (Fig 1 in the original article) from multiply affected families of Georgian Jewish ancestry, as well as targeted sequencing of patients from German ancestry and Turkish ancestry without affected family members. Additionally, they performed sequencing on controls of Georgian Jewish and Turkish ancestry. Through multiple steps of genomic sequencing and analysis of gene products, the authors found that a single gene mutation resulting in the reduced activity of adenosine deaminase 2 (ADA-2) was shared by the affected patients in this study. The autosomal recessive mutations in the ADA-2 encoding gene *CECR1* resulted in a wide spectrum of disease severity among affected individuals in the study, which pointed to other potential contributors to the condition, such as the environment. Of note, a good therapeutic response was seen with tumor necrosis factor inhibitors in 10 of the 20 subjects. They found a high rate of mutation carriers among the Georgian Jewish population (10%), which suggests that there may be many more undiagnosed cases. This important study is a step forward to providing a genetic diagnosis for a potentially fatal disease.

J. Barton, MD

PART TWO

INFECTIOUS DISEASE

NANCY M. KHARDORI, MD, PHD

11 Bacterial Infections

FDA Moves to Curb Antibiotic Use in Livestock
Kuehn BM
JAMA 311:347-348, 2014

Background.—In the effort to reduce the use of medically important antibiotics, the US Food and Drug Administration (FDA) has asked the companies that produce antibiotics for use in livestock to voluntarily change their labels to indicate they are no longer FDA-approved for growth promotion and their use must be overseen by a veterinarian. This would make it illegal for livestock producers to routinely add subtherapeutic doses of these antibiotics to animal feed to enhance growth. Such a move is a major step toward ensuring that antimicrobial agents maintain their effectiveness against human disease.

Proposed Changes.—The change in labeling would be phased in over the course of 3 years and would end the practice of adding low doses of medically useful antibiotics to the food or water of livestock to help them grow faster. Companies have been given 90 days to submit plans for implanting the changes. This practice has been tied to the development of antibiotic resistance and has been widely criticized. Livestock producers have been able to purchase antibiotics over the counter without the oversight of a veterinarian for use as growth promoters, but the change would end that. Many countries, such as the European Union and South Korea, have banned the practice of using antibiotics to enhance growth. The effort to enlist the cooperation of drug makers and animal production facilities is designed to implement the changes more efficiently and without lengthy legal skirmishes. Livestock producers will still be able to add some antimicrobials as growth promoters. However, the proposed change narrows the circumstances classified as acceptable for using medically important antibiotics for preventing disease, stating that the animals must be at risk for a specific agent and treated with an antibiotic that targets that agent for a designated period of time.

Reactions.—The Infectious Diseases Society of America (IDSA) supports this step by the FDA but has some misgivings. The IDSA is disappointed that the changes are not mandatory and has encouraged the FDA to act decisively if the drug manufacturers do not respond quickly. Urgent concerns about the loss of antibiotic effectiveness may spur companies to sign on to the initiative.

Conclusions.—The United States is moving closer to regulating the use of antibiotics for animals but further steps are still needed. To ensure that antibiotics will remain useful for the prevention and treatment of human disease requires not just the reduction in their use for medical conditions but also a change in attitude. Antibiotics should be the absolutely last option whether it is for humans or animals.

▶ It has been standard practice in the United States for livestock producers to routinely add subtherapeutic doses of medically important antibiotics to animal feed and water to promote faster growth. Resistance follows antibiotic use anywhere, especially when used in subtherapeutic/subinhibitory concentrations. There is good evidence that antibiotic resistance on farms makes its way into the food supply and eventually to the human colonizing and pathogenic bacteria. The European Union and South Korea have banned this practice.

In April 2012, the US Food and Drug Administration (FDA) published a draft proposal as a step toward reducing the use of medically important antibiotics as growth promoters in livestock. The latest version of this proposal was released in December 2013. This is considered a major step forward to ensure that antimicrobials maintain their effectiveness. The proposal hinges on the cooperation of antibiotic manufacturers and the animal production industry. Livestock producers have been able to buy antibiotics, including some commonly used in human infections (tetracyclines, penicillins, macrolides), over the counter for use as growth promoters without veterinary oversight. The FDA chose to work with the drug makers and animal production industry to implement the changes. Once the manufacturers make label changes, it will be illegal for livestock producers to use these products for growth promotion or for veterinarians to prescribe them for nonmedical uses. Products like ionophores that are not used to treat humans will still be allowed to be used as growth promoters. The FDA gave companies 90 days to submit their plans to implement the changes and is allowing a 3-year phase in of the changes to give the livestock industry time to find alternatives to using medically important bacteria as growth promoters. Some producers have already made changes in response to demands from major fast food chains.

N. Khardori, MD

Bacterial Meningitis in Adults After Splenectomy and Hyposplenic States

Adriani KS, Brouwer MC, van der Ende A, et al (Academic Med Ctr, Amsterdam, the Netherlands)

Mayo Clin Proc 88:571-578, 2013

Objective.—To examine the occurrence, disease course, prognosis, and vaccination status of patients with community-acquired bacterial meningitis with a history of splenectomy or functional hyposplenia.

Patients and Methods.—Patients with bacterial meningitis proven by cerebrospinal fluid culture were prospectively included in a nationwide cohort study between March 1, 2006, and September 1, 2011. Splenectomy or diseases associated with functional hyposplenia were scored for all patients. Vaccination status, clinical features, and outcome of patients with a history of splenectomy or functional hyposplenia were analyzed and compared with patients with normal spleen function.

Results.—Twenty-four of 965 patients (2.5%) had an abnormal splenic function: 16 had a history of splenectomy and 8 had functional hyposplenia. All patients had pneumococcal meningitis. Pre-illness vaccination status could be retrieved for 19 of 21 patients (90%), and only 6 patients (32%) were adequately vaccinated against pneumococci. Pneumococcal serotype was known in 21 patients; 52% of pneumococcal isolates had a serotype included in the 23-valent vaccine. Vaccine failure occurred in 3 patients. Splenectomized patients more often presented with signs of septic shock compared with patients with a normal spleen (63% vs 24%; $P = .02$). Outcome was unfavorable in 14 patients (58%), and 6 patients died (25%).

Conclusion.—Splenectomy or functional hyposplenia is an uncommon risk factor for bacterial meningitis but results in a high rate of mortality and unfavorable outcome. Most patients were not adequately vaccinated against Streptococcus pneumoniae.

▶ Bacterial meningitis remains a cause of high morbidity and mortality. *Streptococcus pneumoniae* is the etiologic pathogen in 70% of community-acquired cases of bacterial meningitis with a case fatality rate of 16% to 37% and neurologic sequelae in 30% to 52% of survivors.[1,2] Loss of splenic function is an important acquired cause of increased susceptibility to pneumococcal infection. These patients should be vaccinated, and if the immune response to vaccine is insufficient, they should receive antibiotic prophylaxis.

This article reports on a prospective, nationwide cohort study, including the occurrence, disease course, prognosis, and vaccination status of adult patients with asplenia or hyposplenia and community-acquired bacterial meningitis. Between 2000 and 2011, 965 patients were diagnosed with bacterial meningitis. Of these, 2.5% had abnormal splenic function, 16 patients with history of splenectomy, and 8 had functional hyposplenia. All of these patients had pneumococcal meningitis. The proportion of patients with splenic dysfunction in this cohort was lower than reported in earlier retrospective studies. However, the study did show a high rate of mortality and unfavorable outcome (58.3%) in patients with splenic dysfunction. Less than one-third of patients had received recommended vaccination against *S. pneumoniae*.

Because a substantial portion of episodes was caused by serotypes not included in the vaccines and vaccine failures occur in these patients, increased awareness among patients and their physicians and preventive measures are needed to reduce mortality and morbidity. Patients should be educated about the signs and symptoms of early meningitis and told to seek immediate medical attention should they arise. The physician should make obtaining the splenic function status a part of routine history taking.

N. Khardori, MD

References

1. Brouwer MC, Tunkel AR, van de Beek D. Epidemiology, diagnosis, and antimicrobial treatment of acute bacterial meningitis. *Clin Microbiol Rev.* 2010;23:467-492.
2. van de Beek D, de Gans J, Spanjaard L, Weisfelt M, Reitsma JB, Vermeulen M. Clinical features and prognostic factors in adults with bacterial meningitis. *N Engl J Med.* 2004;351:1849-1859.

Cluster of Macrolide-Resistant *Mycoplasma pneumoniae* Infections in Illinois in 2012

Tsai V, Pritzker BB, Diaz MH, et al (Illinois Dept of Public Health, Chicago; Lake Forest Pediatric Associates, Ltd, IL; Ctrs for Disease Control and Prevention, Atlanta, GA)

J Clin Microbiol 51:3889-3892, 2013

Macrolide-resistant *Mycoplasma pneumoniae* is an increasing problem worldwide but is not well documented in the United States. We report a cluster of macrolide-resistant *M. pneumoniae* cases among a mother and two daughters.

▶ The macrolide class of antibiotics is the first choice for treatment of *Mycoplasma pneumoniae* infections. This class is the optimal choice for children because the other active classes, such as tetracyclines and fluoroquinolones, are not approved and/or recommended options. In the past decade, reports of macrolide-resistant *M. pneumoniae* isolates have increased globally. The expanded use of improved microbiological diagnostic methods has likely contributed to this. The reports have implicated macrolide-resistant isolates in individual cases, family clusters, and outbreaks in the United States and other countries with a prevalence of 8% to 27%.[1,2]

This report describes an intrafamilial cluster of macrolide-resistant *M. pneumoniae* infections in Illinois in 2012. The mother and 8- and 10-year-old daughters developed pneumonia that did not respond to macrolides and Cefdinir. Polymerase chain reaction (PCR) for *M. pneumoniae* was positive in all 3 patients. The mother and the 10-year-old responded to levofloxacin and doxycycline, respectively. The course of illness in these patients was 17 days and 11 days, respectively. The 8-year-old did not respond to azithromycin, and the course of illness was 24 days. Nasopharyngeal specimens (NP) from the 10-year-old at the point of care was positive for *M. pneumoniae* by qualitative PCR. Two of these specimens were sent to the Centers for Disease Control and Prevention for qualitative PCR, culture, and macrolide susceptibility testing. Both NP specimens and the corresponding culture isolates were tested for macrolide resistance using a qualitative PCR with light upon extension chemistry and high-resolution melt analysis to identify single-base mutations in the 23S ribosomal RNA gene that confers resistance to macrolide antibiotics. This report further highlights the need for increased awareness among clinicians of circulating macrolide-resistant *M. pneumoniae* strains and its transmission among close contacts. Early detection of resistance by reliable diagnostic tests for rapid identification and antimicrobial susceptibility testing and public health surveillance are both warranted.

N. Khardori, MD

References

1. Li X, Atkinson TP, Hagood J, Makris C, Duffy LB, Waites KB. Emerging macrolide resistance in Mycoplasma pneumoniae in children: detection and characterization of resistant isolates. *Pediatr Infect Dis J*. 2009;28:693-696.
2. Cao B, Zhao CJ, Yin YD, et al. High prevalence of macrolide resistance in Mycoplasma pneumoniae isolates from adult and adolescent patients with respiratory tract infection in China. *Clin Infect Dis*. 2010;51:189-194.

Escherichia coli **O157:H7 Infections Associated With Consumption of Locally Grown Strawberries Contaminated by Deer**

Laidler MR, Tourdjman M, Buser GL, et al (Oregon Public Health Division, Portland; et al)

Clin Infect Dis 57:1129-1134, 2013

Background.—An outbreak of *Escherichia coli* O157:H7 was identified in Oregon through an increase in Shiga toxin–producing *E. coli* cases with an indistinguishable, novel pulsed-field gel electrophoresis (PFGE) subtyping pattern.

Methods.—We defined confirmed cases as persons from whom *E. coli* O157:H7 with the outbreak PFGE pattern was cultured during July–August 2011, and presumptive cases as persons having a household relationship with a case testing positive for *E. coli* O157:H7 and coincident diarrheal illness. We conducted an investigation that included structured hypothesis-generating interviews, a matched case-control study, and environmental and traceback investigations.

Results.—We identified 15 cases. Six cases were hospitalized, including 4 with hemolytic uremic syndrome (HUS). Two cases with HUS died. Illness was significantly associated with strawberry consumption from roadside stands or farmers' markets (matched odds ratio, 19.6; 95% confidence interval, 2.9–∞). A single farm was identified as the source of contaminated strawberries. Ten of 111 (9%) initial environmental samples from farm A were positive for *E. coli* O157:H7. All samples testing positive for *E. coli* O157:H7 contained deer feces, and 5 tested farm fields had $\geq$1 sample positive with the outbreak PFGE pattern.

Conclusions.—The investigation identified fresh strawberries as a novel vehicle for *E. coli* O157:H7 infection, implicated deer feces as the source of contamination, and highlights problems concerning produce contamination by wildlife and regulatory exemptions for locally grown produce. A comprehensive hypothesis-generating questionnaire enabled rapid identification of the implicated product. Good agricultural practices are key barriers to wildlife fecal contamination of produce.

▶ The major reservoirs of *Escherichia Coli* O157:H7 are ruminant animals including cattle, sheep, goat, and deer. Infection caused by *E. Coli* O157:H7 can range from asymptomatic carriage to bloody diarrhea with severe abdominal cramping, hemolytic uremic syndrome (HUS), and death.[1] Infections are transmitted by fecally contaminated water or food (especially meat or produce), by person-to-person spread, and through contact with colonized animals and their environment. Lettuce, spinach, and other ground crops are well-documented sources of infection. Hepatitis A virus and norovirus, both viruses with humans as reservoirs, have been reported to be transmitted by strawberries. None of the berries including strawberries has previously been identified as a vehicle for *E. coli* O157:H7. Consumption or handling of deer or elk meat has been identified as a cause of *E. coli* O157:H7 infection.

This article reports an outbreak of *E. coli* O157:H7 infection with 15 identified cases of which 6 were hospitalized and 7 developed HUS. A comprehensive hypothesis-generating questionnaire was used to investigate the outbreak. Strawberry consumption and shopping at roadside stands and farmers markets were flagged in the interviews. These were quickly corroborated by a case-control study and traceback. Strawberries as a previously unsuspected vehicle for *E. coli* O157:H7 were identified within days of the initial report through matching isolates by pulse field gel electrophoresis. Foodborne outbreaks of infectious disease are likely to continue and are related to local as well as imported food vehicles. Rapid point source identification using standardized exposure elements in questionnaires such as the one used in this study can limit morbidity, mortality, and economic loss.

N. Khardori, MD

Reference

1. Pennington H. *Escherichia coli* O157. *Lancet.* 2010;376:1428-1435.

Clinical Outcomes with Rapid Detection of Methicillin-Resistant and Methicillin-Susceptible *Staphylococcus aureus* Isolates from Routine Blood Cultures

Nicolsen NC, LeCroy N, Alby K, et al (UNC Health Care, Chapel Hill, NC; et al)
J Clin Microbiol 51:4126-4129, 2013

Staphylococcus aureus is a common cause of bacteremia, with a substantial impact on morbidity and mortality. Because of increasing rates of methicillin-resistant *Staphylococcus aureus*, vancomycin has become the standard empirical therapy. However, beta-lactam antibiotics remain the best treatment choice for methicillin-susceptible strains. Placing patients quickly on the optimal therapy is one goal of antimicrobial stewardship. This retrospective, observational, single-center study compared 33 control patients utilizing only traditional full-susceptibility methodology to 22 case patients utilizing rapid methodology with CHROMagar medium to detect and differentiate methicillin-resistant and methicillin-susceptible *Staphylococcus aureus* strains hours before full susceptibilities were reported. The time to targeted therapy was statistically significantly different between control patients (mean, 56.5 ± 13.6 h) and case patients (44.3 ± 17.9 h) ($P = 0.006$). Intensive care unit status, time of day results emerged, and patient age did not make a difference in time to targeted therapy, either singly or in combination. Neither length of stay ($P = 0.61$) nor survival ($P = 1.0$) was statistically significantly different. Rapid testing yielded a significant result, with a difference of 12.2 h to targeted therapy. However, there is still room for improvement, as the difference in time to susceptibility test result between the full traditional methodology and CHROMagar was even larger (26.5 h). This study supports the hypothesis that rapid testing plays a role in antimicrobial stewardship by getting patients on targeted therapy faster.

► Bacteremia caused by *Staphylococcus aureus* is associated with a high incidence of morbidity and mortality.[1] Some studies have found that methicillin-resistant *S aureus* (MRSA) bacteremia causes a significantly higher mortality rate than that caused by methicillin-susceptible *S aureus* (MSSA).[2] Based on the increasing rates of MRSA in the hospitals and communities, vancomycin has been standard presumptive therapy for gram-positive bacteremias until methicillin resistance is excluded. Once susceptibility testing is available, appropriate targeted therapy for MRSA and MSSA bacteremia differ. For MSSA bacteremia, oxacillin, nafcillin, and first-generation cephalosporin like cefazolin have shown superiority over vancomycin,[3] and for MRSA, Vancomycin may be ineffective if MICS are higher than 1. Placing patients on appropriate targeted therapy is delayed by the time it takes for conventional methods to identify and determine antimicrobial susceptibilities.

This retrospective, observational, single-center study reports a culture-based rapid susceptibility screen (CHROMagar) and its impact on the overall patient care. The clinical endpoints were time to targeted therapy, length of stay, and survival. There was a significant decrease (12.2 h) in the time to targeted therapy attributable to the utilization of the CHROMagar method. Studies like this bring to focus the value of rapid testing in infectious disease. Many tests, including molecular methodologies are available for the rapid determination MRSA versus MSSA in positive blood cultures. Any institution's choice of the test depends on a number of factors including cost. However, collaboration between the laboratory and clinicians is needed to find the most optimal way of improving the treatment strategies for *S aureus* bacteremia. Earlier use of targeted therapy should be seen as having a significant role in antimicrobial stewardship.

N. Khardori, MD

References

1. van Hal SJ, Jensen SO, Vaska VL, Espedido BA, Paterson DL, Gosbell IB. Predictors of mortality in *Staphylococcus aureus* bacteremia. *Clin Microbiol Rev.* 2012; 25:362-386.

2. Blot SI, Vandewoude KH, Hoste EA, Colardyn FA. Outcome and attributable mortality in critically ill patients with bacteremia involving methicillin-susceptible and methicillin-resistant *Staphylococcus aureus*. *Arch Intern Med*. 2002;162:2229-2235.
3. Schweizer ML, Furuno JP, Harris AD, et al. Comparative effectiveness of nafcillin or cefazolin versus vancomycin in methicillin-susceptible *Staphylococcus aureus* bacteremia. *BMC Infect Dis*. 2011;11:279-285.

Laboratory Diagnosis of *Clostridium difficile* Infections: There Is Light at the End of the Colon

Brecher SM, Novak-Weekley SM, Nagy E (VA Boston Healthcare System, West Roxbury, MA; Southern California Permanente Med Group, North Hollywood, CA; Univ of Szeged, Hungary)
Clin Infect Dis 57:1175-1181, 2013

Single molecular or multistep assays (glutamate dehydrogenase, toxin A/B, ± molecular) are recommended for the diagnosis of CDI in patients with clinically significant diarrhea. Rapid and accurate tests can improve resource allocations and improve patient care. Enzyme immunoassay (EIA) for toxins A/B is too insensitive for use as a stand-alone assay. This guideline will examine the use of molecular tests and multitest algorithms for the diagnosis of *Clostridium difficile* infection (CDI). These new tests, alone or in a multistep algorithm consisting of >1 assay, are more expensive than the older EIA assays; however, rapid and accurate testing can save money overall by initiating appropriate treatment and infection control protocols sooner and by possibly reducing length of hospital stay. We recommend testing only unformed stool in patients with clinically significant diarrhea by a molecular method or by a 2- to 3-step algorithm (Tables 1, 3 and 7).

▶ Diagnostic testing for *Clostridium difficile* infection (CDI) has expanded and improved dramatically in the last 3 years. In the past, enzyme immunoassays (EIAs) for toxin A/B were done as a stand-alone test. This practice has changed to the use of a molecular assay (polymerase chain reaction/loop-mediated

TABLE 1.—Risk Assessment: Does My Patient Have *Clostridium difficile* Infection?

Risk Factor	Significance	Comment
Currently on antibiotics	High	Certain antibiotics have greater risk than others
Antibiotics in last 2 mo[45]	Moderate	All recent antibiotic use important
≥3 UF BMs per 24 h	Case definition	As CDI severity increases, number of UF BMs increases
Leukocytosis	High	As CDI severity increases, WBC usually increases
Creatinine ≥1.5 times premorbid level	Moderate	Renal disease associated with CDI
Decreasing albumin	Moderate	Protein loss associated with CDI

Abbreviations: BM, bowel movement; CDI, *Clostridium difficile* infection; UF, unformed; WBC, white blood cell.
Editor's Note: Please refer to original journal article for full references.

TABLE 3.—Performance Characteristics: Results for Different Testing Strategies

Assay(s)	Sensitivity,%	Specificity,%	References[a]
Toxin A/B alone	32–98.7	84–100	[16, 23, 46–50]
GDH and toxin A/B EIA	41–92	94–100	[24, 46, 51]
GDH/toxin A/B EIA and molecular	68–100	97–100	[26, 27, 51]
Molecular alone	73–100	91–100	[27, 46, 51–56]

Abbreviations: EIA, enzyme immunoassay; GDH, glutamate dehydrogenase.
Editor's Note: Please refer to original journal article for full references.
[a]Reference list is not inclusive of all published studies.
Reprinted from Brecher SM, Novak-Weekley SM, Nagy E. Laboratory Diagnosis of Clostridium difficile Infections: There Is Light at the End of the Colon. Clin Infect Dis. 2013;57:1175-1181, by permission of the Infectious Diseases Society of America.

TABLE 7.—Summary and Recommendations

Test only loose (Brecher guidelines) or liquid stool specimens
Only test stool from patients with clinically significant diarrhea
Perform a single molecular test or a 2- to 3-step algorithm
Test 1 stool sample per patient per week unless there are clinically compelling reasons to test another sample
Do not perform a test of cure
Create a *Clostridium difficile* infection management team

Reprinted from Brecher SM, Novak-Weekley SM, Nagy E. Laboratory Diagnosis of Clostridium difficile Infections: There Is Light at the End of the Colon. Clin Infect Dis. 2013;57:1175-1181, by permission of the Infectious Diseases Society of America.

isothermal amplification) or a multistep assay (glutamate dehydrogenase), toxin A/b =/- molecular. The algorithm approach is cost saving because it decreases the number of specimens tested by currently expensive molecular assay.

This practice guideline gives a step-by-step reasoning and approach to the laboratory diagnosis of CDI. Table 1 gives the risk assessment for initiating testing for CDI. They recommend testing only unformed stool in patients with clinically significant diarrhea (CDI defined as ≥3 unformed stool samples within 24 hours in patients who also have risk factors as noted in Table 1). Table 3 shows the performance characteristic for different testing strategies. Summary recommendations are given in Table 7. It is likely that as they become more universally available and less expensive, molecular tests will replace multistep algorithms for the diagnosis of CDI.

N. Khardori, MD

An Ongoing National Intervention to Contain the Spread of Carbapenem-Resistant Enterobacteriaceae

Schwaber MJ, Carmeli Y (Natl Ctr for Infection Control, Tel Aviv, Israel)
Clin Infect Dis 58:697-703, 2014

In 2007, the Israel Ministry of Health initiated a nationwide intervention aimed at containing the spread of carbapenem-resistant Enterobacteriaceae (CRE), primarily manifested by the rapid dissemination of a single clone of *Klebsiella pneumoniae*. Data were gathered from acute and long-term care facilities, and ward-based mandatory guidelines for carrier isolation, patient and staff cohorting, and active surveillance were issued. Guidelines were issued to the microbiology laboratories delineating procedures for identifying CRE and carbapenemase production. A protocol for ruling out continued carriage in known carriers was established. Compliance with national guidelines was overseen via site visits at healthcare facilities, routine reporting of carrier census and isolation status, and the establishment of a network of communications to facilitate reporting on identified carriage, contact tracing and screening, and outbreak investigations. During the intervention, nosocomial CRE acquisition in acute care declined from a monthly high of 55.5 to an annual low of 4.8 cases per 100 000 patient-days ($P < .001$) (Fig 3).

▶ The emergence and spread of carbapenem-resistant Enterobacteriaceae (CRE) including *Klebsiella pneumoniae* and *Escherichia coli* in the last few years has become a major challenge because of the absolute paucity of effective and/or safe agents available currently. The crude mortality rate from these infections ranges from 46% to 70% with attributable mortality of 50% for bacteremia.[1]

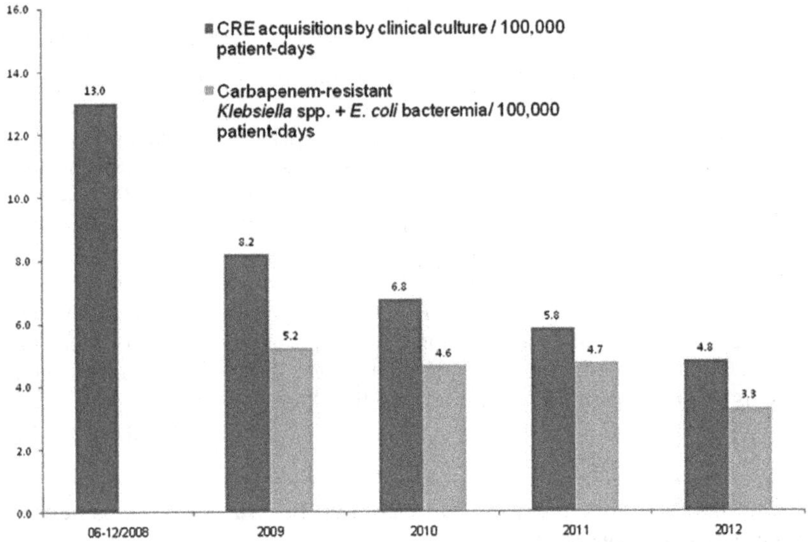

FIGURE 3.—Annual nosocomial incidence of carbapenem-resistant Enterobacteriaceae (CRE) detected by clinical culture and annual incidence of bacteremia per 100 000 patient-days in acute care hospitals. The blue bars represent annual incidence of nosocomial CRE detected by clinical culture per 100 000 patient-days in acute care hospitals, as determined by the daily census reports. The red bars represent incidence of bacteremia caused by carbapenemresistant *Klebsiella* species and *Escherichia coli* per 100 000 patient-days in acute care hospitals, as determined by monthly reporting of single-patient incidence of bacteremia caused by these pathogens. (Reprinted from Schwaber MJ, Carmeli Y. An ongoing national intervention to contain the spread of carbapenem-resistant enterobacteriaceae. *Clin Infect Dis.* 2014;58:697-703, by permission of the Infectious Diseases Society of America.)

This report from Israel using a multifaceted and comprehensive approach can serve as a model showing that even when CRE has become endemic, its spread can be contained, and safety in the health care setting can be re-established. It also serves as a warning and a tool for nations in which CRE is still rare or absent. A proactive centralized plan for detection and isolation of CRE would be optimal. In this report of a nationwide intervention with focus on both the laboratory testing and transmission prevention of CRE in both acute care hospitals and long-term care facilities, resulted in local and overall dramatic reduction in infections caused by CRE. The monthly CRE acquisition rates in acute care hospitals decreased from 55.5 per 100 000 patients to 11.7 over 1 year. The incidence further declined to an annual low of 4.8 per 100 000 patient days in 2012. The success of the intervention resulted in decline of 37% in bacteremia caused by carbapenem-resistant *Klebsiella* species and *E coli* (Fig 3).

N. Khardori, MD

Reference

1. Ben-David D, Kordevani R, Keller N, et al. Outcome of carbapenem resistant Klebsiella pneumoniae bloodstream infections. *Clin Microbiol Infect.* 2012;18: 54-60.

Distinguishing Community-Associated From Hospital-Associated *Clostridium difficile* Infections in Children: Implications for Public Health Surveillance

Tschudin-Sutter S, Tamma PD, Naegeli AN, et al (Johns Hopkins Univ School of Medicine, Baltimore, MD)

Clin Infect Dis 57:1665-1672, 2013

Background.—Children are increasingly recognized as being at risk for *C. difficile* infection (CDI), even without prior exposure to antibiotics or the healthcare environment. We aimed to distinguish risk factors, clinical course, and outcomes between healthcare facility-associated (HA) and community-associated (CA) CDI.

Methods.—This was a retrospective, observational cohort study conducted at the Johns Hopkins Children's Center, Baltimore, Maryland. All inpatients, aged ≥1 year, hospitalized from July 2003 to July 2012 and diagnosed with CDI based on clinical characteristics and confirmatory laboratory testing were included. The main outcome was CDI, categorized as HA-CDI, CA-CDI, and "indeterminate" (classified as disease onset in the community, 4–12 weeks from hospital discharge).

Results.—Two hundred two pediatric inpatients were diagnosed with CDI, of whom 38 had CA-CDI, 144 had HA-CDI, and 20 had indeterminate CDI. Children with indeterminate CDI had baseline characteristics similar to those identified for HA-CDI. Children hospitalized with CA-CDI were less likely to have comorbidities (odds ratio [OR], 0.14; 95% confidence interval [CI], .03–.65; $P = .013$), to have been exposed to antibiotics (OR, 0.17; 95% CI, .07–.44; $P < .001$), or prior surgeries (OR,

0.03; 95% CI, .00–.24; $P = .001$), compared to children with HA-CDI. Compared with HA-CDI, children with CA-CDI had a trend toward more episodes of septic shock ($P = .07$), toxic megacolon ($P = .04$), and recurrences ($P = .04$).

Conclusions.—In a hospitalized cohort, CA-CDI is more often seen in previously healthy children without antibiotic exposure or comorbid conditions and has more frequent complications and recurrences compared to HA-CDI. For surveillance purposes, "indeterminate" CDI should be allocated to HA-CDI rather than CA-CDI.

► The incidences of *Clostridium difficile* infection (CDI), including hospital admissions due to CDI and the number of hospital-acquired cases, has steadily increased in the past decade.[1] CDI in hospitalized children has recently been associated with increased mortality, longer hospital stay, and increased cost. For surveillance purposes, CDI is considered health care facility-associated (HA-CDI) when symptom onset occurs during hospitalization (48 hours after admission) or up to 4 weeks after discharge. It is classified as "Indeterminate" if symptom onset is between 4 and 12 weeks after discharge. It is recommended not to differentiate these from community-associated CDI (CA-CDI), defined as symptom onset in the community or during the first 48 hours of admission and no previous admission to a health care facility in the past 12 weeks.[2]

This was a retrospective, observational cohort study to distinguish risk factors and clinical outcomes of children with HA-CDI and CA-CDI and to clarify where indeterminate disease cases fall. Among more than 200 hospitalized children with CDI, those with CA-CDI were less likely to have comorbid conditions, exposure to antibiotics, or surgical procedures 30 days before disease onset compared with those with HA-CDI. However, CA-CDI trended toward more severe CDI-related complications including septic shock and toxic megacolon. Recurrences were more common with CA-CDI than HA-CDI. The risk profiles of children with indeterminate CDI were more like those identified for HA-CDI, suggesting their inclusion with HA-CDI for surveillance purposes. Among children with CA-CDI, 84% had contact with the health care system as outpatients in the 3 months before onset of disease. No antibiotic exposure was noted in approximately 30% of children who developed CA-CDI. Exposure to gastric acid suppression was seen in 56% of CDI patients and more likely in HA-CDI than CA-CDI cases. The data point to factors other than antibiotics, recent surgery, and the presence of comorbid conditions as responsible for driving the increasing rates of CA-CDI. Among these are the circulation of more virulent strains such as polymerase chain reaction (PCR) ribotype 027, which would also explain the higher proportions of complication and recurrences in CA-CDI in this study cohort. A new hypovirulent strain of *C. difficile* (PCR ribotype 078), affecting a younger population and more frequently associated with CA-CDI, has been reported from the Netherlands.[3] In otherwise healthy children, even without recent exposure to antibiotics, CDI should be considered in the presence of relevant clinical symptoms.

N. Khardori, MD

References

1. Schutze GE, Willoughby RE. *Clostridium difficile* infection in infants and children. *Pediatrics.* 2013;131:196-200.
2. McDonald LC, Coignard B, Dubberke E, Song X, Horan T, Kutty PK. Recommendations for surveillance of *Clostridium difficile*—associated disease. *Infect Control Hosp Epidemiol.* 2007;28:140-145.
3. Goorhuis A, Bakker D, Corver J, et al. Emergence of *Clostridium difficile* infection due to a new hypervirulent strain, polymerase chain reaction ribotype 078. *Clin Infect Dis.* 2008;47:1162-1170.

Spinal epidural abscesses: risk factors, medical versus surgical management, a retrospective review of 128 cases

Patel AR, Alton TB, Bransford RJ, et al (Univ of Washington, Seattle)
Spine J 14:326-330, 2014

Background Context.—Spinal epidural abscess (SEA) is a rare, serious and increasingly frequent diagnosis. Ideal management (medical vs. surgical) remains controversial.

Purpose.—The purpose of this study is to assess the impact of risk factors, organisms, location and extent of SEA on neurologic outcome after medical management or surgery in combination with medical management.

Study Design.—Retrospective electronic medical record (EMR) review.

Patient Sample.—We included 128 consecutive, spontaneous SEA from a single tertiary medical center, from January 2005 to September 11. There were 79 male and 49 female with a mean age of 52.9 years (range, 22–83).

Outcome Measures.—Patient demographics, presenting complaints, radiographic features, pre/post-treatment neurologic status (ASIA motor score [MS] 0–100), treatment (medical vs. surgical) and clinical follow-up were recorded. Neurologic status was determined before treatment and at last available clinical encounter. Imaging studies reviewed location/extent of pathology.

Methods.—Inclusion criteria were a diagnosis of a bacterial SEA based on radiographs and/or intraoperative findings, age greater than 18 years, and adequate EMR. Exclusion criteria were postinterventional infections, Pott's disease, isolated discitis/osteomyelitis, treatment initiated at an outside facility, and imaging suggestive of a SEA but negative intraoperative findings/cultures.

Results.—The mean follow-up was 241 days. The presenting chief complaint was site-specific pain (100%), subjective fevers (50%), and weakness (47%). In this cohort, 54.7% had lumbar, 39.1% thoracic, 35.9% cervical, and 23.4% sacral involvement spanning an average of 3.85 disc levels. There were 36% ventral, 41% dorsal, and 23% circumferential infections. Risk factors included a history of IV drug abuse (39.1%), diabetes mellitus (21.9%), and no risk factors (22.7%). Pathogens were methicillin-sensitive *Staphylococcus aureus* (40%) and methicillin-resistance *S aureus* (30%).

Location, SEA extent, and pathogen did not impact MS recovery. Fifty-one patients were treated with antibiotics alone (group 1), 77 with surgery and antibiotics (group 2). Within group 1, 21 patients (41%) failed medical management (progressive MS loss or worsening pain) requiring delayed surgery (group 3). Irrespective of treatment, MS improved by 3.37 points. Thirty patients had successful medical management (MS: pretreatment, 96.5; post-treatment, 96.8). Twenty-one patients failed medical therapy (41%; MS: pretreatment, 99.86, decreasing to 76.2 [mean change, −23.67 points], postoperative improvement to 85.0; net deterioration, −14.86 points). This is significantly worse than the mean improvement of immediate surgery (group 2; MS: pretreatment, 80.32; post-treatment, 89.84; recovery, 9.52 points). Diabetes mellitus, C-reactive protein greater than 115, white blood count greater than 12.5, and positive blood cultures predict medical failure: None of four parameters, 8.3% failure; one parameter, 35.4% failure; two parameters, 40.2% failure; and three or more parameters, 76.9% failure.

Conclusion.—Early surgery improves neurologic outcomes compared with surgical treatment delayed by a trial of medical management. More than 41% of patients treated medically failed management and required surgical decompression. Diabetes, C-reactive protein greater than 115, white blood count greater than 12.5, and bacteremia predict failure of medical management. If a SEA is to be treated medically, great caution and vigilance must be maintained. Otherwise, early surgical decompression, irrigation, and debridement should be the mainstay of treatment.

▶ The rates of spinal epidural abscess (SEA) have doubled in the past 20 years.[1] The source of infection is hematogenous spread in 50% of cases, contiguous spread in 33%, and unknown in the remaining cases. Spinal cord injury is believed to be the result of ischemia from direct compression and/or disruption of vascular supply from septic thrombophlebitis. Neurologic function at presentation determines the clinical outcome. Many groups endorse early operative decompression and intravenous antibiotic(s) as the treatment of choice because it is difficult to predict who will experience deterioration in neurologic function. However, contradictory arguments stemming from small studies have been published, some favoring medical management only in neurologically intact patients and urgent surgical decompression when neurologic deterioration occurs. Because severe neurologic deficits can occur after failed medical management, randomized controlled trials cannot be performed to determine the optimal management strategy. Early diagnosis of SEA is critical because treatment delay can have devastating consequences. Early diagnosis depends on awareness of risk factors and high index of suspicion.

This is a retrospective review of electronic medical records of 128 consecutive, spontaneous SEAs over a 6-year period. The impact of risk factors, infecting organism, and location and size of SEA on neurologic outcome is compared between patients who initially received medical management only and those who underwent surgery in addition to medical management. The risk factors that predicted failure of medical management were diabetes mellitus, white blood cell count greater than 12.5, blood cultures with growth, and C-reactive protein greater than 115. *Staphylococcus aureus* was the causative organism in 70% of cases, of which 30% were methicillin resistant. The baseline rate of failure of medical management without any risk factors was 8.3%. It increased to 35.4%, 40.2%, and 76.9% in the presence of 1, 2, and 3 or more risk factors, respectively. Overall, more than 41% of patients failed medical management and required surgical decompression. These results strongly favor early surgical decompression, irrigation, and debridement of SEA.

N. Khardori, MD

Reference

1. Darouiche RO. Spinal epidural abscess. *N Engl J Med.* 2006;355:2012-2020.

12 Human Immunodeficiency Virus

Are We Prepped for Preexposure Prophylaxis (PrEP)? Provider Opinions on the Real-World Use of PrEP in the United States and Canada

Karris MY, Beekmann SE, Mehta SR, et al (Univ of California San Diego, La Jolla; Univ of Iowa Carver College of Medicine)

Clin Infect Dis 58:704-712, 2014

Background.—Preexposure prophylaxis (PrEP) with tenofovir disoproxil fumarate and emtricitabine (Truvada) has demonstrated efficacy in placebo-controlled clinical trials involving men who have sex with men, high-risk heterosexuals, serodiscordant couples, and intravenous drug users. To assist in the real-world provision of PrEP, the Centers for Disease Control and Prevention (CDC) has released guidance documents for PrEP use.

Methods.—Adult infectious disease physicians were surveyed about their opinions and current practices of PrEP through the Emerging Infections Network (EIN). Geographic information systems analysis was used to map out provider responses across the United States.

Results.—Of 1175 EIN members across the country, 573 (48.8%) responded to the survey. A majority of clinicians supported PrEP but only 9% had actually provided it. Despite CDC guidance, PrEP practices were variable and clinicians reported many barriers to its real-world provision.

Conclusions.—The majority of adult infectious disease physicians across the United States and Canada support PrEP but have vast differences of opinion and practice, despite the existence of CDC guidance documents. The success of real-world PrEP will likely require multifaceted programs addressing barriers to its provision and will be assisted with the development of comprehensive guidelines for real-world PrEP.

▶ Clinical trials of high-risk men who have sex with men, HIV-discordant couples, heterosexual persons in areas of high HIV incidence, and intravenous drug users have shown that preexposure prophylaxis (PrEP) decreases the risk of acquiring HIV infection.[1-3] However, the results of female PrEP in 2 studies were not promising, raising concerns about the feasibility and efficacy of real-world PrEP. The Centers for Disease Control and Prevention (CDC) has published guidance documents on how to determine eligibility, begin treatment, follow-up, and discontinue PrEP.[4]

Following the US Food and Drug Administration approval of Truvada for PrEP, strong support was shown for PrEP. This study is the largest survey to date of infectious disease physicians' opinions about and practices of PrEP across the United States and Canada.

It is interesting that despite the support for the concept and availability of the CDC guidance documents, great variability exists in the real-world practice of PrEP. The uptake and practice of PrEP are still low, and perceptions persist that multiple barriers exist to adequately provide PrEP. Concerns about risk compensation (ie, practice of higher risk behaviors) negating the benefit of PrEP, resource intensiveness and lack of cost-effectiveness were cited as some of the barriers. These findings highlight the importance of future studies that specifically address the efficacy and risk compensation, which will be determined by the ongoing open-label PrEP studies and future studies of real-world PrEP implementation.

N. Khardori, MD

References

1. Grant RM, Lama JR, Anderson PL, et al. Preexposure chemoprophylaxis for HIV prevention in men who have sex with Men. *N Engl J Med.* 2010;363:2587-2599.
2. Thigpen MC, Kebaabetswe PM, Paxton LA, et al. Antiretroviral preexpsoure prophylaxis for heterosexual HIV transmission in Botswana. *N Engl J Med.* 2012; 367:423-434.
3. Centers for Disease Control and Prevention (CDC). Update to interim guidance for preexposure prophylaxis (PrEP) for the prevention of HIV infection: PrEP for injecting drug users. *MMWR Morb Mortal Wkly Rep.* 2013;62:463-465.
4. Centers for Disease Control and Prevention (CDC). Interim guidance for clinicians considering the use of preexposure prophylaxis for the prevention of HIV infection in heterosexually active adults. *MMWR Morb Mortal Wkly Rep.* 2012;61:586-589.

Antiretroviral Therapy for Prevention of HIV Transmission in HIV-Discordant Couples

Anglemyer A, Horvath T, Rutherford G (Univ of California, San Francisco)
JAMA 310:1619-1620, 2013

Clinical Question.—Does treating the HIV-infected partner in a serodiscordant couple reduce the risk of HIV transmission to the uninfected partner?

Bottom Line.—Compared with serodiscordant couples without treatment, couples in which the infected partner is treated with antiretroviral therapy have a lower risk of HIV transmission.

▶ In spite of effective treatments and control method for HIV infection, the transmission of the virus is ongoing globally. Antiretroviral therapy (ART) prevents perinatal transmission to newborns.[1] It is estimated that in Africa up to half of new infections occur in stable discordant couples where one member is

HIV infected and the other is not.[2] Observation studies suggest that transmission in this setting can be prevented if the infected partner is taking ART.

This clinical evidence synopsis summarizes the findings of 9 observational studies and a randomized clinical trial (RCT). The RCT included asymptomatic HIV-infected patients with CD4 cell count of 350 to 500 with uninfected partners. This group was subdivided into those receiving ART and those whose treatment was delayed until their CD4 count was less than 350.[3] The evidence synopsis uses incident HIV infection as the primary outcome and adverse events as the secondary outcome. The RCT confirms the suspected benefit to the uninfected partner seen in observational studies. A more recent retrospective observational cohort study from China lends further support to the intervention and suggests it to be a feasible public health prevention strategy in developing countries.[4] The durability of protection, the balance of benefits and adverse events associated with earlier therapy, long-term adherence and transmission of ART-resistant strains to partners all remain questions at this point.

In the United States, guidelines from the International Antiretroviral Society recommend initiating antiretroviral therapy regardless of CD4 cell counts for the patient's benefit.[5] The World Health Organization recommended in 2012 that the partners in discordant couples living with HIV infection be offered antiretroviral therapy regardless of CD4 cell count. The recent report of clearance of HIV infection in a newborn (given ART soon after birth) sustained after cessation of therapy adds a new dimension to the benefits of ART.

N. Khardori, MD

References

1. Siegfried N, van der Merwe L, Brocklehurst P, Sint TT. Antiretrovirals for reducing the risk of mother-to-child transmission of HIV infection. *Cochrane Database Syst Rev.* 2011;(7):CD003510.
2. Coburn BJ, Gerberry DJ, Blower S. Quantification of the role of discordant couples in driving incidence of HIV in sub-Saharan Africa. *Lancet Infect Dis.* 2011; 11:263-264.
3. Cohen MS, Chen YQ, McCauley M, et al. HPTN 052 Study Team. Prevention of HIV-1 infection with early antiretroviral therapy. *N Engl J Med.* 2011;365:493-505.
4. Jia Z, Mao Y, Zhang F, et al. Antiretroviral therapy to prevent HIV transmission in serodiscordant couples in China (2003—11): a national observational cohort study. *Lancet.* 2013;382:1195-1203.
5. Thompson MA, Aberg JA, Hoy JF, et al. Antiretroviral treatment of adult HIV infection: 2012 recommendations of the International Antiviral Society-USA panel. *JAMA.* 2012;308:387-402.

Absence of Detectable HIV-1 Viremia after Treatment Cessation in an Infant

Persaud D, Gay H, Ziemniak C, et al (Johns Hopkins Univ School of Medicine, Baltimore, MD; Univ of Mississippi Med Ctr, Jackson; et al)
N Engl J Med 369:1828-1835, 2013

An infant born to a woman with human immunodeficiency virus type 1 (HIV-1) infection began receiving antiretroviral therapy (ART) 30 hours after birth owing to high-risk exposure. ART was continued when detection of HIV-1 DNA and RNA on repeat testing met the standard diagnostic criteria for infection. After therapy was discontinued (when the child was 18 months of age), levels of plasma HIV-1 RNA, proviral DNA in peripheral-blood mononuclear cells, and HIV-1 antibodies, as assessed by means of clinical assays, remained undetectable in the child through 30 months of age. This case suggests that very early ART in infants may alter the establishment and long-term persistence of HIV-1 infection.

▶ Of the estimated 70 million persons who have acquired HIV-1 infection since the beginning of the epidemic, a cure has been documented in one person known as make *"the"* ROM *Berlin Patient.*[1] After chemotherapy, radiation therapy and stem cell transplantation for acute myelogenous leukemia cleared the long-lived, replication-competent HIV-1 reservoirs sufficiently to prevent the discontinuation of antiretroviral therapy (ART) without subsequent viral rebound. A few cases of transient HIV infection in infants have been reported.[2] However, laboratory contamination or sample mislabeling in these cases could not be ruled out by forensic and phylogenic studies.

This brief report describes an infant born at 35 weeks of gestation to a mother who had not received any prenatal care. The mother had HIV infection diagnosed during delivery. The baby was born before antiretroviral prophylaxis could be administered to the mother. The antiretroviral therapy regimen of Zidovudine, lamivudine, and nevirapine was initiated in the infant at 30 hours of age and continued based on detection of HIV DNA and RNA on repeat testing. The infant was lost to follow-up between 18 and 23 months of age. At 23 months, the reports from mother and the pharmacy indicated that ART had been discontinued between 15 and 18 months of age. Table 1 in the original article shows laboratory test results and antiretroviral therapy received by mother and the infant between delivery and 26 months after. The infant's HIV-1 RNA was undetectable in the blood at 29 days and at 23 and 24 months of age. Repeat HIV-1 DNA polymerase chain reaction and HIV-1 antibody test at 24 months of age were negative. The last reported results at 30 months showed undetectable HIV-1 RNA and antibody. The CD4 percentage was normal for age at the time points as was growth and development. This case shows the potential of early ART in infants for arresting the establishment and persistence of HIV-1 infection.

The positive impact of early ART in newborns is further substantiated by a recent second report. The infant was born to a mother with untreated HIV infection, started on combination ART just 4 hours after birth, and had no detectable viral load by 11 days of age. The infant was HIV free at 5 months. The infant in the first report was 36 months old at the time of publication and had no detectable level of HIV-1 RNA at least 18 months after the cessation of ART.

N. Khardori, MD

References

1. Hutter G, Nowak D, Mossner M, et al. Long-term control of HIV by CCR5 Delta32/Delta32 stem-cell transplantation. *N Engl J Med.* 2009;360: 692-698.
2. Roques PA, Gras G, Parnet-Mathieu F, et al. Clearance of HIV infection in 12 perinatally infected children: clinical, virological and immunological data. *AIDS.* 1995;9:F19-F26.

13 Vaccines

Acellular pertussis vaccines protect against disease but fail to prevent infection and transmission in a nonhuman primate model

Warfel JM, Zimmerman LI, Merkel TJ (Ctr for Biologies Evaluation and Res, Bethesda, MD)

Proc Natl Acad Sci U S A 111:787-792, 2014

Pertussis is a highly contagious respiratory illness caused by the bacterial pathogen *Bordetella pertussis*. Pertussis rates in the United States have been rising and reached a 50-y high of 42,000 cases in 2012. Although pertussis resurgence is not completely understood, we hypothesize that current acellular pertussis (aP) vaccines fail to prevent colonization and transmission. To test our hypothesis, infant baboons were vaccinated at 2, 4, and 6 mo of age with aP or whole-cell pertussis (wP) vaccines and challenged with *B. pertussis* at 7 mo. Infection was followed by quantifying colonization in nasopharyngeal washes and monitoring leukocytosis and symptoms. Baboons vaccinated with aP were protected from severe pertussis-associated symptoms but not from colonization, did not clear the infection faster than naïve animals, and readily transmitted *B. pertussis* to unvaccinated contacts. Vaccination with wP induced a more rapid clearance compared with naïve and aP-vaccinated animals. By comparison, previously infected animals were not colonized upon secondary infection. Although all vaccinated and previously infected animals had robust serum antibody responses, we found key differences in T-cell immunity. Previously infected animals and wP-vaccinated animals possess strong B. *pertussis*-specific T helper 17 (Th17) memory and Th1 memory, whereas aP vaccination induced a Th1/Th2 response instead. The observation that aP, which induces an immune response mismatched to that induced by natural infection, fails to prevent colonization or transmission provides a plausible explanation for the resurgence of pertussis and suggests that optimal control of pertussis will require the development of improved vaccines.

▶ After the inactivated whole-cell pertussis (wP) vaccines were introduced during the 1940s in the United States, a precipitous decrease in the incidence of pertussis was noted.[1] A resurgence began during the wP vaccine era, but the pace has increased significantly since the replacement of wP by acellular pertussis (aP) in the 1990s.[2] Recent observational studies concluded that children primed with aP vaccine had a 2- to 5-fold greater risk of pertussis diagnosis compared with children primed with wP.

This study in nonhuman primates provides scientific evidence showing that animals vaccinated with wP cleared infection by a direct challenge twice as fast as animals vaccinated with aP. Neither vaccine prevented colonization or immunity from a previous infection. The second hypothesis for resurgence of pertussis is the shorter duration of immunity induced by aP. This waning of immunity has been demonstrated in recent cohort and case-control studies. These studies show that 5 years after the fifth aP dose, children are up to 15-fold more likely to acquire pertussis compared with the first year after vaccination.

This study tested the hypothesis that current aP pertussis vaccines do not prevent colonization and transmission. Using an infant baboon model, the investigators show that natural infection, wP, and aP all induce high antibody levels. Earlier studies suggest that aP vaccination induces Th2 or mixed Th2/Th1 responses, whereas wP vaccination and natural infection induce a Th1 response.[3] This study shows that natural infection induces a robust Th17 and Th1 immunity. Th17 memory is mediated by a recently identified T cell that specializes in controlling extracellular bacterial infections at mucosal surfaces. wP vaccination in animals that cleared infection faster than naive and aP-vaccinated animals showed similar but weaker T-cell responses. To achieve high levels of protection and optimal herd immunity, the vaccines should effectively block pertussis infection, colonization, and transmission.

N. Khardori, MD

References

1. Libster R, Edwards KM. Re-emergence of pertussis: what are the solutions? *Expert Rev Vaccines*. 2012;11:1331-1346.
2. Clark TA, Messonnier NE, Hadler SC. Pertussis control: time for something new? *Trends Microbiol.* 2012;20:211-213.
3. Higgs R, Higgins SC, Ross PJ, Mills KH. Immunity to the respiratory pathogen Bordetella pertussis. *Mucosal Immunol.* 2012;5:485-500.

Effects of Immunocompromise and Comorbidities on Pneumococcal Serotypes Causing Invasive Respiratory Infection in Adults: Implications for Vaccine Strategies

Luján M, Burgos J, Gallego M, et al (Universitat Autònoma de Barcelona, Spain)
Clin Infect Dis 57:1722-1730, 2013

Background.—The 13-valent pneumococcal conjugate vaccine (PCV13) has recently been approved for use in immunocompromised adults. However, it is unclear whether there is an association between specific underlying conditions and infection by individual serotypes. The objective was to determine the prevalence of serotypes covered by PCV13 in a cohort of patients with invasive pneumococcal disease of respiratory origin and to determine whether there are specific risk factors for each serotype.

Methods.—An observational study of adults hospitalized with invasive pneumococcal disease in 2 Spanish hospitals was conducted during the period 1996–2011. A multinomial regression analysis was performed to identify conditions associated with infection by specific serotypes (grouped according their formulation in vaccines and individually).

Results.—A total of 1094 patients were enrolled; the infecting serotype was determined in 993. In immunocompromised patients, 64% of infecting serotypes were covered by PCV13. After adjusting for age, smoking, alcohol abuse, and nonimmunocompromising comorbidities, the group of serotypes not included in either PCV13 or PPV23 were more frequently isolated in patients with immunocompromising conditions and cardiopulmonary comorbidities. Regarding individual serotypes, 6A, 23F, 11A, and 33F were isolated more frequently in patients with immunocompromise and specifically in some of their subgroups. The subgroup analysis showed that serotype10A was also associated with HIV infection.

Conclusions.—Specific factors related to immunocompromise seem to determine the appearance of invasive infection by specific pneumococcal serotypes. Although the coverage of serotypes in the 13-valent conjugate pneumococcal vaccine (PCV13) was high, some non-PCV13-emergent serotypes are more prevalent in immunocompromised patients.

▶ Infections caused by *Streptococcus pneumoniae* remain a major cause of morbidity and mortality globally. *S pneumoniae* is the leading cause of community-acquired pneumonia in adults.[1] Active immunization with 23-valent pneumococcus polysaccharide vaccine (PPV23) has been available since 1983. However, the effectiveness in children, the immunocompromised, and the elderly is suboptimal.[2] Pneumococcal conjugate vaccines (PCVs) are more immunogenic in children and immunocompromised adults. The introduction of PCV7 for children in 2000 has led to a significant reduction of pneumococcal disease in children and indirectly in adults. This impact has reinforced the hypothesis that children are both reservoirs and vectors for adult pneumococcal disease. The Advisory Committee on Immunization Practices recommended the routine use of 13-valent pneumococcal conjugate vaccine (PCV13) for immunocompromised adults in 2012. The protective effect of PCV13 can be impacted by age, comorbidities, and infection by individual pneumococcal serotypes.

This is an observational study of adult patients hospitalized with invasive pneumococcal disease in Spain from 1996 to 2011. Pneumococcal serotypes not covered by PPV23 and PVC13 were more frequently isolated in patients with cardiorespiratory comorbidities and immunocompromise. The 3 serotypes (10A, 11A, and 33F) that are not included in the PCV13 were the most frequently isolated in immunocompromised patients even though their prevalence among the entire cohort was low. Individual serotypes have been reported to have different clinical manifestations and lead to different outcomes. Some serotypes are more likely to cause oro-pharyngeal colonization and others cause bacteremia more commonly. The incidence of invasive pneumococcal disease in immunocompromised patients can be greater than 20 times higher than those without high-risk medical conditions. Only half of the cases of invasive disease in 2010 among immunocompromised patients were caused by serotypes in PCV13. The emergence of pneumococcal serotypes that are not included in commercially available vaccines and their association with specific underlying host conditions needs to be monitored.

N. Khardori, MD

References

1. Ardanuy C, Tubau F, Pallares R, et al. Epidemiology of invasive pneumococcal disease among adult patients in Barcelona before and after pediatric 7-valent pneumococcal conjugate vaccine introduction 1997–2007. *Clin Infect Dis.* 2009;48: 57-64.
2. Lynch JP III, Zhanel GG. Streptococcus pneumoniae: epidemiology and risk factors, evolution of antimicrobial resistance, and impact of vaccines. *Curr Opin Pulm Med.* 2010;16:217-225.

Safety and Immunogenicity of A Vero Cell Culture–Derived Whole-Virus Influenza A(H5N1) Vaccine in a Pediatric Population

van der Velden MVW, Fritz R, Pöllabauer EM, et al (Baxter BioScience, Vienna, Austria; Baxter BioScience, Orth/Donau, Austria; et al)
J Infect Dis 209:12-23, 2014

Background.—Children are highly vulnerable to infection with novel influenza viruses. It is essential to develop candidate pandemic influenza vaccines that are safe and effective in the pediatric population.

Methods.—Infants and children aged 6–35 months and 3–8 years, respectively, were randomized to receive 2 immunizations with a 7.5-µg or 3.75-µg hemagglutinin (HA) dose of a nonadjuvanted whole-virus A/Vietnam(H5N1) vaccine; adolescents aged 9–17 years received a 7.5-µg dose only. A subset of participants received a booster immunization with an A/Indonesia(H5N1) vaccine approximately 1 year later. HA and neuraminidase antibody responses were assessed.

Results.—Vaccination was safe and well tolerated; adverse reactions were transient and predominantly mild. Two immunizations with the 7.5-µg dose of A/Vietnam vaccine induced virus microneutralization (MN) titers of ≥1:20 against the A/Vietnam strain in 68.8%–85.4% of participants in the different age groups. After the booster, 93.1%–100% of participants achieved MN titers of ≥1:20 against the A/Vietnam and A/Indonesia strains. Neuraminidase-inhibiting antibodies were induced in ≥90% of participants after 2 immunizations with the 7.5 µg A/Vietnam vaccine and in 100% of participants after the booster.

Conclusions.—A whole-virus influenza A(H5N1) vaccine is suitable for prepandemic or pandemic immunization in a pediatric population.

Clinical Trials Registration.—NCT01052402.

▶ Highly pathogenic avian influenza A (H5N1) causes sporadic but severe zoonotic infections with a case fatality rate around 60%.[1] There is limited evidence of human-to-human transmission at this point. However, based on experimental data, only some mutations are required for H5N1 to adapt to aerosol transmission between mammals.[2] Surveillance studies indicate that mammalian adaptation is occurring in nature.[3] The emergence of an H5N1 influenza A virus that is able to spread between humans would be expected to result in a severe pandemic. The pediatric population is at particular risk of infection with a novel influenza virus partly because of a lack of heterosubtypic immunity from the absence of repeated exposures to influenza viruses. The highest incidence of infection during the 2009 H1N1 pandemic was reported in children. Also, about half of the reported cases caused by H5N1 have occurred in the pediatric population. Children play a central role in transmission of influenza because they shed large amounts of virus over prolonged periods.

A Vero cell culture-derived, nonadjuvanted (NA) whole virus H5N1 influenza A vaccine has been found to be immunogenic and safe in adults and elderly populations in multiple clinical studies.[4]

In this study, the safety and immunogenicity of this vaccine in the pediatric population is reported. It was found to be safe, immunogenic, and well tolerated in healthy infants, children, and adolescents age 6 months to 17 years. Functional antibody responses were induced to both hemagglutinin and NA, which primed for robust cross-clade neutralizing antibody responses after boosting with a heterologous vaccine about 1 year later. NA antibodies have been found to be an independent correlate of protection and the only predictor of disease amelioration in infected humans. These data support the use of this vaccine in both prepandemic and pandemic vaccination programs for the pediatric populations.

N. Khardori, MD

References

1. *Cumulative Number of Confirmed Humans Cases of Avian Influenza A (H5N1) Reported to WHO*. Geneva, Switzerland: WHO; 2012, http://www.who.int/influenza/human_animal_interface/H5N1_cumulative_table_archives/en/index.html. Accessed October 1, 2013.
2. Herfst S, Schrauwen EJ, Linster M, et al. Airborne transmission of influenza A/H5N1 virus between ferrets. *Science*. 2012;336:1534-1541.
3. Watanabe Y, Ibrahim MS, Ellakany HF, et al. Acquisition of human-type receptor binding specificity by new H5N1 influenza virus sublineages during their emergence in birds in Egypt. *PLoS Pathog*. 2011;7:e1002068.
4. Barrett PN, Portsmouth D, Ehrlich HJ. Vero cell culture-derived pandemic influenza vaccines: preclinical and clinical development. *Expert Rev Vaccines*. 2012; 30:6127-6135.

A Multi-Component Meningococcal Serogroup B Vaccine (4CMenB): The Clinical Development Program

O'Ryan M, Stoddard J, Toneatto D, et al (Universidad de Chile, Santiago; Novartis Vaccines and Diagnostics, Cambridge, MA)

Drugs 74:15-30, 2014

Recently approved in Europe and Australia, the multi-component meningococcal B vaccine, 4CMenB (Bexsero®, Novartis Vaccines and

Diagnostics), contains three surface-exposed recombinant proteins (fHbp, NadA, and NHBA) and New Zealand strain outer membrane vesicles (NZ OMV) with PorA 1.4 antigenicity. This comprehensive review of the 4CMenB clinical development program covers pivotal phase I/IIb/III studies in over 7,000 adults, adolescents, and infants. The immunological correlate for clinical protection used was human complement-mediated serum bactericidal activity titers ≥4 or 5 against indicator strains for individual antigens. Based on achievement of protective titers, a four-dose schedule (three primary doses and one booster dose) for infants and a two-dose schedule for adolescents provided the best results. Observed increases in injection site pain/tenderness and fever in infants, and injection site pain, malaise, and headache in adolescents compared with routine vaccines, were mostly mild to moderate; frequencies of rare events (Kawasaki disease, juvenile arthritis) were not significantly different from non-vaccinated individuals. 4CMenB is conservatively estimated to provide 66–91 % coverage against meningococcal serogroup B strains worldwide.

▶ The successful introduction of safe and effective conjugate vaccines (serogroups ACWY, serogroup C, and serogroup A) against invasive meningococcal disease (IMD) into childhood vaccination programs in various parts of the world has raised the awareness of the need for vaccination against the remaining serogroup B (MenB). Substantial mortality has been documented throughout the world from laboratory-confirmed cases of MenB disease. In the United States, vaccination of adolescents against serogroups A, C, W, and Y is routinely recommended. The cases of IMD in the United States are attributed equally to serogroups B, C, and Y.[1] The development of a vaccine against serogroup B has been complicated by poor immunogenicity of MenB capsular polysaccharide and antigenic diversity of its surface proteins. The use of protein-based meningococcal vaccine derived from meningococcal outer membrane vesicles (OMVs) to control regional outbreaks caused by specific MenB strains has paved the way for development of vaccines with broad coverage against diverse disease-causing strains.[2]

This review discusses the clinical development program for a multicomponent meningococcal serogroup B vaccine (4CMenB). This vaccine, now licensed in Europe and Australia, contains 3 recombinant antigens, fHbp (factor H binding protein), NadA (Neisserial adhesin A), and NHBAC (Neisseria heparin-binding antigen) combined with OMVs from MenB strain NZ98/254. This vaccine provides broad protection against circulating heterologous strains of MenB. It has proven immunogenic in adults, adolescents, and young infants. The tolerability profile in the most susceptible age groups is well characterized. Concomitant use with DTaP-HBV-IPV/Hib, Pcv7, MMRV, and rotavirus vaccines does not interfere with immunogenicity of any of the vaccines. This is the first vaccine against IMD caused by heterologous serogroup B strains.

N. Khardori, MD

References

1. Centers for Disease Control and Prevention. *Active Bacterial core Surveillance Report, Emerging Infections Program Network, Neisseria Meningitidis*, http://www.cdc.gov/abcs/reports-findings/surreports/mening08.html; 2008. Accessed August 14, 2012.
2. Holst J, Martin D, Arnold R, et al. Properties and clinical performance of vaccines containing outer membrane vesicles from Neisseria meningitidis. *Vaccine*. 2009; 27:B3-B12.

14 Viral Infections

Transmission and evolution of the Middle East respiratory syndrome coronavirus in Saudi Arabia: a descriptive genomic study

Cotten M, Watson SJ, Kellam P, et al (Wellcome Trust Sanger Inst, Hinxton, UK; et al)

Lancet 382:1993-2002, 2013

Background.—Since June, 2012, Middle East respiratory syndrome coronavirus (MERS-CoV) has, worldwide, caused 104 infections in people including 49 deaths, with 82 cases and 41 deaths reported from Saudi Arabia. In addition to confirming diagnosis, we generated the MERS-CoV genomic sequences obtained directly from patient samples to provide important information on MERS-CoV transmission, evolution, and origin.

Methods.—Full genome deep sequencing was done on nucleic acid extracted directly from PCR-confirmed clinical samples. Viral genomes were obtained from 21 MERS cases of which 13 had 100%, four 85–95%, and four 30–50% genome coverage. Phylogenetic analysis of the 21 sequences, combined with nine published MERS-CoV genomes, was done.

Findings.—Three distinct MERS-CoV genotypes were identified in Riyadh. Phylogeographic analyses suggest the MERS-CoV zoonotic reservoir is geographically disperse. Selection analysis of the MERS-CoV genomes reveals the expected accumulation of genetic diversity including changes in the S protein. The genetic diversity in the Al-Hasa cluster suggests that the hospital outbreak might have had more than one virus introduction.

Interpretation.—We present the largest number of MERS-CoV genomes (21) described so far. MERS-CoV full genome sequences provide greater detail in tracking transmission. Multiple introductions of MERS-CoV are identified and suggest lower R_0 values. Transmission within Saudi Arabia is consistent with either movement of an animal reservoir, animal products, or movement of infected people. Further definition of the exposures responsible for the sporadic introductions of MERS-CoV into human populations is urgently needed.

▶ Middle East respiratory syndrome (MERS) is a newly described disease in humans. It was first reported from Saudi Arabia in a patient who died from a severe respiratory illness.[1] In the following 12 months, 114 laboratory-confirmed cases of MERS-coronavirus (MERS-CoV) infections with 54 deaths were reported to the World Health Organization. All cases are directly or indirectly linked to 1 of the 4 countries in the Middle East (Saudi Arabia, Jordan, Qatar, and the United Arab Emirates). Most cases (90 cases and 44 deaths) have been reported from Saudi Arabia and have occurred as sporadic, family, or hospital clusters. Human-to-human transmission has been documented in England, France, Tunisia, Italy, and Saudi Arabia. Coronavirus family, which includes severe acute respiratory syndrome coronavirus (SARS-CoV) described in 2002, infects birds and mammals. The source of SARS-CoV infection for humans is probably bats.

Not much is known at this point about the molecular evolution of MERS-CoV and its relationship to virus transmission. This study reports the genetic analysis of MERS-CoV genomes obtained directly from 21 patients with MERS from Saudi Arabia and assesses the spatiotemporal distribution of the causative MERS-CoV in Saudi Arabia. The findings show that at least 2 distinct lineages were circulating in Riyadh in October 2012, and transmission patterns in the epidemic are consistent with both human-to-human transmission and sporadic zoonotic events. Calculations with the larger set of MERS-CoV sequences provided an estimate of the emergence of MERS-CoV in July 2011. Analysis of short sequences suggested that the MERS-CoV may have an ancestor in bats. MERS-CoV has not yet been identified in any animal sources, and the evolutionary rate from this study shows a substantial period, as these viruses shared a common ancestor suggesting the possibility of an intermediary host as the source of human infection.

N. Khardori, MD

Reference

1. Zaki AM, van Boheemen S, Bestebroer TM, Osterhaus AD, Fouchier RA. Isolation of a novel coronavirus from a man with pneumonia in Saudi Arabia. *N Engl J Med.* 2012;367:1814-1820.

A common solution to group 2 influenza virus neutralization

Friesen RHE, Lee PS, Stoop EJM, et al (Crucell Vaccine Inst, Leiden, The Netherlands; The Scripps Res Inst, La Jolla, CA; et al)

Proc Natl Acad Sci U S A 111:445-450, 2014

The discovery and characterization of broadly neutralizing antibodies (bnAbs) against influenza viruses have raised hopes for the development of monoclonal antibody (mAb)-based immunotherapy and the design of universal influenza vaccines. Only one human bnAb (CR8020) specifically recognizing group 2 influenza A viruses has been previously characterized that binds to a highly conserved epitope at the base of the hemagglutinin (HA) stem and has neutralizing activity against H3, H7, and H10 viruses. Here, we report a second group 2 bnAb, CR8043, which was derived from a different germ-line gene encoding a highly divergent amino acid sequence. CR8043 has in vitro neutralizing activity against H3 and H10 viruses and protects mice against challenge with a lethal dose of H3N2 and H7N7 viruses. The crystal structure and EM reconstructions of the

CR8043-H3 HA complex revealed that CR8043 binds to a site similar to the CR8020 epitope but uses an alternative angle of approach and a distinct set of interactions. The identification of another antibody against the group 2 stem epitope suggests that this conserved site of vulnerability has great potential for design of therapeutics and vaccines.

► The 2 major hurdles to the control of annual epidemic and pandemic influenza are the suboptimal protective efficacy of the vaccine in the groups at the highest risk and the need for update to the vaccines annually because of to strain specificity of the neutralizing protective antibody. The recent discovery and characterization of broadly neutralizing antibodies (6nAbs) against influenza viruses are the most hopeful steps toward the design of universal influenza vaccines and development of monoclonal antibody (mAb)-based immunotherapy. The human 6nAbs recognize nearly invariant epitopes of influenza A viruses and would cross the barrier between groups and subtypes. So far, only one, 6nAb CR8020 has been structurally characterized.[1]

In this study, a second 6nAb, CR8043 was isolated from the same donor as CR8020 and has broadly neutralizing activity against group 2 influenza virus subtypes. Both these broadly neutralizing antibodies interfere with virus infectivity by inhibiting HA0 maturation as well as the ph-triggered conformational rearrangements in hemagglutinin (HA) that are required for membrane fusion. These antibodies bind to the membrane-proximal HA stem region rather than the immunodominant HA head region, which has high mutation rates. The influenza antibodies elicited by currently available vaccines target the HA head and are typically only effective against strains closely related to the vaccine strain. CR8043 protects mice against lethal challenge with H3 and H7 viruses and has in vitro activity against H3 and H10 viruses.

The identification of this second 6nAb against influenza viruses and its target site pave the way for development of broad-spectrum vaccines and monoclonal antibodies, respectively, for prevention and treatment of a worldwide epidemic and potential pandemic disease.

N. Khardori, MD

Reference

1. Ekiert DC, Friesen RH, Bhabha G, et al. A highly conserved neutralizing epitope on group 2 influenza A viruses. *Science.* 2011;333:843-850.

Efficacy, Safety, and Immunogenicity of an Enterovirus 71 Vaccine in China

Zhu F, Xu W, Xia J, et al (Jiangsu Provincial Ctr for Disease Control and Prevention, Nanjing, China; Chinese Ctr for Disease Control and Prevention, Beijing, China; Fourth Military Med Univ, Xi'an, China; et al)
N Engl J Med 370:818-828, 2014

Background.—Enterovirus 71 (EV71) is one of the major causative agents of outbreaks of hand, foot, and mouth disease or herpangina worldwide. This phase 3 trial was designed to evaluate the efficacy, safety, and immunogenicity of an EV71 vaccine.

Methods.—We conducted a randomized, double-blind, placebo-controlled, multicenter trial in which 10,007 healthy infants and young children (6 to 35 months of age) were randomly assigned in a 1:1 ratio to receive two intramuscular doses of either EV71 vaccine or placebo, 28 days apart. The surveillance period was 12 months. The primary end point was the occurrence of EV71-associated hand, foot, and mouth disease or herpangina.

Results.—During the 12-month surveillance period, EV71-associated disease was identified in 0.3% of vaccine recipients (13 of 5041 children) and 2.1% of placebo recipients (106 of 5028 children) in the intention-to-treat cohort. The vaccine efficacy against EV71-associated hand, foot, and mouth disease or herpangina was 94.8% (95% confidence interval [CI], 87.2 to 97.9; $P < 0.001$) in this cohort. Vaccine efficacies against EV71-associated hospitalization (0 cases vs. 24 cases) and hand, foot, and mouth disease with neurologic complications (0 cases vs. 8 cases) were both 100% (95% CI, 83.7 to 100 and 42.6 to 100, respectively). Serious adverse events occurred in 111 of 5044 children in the vaccine group (2.2%) and 131 of 5033 children in the placebo group (2.6%). In the immunogenicity subgroup (1291 children), an anti-EV71 immune response was elicited by the two-dose vaccine series in 98.8% of participants at day 56. An anti-EV71 neutralizing antibody titer of 1:16 was associated with protection against EV71-associated hand, foot, and mouth disease or herpangina.

Conclusions.—The EV71 vaccine provided protection against EV71-associated hand, foot, and mouth disease or herpangina in infants and young children. (Funded by Sinovac Biotech; ClinicalTrials.gov number, NCT01507857.)

▶ The most common causes of hand, foot, and mouth disease, a common childhood exanthem, are human enterovirus 71 (EV71) and coxsackievirus A16. Epidemics caused by EV71 place children younger than 5 years at increased risk for severe neurologic disease. Over the past decade, there have been an estimated 6 million cases of EV71 infection worldwide, and more than 2000 of these were fatal.[1] The neurologic complications associated with EV71 infection include brainstem encephalitis, acute flaccid paralysis, and aseptic meningitis and can occur in the absence of cutaneous manifestations. EV71-associated aseptic meningitis is usually self-limited. Acute flaccid paralysis mimics poliomyelitis and generally results in permanent paralysis. Brainstem encephalitis is the most severe neurologic manifestation of EV71 infection resulting, in extensive inflammation in the hypothalamus, brainstem, spinal cord, and cerebellar dentate nucleus. Neurogenic pulmonary edema progresses rapidly and is associated with high mortality. Even with aggressive supportive care, most survivors are left with clinically significant neurologic sequelae especially in children younger than 2 years of age. The increasing burden of acute neurologic disease associated with EV71 infection, especially in the Asia-Pacific region, and the lack of effective antiviral therapy has made disease prevention by vaccination a priority. Strategies that are being followed for developing EV71 vaccine include whole virus inactivation, viruslike particles, live attenuated EV71 strain, and cloned subunit vaccines. A phase 3 clinical trial using inactivated whole virus EV71 was completed in 2013.[2]

This article reports on a randomized double-blind placebo-controlled multicenter trial in infants and children (6–35 months of age). Vaccine efficacy against hand, foot, and mouth disease as well as EV71-associated hospitalizations was 100%. In a second study published in the same issue, the inactivated EV71 vaccine was shown to elicit EV71-specific immune responses and afford protection against EV71-associated hand, foot, and mouth disease in children 6 to 71 months of age from a different region of China.[3] In this randomized, double-blind placebo-controlled trial including 12 000 healthy children, the inactivated EV71 vaccine showed 97.6% efficacy for hand, foot, and mouth disease over a 11-month period covering 2 epidemic seasons. The side effects observed in the study population were mild, and serious adverse events were fewer in vaccine recipients than among placebo recipients. If the promise of these 3 EV71 vaccines is realized, their addition to the childhood vaccines will represent a major victory for public health and infectious diseases. The fact that EV71 research and vaccine development have primarily been centered in Asia reflects the predominance of EV71 epidemics in this region and, more important, the increasing importance of Asia as a center of medical research.

N. Khardori, MD

References

1. *A Guide to Clinical Management and Public Health Response for Hand, Foot and Mouth Disease (HFMD)*. Geneva, Switzerland: World Health Organization; 2011. http://www.wpro.who.int/publications/docs/Guidancefortheclinicalmanagementof HFMD.pdf. Accessed May 8, 2014.
2. Zhu FC, Meng FY, Li JX, et al. Efficacy, safety, and immunology of an inactivated alum-adjuvant enterovirus 71 vaccine in children in China: a multicentre, randomised, double-blind, placebo-controlled, phase 3 trial. *Lancet*. 2013;381:2024-2032.
3. Li R, Liu L, Mo Z, et al. An inactivated enterovirus 71 vaccine in healthy children. *N Engl J Med*. 2014;370:829-837.

Helicase–Primase Inhibitor Pritelivir for HSV-2 Infection

Wald A, Corey L, Timmler B, et al (Univ of Washington and Fred Hutchinson Cancer Res Ctr, Seattle; AiCuris, Wuppertal, Germany; et al)
N Engl J Med 370:201-210, 2014

Background.—Pritelivir, an inhibitor of the viral helicase–primase complex, exhibits antiviral activity in vitro and in animal models of herpes simplex virus (HSV) infection. We tested the efficacy and safety of pritelivir in otherwise healthy persons with genital HSV-2 infection.

Methods.—We randomly assigned 156 HSV-2–positive persons with a history of genital herpes to receive one of four doses of oral pritelivir (5,

25, or 75 mg daily, or 400 mg weekly) or placebo for 28 days. Participants obtained daily swabs from the genital area for HSV-2 testing, which was performed with a polymerase-chain-reaction assay. Participants also maintained a diary of genital signs and symptoms. The primary end point was the rate of genital HSV shedding.

Results.—HSV shedding among placebo recipients was detected on 16.6% of days; shedding among pritelivir recipients was detected on 18.2% of days among those receiving 5 mg daily, 9.3% of days among those receiving 25 mg daily, 2.1% of days among those receiving 75 mg daily, and 5.3% of days among those receiving 400 mg weekly. The relative risk of viral shedding with pritelivir, as compared with placebo, was 1.11 (95% confidence interval [CI], 0.65 to 1.87) with the 5-mg daily dose, 0.57 (95% CI, 0.31 to 1.03) with the 25-mg daily dose, 0.13 (95% CI, 0.04 to 0.38) with the 75-mg daily dose, and 0.32 (95% CI, 0.17 to 0.59) with the 400-mg weekly dose. The percentage of days with genital lesions was also significantly reduced, from 9.0% in the placebo group to 1.2% in both the group receiving 75 mg of pritelivir daily (relative risk, 0.13; 95% CI, 0.02 to 0.70) and the group receiving 400 mg weekly (relative risk, 0.13; 95% CI, 0.03 to 0.52). The rate of adverse events was similar in all groups.

Conclusions.—Pritelivir reduced the rates of genital HSV shedding and days with lesions in a dose-dependent manner in otherwise healthy men and women with genital herpes. (Funded by AiCuris; ClinicalTrials.gov number, NCT01047540.)

▶ The nucleoside analogues, acyclovir, famciclovir, fenciclovir and valacyclovir are all efficacious in treatment of herpes simplex virus (HSV) infections. They inhibit the HSV DNA polymerase after phosphorylation by the viral thymidine kinase. In the treatment of genital infections caused by HSV, the nucleoside analogues ameliorate clinical disease but do not abrogate viral shedding leading to only partial reduction in the risk of transmission to sexual partners.[1] Resistance to nucleoside analogues develops occasionally in immunocompromised patients, and the reports have become more frequent in the last few years.[2] Treatment options for acyclovir-resistant HSV are limited because the mechanism of resistance is shared among all nucleoside analogues. Thiazolyl amides, a new class of antiviral agents, inhibit HSV replication by targeting the viral helicase-primase enzyme complex. They do not require activation by phosphorylation (by the viral thymidine kinase) and are active in uninfected cells also. Pritelivir is the first in this class shown to exhibit potent in vitro activity against HSV-1 and HSV-2 isolates, including those resistant to nucleoside analogues. It has shown efficacy in animal studies including a study of genital infection in guinea pigs. In humans, pritelivir was shown to be safe with a terminal half-life up to 80 hours.

This is a proof-of-concept safety and efficacy study to evaluate the effect of 4 different doses of oral pritelivir on mucocutaneous viral shedding in adults with genital HSV-2 infection. A total of 156 HSV-2–positive persons with a history of genital herpes were randomly assigned to receive 1 of the 4 doses (5, 25, or

75 mg daily or 400 mg weekly) of oral pritelivir versus placebo for 25 days. Table 2 in the original article shows virologic and clinical endpoints. Both the frequency of genital HSV shedding and lesions in otherwise healthy subjects with genital HSV-2 infection were significantly reduced. The effect was dose dependent. At a 75-mg daily dose, pritelivir reduced the quantity of HSV in breakthrough shedding by more than 98%. A significant reduction in the number of days of genital lesions at doses of 75 mg daily and 400 mg weekly was observed. No serious adverse events were observed in this study. However, the clinical development of pritelivir was put on hold by the US Food and Drug Administration in May 2013 because of unexplained dermal and hematologic adverse events in a toxicology study of monkeys given doses that were 70 to 900 times higher than the dose of 75 mg in humans.

N. Khardori, MD

References

1. Corey L, Wald A, Patel R, et al. Once-daily valacyclovir to reduce the risk of transmission of genital herpes. *N Engl J Med.* 2004;350:11-20.
2. Reyes M, Shaik NS, Graber JM, et al. Acyclovir-resistant genital herpes among persons attending sexually transmitted disease and human immunodeficiency virus clinics. *Arch Intern Med.* 2003;163:76-80.

15 Nosocomial Infections

Emergence of Colistin-Resistance in Extremely Drug-Resistant *Acinetobacter baumannii* Containing a Novel *pmrCAB* Operon During Colistin Therapy of Wound Infections

Lesho E, Yoon E-J, Mcgann P, et al (Walter Reed Army Inst of Res, Silver Spring, MD; Institut Pasteur, Paris, France)

J Infect Dis 208:1142-1151, 2013

Background.—Colistin resistance is of concern since it is increasingly needed to treat infections caused by bacteria resistant to all other antibiotics and has been associated with poorer outcomes. Longitudinal data from in vivo series are sparse.

Methods.—Under a quality-improvement directive to intensify infection-control measures, extremely drug-resistant (XDR) bacteria undergo phenotypic and molecular analysis.

Results.—Twenty-eight XDR *Acinetobacter baumannii* isolates were longitudinally recovered during colistin therapy. Fourteen were susceptible to colistin, and 14 were resistant to colistin. Acquisition of colistin resistance did not alter resistance to other antibiotics. Isolates had low minimum inhibitory concentrations of an investigational aminoglycoside, belonged to multi-locus sequence type 94, were indistinguishable by pulsed-field gel electrophoresis and optical mapping, and harbored a novel *pmrC1A1B* allele. Colistin resistance was associated with point mutations in the *pmrA1* and/or *pmrB* genes. Additional *pmrC* homologs, designated *eptA-1* and *eptA-2*, were at distant locations from the operon. Compared with colistin-susceptible isolates, colistin-resistant isolates displayed significantly enhanced expression of *pmrC1A1B*, *eptA-1*, and *eptA-2*; lower growth rates; and lowered fitness. Phylogenetic analysis suggested that colistin resistance emerged from a single progenitor colistin-susceptible isolate.

Conclusions.—We provide insights into the in vivo evolution of colistin resistance in a series of XDR *A. baumannii* isolates recovered during therapy of infections and emphasize the importance of antibiotic stewardship and surveillance.

▶ The polymixin class of antibiotics with activity against gram-negative bacteria (GNB) has been available since the 1940s, but because of poor pharmacokinetics and adverse events, they were effectively replaced by various types of betalactam antibiotics until the emergence of bacteria resistant to all other antibiotics emerged.[1] Colistin or polymixin E has become the last resort to treat these extremely drug resistant organisms such as *Acinetobacter baumannii*. The bactericidal activity of colistin is thought to be related to a detergent-like effect and disruption of the outer membrane. A second proposed mechanism involves hydroxyl radical production. Development of resistance to colistin is of grave significance because there are no new antibiotics active against GNB in the pipeline.[2] *A. baumannii*, already resistant to many antibiotics, emerged as an important nosocomial pathogen in the past decade. It has shown propensity to acquire further resistance. There are 2 proposed mechanisms of resistance to colistin in *A. baumannii*: (1) mutations in genes encoding lipid A biosynthesis cause a complete loss of lipopolysaccharide. This results in decreased outer-membrane integrity and increased susceptibility to other antibiotics. (2) The second and the more common mechanism leads to modification of bacterial lipopolysaccharide, which does not result in increased susceptibility to other antibiotics. Colistin resistance has been associated with worse clinical outcomes.

This study provides an in-depth characterization of a longitudinal series of colistin-resistant *A. baumannii* isolates recovered during concurrent colistin therapy in severely wounded patients. It is the result of a quality-improvement initiative authorized by the US Army Medical Command and institutional review boards as a part of measures to intensify and prevent transmission. The data suggest that multiple independent colistin-resistant clones arose from the initial susceptible strains.

Because bacteria in the diagnostic laboratory are tested from single "pure" colonies, subpopulations of *Acinetobacter* with resistance could exist in the same patient and go undetected. This heteroresistance has been described in other bacteria, particularly *Staphylococcus aureus*. Active longitudinal surveillance of clinical isolates and clinical outcomes combined with translational research will allow detection of this type of extremely serious antibiotic resistance.

N. Khardori, MD

References

1. Dalfino L, Puntillo F, Mosca A, et al. High-dose, extended-interval colistin administration in critically ill patients: is this the right dosing strategy? A preliminary study. *Clin Infect Dis*. 2012;54:12720-12726.
2. Boucher HW, Talbot GH, Bradley JS, et al. Bad bugs, no drugs: no ESKAPE! An update from the Infectious Diseases Society of America. *Clin Infect Dis*. 2009;48:1-12.

Effect of Aerosolized Colistin as Adjunctive Treatment on the Outcomes of Microbiologically Documented Ventilator-Associated Pneumonia Caused by Colistin-Only Susceptible Gram-Negative Bacteria

Tumbarello M, De Pascale G, Trecarichi EM, et al (Università Cattolica del Sacro Cuore, Rome, Italy)
Chest 144:1768-1775, 2013

Background.—The increasing frequency of ventilator-associated pneumonia (VAP) caused by colistin-only susceptible (COS) gram-negative bacteria (GNB) is of great concern. Adjunctive aerosolized (AS) colistin can reportedly increase alveolar levels of the drug without increasing systemic toxicity. Good clinical results have been obtained in patients with cystic fibrosis, but conflicting data have been reported in patients with VAP.

Methods.—We conducted a retrospective, 1:1 matched case-control study to evaluate the efficacy and safety of AS plus IV colistin vs IV colistin alone in 208 patients in the ICU with VAP caused by COS *Acinetobacter baumannii, Pseudomonas aeruginosa*, or *Klebsiella pneumoniae.*

Results.—Compared with the IV colistin cohort, the AS-IV colistin cohort had a higher clinical cure rate (69.2% vs 54.8%, $P = .03$) and required fewer days of mechanical ventilation after VAP onset (8 days vs 12 days, $P = .001$). In the 166 patients with posttreatment cultures, eradication of the causative organism was also more common in the AS-IV colistin group (63.4% vs 50%, $P = .08$). No between-cohort differences were observed in all-cause ICU mortality, length of ICU stay after VAP onset, or rates of acute kidney injury (AKI) during colistin therapy. Independent predictors of clinical cure were trauma-related ICU admission ($P = .01$) and combined AS-IV colistin therapy ($P = .009$). Higher mean Simplified Acute Physiology Score II ($P = .002$) and Sequential Organ Failure Assessment ($P = .05$) scores, septic shock ($P < .001$), and AKI onset during colistin treatment ($P = .04$) were independently associated with clinical failure.

Conclusions.—Our results suggest that AS colistin might be a beneficial adjunct to IV colistin in the management of VAP caused by COS GNB.

▶ Ventilator-associated pneumonia (VAP) remains the most common complication in intensive care units (ICUs). VAP affects 10% to 20% of patients receiving mechanical ventilation.[1] Depending on the comorbid conditions and the type of infecting organism, mortality rates vary from 10% to 70%. The proportion of VAP cases caused by multidrug-resistant Gram-negative bacteria (MDR-GNR) such as *Acinetobacter baumannii, Pseudomonas aeruginosa*, and *Klebsiella pneumoniae* have increased in the recent years.[2] The polymyxin class of antibacterials are among the limited treatment choices and often a last resort. This class has not being used much since the availability of newer and safer agents. Polymyxin E or colistin has good in vitro activity against carbapenem-resistant strains of *A. baumannii, P. aeruginosa*, and *Klebsiella pneumoniae*. However, the polycationic/hydrophilic structure of colistin limits its penetration into lung tissue.

Nebulization of antimicrobials such as aminoglycosides and colistin has been used to achieve bactericidal concentrations against MDR-GNR at the alveolar level.[3] The efficacy of this route of administration has been demonstrated in cystic fibrosis. The studies in VAP have been small with conflicting results.

This is a retrospective matched-cohort analysis on a large homogenous patient population with VAP caused by *A. baumannii, P. aeruginosa*, or *K.* pneumoniae that were susceptible to colistin only (COS GNB). The study showed that the addition of aerosolized colistin (1 million IU 3 times a day in a jet or ultrasonic nebulizer) to intravenous colistin significantly shortened the duration of mechanical ventilation and increased clinical cure rates in VAP compared with intravenous colistin monotherapy. There was no increased risk of nephrotoxicity in the dual-route cohort. There was no difference between the groups in post-VAP ICU stays and all-cause ICU mortality. The impact of microbiologic cure rates was borderline.

N. Khardori, MD

References

1. van der Kooi TI, de Boer AS, Mannien J, et al. Incidence and risk factors of device-associated infections and associated mortality at the intensive care in the Dutch surveillance system. *Intensive Care Med.* 2007;33:271-278.
2. Timsit JF, Zahar JR, Chevret S. Attributable mortality of ventilator-associated pneumonia. *Curr Opin Crit Care.* 2011;17:464-471.
3. Wood GC. Aerosolized antibiotics for treating hospital-acquired and ventilator-associated pneumonia. *Expert Rev Anti Infect Ther.* 2011;9:993-1000.

Diverse Sources of *C. difficile* Infection Identified on Whole-Genome Sequencing

Eyre DW, Cule ML, Wilson DJ, et al (Univ of Oxford, UK; et al)
N Engl J Med 369:1195-1205, 2013

Background.—It has been thought that *Clostridium difficile* infection is transmitted predominantly within health care settings. However, endemic spread has hampered identification of precise sources of infection and the assessment of the efficacy of interventions.

Methods.—From September 2007 through March 2011, we performed whole-genome sequencing on isolates obtained from all symptomatic patients with *C. difficile* infection identified in health care settings or in the community in Oxfordshire, United Kingdom. We compared single-nucleotide variants (SNVs) between the isolates, using *C. difficile* evolution rates estimated on the basis of the first and last samples obtained from each of 145 patients, with 0 to 2 SNVs expected between transmitted isolates obtained less than 124 days apart, on the basis of a 95% prediction interval. We then identified plausible epidemiologic links among genetically related cases from data on hospital admissions and community location.

Results.—Of 1250 *C. difficile* cases that were evaluated, 1223 (98%) were successfully sequenced. In a comparison of 957 samples obtained from April 2008 through March 2011 with those obtained from September 2007 onward, a total of 333 isolates (35%) had no more than 2 SNVs from at least 1 earlier case, and 428 isolates (45%) had more than 10 SNVs from all previous cases. Reductions in incidence over time were similar in the two groups, a finding that suggests an effect of interventions targeting the transition from exposure to disease. Of the 333 patients with no more than 2 SNVs (consistent with transmission), 126 patients (38%) had close hospital contact with another patient, and 120 patients (36%) had no hospital or community contact with another patient. Distinct subtypes of infection continued to be identified throughout the study, which suggests a considerable reservoir of *C. difficile.*

Conclusions.—Over a 3-year period, 45% of *C. difficile* cases in Oxfordshire were genetically distinct from all previous cases. Genetically diverse sources, in addition to symptomatic patients, play a major part in *C. difficile* transmission. (Funded by the U.K. Clinical Research Collaboration Translational Infection Research Initiative and others.)

▶ It is generally believed that *Clostridium difficile* infection results from recent acquisition within a health care setting. Horizontal transmission from symptomatic patients forms the basis for recent prevention guidelines.[1] Although person-to-person transmission and contamination of the surroundings by *C. difficile* is well documented, there are multiple other potential sources. The contribution of such sources including patients with asymptomatic colonization, water, food, farm animals, and pets to the disease burden is not clear. Reports of community-associated infection are increasing.[2] A combination of data from hospital admissions and genotyping have shown that less than 25% of new cases can be attributed to hospital-based contact with patients with known *C. difficile* infection.

This study reports on the use of whole-genome sequencing in quantification of the role of symptomatic patients in transmission of C. *difficile* and the variation in transmission over time (3.6 years) in a defined geographic area. The results show that in the majority of cases, *C. difficile* is not transmitted from another symptomatic patient. Only 35% of cases were genetically related to at least 1 previous case; 13% were genetically related and involved hospital ward contact; 19% were genetically related and involved some sort of hospital contact. In 45% of cases, genetic diversity was enough to represent transmission originating from sources other than the symptomatic patients included in the study. The authors explain the reduction in cases in the area studied over the past 5 years to be related to changes in the use of antibiotics rather than the measures to reduce transmission from symptomatic patients. The use of a highly discriminating methodology in this study suggests that many cases of *C. difficile* infection arise from genetically diverse sources. Such methodology allows the identification of genetically related cases in real time and help in targeting prevention measures in case of an epidemiologic link. In addition, the approach permits more sensitive monitoring of infection control performance—that is, focus on genetically related cases rather than all cases. In genetically related cases without an epidemiologic link, novel routes of transmission can be sought.

N. Khardori, MD

References

1. Surawicz CM, Brandt LJ, Binion DG, et al. Guidelines for diagnosis, treatment, and prevention of Clostridium difficile infections. *Am J Gastroenterol.* 2013; 108:478-498.
2. Health Protection Agency. Quarterly epidemiological commentary: mandatory MRSA, MSSA and *E. coli* infection data (up to October–December 2012). http://www.hpa.org.uk/webc/HPAwebFile/HPAweb_C/1284473407318. Accessed May 8, 2014.

16 Tuberculosis

A Trial of Mass Isoniazid Preventive Therapy for Tuberculosis Control

Churchyard GJ, for the Thibela TB Study Team (Univ of the Witwatersrand, Johannesburg, South Africa; et al)

N Engl J Med 370:301-310, 2014

Background.—Tuberculosis is epidemic among workers in South African gold mines. We evaluated an intervention to interrupt tuberculosis transmission by means of mass screening that was linked to treatment for active disease or latent infection.

Methods.—In a cluster-randomized study, we designated 15 clusters with 78,744 miners as either intervention clusters (40,981 miners in 8 clusters) or control clusters (37,763 miners in 7 clusters). In the intervention clusters, all miners were offered tuberculosis screening. If active tuberculosis was diagnosed, they were referred for treatment; if not, they were offered 9 months of isoniazid preventive therapy. The primary outcome was the cluster-level incidence of tuberculosis during the 12 months after the intervention ended. Secondary outcomes included tuberculosis prevalence at study completion.

Results.—In the intervention clusters, 27,126 miners (66.2%) underwent screening. Of these miners, 23,659 (87.2%) started taking isoniazid, and isoniazid was dispensed for 6 months or more to 35 to 79% of miners, depending on the cluster. The intervention did not reduce the incidence of tuberculosis, with rates of 3.02 per 100 person-years in the intervention clusters and 2.95 per 100 person-years in the control clusters (rate ratio in the intervention clusters, 1.00; 95% confidence interval [CI], 0.75 to 1.34; $P = 0.98$; adjusted rate ratio, 0.96; 95% CI, 0.76 to 1.21; $P = 0.71$), or the prevalence of tuberculosis (2.35% vs. 2.14%; adjusted prevalence ratio, 0.98; 95% CI, 0.65 to 1.48; $P = 0.90$). Analysis of the direct effect of isoniazid in 10,909 miners showed a reduced incidence of tuberculosis during treatment (1.10 cases per 100 person-years among miners receiving isoniazid vs. 2.91 cases per 100 person-years among controls; adjusted rate ratio, 0.42; 95% CI, 0.20 to 0.88; $P = 0.03$), but there was a subsequent rapid loss of protection.

Conclusions.—Mass screening and treatment for latent tuberculosis had no significant effect on tuberculosis control in South African gold mines, despite the successful use of isoniazid in preventing tuberculosis during treatment. (Funded by the Consortium to Respond Effectively to the

AIDS TB Epidemic and others; Thibela TB Current Controlled Trials number, ISRCTN63327174.)

▶ Tuberculosis (TB) remains a leading cause of death globally and was estimated to cause 1.4 million deaths in 2011. HIV infection, environmental exposure to dustlike silica, and close living and working conditions in many parts of the world continue to intensify the tuberculosis epidemic.

In a landmark trial in the 1960s, households in Alaska, where TB was epidemic, were randomly selected; preventive therapy with isoniazid for all household members led to 55% decline in TB over 6 years.[1] These findings led to the use of this novel intervention in South African gold miners. In trials in Greenland villages and Tunisian city blocks, the lack of success for this intervention was attributed to an inadequate dose of isoniazid.

This is a cluster-randomized study on 78 744 gold miners in South Africa. The report is on 8 intervention clusters and 7 control clusters. All miners in the intervention clusters were offered tuberculosis screening. They were then referred for treatment of active TB disease or offered 9 months of isoniazid preventive therapy.

Table 2 in the original article shows the overall effect of communitywide isoniazid preventive therapy. The prevalence of TB among intervention (2.35%) and control clusters (2.14%) was similar. The prevalence ratio did not change after adjustment for potential cofounders or when the analysis was restricted only to employees who were in the workforce during the main enrollment period. The incidence of TB was reduced by 58% among employees who started isoniazid prevention during the 9-month treatment period. However, the effect was lost immediately after treatment was discontinued, which is consistent with the limited durability of isoniazid therapy-associated prevention shown among HIV-infected adults in sub-Saharan Africa.[2] The conclusion of the study is that a 9-month course of community-wide isoniazid preventive therapy did not improve TB control in South African gold miners.

Increased vulnerability to TB caused by to HIV infection and silicosis and ongoing transmission of tuberculosis were some of the potential variables in this setting. Such factors would have the same impact on strategies to control TB in other TB-epidemic areas of the world.

N. Khardori, MD

References

1. Comstock GW, Ferebee SH, Hammes LM. A controlled trial of community-wide isoniazid prophylaxis in Alaska. *Am Rev Respir Dis.* 1967;95:935-943.
2. Samandari T, Agizew TB, Nyirenda S, et al. 6-month versus 36-month isoniazid preventive treatment for tuberculosis in adults with HIV infection in Botswana: a randomised, double-blind, placebo-controlled trial. *Lancet.* 2011;377: 1588-1598.

17 Miscellaneous

Advantages of Using Matrix-Assisted Laser Desorption Ionization–Time of Flight Mass Spectrometry as a Rapid Diagnostic Tool for Identification of Yeasts and Mycobacteria in the Clinical Microbiological Laboratory

Chen JHK, Yam W-C, Ngan AHY, et al (Univ of Hong Kong, China)

J Clin Microbiol 51:3981-3987, 2013

Yeast and mycobacteria can cause infections in immunocompromised patients and normal hosts. The rapid identification of these organisms can significantly improve patient care. There has been an increasing number of studies on using matrix-assisted laser desorption ionization–time of flight mass spectrometry (MALDI-TOF MS) for rapid yeast and mycobacterial identifications. However, studies on direct comparisons between the Bruker Biotyper and bioMérieux Vitek MS systems for the identification of yeast and mycobacteria have been limited. This study compared the performance of the two systems in their identification of 98 yeast and 102 mycobacteria isolates. Among the 98 yeast isolates, both systems generated species-level identifications in > 70% of the specimens, of which *Candida albicans* was the most commonly cultured species. At a genus-level identification, the Biotyper system identified more isolates than the Vitek MS system for *Candida* (75/78 [96.2%] versus 68/78 [87.2%], respectively; $P = 0.0426$) and non-*Candida* yeasts (18/20 [90.0%] versus 7/20 [35.0%], respectively; $P = 0.0008$). For mycobacterial identification, the Biotyper system generated reliable identifications for 89 (87.3%) and 64 (62.8%) clinical isolates at the genus and species levels, respectively, from solid culture media, whereas the Vitek MS system did not generate any reliable identification. The MS method differentiated 12/21 clinical species, despite the fact that no differentiation between *Mycobacterium abscessus* and *Mycobacterium chelonae* was found by using 16S rRNA gene sequencing. In summary, the MALDI-TOF MS method provides short turnaround times and a standardized working protocol for the identification of yeast and mycobacteria. Our study demonstrates that MALDI-TOF MS is suitable as a first-line test for the identification of yeast and mycobacteria in clinical laboratories.

▶ The current gold standard laboratory methods for diagnosis of infectious diseases are culture-based, which require 48 hours or longer for preliminary reporting. After that, it can take another 24 to 48 hours for identification and susceptibility testing. Matrix-assisted laser desorption ionization–time of flight mass spectrometry (MALDI-TOF MS) has proven to be a promising tool for the rapid identification of clinical bacterial isolates.[1]

This study reports the use of MALDI-TOF MS for identification of yeasts and mycobacteria in clinical specimens. Some yeast species cannot be clearly differentiated by conventional phenotypic methods, and molecular methods are time-consuming and technically demanding. Species-level identification is essential for differentiating tuberculosis-causing mycobacteria from nontuberculosis mycobacteria (NTM) for epidemiological, public health, and treatment purposes. Conventional phenotypic methods for identification are laborious and time-consuming. Molecular methods, including polymerase chain reaction (PCR) sequencing and PCR hybridization, have become the new gold standard for mycobacterial identification. These methods are highly specific and might shorten the length of diagnostic procedures; a number of species require advanced genotypic methods that are unaffordable to diagnostic laboratories. Several studies have evaluated the use of MALDI-TOF MS in identification of mycobacteria and yeasts.[2,3]

In this study, the investigators compare the performance of 2 MALDI-TOF MS systems for the rapid identification of clinical yeasts and mycobacteria to the species level compared with currently used phenotypic and molecular methods. The turnaround time was shortened by 24 to 72 hours by MALDI-TOF MS. The quick turnaround time and expandability of MALDI-TOF MS identification databases favor this method as a suitable first-line test for the identification of yeast and mycobacteria in clinical samples.

N. Khardori, MD

References

1. Tan KE, Ellis BC, Lee R, Stamper PD, Zhang SX, Carroll KC. Prospective evaluation of a matrix-assisted laser desorption ionization-time of flight mass spectrometry system in a hospital clinical microbiology laboratory for identification of bacteria and yeasts: a bench-by-bench study for assessing the impact on time to identification and cost-effectiveness. *J Clin Microbiol.* 2012;50:3301-3308.
2. Pignone M, Greth KM, Cooper J, Emerson D, Tang J. Identification of mycobacteria by matrix-assisted laser desorption ionization-time-of-flight mass spectrometry. *J Clin Microbiol.* 2006;44:1963-1970.
3. Westblade LF, Jennemann R, Branda JA, et al. Multicenter study evaluating the Vitek MS system for identification of medically important yeasts. *J Clin Microbiol.* 2013;51:2267-2272.

A genetic strategy to identify targets for the development of drugs that prevent bacterial persistence

Kim J-H, O'Brien KM, Sharma R, et al (Weill Cornell Med College, NY; et al)
Proc Natl Acad Sci U S A 110:19095-19100, 2013

Antibacterial drug development suffers from a paucity of targets whose inhibition kills replicating and nonreplicating bacteria. The latter include phenotypically dormant cells, known as persisters, which are tolerant to many antibiotics and often contribute to failure in the treatment of chronic infections. This is nowhere more apparent than in tuberculosis caused by *Mycobacterium tuberculosis*, a pathogen that tolerates many antibiotics once it ceases to replicate. We developed a strategy to identify proteins that *Mycobacterium tuberculosis* requires to both grow and persist and whose inhibition has the potential to prevent drug tolerance and persister formation. This strategy is based on a tunable dual-control genetic switch that provides a regulatory range spanning three orders of magnitude, quickly depletes proteins in both replicating and nonreplicating mycobacteria, and exhibits increased robustness to phenotypic reversion. Using this switch, we demonstrated that depletion of the nicotinamide adenine dinucleotide synthetase (NadE) rapidly killed *Mycobacterium tuberculosis* under conditions of standard growth and nonreplicative persistence induced by oxygen and nutrient limitation as well as during the acute and chronic phases of infection in mice. These findings establish the dual-control switch as a robust tool with which to probe the essentiality of *Mycobacterium tuberculosis* proteins under different conditions, including those that induce antibiotic tolerance, and NadE as a target with the potential to shorten current tuberculosis chemotherapies.

▶ Persistence of nongrowing bacteria, phenotypic variants that are not affected by bactericidal antibiotics, complicate the treatment of many chronic infections. Current genetic approaches to antimicrobial therapy are target-based and do not identify proteins required for growth as well as for the survival and persistence of nongrowing bacteria.

This study sought to address improvement in genetic technology to more closely mimic the kinetics and magnitude of chemical inhibition to facilitate identification of new potential drug targets. They engineered a dual-control (DUC) switch in which a single inducer—anhydrotetracycline (atc) or doxycycline (doxy)—simultaneously triggers transcriptional repression of a target gene and degradation of its encoded protein. This switch can identify proteins required by both replicating and nonreplicating *Mycobacterium tuberculosis*. This approach of combining transcriptional repression with regulated proteolysis has the potential of drastically reducing or overcoming many of the limitations in currently available antimicrobial agents. The regulatory component of the DUC switch has been shown to control gene expression in several bacteria and eukaryotes.[1] It has been a major challenge to add to the current armamentarium of antimicrobial agents, new classes with efficacy against the worsening resistance patterns in major microbial pathogens. It is the persistence of bacteria that ultimately leads to resistance. The Centers for Disease Control and Prevention now estimates that 80% of infections are associated with biofilm formation, especially those persisting on medical devices. A direction to antibiotic development as described in this report promises to be a breakthrough in the management of infectious diseases at large.

N. Khardori, MD

Reference

1. Berens C, Hillen W. Gene regulation by tetracyclines. Constraints of resistance regulation in bacteria shape TetR for application in eukaryotes. *Eur J Biochem.* 2003; 270:3109-3121.

Conjunctivitis: A Systematic Review of Diagnosis and Treatment

Azari AA, Barney NP (Univ of Wisconsin, Madison)

JAMA 310:1721-1729, 2013

Importance.—Conjunctivitis is a common problem.

Objective.—To examine the diagnosis, management, and treatment of conjunctivitis, including various antibiotics and alternatives to antibiotic use in infectious conjunctivitis and use of antihistamines and mast cell stabilizers in allergic conjunctivitis.

Evidence Review.—A search of the literature published through March 2013, using PubMed, the ISI Web of Knowledge database, and the Cochrane Library was performed. Eligible articles were selected after review of titles, abstracts, and references.

Findings.—Viral conjunctivitis is the most common overall cause of infectious conjunctivitis and usually does not require treatment; the signs and symptoms at presentation are variable. Bacterial conjunctivitis is the second most common cause of infectious conjunctivitis, with most uncomplicated cases resolving in 1 to 2 weeks. Mattering and adherence of the eyelids on waking, lack of itching, and absence of a history of conjunctivitis are the strongest factors associated with bacterial conjunctivitis. Topical antibiotics decrease the duration of bacterial conjunctivitis and allow earlier return to school or work. Conjunctivitis secondary to sexually transmitted diseases such as chlamydia and gonorrhea requires systemic treatment in addition to topical antibiotic therapy. Allergic conjunctivitis is encountered in up to 40% of the population, but only a small proportion of these individuals seek medical help; itching is the most consistent sign in allergic conjunctivitis, and treatment consists of topical antihistamines and mast cell inhibitors.

Conclusions and Relevance.—The majority of cases in bacterial conjunctivitis are self-limiting and no treatment is necessary in uncomplicated cases. However, conjunctivitis caused by gonorrhea or chlamydia and conjunctivitis in contact lens wearers should be treated with antibiotics. Treatment for viral conjunctivitis is supportive. Treatment with antihistamines and mast cell stabilizers alleviates the symptoms of allergic conjunctivitis (Fig 2, Table 3).

▶ It is estimated that in the United States, acute conjunctivitis affects 6 million people annually, about 10% of all primary care office visits are related to conjunctivitis, and about 70% of all patients with acute conjunctivitis are initially seen in primary care and urgent care offices[1,2] Allergic conjunctivitis is the most frequent cause, is seen more frequently in spring and summer, and affects 15% to 40% of

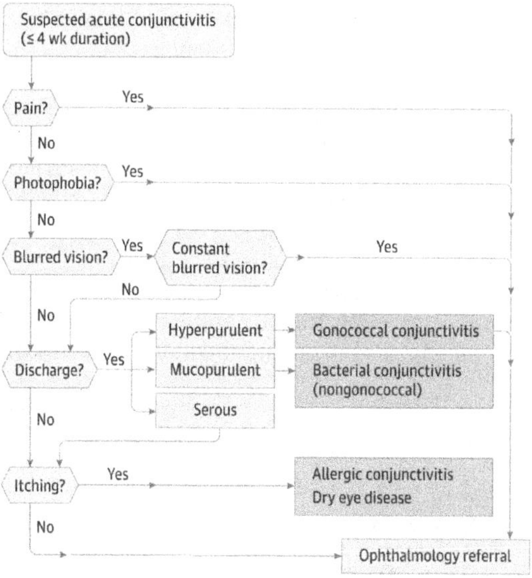

FIGURE 2.—Suggested Algorithm for Clinical Approach to Suspected Acute Conjunctivitis. (Reprinted from Azari AA, Barney NP. Conjunctivitis: a systematic review of diagnosis and treatment. *JAMA.* 2013;310:1721-1729.)

TABLE 3.—Evidence-Based Recommendations in Conjunctivitis

Recommendation	Level of Evidence
Topical antibiotics are effective in reducing the duration of conjunctivitis.	A[19]
Observation is reasonable in most cases of bacterial conjunctivitis (suspected or confirmed) because they often resolve spontaneously and no treatment is necessary.	A[41]
It is reasonable to use any broad-spectrum antibiotics for treating bacterial conjunctivitis.	A[19,41]
In allergic conjunctivitis, use of topical antihistamines and mast cell stabilizers is recommended.	A[52]
Good hand hygiene can be used to decrease the spread of acute viral conjunctivitis.	C[16]
Bacterial cultures can be useful in cases of severely purulent conjunctivitis or cases that are recalcitrant to therapy.	C[16]
It may be helpful to treat viral conjunctivitis with artificial tears, topical antihistamines, or cold compresses.	C[16]
Topical steroids are not recommended for bacterial conjunctivitis.	C[65]

Editor's Note: Please refer to original journal article for full references.

the population. Nonherpetic viral conjunctivitis is the most common cause of infectious conjunctivity and is more prevalent in summer. Bacterial conjunctivitis as the second most common cause is responsible for most (50%–75%) cases in children and is seen more commonly between December and April.

This is a systematic review of diagnosis and treatment of conjunctivitis based on a search of literature published through March 2013. Fig 2 shows an algorithm approach to suspected acute conjunctivitis. The most common cause of viral conjunctivitis is adenovirus. Use of topical antibiotics in viral conjunctivitis should be avoided because of adverse treatment effects. A rapid antigen test to diagnose viral conjunctivitis can help avoid inappropriate use of antibiotics. A total of 60% of culture-proven or clinically suspected bacterial conjunctivitis cases are self-limited without treatment. Topical antibiotics are recommended for contact lens wearers, patients with mucopurulent discharge and eye pain, suspected cases of gonococcal and chlamydial conjunctivitis, and patients with pre-existing ocular surface disease. Table 3 shows evidence-based recommendations for treatment of conjunctivitis. Patients should be referred promptly to an ophthalmologist if they have visual loss, moderate to severe pain, severe purulent discharge, corneal involvement, conjunctival scarring, lack of response to therapy, or recurrent episodes of conjunctivitis or have a history of herpes simplex virus eye disease.

N. Khardori, MD

References

1. Leibowitz HM. The red eye. *N Engl J Med.* 2000;343:345-351.
2. Kaufman HE. Adenovirus advances: new diagnostic and therapeutic options. *Curr Opin Ophthalmol.* 2011;22:290-293.

Infectious Diseases Specialty Intervention Is Associated With Decreased Mortality and Lower Healthcare Costs

Schmitt S, McQuillen DP, Nahass R, et al (Cleveland Clinic, OH; Tufts Univ School of Medicine, Burlington, MA; ID Care, Hillsborough, NJ; et al)
Clin Infect Dis 58:22-28, 2014

Background.—Previous studies, largely based on chart reviews with small sample sizes, have demonstrated that infectious diseases (ID) specialists positively impact patient outcomes. We investigated how ID specialists impact mortality, utilization, and costs using a large claims dataset.

TABLE 3.—Patient and Index Stay Characteristics

Category	No ID Intervention		ID Intervention	
	Number	Percent	Number	Percent
%Male	75 992	46.8	50 012	51.2
%Female	86 473	53.2	47 663	48.8
%Aged <65 y	37 007	22.8	26 326	27.0
%Aged 65–74 y	39 419	24.3	25 574	26.2
%Aged 75–84 y	50 506	31.1	29 080	29.8
%Aged 85+ y	35 533	21.9	16 704	17.1
%Index stays at teaching hospital	83 517	49.0	59 746	58.6
%Index stays with ICU days	41 916	24.6	28 359	27.8

Percentages of cases in the age and gender groups excluded from the denominator 7901 non-ID consult and 4307 ID consult cases where the age and gender of the patient are missing.

Abbreviations: ICU, intensive care unit; ID, infectious diseases.

TABLE 4.—Unadjusted and Risk-Adjusted Outcomes for Stays With and Without Infectious Diseases Interventions

Outcome	Unadjusted Outcomes			Risk-Adjusted Outcomes			
	No ID	ID	OR/%Δ (95% CI)	No ID	ID	*P* Value	OR/%Δ (95% CI)
Index stay length of stay	7.3	11.5	+56.1% (+54.9% to +57.3%)	9.5	9.6	.001	1.3% (+.5% to +2.1%)
Index stay ICU days[a]	5.2	7.9	+54.2% (+51.4% to +57.1%)	6.7	6.4	<.001	−3.7% (−5.5% to −1.9%)
Index stay mortality (%)	10.1	9.7	0.95 (.93 to .98)	10.7	9.8	<.001	0.87 (.83 to .91)
30-day mortality (%)[b]	8.0	8.1	1.02 (.99 to 1.05)	8.7	7.7	<.001	0.86 (.82 to .90)
30-day readmission rate (%)[b]	20.8	23.4	1.17 (1.15 to 1.19)	22.7	22.1	.009	0.96 (.93 to .99)
ACH charges for index stay	$46 974	$86 117	+83.3% (+81.3% to +85.4%)	$65 570	$66 811	<.001	+1.9% (+.9% to +2.8%)
Medicare payments to ACH for index stay	$12 699	$18 802	+48.1% (+46.5% to +50.0%)	$15 850	$15 799	.435	−0.3% (−1.1% to +.5%)
Medicare payments for index stay	$14 188	$21 837	+53.9% (+52.4% to +55.4%)	$18 017	$18 076	.397	+0.3% (−.4% to +1.1%)
Medicare payments for 30-day episode[b]	$6460	$8512	+31.8% (+29.8% to +33.7%)	$7706	$7858	.069	+2.0% (−.2% to +4.1%)

Abbreviations: ACH, acute care hospital; CI, confidence interval; ICU, intensive care unit; ID, infectious diseases; OR, odds ratio; %Δ, percent difference.

[a]Only patients with 1 or more ICU days.

[b]Excludes patients expiring in the hospital.

Reprinted from Schmitt S, McQuillen DP, Nahass R, et al. Infectious Diseases Specialty Intervention Is Associated With Decreased Mortality and Lower Healthcare Costs. Clin Infect Dis. 2014;58:22-28, by permission of the Infectious Diseases Society of America.

TABLE 5.—Risk-Adjusted Outcomes for Stays Receiving Early Versus Late Infectious Diseases Interventions

Outcome	Early ID (within 2 d)	Late ID	*P* Value	OR/%Δ (95% CI)
Index stay length of stay	13.2	13.8	<.001	−3.8% (−4.8% to −2.9%)
Index stay ICU days[a]	7.6	8.1	<.001	−5.1% (−7.7% to −2.4%)
Index stay mortality (%)	7.1	7.5	.122	0.94 (.88 to 1.02)
30-day mortality (%)[b]	8.6	9.6	<.001	0.87 (.82 to .93)
30-day readmission rate (%)[b]	24.6	26.1	<.001	0.92 (.89 to .96)
ACH charges for index stay	$95 135	$98 015	<.001	−2.9% (−4.1% to −1.7%)
Medicare payments to ACH for index stay	$18 111	$18 728	<.001	−3.3% (−4.3% to −2.3%)
Medicare payments for index stay	$21 453	$22 207	<.001	−3.4% (−4.3% to −2.5%)
Medicare payments for 30-day episode[b]	$8739	$9318	<.001	−6.2% (−8.8% to −3.5%)

Abbreviations: ACH, acute care hospital; CI, confidence interval; ICU, intensive care unit; ID, infectious diseases; OR, odds ratio; %Δ, percent difference.

[a]Only patients with 1 or more ICU days.

[b]Excludes patients expiring in the hospital.

Reprinted from Schmitt S, McQuillen DP, Nahass R, et al. Infectious Diseases Specialty Intervention Is Associated With Decreased Mortality and Lower Healthcare Costs. Clin Infect Dis. 2014;58:22-28, by permission of the Infectious Diseases Society of America.

Methods.—We used administrative fee-for-service Medicare claims to identify beneficiaries hospitalized from 2008 to 2009 with at least 1 of 11 infections. There were 101 991 stays with and 170 336 stays without ID interventions. Cohorts were propensity score matched for patient demographics, comorbidities, and hospital characteristics. Regression models compared ID versus non-ID intervention and early versus late ID intervention. Risk-adjusted outcomes included hospital and intensive care unit (ICU) length of stay (LOS), mortality, readmissions, hospital charges, and Medicare payments.

Results.—The ID intervention cohort demonstrated significantly lower mortality (odds ratio [OR], 0.87; 95% confidence interval [CI], .83 to .91) and readmissions (OR, 0.96; 95% CI, .93 to .99) than the non-ID intervention cohort. Medicare charges and payments were not significantly different; the ID intervention cohort ICU LOS was 3.7% shorter (95% CI, −5.5% to −1.9%). Patients receiving ID intervention within 2 days of admission had significantly lower 30-day mortality and readmission, hospital and ICU length of stay, and Medicare charges and payments compared with patients receiving later ID interventions.

Conclusions.—ID interventions are associated with improved patient outcomes. Early ID interventions are also associated with reduced costs for Medicare beneficiaries with select infections (Tables 3-5).

▶ Hospitalized patients often have multiple and complex medical conditions. Consultations by cognitive specialists offer evidence-based recommendations and experience on diagnosis and management of a group of diseases. Infectious disease (ID) specialists provide consultations that give differential diagnosis, appropriate diagnostic methods, and management in patients who may have one or more infectious diseases, which are often severe and complex.[1] They optimize type, duration, route of delivery, and adverse reactions monitoring for antimicrobial therapy. In addition, they facilitate care transition through outpatient parenteral antibiotic therapy, follow-up to resolution, and monitoring for any complications. Published studies with small sample sizes have found an ID consultation leads to more correct diagnoses, shorter lengths of stay, more appropriate therapies, fewer complications, and overall less antibiotic use.

This study uses a large, administrative fee-for-service (Medicare) claims data set to determine how ID specialists impact mortality, utilization, and costs. The data suggest that ID specialists routinely care for a very complex patient population (Table 3); therefore, a risk assessment may be used to compare unadjusted and adjusted outcomes and cost of care. Table 4 shows the unadjusted and risk-adjusted outcomes for stays with and without infectious diseases intervention. An overall positive impact of early versus later ID involvement is shown in Table 5. These results, based on a robust database, show a strong influence on outcomes and cost by ID specialty intervention. This type of data applied to other specialties and clinical syndromes may help guide resource allocation and provide a more comprehensive view of the relative value of various patient care components.

N. Khardori, MD

Reference

1. Petrak RM, Sexton DJ, Butera ML, et al. The value of an infectious disease specialist. *Clin Infect Dis*. 2003;36:1013-1017.

Inhaled Corticosteroids and Risk of Recurrent Pneumonia: A Population-Based, Nested Case-Control Study

Eurich DT, Lee C, Marrie TJ, et al (Univ of Alberta, Edmonton, Canada; Univ of Toronto, Ontario, Canada; Dalhousie Univ, Halifax, Nova Scotia, Canada)

Clin Infect Dis 57:1138-1144, 2013

Background.—Studies have suggested an increased risk of pneumonia with inhaled corticosteroid (ICS) use, although this association is inconsistent. We evaluated the risk of recurrent pneumonia associated with ICS use in a high-risk population of individuals who survived an episode of pneumonia.

Methods.—Clinical and 5-year follow-up data were collected on all adults aged ≥65 years with pneumonia over a period of 2 years. Using a nested case-control design, first cases (patients with recurrent pneumonia ≥30 days after initial episode) and then controls (free of pneumonia and matched on age, sex, and chronic obstructive pulmonary disease [COPD]) were identified. ICS use was classified as never, past (remote, only before initial pneumonia), or current. Our primary outcome measure was recurrent pneumonia assessed using conditional multivariate logistic regression after adjustment of demographics and clinical data.

Results.—During 5 years of follow-up, 653 recurrent pneumonia cases were matched with 6244 controls; mean age was 79 (SD, 8) years, 3577

(52%) were male, 2652 (38%) had COPD, and 2294 (33%) ever used ICS. Overall, 123 of 870 (14%) current ICS users had recurrent pneumonia compared to 395 of 4603 (9%) never-users (adjusted odds ratio, 1.90; 95% confidence interval, 1.45–2.50; $P < .001$; number need to harm = 20). Conversely, there was no association between past (remote) use of ICS and pneumonia: 9% of past users versus 9% never-users ($P = .36$).

Conclusions.—ICS use was associated with a 90% relative increase in the risk of recurrent pneumonia among high-risk pneumonia survivors. This should be considered when prescribing ICS and when deciding which patients might need more intensive follow-up.

▶ The risk factors associated with the development of community-acquired pneumonia (CAP) are numerous and include age, previous pneumonia, asthma, chronic obstructive pulmonary disease, and poor functional status.[1] CAP accounts for one-third of all hospitalizations in older adults and increases the risk of recurrent pneumonia by 2-fold. The role of concomitant medications such as proton pump inhibitors, antipsychotics, and inhaled corticosteroids (ICSs) as risk factors for CAP has recently been a focus.[2] ICSs are widely used in all patient populations with respiratory symptoms. Some trials and meta-analyses of randomized controlled trials have confirmed a 34% to 57% increased risk of CAP with ICS use.[3] However, the current literature is inconclusive.

This study is on a prospective population-based clinical registry that contains comprehensive data on all 6874 patients aged 17 or older with CAP seen in all 7 emergency departments and 6 hospitals serving the Edmonton (Canada) health region between the years 2000 and 2002. CAP in this database is defined as confirmed radiographic findings by the treating physician and at least 2 of the following: cough, pleurisy, shortness of breath, temperature > 38°C, and crackles or bronchial breathing on auscultation. Among this population-based cohort of uniformly high-risk elderly patients who survived an episode of pneumonia, there was a 2-fold relative increase (5% absolute increase) in risk of recurrent pneumonia if they were currently using ICSs. The increased risk was irrespective of whether ICS use started before or after hospitalization for initial pneumonia, suggesting that any current use of ICSs is a risk factor.

A second recent study has shown that people with asthma receiving ICSs are at an increased risk of pneumonia, and high doses pose a greater risk.[4] A third study reported that patients with COPD have a higher incidence of pneumonia if they are using ICSs. As in the second study, the risk was dose-related.[5] The findings in many previous and current studies should be considered when prescribing ICS and are a reason for more intensive follow-up in selected patients.

N. Khardori, MD

References

1. Farr BM, Bartlett CL, Wadsworth J, Miller DL. Risk factors for community-acquired pneumonia diagnosed upon hospital admission. British Thoracic Society Pneumonia Study Group. *Respir Med.* 2000;94:954-963.

2. Eurich DT, Sadowski CA, Simpson SH, Marrie TJ, Majumdar SR. Recurrent community-acquired pneumonia in patients starting acid-suppressing drugs. *Am J Med.* 2010;123:47-53.
3. Singh S, Loke YK. Risk of pneumonia associated with long-term use of inhaled corticosteroids in chronic obstructive pulmonary disease: a critical review and update. *Curr Opin Pulm Med.* 2010;16:118-122.
4. McKeever T, Harrison TW, Hubbard R, Shaw D. Inhaled corticosteroids and the risk of pneumonia in people with asthma: a case-control study. *Chest.* 2013;144: 1788-1794.
5. Suissa S, Patenaude V, Lapi F, Ernst P. Inhaled corticosteroids in COPD and the risk of serious pneumonia. *Thorax.* 2013;68:1029-1036.

A Novel Prion Disease Associated with Diarrhea and Autonomic Neuropathy

Mead S, Gandhi S, Beck J, et al (Univ College London (UCL) Inst of Neurology, UK; et al)

N Engl J Med 369:1904-1914, 2013

Background.—Human prion diseases, although variable in clinicopathological phenotype, generally present as neurologic or neuropsychiatric conditions associated with rapid multifocal central nervous system degeneration that is usually dominated by dementia and cerebellar ataxia. Approximately 15% of cases of recognized prion disease are inherited and associated with coding mutations in the gene encoding prion protein (*PRNP*). The availability of genetic diagnosis has led to a progressive broadening of the recognized spectrum of disease.

Methods.—We used longitudinal clinical assessments over a period of 20 years at one hospital combined with genealogical, neuropsychological, neurophysiological, neuroimaging, pathological, molecular genetic, and biochemical studies, as well as studies of animal transmission, to characterize a novel prion disease in a large British kindred. We studied 6 of 11 affected family members in detail, along with autopsy or biopsy samples obtained from 5 family members.

Results.—We identified a *PRNP* Y163X truncation mutation and describe a distinct and consistent phenotype of chronic diarrhea with autonomic failure and a length-dependent axonal, predominantly sensory, peripheral polyneuropathy with an onset in early adulthood. Cognitive decline and seizures occurred when the patients were in their 40s or 50s. The deposition of prion protein amyloid was seen throughout peripheral organs, including the bowel and peripheral nerves. Neuropathological examination during end-stage disease showed the deposition of prion protein in the form of frequent cortical amyloid plaques, cerebral amyloid angiopathy, and tauopathy. A unique pattern of abnormal prion protein fragments was seen in brain tissue. Transmission studies in laboratory mice were negative.

Conclusions.—Abnormal forms of prion protein that were found in multiple peripheral tissues were associated with diarrhea, autonomic failure, and neuropathy. (Funded by the U.K. Medical Research Council and others.)

▶ Prions are transmissible agents thought to comprise misfolded and aggregated forms of the normal cell-surface prion protein. Propagation of prions is thought to occur by means of seeded protein polymerization, a process involving the binding and templated misfolding of normal cellular prion protein. The prion diseases described in humans are neurodegenerative disorders that may be inherited or acquired or may occur spontaneously as in sporadic Creutzfeldt-Jakob disease.[1] The inherited prion diseases are caused by mutations in the gene-encoding prion protein (PRNP) and are autosomal dominant. They are classified into overlapping neurologic syndromes called Gerstmann-Straussler Scheinker (GSS) syndrome, fatal familial insomnia, and familial Creutzfeldt-Jakob disease.

This article describes a prion protein disease characterized by diarrhea and autonomic neuropathy. Multiple modalities including animal transmission studies were used to study 6 of 11 affected family members in detail. The studies started with a patient who donated his brain to the Bank for Neurological Diseases, London, to study the cause of neuropathy in his family. The clinical syndrome consisted of chronic diarrhea starting in their 30s followed by a mixed, predominantly sensory and autonomic neuropathy. Patients had received diagnoses of irritable bowel syndrome and Crohn disease. Some patients developed bladder denervation and urinary retention and impotence. Others developed postural hypotension, which responded to mineralocorticoid therapy. As the disease advanced, some patients had weight loss, vomiting, and severe diarrhea warranting parenteral feeding in 2 of them. The onset of seizures and cognitive deficits occurred when patients were in their 40s and 50s. They died between 40 and 70 years of age. Average lifespan was 57 years. The disorder was shown to be associated with a Y163X mutation in PRNP, a nonneurologic presentation, widespread deposition of prion protein amyloid in systemic organs including the bowel and peripheral nerves, and slow disease progression. Neuropathology showed deposition of prion protein in the form of cortical amyloid plaques, cerebral amyloid angiopathy, and tauopathy. Murine model studies did not show experimental transmissibility. Based on their elegant and extensive study of this disease, the authors recommend that PRNP analysis be considered in the investigation of unexplained chronic diarrhea associated with a neuropathy or an unexplained syndrome similar to familial amyloid polyneuropathy.

N. Khardori, MD

Reference

1. Collinge J. Prion diseases of humans and animals: their causes and molecular basis. *Annu Rev Neurosci.* 2001;24:519-550.

PART THREE

HEMATOLOGY AND ONCOLOGY

COLLEEN A. LAWTON, MD

18 Gynecologic Cancers

ACR Appropriateness Criteria Staging and Follow-up of Ovarian Cancer
Mitchell DG, Javitt MC, Glanc P, et al (Thomas Jefferson Univ Hosp, Philadelphia, PA; Walter Reed Natl Military Med Ctr, Bethesda, MA; Sunnybrook Health Sciences Centre, Toronto, Ontario, Canada; et al)
J Am Coll Radiol 10:822-827, 2013

Imaging is used to detect and characterize adnexal masses and to stage ovarian cancer both before and after initial treatment, although the role for imaging in screening for ovarian cancer has not been established. CT and MRI have been used to determine the resectability of tumors, the candidacy of patients for effective cytoreductive surgery, the need for postoperative chemotherapy if debulking is suboptimal, and the need for referral to a gynecologic oncologist. Radiographic studies such as contrast enema and urography have been replaced by CT and other cross-sectional imaging for staging ovarian cancer. Contrast-enhanced CT is the procedure of choice for preoperative staging of ovarian cancer. MRI without and with contrast may be useful after equivocal CT, but is usually not the best initial procedure for ovarian cancer staging. Fluorine-18-2-fluoro-2-deoxy-D-glucose—PET/CT may not be needed preoperatively, but its use is appropriate for detecting and defining post-treatment recurrence. Ultrasound is useful for evaluating adnexal disease, but has limited utility for staging ovarian cancer.

The ACR Appropriateness Criteria are evidence-based guidelines for specific clinical conditions that are reviewed every 2 years by a multidisciplinary expert panel. The guideline development and review include an extensive analysis of current medical literature from peer-reviewed journals and the application of a well-established consensus methodology (modified Delphi) to rate the appropriateness of imaging and treatment procedures by the panel. In those instances where evidence is lacking or not definitive, expert opinion may be used to recommend imaging or treatment.

▶ Ovarian cancer is often referred to as the "silent killer" because there is really no easy way to screen for it, and by the time patients have symptoms, it is often advanced and, therefore, not easily cured.

Once diagnosed, it is imperative to have accurate staging to select the best form of treatment. Usually computed tomography is used for such staging with some use of magnetic resonance imaging. Assuming that resection is possible, this is the next appropriate step followed by chemotherapy plus or minus radiation therapy pending the stage and amount of residual disease.

After primary treatment is completed, the patient needs appropriate and close follow-up. This includes the use of laboratory values such as CA125 and other diagnostic tests. These "appropriateness criteria" defined by an expert panel of gynecologic oncologists and radiation oncologists are helpful to guide both ovarian cancer survivors and their physicians in the best and most up-to-date follow-up processes.

With the coming Center for Medicaid and Medicare Services mandate of survivorship plans and protocols, these types of criteria will provide the basic tools needed to correctly develop such protocols.

C. A. Lawton, MD

19 Breast Cancer

Prognosis of Women With Primary Breast Cancer Diagnosed During Pregnancy: Results From an International Collaborative Study

Amant F, von Minckwitz G, Han SN, et al (Univ Hosp Leuven, Belgium; German Breast Group, Neu-Isenburg, Germany)

J Clin Oncol 31:2532-2539, 2013

Purpose.—We aimed to determine the prognosis of patients with breast cancer diagnosed during pregnancy (BCP).

Patients and Methods.—In this cohort study, a multicentric registry of patients with BCP (from Cancer in Pregnancy, Leuven, Belgium, and GBG 29/BIG 02-03) compiled pro- and retrospectively between 2003 and 2011 was compared with patients who did not have associated pregnancies, using an age limit of 45 years. Patients with a diagnosis postpartum were excluded. The main analysis was performed using Cox proportional hazards regression of disease-free survival (DFS) and overall survival (OS) on exposure (pregnant or not), adjusting for age, stage, grade, hormone receptor status, human epidermal growth factor 2 status, histology, type of chemotherapy, use of trastuzumab, radiotherapy, and hormone therapy.

Results.—The registry contained 447 women with BCP, mainly originating from Germany and Belgium, of whom 311 (69.6%) were eligible for analysis. The nonpregnant group consisted of 865 women. Median age was 33 years for the pregnant and 41 years for the nonpregnant patients. Median follow-up was 61 months. The hazard ratio of pregnancy was 1.34 (95% CI, 0.93 to 1.91; P=.14) for DFS and 1.19 (95% CI, 0.73 to 1.93; P=.51) for OS. Cox regression estimated that the 5-year DFS rate for pregnant patients would have increased from 65% to 71% if these patients had not been pregnant. Likewise, the 5-year OS rate would have increased from 78% to 81%.

Conclusion.—The results show similar OS for patients diagnosed with BCP compared with nonpregnant patients. This information is important when patients are counseled and supports the option to start treatment with continuation of pregnancy.

▶ It is well documented scientifically that younger age at diagnosis for breast cancer patients is associated with a poorer prognosis. It has also been well shown that breast cancer has a hormonal dependency such that estrogen supplementation in patients with a history of breast cancer is not recommended. Thus, serious concern is raised for women diagnosed with breast cancer during pregnancy, because pregnancy is associated with younger age and an elevated estrogen state. These data looking at the prognosis for women with breast cancer diagnosed during pregnancy is critical for women in such a situation. Many women in this predicament have been faced with an urging to terminate the pregnancy (clearly a heart-wrenching decision) to increase the chances of their own survival. These data looking at breast cancer patients diagnosed at fewer than 45 years of age support a decrease in concern for patients who are diagnosed while pregnant. These authors found a similar overall survival for patients regardless of pregnancy status in this analysis from Western Europe. Despite a younger median age for the pregnant group of women (33 years vs 41 years), the overall survival at a median follow-up of just over 5 years was similar. Certainly these data offer some comfort for women diagnosed with breast cancer during pregnancy.

C. A. Lawton, MD

Randomized Trial of Pentoxifylline and Vitamin E vs Standard Follow-up After Breast Irradiation to Prevent Breast Fibrosis, Evaluated by Tissue Compliance Meter

Jacobson G, Bhatia S, Smith BJ, et al (Univ of Iowa Hosps and Clinics)
Int J Radiat Oncol Biol Phys 85:604-608, 2013

Purpose.—To conduct a randomized clinical trial to determine whether the combination of pentoxifylline (PTX) and vitamin E given for 6 months after breast/chest wall irradiation effectively prevents radiation-induced fibrosis (RIF).

Methods and Materials.—Fifty-three breast cancer patients with localized disease were enrolled and randomized to treatment with oral PTX 400 mg 3 times daily and oral vitamin E 400 IU daily for 6 months after radiation (n = 26), or standard follow up (n = 27). Tissue compliance meter (TCM) measurements were obtained at 18 months to compare tissue compliance in the irradiated and untreated breast/chest wall in treated subjects and controls. Measurements were obtained at 2 mirror image sites on each breast/chest wall, and the average difference in tissue compliance was scored. Differences in TCM measurements were compared using a *t* test. Subjects were followed a minimum of 2 years for local recurrence, disease-free survival, and overall survival.

Results.—The mean difference in TCM measurements in the 2 groups was 0.88 mm, median of 1.00 mm (treated) and 2.10 mm, median of 2.4 mm (untreated). The difference between the 2 groups was significant ($P = .0478$). Overall survival (100% treated, 90.6% controls at 5 years) and disease-free survival (96.2% treated, 86.8% controls at 5 years) were not significantly different in the 2 groups.

Conclusions.—This study of postirradiation breast cancer patients treated with PTX/vitamin E or standard follow-up indicated a significant difference in radiation-induced fibrosis as measured by TCM. There was no observed impact on local control or survival within the first 2 years of follow-up. The treatment was safe and well tolerated. Pentoxifylline/vitamin E may be clinically useful in preventing fibrosis after radiation in high-risk patients.

▶ The defining benefit of breast-conservation therapy for breast cancer patients is the cosmesis issue. The vast majority of patients with breast cancer naturally want the affected breast to look and feel as close to the pretreatment breast as possible, so methods to increase cosmesis for these patients are especially important to radiation oncologists. Yet cosmesis is unquestionably subjective endpoint. Therefore, any way to quantify this outcome in a more objective way is a benefit.

This trial, which randomized breast cancer patients to pentoxifylline and vitamin E, versus standard follow-up was able to assess 1 aspect of cosmesis with increased objectivity through the use of a tissue compliance meter. Increased tissue compliance is seen in patients with less radiation-induced fibrosis and is correlated with improved cosmesis with regard to both visual and palpable aspects of cosmesis. The results of this trial suggest a benefit to the use of pentoxifylline and vitamin E in postradiation breast cancer patients. Certainly a larger cohort of patients and longer follow-up would increase the likelihood of verifying the benefit of these supplements for breast cancer patients who are treated with breast-conserving therapy.

C. A. Lawton, MD

The American Brachytherapy Society consensus statement for accelerated partial breast irradiation

Shah C, Vicini F, Wazer DE, et al (Washington Univ School of Medicine, Saint Louis, MO; Michigan Healthcare Professionals/21st Century Oncology, Farmington Hills; Tufts Univ School of Medicine, Boston, MA; et al)

Brachytherapy 12:267-277, 2013

Purpose.—To develop clinical guidelines for the quality practice of accelerated partial breast irradiation (APBI) as part of breast-conserving therapy for women with early-stage breast cancer.

Methods and Materials.—Members of the American Brachytherapy Society with expertise in breast cancer and breast brachytherapy in particular devised updated guidelines for appropriate patient evaluation and selection based on an extensive literature search and clinical experience.

Results.—Increasing numbers of randomized and single and multi-institution series have been published documenting the efficacy of various APBI modalities. With more than 10-year followup, multiple series have documented excellent clinical outcomes with interstitial APBI. Patient selection for APBI should be based on a review of clinical and pathologic factors by the clinician with particular attention paid to age (≥50 years old), tumor size (≤3 cm), histology (all invasive subtypes and ductal carcinoma *in situ*), surgical margins (negative), lymphovascular space invasion (not present), and nodal status (negative). Consistent dosimetric guidelines should be used to improve target coverage and limit potential for toxicity following treatment.

Conclusions.—These guidelines have been created to provide clinicians with appropriate patient selection criteria to allow clinicians to use APBI in a manner that will optimize clinical outcomes and patient satisfaction. These guidelines will continue to be evaluated and revised as future publications further stratify optimal patient selection.

▶ The ability for women who have breast cancer to keep their breast intact via lumpectomy and postoperative whole breast radiation therapy was one of the largest cancer breakthroughs in the 20th century in terms of increasing the quality of life for breast cancer patients. Based on numerous prospective randomized trials comparing this technique to standard modified radical mastectomy has proven its equivalence to this mutilating surgery. The standard approach for postlumpectomy radiation therapy is approximately 6 weeks in duration, with daily radiation to the whole breast for approximately 5 of those weeks then a boost to the tumor bed for the final week. This time commitment can be a real challenge for many women, especially if they do not have a radiation facility close to home. Alternate radiation therapy options have been studied, one of which is accelerated partial breast irradiation (APBI). This alternative form of postlumpectomy radiation therapy can be performed as an interstitial implant and as such has been studied via multiple single and multi-institutional trials. Although this approach is not ideal for all breast cancer patients, this article represents an excellent outline of patients who would be best suited for this approach. Based on the current science in this area, these authors have encouraged patients and their radiation oncologists to carefully consider this approach with special attention paid to age, tumor size, histologic subtypes, lymphovascular space invasion, and nodal status.

C. A. Lawton, MD

Interim Cosmetic and Toxicity Results From RAPID: A Randomized Trial of Accelerated Partial Breast Irradiation Using Three-Dimensional Conformal External Beam Radiation Therapy

Olivotto IA, Whelan TJ, Parpia S, et al (British Columbia Cancer Agency, Vancouver, Canada; McMaster Univ, Hamilton, Ontario, Canada; et al)
J Clin Oncol 31:4038-4045, 2013

Purpose.—To report interim cosmetic and toxicity results of a multicenter randomized trial comparing accelerated partial-breast irradiation (APBI) using three-dimensional conformal external beam radiation therapy (3D-CRT) with whole-breast irradiation (WBI).

Patients and Methods.—Women age > 40 years with invasive or in situ breast cancer ≤ 3 cm were randomly assigned after breast-conserving surgery to 3D-CRT APBI (38.5 Gy in 10 fractions twice daily) or WBI (42.5 Gy in 16 or 50 Gy in 25 daily fractions ± boost irradiation). The primary outcome was ipsilateral breast tumor recurrence (IBTR). Secondary outcomes were cosmesis and toxicity. Adverse cosmesis was defined as a fair or poor global cosmetic score. After a planned interim cosmetic analysis, the data, safety, and monitoring committee recommended release of results. There have been too few IBTR events to trigger an efficacy analysis.

Results.—Between 2006 and 2011, 2,135 women were randomly assigned to 3D-CRT APBI or WBI. Median follow-up was 36 months. Adverse cosmesis at 3 years was increased among those treated with APBI compared with WBI as assessed by trained nurses (29% *v* 17%; $P < .001$), by patients (26% *v* 18%; $P = .0022$), and by physicians reviewing digital photographs (35% *v* 17%; $P < .001$). Grade 3 toxicities were rare in both treatment arms (1.4% *v* 0%), but grade 1 and 2 toxicities were increased among those who received APBI compared with WBI ($P < .001$).

Conclusion.—3D-CRT APBI increased rates of adverse cosmesis and late radiation toxicity compared with standard WBI. Clinicians and patients are cautioned against the use of 3D-CRT APBI outside the context of a controlled trial.

▶ Breast-conserving treatment with lumpectomy and postoperative radiation therapy was a great advance in organ preservation for tens of thousands with breast cancer. The ability to have such treatment and remain active (working and leading fairly normal lives) is a big improvement over traditional mastectomy and breast reconstruction. Yet there is the burden of 5 to 6 weeks of daily radiation therapy. So naturally, with the advent of favorable results in randomized trials of hypofractionation, this burden has lessened some.

Hypofractionation and/or accelerated fractionation has been approached with caution for many cancers treated primarily with radiation because of the concern for late toxicity. Thus, this type of data is critically important for breast cancer patients because good cosmesis is one of the important end points of breast-conserving therapy. Given the results seen in this randomized trial, the caution that the authors suggest should be heeded. Obviously, more data are needed to verify or refute these findings. We look forward to such data.

C. A. Lawton, MD

Incidence of Breast Cancer With Distant Involvement Among Women in the United States, 1976 to 2009

Johnson RH, Chien FL, Bleyer A, et al (Univ of Washington, Seattle; Central Oregon and Oregon Health and Science Univ, Portland)

JAMA 309:800-805, 2013

Importance.—Evidence from the US National Cancer Institute Surveillance, Epidemiology, and End Results (SEER) database suggests that the incidence of advanced breast cancer in young women is increasing.

Objective.—To quantify this trend and analyze it as a function of stage at diagnosis, race/ethnicity, residence, and hormone receptor status.

Design, Setting, and Patients.—Breast cancer incidence, incidence trends, and survival rates as a function of age and extent of disease at diagnosis were obtained from 3 SEER registries that provide data spanning 1973-2009, 1992-2009, and 2000- 2009. SEER defines *localized* as disease confined to the breast, *regional* to contiguous and adjacent organ spread (eg, lymph nodes, chest wall), and *distant disease* to remote metastases (bone, brain, lung, etc).

Main Outcome Measure.—Breast cancer incidence trends in the United States.

Results.—In the United States, the incidence of breast cancer with distant involvement at diagnosis increased in 25- to 39-year-old women from 1.53 (95% CI, 1.01 to 2.21) per 100 000 in 1976 to 2.90 (95% CI, 2.31 to 3.59) per 100 000 in 2009. This is an absolute difference of 1.37 per 100 000, representing an average compounded increase of 2.07% per year (95% CI, 1.57% to 2.58%; $P < .001$) over the 34-year interval. No other age group or extent-of-disease subgroup of the same age range had a similar increase. For 25- to 39-year-olds, there was an increased incidence in distant disease among all races and ethnicities evaluated, especially non-Hispanic white and African American, and this occurred in both metropolitan and nonmetropolitan areas. Incidence for women with estrogen receptor–positive subtypes increased more than for women with estrogen receptor–negative subtypes.

Conclusion and Relevance.—Based on SEER data, there was a small but statistically significant increase in the incidence of breast cancer with distant involvement in the United States between 1976 and 2009 for women aged 25 to 39 years, without a corresponding increase in older women.

▶ Breast cancer continues to be a major health problem in the United States with more than 38 000 deaths annually. Screening for breast cancer, although somewhat controversial, usually begins at age 40. We know that young age is an independent adverse predictor of outcome for breast cancer patients. There is concern that women who develop breast cancer at a younger age (ie, less than 40 years of age) have a higher risk of being diagnosed with distant disease, and thus they carry additional risk of death from the disease. These authors have used SEER (US Surveillance, Epidemiology, and End Results) data to assess trends in disease status based on age of diagnosis. The fact that they found a statistically significant increase in incidence of breast cancer with distant disease in women in the United States aged 25 to 39 compared with older women is of real concern. If corroborated with other data, it will be important to try to understand the causes of this more aggressive breast cancer. We need to understand these aggressive cancers in young women to know how better to screen for them such that we find the disease before it metastasizes.

C. A. Lawton, MD

20 Prostate Cancer

Long-Term Functional Outcomes after Treatment for Localized Prostate Cancer

Resnick MJ, Koyama T, Fan K-H, et al (Vanderbilt Univ, Nashville, TN; et al)

N Engl J Med 368:436-445, 2013

Background.—The purpose of this analysis was to compare long-term urinary, bowel, and sexual function after radical prostatectomy or external-beam radiation therapy.

Methods.—The Prostate Cancer Outcomes Study (PCOS) enrolled 3533 men in whom prostate cancer had been diagnosed in 1994 or 1995. The current cohort comprised 1655 men in whom localized prostate cancer had been diagnosed between the ages of 55 and 74 years and who had undergone either surgery (1164 men) or radiotherapy (491 men). Functional status was assessed at baseline and at 2, 5, and 15 years after diagnosis. We used multivariable propensity scoring to compare functional outcomes according to treatment.

Results.—Patients undergoing prostatectomy were more likely to have urinary incontinence than were those undergoing radiotherapy at 2 years (odds ratio, 6.22; 95% confidence interval [CI], 1.92 to 20.29) and 5 years (odds ratio, 5.10; 95% CI, 2.29 to 11.36). However, no significant between-group difference in the odds of urinary incontinence was noted at 15 years. Similarly, although patients undergoing prostatectomy were more likely to have erectile dysfunction at 2 years (odds ratio, 3.46; 95% CI, 1.93 to 6.17) and 5 years (odds ratio, 1.96; 95% CI, 1.05 to 3.63), no significant between-group difference was noted at 15 years. Patients undergoing prostatectomy were less likely to have bowel urgency at 2 years (odds ratio, 0.39; 95% CI, 0.22 to 0.68) and 5 years (odds ratio, 0.47; 95% CI, 0.26 to 0.84), again with no significant between-group difference in the odds of bowel urgency at 15 years.

Conclusions.—At 15 years, no significant relative differences in disease-specific functional outcomes were observed among men undergoing prostatectomy or radiotherapy. Nonetheless, men treated for localized prostate cancer commonly had declines in all functional domains during 15 years of follow-up. (Funded by the National Cancer Institute.)

▶ As radiation oncologists, we have all been told by our urologic counterparts that although the radiation therapy options of external beam and/or brachytherapy may be equal in terms of prostate cancer control and survival, surgery over time remains the less toxic option. Without good data to refute this ideation, it has been difficult to address.

There have been multiple studies (mostly retrospective, single-institution or Surveillance Epidemiology End Results based) suggesting that in fact radiation therapy may not be associated with worse outcomes for our patients than radical retropubic prostatectomy (RRP) in terms of quality of life. Yet without standardized patient reported outcomes, none of the previous data were met with anything except skepticism. The other pushback we radiation oncologists get from our surgical colleagues is that there may not be quality-of-life differences at early time points such as 3 to 5 years but it is at the 10-plus-year time frame when the surgeons will argue quality-of-life benefits of surgery over radiation.

These data, which are the result of patient-reported outcomes, tells us that all patients have their quality of life affected either with RRP or radiation therapy for localized prostate cancer. The data are from 2-, 5-, and 15-year follow-up, so it clearly addresses the long-term issues that these patients face. At the 15-year time point, men with RRP were statistically more likely to wear pads because of incontinence issues compared with the radiation-therapy group. Sexual functioning, although negatively affected by both surgery and radiation, was not different between the 2 modalities. Finally gastrointestinal functioning in terms of "bother" was statistically worse for the radiation group.

These data should be used to help men make the best choice for the care of their localized prostate cancer.

C. A. Lawton, MD

Abiraterone in Metastatic Prostate Cancer without Previous Chemotherapy

Ryan CJ, for the COU-AA-302 Investigators (Univ of California, San Francisco)

N Engl J Med 368:138-148, 2013

Background.—Abiraterone acetate, an androgen biosynthesis inhibitor, improves overall survival in patients with metastatic castration-resistant prostate cancer after chemotherapy. We evaluated this agent in patients who had not received previous chemotherapy.

Methods.—In this double-blind study, we randomly assigned 1088 patients to receive abiraterone acetate (1000 mg) plus prednisone (5 mg twice daily) or placebo plus prednisone. The coprimary end points were radiographic progression-free survival and overall survival.

Results.—The study was unblinded after a planned interim analysis that was performed after 43% of the expected deaths had occurred. The median radiographic progressionfree survival was 16.5 months with abiraterone–prednisone and 8.3 months with prednisone alone (hazard ratio for abiraterone–prednisone vs. prednisone alone, 0.53; 95% confidence interval [CI], 0.45 to 0.62; $P < 0.001$). Over a median follow-up period of 22.2 months, overall survival was improved with abiraterone–prednisone (median not reached, vs. 27.2 months for prednisone alone; hazard ratio, 0.75; 95% CI, 0.61 to 0.93; $P = 0.01$) but did not cross the efficacy boundary. Abiraterone—prednisone showed superiority over prednisone alone with respect to time to initiation of cytotoxic chemotherapy, opiate use for cancer-related pain, prostate-specific antigen progression, and decline in performance status. Grade 3 or 4 mineralocorticoid- related adverse events and abnormalities on liver-function testing were more common with abiraterone—prednisone.

Conclusions.—Abiraterone improved radiographic progression-free survival, showed a trend toward improved overall survival, and significantly delayed clinical decline and initiation of chemotherapy in patients with metastatic castration-resistant prostate cancer. (Funded by Janssen Research and Development, formerly Cougar Biotechnology; ClinicalTrials.gov number, NCT00887198.)

▶ Prostate cancer continues to claim the lives of more than 33 000 men in the United States annually. For patients who develop metastatic disease, the standard of care is hormone therapy in terms of an luteinizing hormone releasing hormone agonist and an antiandrogen (otherwise known as total androgen suppression). This standard of care, although temporarily effective, will result in patients becoming castration-resistant with time. Once this happens, death commonly occurs within 2 to 4 years. Therefore, the next steps to help delay death yet preserve quality of life become important.

Taxol-based chemotherapeutic regimens have become a routine option for these patients, yet there are real quality-of-life issues with the addition of cytotoxic chemotherapy. Thus, second-line hormone therapy agents are of particular interest to patients and their oncologists. Abiraterone acetate is an androgen biosynthesis inhibitor that has been shown to increase overall survival in patients with metastatic castrate resistant prostate cancer who have already had chemotherapy. Whether this drug would work well for castration-resistant prostate cancer patients before their receiving chemotherapy is a reasonable question to ask.

This randomized double-blind trial has asked the correct question for these patients: abiraterone plus prednisone vs prednisone alone. The results show a benefit to the use of abiraterone in patients with asymptomatic or mildly symptomatic metastatic castrate resistant prostate cancer who have not yet had prior chemotherapy. Both quantity of life and quality of life were positively affected.

C. A. Lawton, MD

Intermittent versus Continuous Androgen Deprivation in Prostate Cancer

Hussain M, Tangen CM, Berry DL, et al (Univ of Michigan, Ann Arbor; Southwest Oncology Group Statistical Ctr, Seattle, WA; Dana—Farber Cancer Inst, Boston, MA; et al)

N Engl J Med 368:1314-1325, 2013

Background.—Castration resistance occurs in most patients with metastatic hormone-sensitive prostate cancer who are receiving androgen-deprivation therapy. Replacing androgens before progression of the disease is hypothesized to prolong androgen dependence.

Methods.—Men with newly diagnosed, metastatic, hormone-sensitive prostate cancer, a performance status of 0 to 2, and a prostate-specific antigen (PSA) level of 5 ng per milliliter or higher received a luteinizing hormone–releasing hormone analogue and an antiandrogen agent for 7 months. We then randomly assigned patients in whom the PSA level fell to 4 ng per milliliter or lower to continuous or intermittent androgen deprivation, with patients stratified according to prior or no prior hormonal therapy, performance status, and extent of disease (minimal or extensive). The coprimary objectives were to assess whether intermittent therapy was noninferior to continuous therapy with respect to survival, with a one-sided test with an upper boundary of the hazard ratio of 1.20, and whether quality of life differed between the groups 3 months after randomization.

Results.—A total of 3040 patients were enrolled, of whom 1535 were included in the analysis: 765 randomly assigned to continuous androgen deprivation and 770 assigned to intermittent androgen deprivation. The median follow-up period was 9.8 years. Median survival was 5.8 years in the continuous-therapy group and 5.1 years in the intermittent-therapy group (hazard ratio for death with intermittent therapy, 1.10; 90% confidence interval, 0.99 to 1.23). Intermittent therapy was associated with better erectile function and mental health ($P < 0.001$ and $P = 0.003$, respectively) at month 3 but not thereafter. There were no significant differences between the groups in the number of treatment-related high-grade adverse events.

Conclusions.—Our findings were statistically inconclusive. In patients with metastatic hormone-sensitive prostate cancer, the confidence interval for survival exceeded the upper boundary for noninferiority, suggesting that we cannot rule out a 20% greater risk of death with intermittent therapy than with continuous therapy, but too few events occurred to rule out significant inferiority of intermittent therapy. Intermittent therapy resulted in small improvements in quality of life. (Funded by the National Cancer Institute and others; ClinicalTrials.gov number, NCT00002651.)

▶ We have known since the 1940s that prostate cancer responds to androgen deprivation thanks to the work of Drs Huggins and Hodges. For decades, the androgen deprivation came in the form of orchiectomy, which is not only permanent from a therapeutic maneuver perspective but often devastating from a psychological perspective.

The next step in the androgen-deprivation story was the use of estrogens, most notably in the form of diethylstilbestrol. Although this, too, was useful from the perspective of prostate cancer response, it resulted in many unexpected cardiovascular events such that its use had to be stopped.

The current "androgen-deprivation" maneuver comes in the form of Luteinizing-hormone- releasing hormone agonists, which is often combined with antiandrogen oral medication. These medications, although effective in controlling prostate cancer, have their own significant toxicities. Because of these toxicities, patients with metastatic prostate cancer who need these drugs would of course prefer not to take them continuously and indefinitely. So trials such as the one presented here are critical for these patients.

The findings were inconclusive according to the publication. But practically, with a median follow-up of 9.8 years and a median survival difference of 0.7 months (5.8 years vs 5.1 years), patients can now be comforted that if they choose intermittent therapy for whatever reason, they will not unquestionably have done the wrong thing.

C. A. Lawton, MD

Short-term Androgen-Deprivation Therapy Improves Prostate Cancer-Specific Mortality in Intermediate-Risk Prostate Cancer Patients Undergoing Dose-Escalated External Beam Radiation Therapy

Zumsteg ZS, Spratt DE, Pei X, et al (Memorial Sloan-Kettering Cancer Ctr, NY)

Int J Radiat Oncol Biol Phys 85:1012-1017, 2013

Purpose.—We investigated the benefit of short-term androgen-deprivation therapy (ADT) in patients with intermediate-risk prostate cancer (PC) receiving dose-escalated external beam radiation therapy.

Methods and Materials.—The present retrospective study comprised 710 intermediate-risk PC patients receiving external beam radiation therapy with doses of ≥81 Gy at a single institution from 1992 to 2005, including 357 patients receiving neoadjuvant and concurrent ADT. Prostate-specific antigen recurrence-free survival (PSA-RFS) and distant metastasis (DM) were compared using the Kaplan-Meier method and Cox proportional hazards models. PC-specific mortality (PCSM) was assessed using competing-risks analysis.

Results.—The median follow-up was 7.9 years. Despite being more likely to have higher PSA levels, Gleason score 4 + 3 = 7, multiple National Comprehensive Cancer Network intermediate-risk factors, and older age ($P \leq .001$ for all comparisons), patients receiving ADT had improved PSA-RFS (hazard ratio [HR], 0.598; 95% confidence interval [CI], 0.435-0.841; $P = .003$), DM (HR, 0.424; 95% CI, 0.219-0.819; $P = .011$), and PCSM (HR, 0.380; 95% CI, 0.157-0.921; $P = .032$) on univariate analysis. Using multivariate analysis, ADT was an even stronger predictor of improved PSA-RFS (adjusted HR [AHR], 0.516; 95% CI, 0.360-0.739; $P < .001$), DM (AHR, 0.347; 95% CI, 0.176-0.685; $P = .002$), and PCSM (AHR, 0.297; 95% CI, 0.128-0.685; $P = .004$). Gleason score 4 + 3 = 7 and ≥50% positive biopsy cores were other independent predictors of PCSM.

Conclusions.—Short-term ADT improves PSA-RFS, DM, and PCSM in patients with intermediate-risk PC undergoing dose-escalated external beam radiation therapy.

▶ It has been well documented by a prospective phase III randomized trial that patients who have high-risk prostate cancer (defined as Gleason Score 8–10, and/or clinical T3–T4 disease) benefit from androgen deprivation in addition to external beam radiation therapy. Also well studied via prospective phase III randomized trials is the benefit of dose escalation in controlling the disease, especially for patients with intermediate-risk disease (defined as prostate-specific antigen >10 and/or Gleason Score 7 and/or clinical T2b–T2c disease). Yet for intermediate risk patients, it is not know whether, in addition to dose escalation, they might benefit from androgen deprivation.

The current Radiation Therapy and Oncology Group (RTOG) trial 08-15 is asking this very question in a phase III prospective randomized way. The trial continues to accrue, and results from the trial will not be available for years. So data such as those reported in this article are particularly helpful for patients who either are ineligible for RTOG 08-15 or simply do not want to participate in such a trial.

The addition of 4 to 6 months of neoadjuvant and concurrent androgen deprivation consisting of a luteinizing hormone releasing hormone agonist plus or minus an antiandrogen for the first month appears to improve the incidence of distant metastasis and prostate cancer-specific survival. Of course, we will only have the final answer to this question with the results from randomized prospective trials, but in the interim, these data help radiation oncologists make more educated decisions about androgen deprivation for their intermediate-risk patients.

C. A. Lawton, MD

The REDUCE Follow-Up Study: Low Rate of New Prostate Cancer Diagnoses Observed During a 2-Year, Observational, Followup Study of Men Who Participated in the REDUCE Trial

Grubb RL, Andriole GL, Somerville MC, et al (Washington Univ School of Medicine in St Louis, MO; GlaxoSmithKline, Research Triangle Park, NC; et al)
J Urol 189:871-877, 2013

Purpose.—The primary objective of the REDUCE (REduction by DUtasteride of prostate Cancer Events) Follow-Up Study was to collect data on the occurrence of newly diagnosed prostate cancers for 2 years beyond the 4-year REDUCE study.

Materials and Methods.—The 4-year REDUCE study evaluated prostate cancer risk reduction in men taking dutasteride. This 2-year observational study followed men from REDUCE with a clinic visit shortly after study conclusion and with up to 2 annual telephone calls during which patient reported data were collected regarding prostate cancer events, chronic medication use, prostate specific antigen levels and serious adverse events. No study drug was provided and all biopsies during the 2-year followup were performed for cause. The primary objective was to collect data on the occurrence of new biopsy detectable prostate cancers. Secondary end points included assessment of Gleason score and serious adverse events.

Results.—A total of 2,751 men enrolled in the followup study with numbers similar to those of the REDUCE former treatment groups (placebo and dutasteride). Few new prostate cancers were detected during the 2-year followup period in either former treatment group. A greater number of cancers were detected in the former dutasteride group than in the former placebo group (14 vs 7 cases). No Gleason score 8–10 prostate cancers were detected in either former treatment group based on central pathology review. No new safety issues were identified during the study.

Conclusions.—Two years of followup of the REDUCE study cohort demonstrated a low rate of new prostate cancer diagnoses in the former placebo and dutasteride treated groups. No new Gleason 8–10 cancers were detected.

▶ Given that prostate cancer will claim the lives of more than 33 000 men in the United States this year, efforts to decrease its incidence are critical. Two studies conducted in the past decade looked at 2 different, but related, drugs—dutasteride and finasteride—to evaluate their potential to decrease prostate cancer incidence. Both drugs did in fact reduce the incidence of prostate cancer by more than 20% compared with placebo arms. This was good news for certain potential prostate cancer patients. Unfortunately, this benefit came with a downside. In both trials, the patients treated with the 5-alpha reductase inhibitors (5-ARIs) were found to have an increase in the number of high-grade (Gleason score 8–10) cancers. The next obvious question that thankfully was addressed by this follow-up study is, with further follow-up, would there be more of these high-grade cancers in the patients on the treatment arm? More good news is found in these data, which look at 2 additional years of follow-up. There were no additional high-risk prostate cancers found in the treated group and no difference in the number of low-grade prostate cancers found between the treated and placebo groups.

The question, of course, remains as to the potential benefit of this class of drugs in helping to prevent prostate cancer. Until we better understand the etiology of the development of the high-grade cancers in patients treated with 5-ARIs, they should be used with caution.

C. A. Lawton, MD

Results from the Quality Research in Radiation Oncology (QRRO) survey: Evaluation of dosimetric outcomes for low-dose-rate prostate brachytherapy

Zelefsky MJ, Cohen GN, Bosch WR, et al (Memorial Sloan—Kettering Cancer Ctr, NY; Washington Univ, St Louis, MO; et al)

Brachytherapy 12:19-24, 2013

Purpose.—We report on quality of dose delivery to target and normal tissues from low-dose-rate prostate brachytherapy using postimplantation dosimetric evaluations from a random sample of U.S. patients.

Methods and Materials.—Nonmetastatic prostate cancer patients treated with external beam radiotherapy or brachytherapy in 2007 were randomly sampled from radiation oncology facilities nationwide. Of 414 prostate cancer cases from 45 institutions, 86 received low-dose-rate brachytherapy. We collected the 30-day postimplantation CT images of these patients and 10 test cases from two other institutions. Scans were downloaded into a treatment planning system and prostate/ rectal contours were redrawn. Dosimetric outcomes were reanalyzed and compared with calculated outcomes from treating institutions.

Results.—Median prostate volume was 33.4 cm^3. Reevaluated median V_{100}, D_{90}, and V_{150} were 91.1% (range, 45.5–99.8%), 101.7% (range, 59.6–145.9%), and 53.9% (range, 15.7–88.4%), respectively. Low gland coverage included 27 patients (39%) with a D_{90} lower than 100% of the prescription dose (PD), 12 of whom (17% of the entire group) had a D_{90} lower than 80% of PD. There was no correlation between D_{90} coverage and prostate volume, number of seeds, or implanted activity. The median V_{100} for the rectum was 0.3 cm^3 (range, 0–4.3 cm^3). No outcome differences were observed according to the institutional strata. Concordance between reported and reevaluated D_{90} values (defined as within ±10%) was observed in 44 of 69 cases.

Conclusions.—Central review of postimplantation CT scans to assess the quality of prostate brachytherapy is feasible. Most patients achieved excellent dosimetric outcomes, yet 17% had less than optimal target coverage by the PD. There was concordance between submitted target-coverage parameters and central dosimetric review in 64% of implants. These findings will require further validation in a larger cohort of patients.

▶ Prostate low-dose-rate (LDR) brachytherapy as monotherapy remains one of the most clinically and cost-effective approaches for patients with organ-confined prostate cancer. The procedure has been validated as being performed effectively in an Radiation Therapy Oncology Group (RTOG) trial (98-05) that helped confirm the procedure can correctly and effectively be carried out in many centers across the United States. Yet the centers involved in the National Cooperative Groups may or may not be representative of the treatment with this modality across our country.

Most centers—large and small, academic and community based—are performing this procedure given its clinical and cost-effectiveness. Yet exactly what results are found if one polls "the average" cancer treatment facility is not known. Is it easy to do quality prostate LDR brachytherapy in our "average" cancer treatment facility in the United States? The RTOG trial cannot answer this because they are selected centers that have jumped through quality-assurance hoops not required of other centers. So the real way to address this question and many others like it is through voluntary participation in data collection, as was done via the Quality Research in Radiation Oncology (QRRO) group or through a registry format. The QRRO group and its participants are to be commended for the reporting of this data. It helps verify that this procedure is in fact being done correctly in many centers across the United States. The challenge, of course, is that these data are only a snippet of the big picture.

Registries such as those already developed in cardiology, for example (where tens of thousands of patients and their procedures are documented and reviewed for quality metrics and outcomes) is the only way to effectively evaluate medical procedures such as prostate LDR brachytherapy. If behooves us as a specialty to work toward this goal to validate prostate LDR brachytherapy and virtually all of the procedures that we do for our cancer patients. Registry data will help us verify that our treatment is of value to our patients in terms of medical outcomes including quality of life and cost.

C. A. Lawton, MD

ACR Appropriateness Criteria Prostate Cancer—Pretreatment Detection, Staging, and Surveillance

Eberhardt SC, Carter S, Casalino DD, et al (Univ of New Mexico, Albuquerque; Northwestern Univ, Chicago, IL; et al)

J Am Coll Radiol 10:83-92, 2013

Prostate cancer is the most common noncutaneous male malignancy in the United States. The use of serum prostate-specific antigen as a screening tool is complicated by a significant fraction of nonlethal cancers diagnosed by biopsy. Ultrasound is used predominately as a biopsy guidance tool. Combined rectal examination, prostate-specific antigen testing, and histology from ultrasound-guided biopsy provide risk stratification for locally advanced and metastatic disease. Imaging in low-risk patients is unlikely to guide management for patients electing up-front treatment. MRI, CT, and bone scans are appropriate in intermediate-risk to high-risk patients to better assess the extent of disease, guide therapy decisions, and predict outcomes. MRI (particularly with an endorectal coil and multiparametric functional imaging) provides the best imaging for cancer detection and staging. There may be a role for prostate MRI in the context of active surveillance for low-risk patients and in cancer detection for undiagnosed clinically suspected cancer after negative biopsy results.

The ACR Appropriateness Criteria are evidence-based guidelines for specific clinical conditions that are reviewed every 2 years by a multidisciplinary expert panel. The guideline development and review include an extensive analysis of current medical literature from peer-reviewed journals and the application of a well-established consensus methodology (modified Delphi) to rate the appropriateness of imaging and treatment procedures by the panel. In those instances in which evidence is lacking or not definitive, expert opinion may be used to recommend imaging or treatment.

▶ The American College of Radiology (ACR) Appropriateness Criteria have been developed for a number of malignancies, and the process for the development of the criteria is well documented and fairly exhaustive. An expert panel for the disease to be considered is convened, and a "complete" literature review is performed. Based on the literature review and input from the expert panel, a guideline is developed and reviewed every 2 years to try to keep the document current and therefore valid.

Given the changes in the recommendations for prostate cancer regarding screening, it is timely that this guideline was published. Certainly one benefit of this guideline is the recommendation (or lack thereof) for imaging tests pending the risk category of the prostate cancer. It is quite clear, for example, that patients with low-risk disease do not need "staging" imaging and that high-risk patients do. Yet how does one factor in the latest magnetic resonance imaging (MRI) sequences that can be obtained with endorectal coil? The relatively exhaustive addressing of MRI use as well as other imaging is the main message and benefit of this guideline.

C. A. Lawton, MD

Effect of Soy Protein Isolate Supplementation on Biochemical Recurrence of Prostate Cancer After Radical Prostatectomy: A Randomized Trial

Bosland MC, Kato I, Zeleniuch-Jacquotte A, et al (Univ of Illinois at Chicago; New York Univ School of Medicine; et al)

JAMA 310:170-178, 2013

Importance.—Soy consumption has been suggested to reduce risk or recurrence of prostate cancer, but this has not been tested in a randomized trial with prostate cancer as the end point.

Objective.—To determine whether daily consumption of a soy protein isolate supplement for 2 years reduces the rate of biochemical recurrence of prostate cancer after radical prostatectomy or delays such recurrence.

Design, Setting, and Participants.—Randomized, double-blind trial conducted from July 1997 to May 2010 at 7 US centers comparing daily consumption of a soy protein supplement vs placebo in 177 men at high risk of recurrence after radical prostatectomy for prostate cancer. Supplement intervention was started within 4 months after surgery and continued for up to 2 years, with prostate-specific antigen (PSA) measurements made at 2-month intervals in the first year and every 3 months thereafter.

Intervention.—Participants were randomized to receive a daily serving of a beverage powder containing 20 g of protein in the form of either soy protein isolate (n = 87) or, as placebo, calcium caseinate (n = 90).

Main Outcomes and Measures.—Biochemical recurrence rate of prostate cancer (defined as development of a PSA level of ≥0.07 ng/mL) over the first 2 years following randomization and time to recurrence.

Results.—The trial was stopped early for lack of treatment effects at a planned interim analysis with 81 evaluable participants in the intervention group and 78 in the placebo group. Overall, 28.3% of participants developed biochemical recurrence within 2 years of entering the trial (close to the a priori predicted recurrence rate of 30%). Among these, 22 (27.2%) occurred in the intervention group and 23 (29.5%) in the placebo group. The resulting hazard ratio for active treatment was 0.96 (95% CI, 0.53-1.72; log-rank P = .89). Adherence was greater than 90% and there were no apparent adverse events related to supplementation.

Conclusion and Relevance.—Daily consumption of a beverage powder supplement containing soy protein isolate for 2 years following radical prostatectomy did not reduce biochemical recurrence of prostate cancer in men at high risk of PSA failure.

Trial Registration.—clinicaltrials.gov Identifier: NCT00765479.

▶ It has been well documented since the 1940s and the pioneering work of Drs Huggins and Hodges that prostate cancer has a hormonal dependency. This hormonal dependency has been used in the treatment of this disease through the use of androgen deprivation as monotherapy in the case of metastatic disease and in combination with radiation for patients with high-risk disease.

The potential benefit of androgen deprivation in combination with surgery for localized prostate cancer has also been studied extensively. Several randomized trials of preoperative androgen deprivation have failed to show a benefit to this method over surgery alone.

Soy and soy foods have been thought to be a potential preventative (hormonally driven) dietary option for prostate cancer patients. It has been postulated that the increase in soy in the diets of men in Asian countries could help to explain the low incidence of prostate cancer in those countries. These authors studied the effects of soy protein in the diet of postoperative prostate cancer patients in a double-blinded manner. The results show no effect of increased dietary soy on the biochemical disease-free survival of postoperative prostate cancer patients. These results mimic the findings of the use of androgen deprivation preoperatively in these patients. Why these hormonal maneuvers work with radiation and not with surgery is an interesting question that needs further study. It would also be of great interest to do this soy protein supplement study on prostate cancer patients who receive radiation as their primary mode of treatment.

C. A. Lawton, MD

Use of Advanced Treatment Technologies Among Men at Low Risk of Dying From Prostate Cancer

Jacobs BL, Zhang Y, Schroeck FR, et al (Univ of Michigan, Ann Arbor; et al)
JAMA 309:2587-2595, 2013

Importance.—The use of advanced treatment technologies (ie, intensity-modulated radiotherapy [IMRT] and robotic prostatectomy) for prostate cancer is increasing. The extent to which these advanced treatment technologies have disseminated among patients at low risk of dying from prostate cancer is uncertain.

Objective.—To assess the use of advanced treatment technologies, compared with prior standards (ie, traditional external beam radiation treatment [EBRT] and open radical prostatectomy) and observation, among men with a low risk of dying from prostate cancer.

Design, Setting, and Patients.—Using Surveillance, Epidemiology, and End Results (SEER)-Medicare data, we identified a retrospective cohort of men diagnosed with prostate cancer between 2004 and 2009 who underwent IMRT (n = 23 633), EBRT (n = 3926), robotic prostatectomy (n = 5881), open radical prostatectomy (n = 6123), or observation (n = 16 384). Follow-up data were available through December 31, 2010.

Main Outcomes and Measures.—The use of advanced treatment technologies among men unlikely to die from prostate cancer, as assessed by low-risk disease (clinical stage ≤T2a, biopsy Gleason score ≤6, and prostate-specific antigen level ≤10 ng/mL), high risk of noncancer mortality (based on the predicted probability of death within 10 years in the absence of a cancer diagnosis), or both.

Results.—In our cohort, the use of advanced treatment technologies increased from 32% (95% CI, 30%-33%) to 44% (95% CI, 43%-46%) among men with low-risk disease ($P < .001$) and from 36% (95% CI, 35%-38%) to 57% (95% CI, 55%-59%) among men with high risk of noncancer mortality ($P < .001$). The use of these advanced treatment technologies among men with both low-risk disease and high risk of noncancer mortality increased from 25% (95% CI, 23%-28%) to 34% (95% CI, 31%-37%) ($P < .001$). Among all patients diagnosed in SEER, the use of advanced treatment technologies for men unlikely to die from prostate cancer increased from 13% (95% CI, 12%-14%), or 129.2 per 1000 patients diagnosed with prostate cancer, to 24% (95% CI, 24%-25%), or 244.2 per 1000 patients diagnosed with prostate cancer ($P < .001$).

Conclusion and Relevance.—Among men diagnosed with prostate cancer between 2004 and 2009 who had low-risk disease, high risk of noncancer mortality, or both, the use of advanced treatment technologies has increased.

▶ With the discovery of prostate-specific antigen (PSA) as a screening tool for prostate cancer, its incidence rose significantly starting in the early 1990s. Yet it is now well understood that many men diagnosed by PSA elevation have "low-risk" disease (ie, PSA < 10, Gleason score < 6, and T stage < T2a), which often requires no treatment but only monitoring.

During this same time period and especially before the clear understanding that many of these cancers did not need radical treatment, both surgeons and radiation oncologists were working to improve surgery and radiation therapy to make it less toxic. Thus, IMRT (the radiation advance) and robotic prostatectomy (the surgical advance) were developed and are "sold" as less toxic than their traditional counterparts. However, they are more expensive. That incremental expense and utilization, when they are not absolutely necessary, could result in billions of health care dollars wasted.

This article is an analysis of Surveillance Epidemiology and End Results–Medicare database looking at this costly question. The authors found significant "overtreatment" of patients with low-risk disease by both intensity-modulated radiation therapy and robotic surgery. Vigilance is needed by all oncologists to stop this wasteful spending of health care dollars.

C. A. Lawton, MD

Comparative Effectiveness of Intensity-Modulated Radiotherapy and Conventional Conformal Radiotherapy in the Treatment of Prostate Cancer After Radical Prostatectomy

Goldin GH, Sheets NC, Meyer A-M, et al (Univ of North Carolina at Chapel Hill)

JAMA Intern Med 173:1136-1143, 2013

Importance.—Comparative effectiveness research of prostate cancer therapies is needed because of the development and rapid clinical adoption of newer and costlier treatments without proven clinical benefit. Radiotherapy is indicated after prostatectomy in select patients who have adverse pathologic features and in those with recurrent disease.

Objectives.—To examine the patterns of use of intensitymodulated radiotherapy (IMRT), a newer, more expensive technology that may reduce radiation dose to adjacent organs compared with the older conformal radiotherapy (CRT) in the postprostatectomy setting, and to compare disease control and morbidity outcomes of these treatments.

Design and Setting.—Data from the Surveillance, Epidemiology, and End Results–Medicare–linked database were used to identify patients with a diagnosis of prostate cancer who had received radiotherapy within 3 years after prostatectomy.

Participants.—Patients who received IMRT or CRT.

Main Outcomes and Measures.—The outcomes of 457 IMRT and 557 CRT patients who received radiotherapy between 2002 and 2007 were compared using their claims through 2009. We used propensity score methods to balance baseline characteristics and estimate adjusted incidence rate ratios (RRs) and their 95% CIs for measured outcomes.

Results.—Use of IMRT increased from zero in 2000 to 82.1% in 2009. Men who received IMRT vs CRT showed no significant difference in rates of long-term gastrointestinal morbidity (RR, 0.95; 95% CI, 0.66-1.37), urinary nonincontinent morbidity (0.93; 0.66-1.33), urinary incontinence (0.98; 0.71-1.35), or erectile dysfunction (0.85; 0.61-1.19). There was no significant difference in subsequent treatment for recurrent disease (RR, 1.31; 95% CI, 0.90-1.92).

Conclusions and Relevance.—Postprostatectomy IMRT and CRT achieved similar morbidity and cancer control outcomes. The potential clinical benefit of IMRT in this setting is unclear. Given that IMRT is more expensive, its use for postprostatectomy radiotherapy may not be cost-effective compared with CRT, although formal analysis is needed.

▶ The role of postoperative radiation therapy has expanded with the results of the Southwestern Oncology Group (SWOG) trial showing a survival advantage to its use in pathologic T3 patients. Thus, understanding the safest and most effective way to deliver prostate bed radiation therapy is important not only to patients but also to the payers.

Traditionally, 3-dimensional (3D) conformal radiation therapy was used to treat such cases until intensity modulated radiation therapy (IMRT) was developed. Supporters of IMRT over 3D in these cases cite their ability to spare critical organs, especially the rectum, as justification for the IMRT. Yet solid clinical data are lacking to compare these 2 treatment methodologies. Furthermore, a prospective trial to answer the question of IMRT versus 3D in prostate bed irradiation would take a decade or more to perform and get results.

Comparative effectiveness research such as the data reported in this article needs to be performed to try to answer this and other important questions. The source of the data for this report was the SEER-Medicare database. These data have inherent biases, and thus, the answer that there is no difference in terms of toxicity between IMRT and 3D is not the final answer. Further work needs to be done by other data sources to try to confirm or refute these results given the magnitude of patients whose prostate cancer postoperatively will require radiation therapy.

C. A. Lawton, MD

African American Men With Very Low–Risk Prostate Cancer Exhibit Adverse Oncologic Outcomes After Radical Prostatectomy: Should Active Surveillance Still Be an Option for Them?

Sundi D, Ross AE, Humphreys EB, et al (Johns Hopkins Univ, Baltimore, MD)
J Clin Oncol 31:2991-2997, 2013

Purpose.—Active surveillance (AS) is a treatment option for men with very low–risk prostate cancer (PCa); however, favorable outcomes achieved for men in AS are based on cohorts that under-represent African American (AA) men. To explore whether race-based health disparities exist among men with very low–risk PCa, we evaluated oncologic outcomes of AA men with very low–risk PCa who were candidates for AS but elected to undergo radical prostatectomy (RP).

Patients and Methods.—We studied 1,801 men (256 AA, 1,473 white men, and 72 others) who met National Comprehensive Cancer Network criteria for very low–risk PCa and underwent RP. Presenting characteristics, pathologic data, and cancer recurrence were compared among the groups. Multivariable modeling was performed to assess the association of race with upgrading and adverse pathologic features.

Results.—AA men with very low–risk PCa had more adverse pathologic features at RP and poorer oncologic outcomes. AA men were more likely to experience disease upgrading at prostatectomy (27.3% *v* 14.4%; $P < .001$), positive surgical margins (9.8% *v* 5.9%; $P = .02$), and higher Cancer of the Prostate Risk Assessment Post-Surgical scoring system (CAPRA-S) scores. On multivariable analysis, AA race was an independent predictor of adverse pathologic features (odds ratio, [OR], 3.23; $P = .03$) and pathologic upgrading (OR, 2.26; $P = .03$).

Conclusion.—AA men with very low–risk PCa who meet criteria for AS but undergo immediate surgery experience significantly higher rates of upgrading and adverse pathology than do white men and men of other races. AA men with very low–risk PCa should be counseled about increased oncologic risk when deciding among their disease management options.

▶ The use of screening PSA has resulted in an increase in biopsies and resultant diagnosis of many men in the United States with low-risk prostate cancer (prostate-specific antigen [PSA] < 10 ng/mL, Gleason score < 6, and clinical T stage < T2a). Given the low likelihood that low-risk prostate cancer will cause harm or kill a man over his life span, active surveillance is encouraged as a reasonable approach for these patients. Furthermore, there is an National Comprehensive Cancer Network category of "very low-risk" prostate cancer defined as PSA < 10, PSA density < 0.15 ng/mL/cm^3, clinical stage < T1c, Gleason sum < 6, positive core < 2, and cancer involvement of < 50% for which active surveillance is the preferred option for patients with a life expectancy < 20 years.

The science supporting these recommendations is strong for Caucasian patients because the majority of men studied to date meeting these criteria were Caucasian. We know that African American men die of prostate cancer more often than their Caucasian counterparts. So should the recommendations for low-risk disease and very low-risk prostate cancer for African American patients be the same? This data would suggest that it should not. Certainly this is hypothesis generating, and we need more studies to refute or support these findings. While we await such data, we need to rethink the messaging that we give our African American patients who have low-risk and very low-risk prostate cancer regarding their best treatment options.

C. A. Lawton, MD

Agent Orange as a Risk Factor for High-Grade Prostate Cancer

Ansbaugh N, Shannon J, Mori M, et al (Oregon Health and Science Univ, Portland; Oregon Health and Science Univ Knight Cancer Inst, Portland; et al)
Cancer 119:2399-2404, 2013

Background.—Agent Orange (AO) exposure (AOe) is a potential risk factor for the development of prostate cancer (PCa). However, it is unknown whether AOe specifically increases the risk of lethal PCa. The objective of this study was to determine the association between AOe and the risk of detecting high-grade PCa (HGPCa) (Gleason score ≥7) on biopsy in a US Veteran cohort.

Methods.—Risk factors included clinicodemographic and laboratory data from veterans who were referred for an initial prostate biopsy. Outcomes were defined as the presence versus the absence of PCa, HGPCa, or low-grade PCa (LGPCa) (Gleason score ≤6) in biopsy specimens. Risk among AOe veterans relative to unexposed veterans was estimated using multivariate logistic regression. Separate models were used to determine whether AOe was associated with an increased risk of PCa, HGPCa, or LGPCa.

Results.—Of 2720 veterans who underwent biopsy, PCa was diagnosed in 896 veterans (32.9%), and 459 veterans (16.9%) had HGPCa. AOe was associated with a 52% increase in the overall risk of detecting PCa (adjusted odds ratio, 1.52; 95% confidence interval, 1.07-2.13). AOe did not confer an increase in the risk of LGPCa (adjusted odds ratio, 1.24; 95% confidence interval, 0.81-1.91), although a 75% increase in the risk of HGPCa was observed (adjusted odds ratio, 1.75; 95% confidence interval, 1.12-2.74). AOe was associated with a 2.1-fold increase (95% confidence interval, 1.22-3.62; $P < .01$) in the risk of detecting PCa with a Gleason score ≥8.

Conclusions.—The current results indicated that an increased risk of PCa associated with AOe is driven by an increased risk of HGPCa in men who undergo an initial prostate biopsy. These findings may aid in improved PCa screening for Vietnam-era veterans.

▶ Our veterans have been exposed to a number of chemicals over the years while in combat. Agent Orange was one such chemical used extensively in the Vietnam War as a defoliate. The goal of using this compound in both pure and contaminated forms was to kill foliage and thus decrease cover for the guerilla warfare, which was common during that war. Unfortunately, the rampant use of this chemical resulted in birth defects and an increase in many forms of cancers, including soft tissue sarcomas, prostate cancer, and others.

The question of whether the increase in prostate cancers associated with Agent Orange was an increase in fatal cancers (ie, those with higher Gleason scores) or less aggressive and therefore less likely to be fatal cancer has yet to be determined. These data looking at veterans who underwent prostate biopsy showed that exposure to Agent Orange did confer a higher risk of being diagnosed with high-grade prostate cancer. This is important from a perspective of screening. Clearly the veterans exposed to Agent Orange need regular screening for this disease. We owe it to these men who put their lives on the line for our freedom because they now face an increase in a potentially fatal disease, which if caught early could be cured.

C. A. Lawton, MD

Association of Testosterone Therapy With Mortality, Myocardial Infarction, and Stroke in Men With Low Testosterone Levels

Vigen R, O'Donnell CI, Barón AE, et al (The Univ of Texas at Southwestern Med Ctr, Dallas; VA Eastern Colorado Health Care System, Denver, CO)

JAMA 310:1829-1836, 2013

Importance.—Rates of testosterone therapy are increasing and the effects of testosterone therapy on cardiovascular outcomes and mortality are unknown. A recent randomized clinical trial of testosterone therapy in men with a high prevalence of cardiovascular diseases was stopped prematurely due to adverse cardiovascular events raising concerns about testosterone therapy safety.

Objectives.—To assess the association between testosterone therapy and all-cause mortality, myocardial infarction (MI), or stroke among male veterans and to determine whether this association is modified by underlying coronary artery disease.

Design, Setting, and Patients.—A retrospective national cohort study of men with low testosterone levels (<300 ng/dL) who underwent coronary angiography in the Veterans Affairs (VA) system between 2005 and 2011.

Main Outcomes and Measures.—Primary outcome was a composite of all-cause mortality, MI, and ischemic stroke.

Results.—Of the 8709 men with a total testosterone level lower than 300 ng/dL, 1223 patients started testosterone therapy after a median of 531 days following coronary angiography. Of the 1710 outcome events, 748 men died, 443 had MIs, and 519 had strokes. Of 7486 patients not receiving testosterone therapy, 681 died, 420 had MIs, and 486 had strokes. Among 1223 patients receiving testosterone therapy, 67 died, 23 had MIs, and 33 had strokes. At 3 years after coronary angiography, the Kaplan-Meier estimated cumulative percentages with events were 19.9%in the no testosterone therapy group vs 25.7% in the testosterone therapy group, with an absolute risk difference of 5.8% (95% CI, −1.4% to 13.1%). In Cox proportional hazards models adjusting for the presence of coronary artery disease, testosterone therapy use as a time-varying covariate was associated with increased risk of adverse outcomes (hazard ratio, 1.29; 95% CI, 1.04 to 1.58). There was no significant difference in the effect size of testosterone therapy among those with and without coronary artery disease (test for interaction, $P = .41$).

Conclusions and Relevance.—Among a cohort of men in the VA health care system who underwent coronary angiography and had a low serum testosterone level, the use of testosterone therapy was associated with increased risk of adverse outcomes. These findings may inform the discussion about the potential risks of testosterone therapy.

▶ There is a nonstop badgering of advertisements on television and radio pushing men to consider having their testosterone level checked for erectile dysfunction, fatigue, and beyond. The advertising is selling testosterone supplementation to help men regain their "strength and manhood." Yet what is the real cost of such treatment in terms of both cardiovascular risk and cancer risk. The answer is that we don't know for sure. These data are a glimpse at what could be some of the adverse events associated with testosterone supplementation.

Clearly, based on these data, men with underlying coronary artery disease and low testosterone should only consider testosterone supplementation with a great deal of caution. These same types of data are sorely needed for our prostate cancer patients who, due to age or previous androgen deprivation, are left with low testosterone levels and the accompanying side effects. However, just as with the coronary artery disease group of patients, our prostate cancer patients need to approach testosterone supplementation with caution. We truly need to study this further to know whether it is safe to consider testosterone supplementation for both heart disease patients and prostate cancer patients. The advertising pushing the "need" to regain normal testosterone levels does not equate to the safe use of such supplements.

C. A. Lawton, MD

Alpha Emitter Radium-223 and Survival in Metastatic Prostate Cancer

Parker C, for the ALSYMPCA Investigators (Royal Marsden Natl Health Service Foundation Trust and Inst of Cancer Res, Sutton, UK; et al)

N Engl J Med 369:213-223, 2013

Background.—Radium-223 dichloride (radium-223), an alpha emitter, selectively targets bone metastases with alpha particles. We assessed the efficacy and safety of radium-223 as compared with placebo, in addition to the best standard of care, in men with castration-resistant prostate cancer and bone metastases.

Methods.—In our phase 3, randomized, double-blind, placebo-controlled study, we randomly assigned 921 patients who had received, were not eligible to receive, or declined docetaxel, in a 2:1 ratio, to receive six injections of radium-223 (at a dose of 50 kBq per kilogram of body weight intravenously) or matching placebo; one injection was administered every 4 weeks. In addition, all patients received the best standard of care. The primary end point was overall survival. The main secondary efficacy end points included time to the first symptomatic skeletal event and various biochemical end points. A prespecified interim analysis, conducted when 314 deaths had occurred, assessed the effect of radium-223 versus placebo on survival. An updated analysis, when 528 deaths had occurred, was performed before crossover from placebo to radium-223.

Results.—At the interim analysis, which involved 809 patients, radium-223, as compared with placebo, significantly improved overall survival (median, 14.0 months vs. 11.2 months; hazard ratio, 0.70; 95% confidence interval [CI], 0.55 to 0.88; two-sided $P = 0.002$). The updated analysis involving 921 patients confirmed the radium-223 survival benefit (median, 14.9 months vs. 11.3 months; hazard ratio, 0.70; 95% CI, 0.58 to 0.83; $P < 0.001$). Assessments of all main secondary efficacy end points also showed a benefit of radium-233 as compared with placebo. Radium-223 was associated with low myelosuppression rates and fewer adverse events.

Conclusions.—In this study, which was terminated for efficacy at the prespecified interim analysis, radium-223 improved overall survival. (Funded by Algeta and Bayer HealthCare Pharmaceuticals; ALSYMPCA ClinicalTrials.gov number, NCT00699751.)

▶ Given that more than 34 000 men are predicted to die of prostate cancer this year, anything that we can do to try to delay that end seems to be laudable. We know that hormone therapy in the form of androgen deprivation is the first step for these patients once metastatic disease has been found. The next step, after androgen independence, includes several options from the androgen biosynthesis inhibitors to chemotherapy. Many other systemic options are being studied, but these data show that systemic radiation also plays a role.

This study represents a fine example of global collegiality in that 19 countries participated in this double-blind trial showing the survival benefit of this radiopharmaceutical. Not only was survival improved by approximately 3 months, but the toxicity was very low. This study and its findings of a survival benefit with minimal toxicity offer a new nonchemotherapy option for our metastatic prostate cancer patients. In addition, patients had significant pain improvement with this radiopharmaceutical, thus improving their quality of life.

Each of the systemic options available for metastatic prostate cancer patients including Radium 223 helps to transform this condition to one of a chronic illness. This is certainly a positive step for these cancer patients.

C. A. Lawton, MD

Urologists' Use of Intensity-Modulated Radiation Therapy for Prostate Cancer

Mitchell JM (Georgetown Univ, Washington, DC)

N Engl J Med 369:1629-1637, 2013

Background.—Some urology groups have integrated intensity-modulated radiation therapy (IMRT), a radiation treatment with a high reimbursement rate, into their practice. This is permitted by the exception for in-office ancillary services in the federal prohibition against self-referral. I examined the association between ownership of IMRT services and use of IMRT to treat prostate cancer.

Methods.—Using Medicare claims from 2005 through 2010, I constructed two samples: one comprising 35 self-referring urology groups in private practice and a matched control group comprising 35 non–self-referring urology groups in private practice, and the other comprising non–self-referring urologists employed at 11 National Comprehensive Cancer Network centers matched with 11 self-referring urology groups in private practice. I compared the use of IMRT in the periods before and during ownership and used a difference-in-differences analysis to evaluate changes in IMRT use according to self-referral status.

Results.—The rate of IMRT use by self-referring urologists in private practice increased from 13.1 to 32.3%, an increase of 19.2 percentage points ($P < 0.001$). Among non–self-referring urologists, the rate of IMRT use increased from 14.3 to 15.6%, an increase of 1.3 percentage points ($P = 0.05$). The unadjusted difference-indifferences effect was 17.9 percentage points ($P < 0.001$). The regression-adjusted increase in IMRT use associated with self-referral was 16.4 percentage points ($P < 0.001$). The rate of IMRT use by urologists working at National Comprehensive Cancer Network centers remained stable at 8.0% but increased by 33.0 percentage points among the 11 matched self-referring urology groups. The regression-adjusted difference-in-differences effect was 29.3 percentage points ($P < 0.001$).

Conclusions.—Urologists who acquired ownership of IMRT services increased their use of IMRT substantially more than urologists who did not own such services. Allowing urologists to self-refer for IMRT may contribute to increased use of this expensive therapy. (Funded by the American Society for Radiation Oncology.)

▶ The Stark Law was passed several years ago to stop physicians from ordering treatments and advanced lab and x-ray tests when they own such equipment and therefore profited by ordering such, often when it was not medically indicated. Exceptions to the Stark Law were approved (for ancillary services) to avoid disrupting good patient care when a simple x-ray (plain film) or labs (provided in the doctor's office) would improve and foster good patient care. Unfortunately, 1 of the exceptions to the Stark Law was radiation therapy services. It is quite clear that radiation therapy is not ancillary to any service and is a stand-alone treatment for many cancers requiring extensive planning to be executed correctly. Yet under the "law," radiation therapy is exempt, and thus physicians such as urologists can own such equipment and direct patients to radiation therapy without fully disclosing their financial association.

Dr Mitchell's study looks at these types of practices to see if becoming an investor in such changes the treatment recommendations for patients. Sadly, these data show that urologists who acquire ownership in radiation therapy services (in this case, intensity-modulated radiation therapy) increase their utilization of such substantially more than urologists who do not own such services. This result shows that personal gain can get in the way of quality patient care and thus should be stopped. Over treatment of prostate cancer patients who may not require any treatment at all or not providing all of the treatment options for a patient can easily occur when financial gain is on the line.

C. A. Lawton, MD

Treatment of Prostate Cancer With Intermittent Versus Continuous Androgen Deprivation: A Systematic Review of Randomized Trials

Niraula S, Le LW, Tannock IF (Cancer Care Manitoba and Univ of Manitoba, Winnipeg; Princess Margaret Hosp and Univ of Toronto, Ontario, Canada)

J Clin Oncol 31:2029-2036, 2013

Purpose.—Uncertainty exists regarding benefits of intermittent androgen deprivation (IAD) compared with continuous androgen deprivation (CAD) for treatment of prostate cancer. On the basis of a systematic review of evidence, our aim was to formulate a recommendation for either IAD or CAD to treat relapsing, locally advanced, or metastatic prostate cancer.

Methods.—We searched literature published up to September 2012 from MEDLINE, EMBASE, the Cochrane Library, and major conference proceedings. We included randomized controlled trials comparing IAD and

CAD if they reported overall survival (OS) or biochemical/radiologic time to disease progression.

Results.—Nine studies with 5,508 patients met our criteria. There were no significant differences in time-to-event outcomes between the groups in any studies. The pooled hazard ratio (HR) for OS was 1.02 (95% CI, 0.94 to 1.11) for IAD compared with CAD, and the HR for progression-free survival was 0.96 (95% CI, 0.76 to 1.20). More prostate cancer–related deaths with IAD tended to be balanced by more deaths not related to prostate cancer with CAD. Superiority of IAD for sexual function, physical activity, and general well-being was observed in some trials. Median cost savings with IAD was estimated to be 48%.

Conclusion.—There is fair evidence to recommend use of IAD instead of CAD for the treatment of men with relapsing, locally advanced, or metastatic prostate cancer who achieve a good initial response to androgen deprivation. This recommendation is based on evidence against superiority of either strategy for time-to-event outcomes and substantial decrease with IAD in exposure to androgen deprivation, resulting in less cost, inconvenience, and potential toxicity.

▶ It has been know since the 1940s with the discovery by Drs Huggin and Hodges that prostate cancer is hormone sensitive. Thus, androgen deprivation in the form of orchiectomy or more recently luteinizing hormone releasing hormone agonist is the mainstay of treatment for patients with metastatic disease. In addition, it is often part of the treatment in patients with locally advanced disease.

These hormonal manipulations, although helpful from a prostate cancer control perspective, are toxic. Weight gain, muscle mass loss, bone loss, hot flashes, and sexual dysfunction can be seen in most patients treated with androgen deprivation. Given these toxicities, if one could mitigate some of them via intermittent versus continuous androgen deprivation, it could significantly improve the patient's quality of life.

Several trials have looked at this question, and the results are conflicting. The significance of this article is that it is a meta-analysis of 9 randomized controlled trials comparing intermittent versus continuous androgen deprivation in prostate cancer patients. This analysis revealed that there is reasonable evidence to consider intermittent androgen deprivation over continuous androgen deprivation for patients whose initial response to androgen deprivation was good.

This result will likely improve the quality of life for thousands of men with metastatic prostate cancer and should be strongly considered as the standard of care.

C. A. Lawton, MD

Association Between Exercise and Primary Incidence of Prostate Cancer: Does Race Matter?

Singh AA, Jones LW, Antonelli JA, et al (Duke Univ Med Ctr, Durham, NC; et al)

Cancer 119:1338-1343, 2013

Background.—Exercise is a modifiable lifestyle risk factor associated with prostate cancer risk reduction. However, whether this association is different as a function of race is unclear. In the current study, the authors attempted to characterize the link between exercise and prostate cancer (CaP) in white and black American men.

Methods.—Using a prospective design, 307 men (164 of whom were white and 143 of whom were black) who were undergoing prostate biopsy completed a self-reported survey that assessed exercise behavior (metabolic equivalent [MET] hours per week). Crude and adjusted logistic regression analyses were used to estimate the risk of prostate cancer controlling for age, body mass index, digital rectal examination findings, previous biopsy, Charlson comorbidity score, and family history of CaP stratified by self-reported race.

Results.—There was no significant difference noted with regard to the amount of exercise between racial groups ($P = .12$). Higher amounts of MET hours per week were associated with a decreased risk of CaP for white men in both crude ($P = .02$) and adjusted ($P = .04$) regression models. Among whites, men who exercised ≥ 9 MET hours per week were less likely to have a positive biopsy result compared with men exercising < 9 MET hours per week (odds ratio, 0.47; 95% confidence interval, 0.22-0.99 [$P = .047$]). There was no association noted between MET hours per week and risk of CaP among black men in both crude ($P = .79$) and adjusted ($P = .76$) regression models.

Conclusions.—In a prospective cohort of men undergoing biopsy, increased exercise, measured as MET hours per week, was found to be associated with CaP risk reduction among white but not black men. Investigating race-specific mechanisms by which exercise modifies CaP risk and why these mechanisms disfavor black men in particular are warranted.

▶ Prostate cancer incidence in the United States is one of the highest in the world. Factors such as high-fat diets and low exercise have been suggested as potential causes for this increased incidence in our country. Countries such as Japan and Africa have some of the lowest incidences of prostate cancer and are associated with diets low in animal fat and higher exercise patterns relative to the United States.

Given the high incidence of prostate cancer in our country, methods to decrease this need to be considered. One method studied here is to increase exercise. The good news is that increasing exercise was associated with a decrease in prostate cancer found on biopsy of the men studied in this trial. Unfortunately, when evaluated by race, only the white men benefited.

We know that African American men are diagnosed at higher stages of prostate cancer compared with their white counterparts in the United States. We also know that stage-for-stage, black men can do as well as white men when treated appropriately. So we must look for other potential maneuvers for our African American men to decrease their risk of developing this disease. A next obvious approach is to try low-fat diets. This is not an easy task because our country is loaded with high-fat fast-food items that are all too conveniently available. But we owe it to our African American men, and really to all men, to teach them how to eat less fat because it will definitely prevent heart disease (our number 1 killer) and needs to be assessed regarding the effect of low-fat diets on prostate cancer incidence.

C. A. Lawton, MD

21 Colorectal Cancer

Long-Term Colorectal-Cancer Incidence and Mortality after Lower Endoscopy

Nishihara R, Wu K, Lochhead P, et al (Dana–Farber Cancer Inst and Harvard Med School, Boston, MA; Harvard School of Public Health, Boston, MA; et al)

N Engl J Med 369:1095-1105, 2013

Background.—Colonoscopy and sigmoidoscopy provide protection against colorectal cancer, but the magnitude and duration of protection, particularly against cancer of the proximal colon, remain uncertain.

Methods.—We examined the association of the use of lower endoscopy (updated biennially from 1988 through 2008) with colorectal-cancer incidence (through June 2010) and colorectal-cancer mortality (through June 2012) among participants in the Nurses' Health Study and the Health Professionals Follow-up Study.

Results.—Among 88,902 participants followed over a period of 22 years, we documented 1815 incident colorectal cancers and 474 deaths from colorectal cancer. With endoscopy as compared with no endoscopy, multivariate hazard ratios for colorectal cancer were 0.57 (95% confidence interval [CI], 0.45 to 0.72) after polypectomy, 0.60 (95% CI, 0.53 to 0.68) after negative sigmoidoscopy, and 0.44 (95% CI, 0.38 to 0.52) after negative colonoscopy. Negative colonoscopy was associated with a reduced incidence of proximal colon cancer (multivariate hazard ratio, 0.73; 95% CI, 0.57 to 0.92). Multivariate hazard ratios for death from colorectal cancer were 0.59 (95% CI, 0.45 to 0.76) after screening sigmoidoscopy and 0.32 (95% CI, 0.24 to 0.45) after screening colonoscopy. Reduced mortality from proximal colon cancer was observed after screening colonoscopy (multivariate hazard ratio, 0.47; 95% CI, 0.29 to 0.76) but not after sigmoidoscopy. As compared with colorectal cancers diagnosed in patients more than 5 years after colonoscopy or without any prior endoscopy, those diagnosed in patients within 5 years after colonoscopy were more likely to be characterized by the CpG island methylator phenotype (CIMP) (multivariate odds ratio, 2.19; 95% CI, 1.14 to 4.21) and microsatellite instability (multivariate odds ratio, 2.10; 95% CI, 1.10 to 4.02).

Conclusions.—Colonoscopy and sigmoidoscopy were associated with a reduced incidence of cancer of the distal colorectum; colonoscopy was also associated with a modest reduction in the incidence of proximal colon cancer. Screening colonoscopy and sigmoidoscopy were associated with reduced colorectal-cancer mortality; only colonoscopy was associated with reduced mortality from proximal colon cancer. Colorectal cancer diagnosed within 5 years after colonoscopy was more likely than cancer diagnosed after that period or without prior endoscopy to have CIMP and microsatellite instability. (Funded by the National Institutes of Health and others.)

▶ Colon cancer kills tens of thousands of patients annually and needs to be screened for if we expect to decrease these deaths. How to screen (sigmoidoscopy vs colonoscopy) and how often to screen remains a question.

Published data have shown that sigmoidoscopy decreases the incidence of rectal sigmoid cancers and thus decreases the mortality from them. The question of the impact of screening colonoscopy on the incidence and mortality of more proximal colon cancers remains. These data help answer the question regarding the potential benefit of colonoscopy relative to sigmoidoscopy. These authors have shown that colonoscopy does decrease the incidence of both proximal and distal colon cancers and also decreases the mortality related to both. It also helps to establish the role of colonoscopy over sigmoidoscopy. Although these data do help clarify the question of the benefit of colonoscopy, the timing remains in question. Currently for patients with a family history of colon cancer who have a negative colonoscopy after age 50, the next recommended procedure is 10 years later. These data support that recommendation. But for patients with a family history of colon cancer or a history of a "high-risk" adenoma from previous colonoscopies, these data suggest that the 5-year interval between colonoscopies may be too long. We await further data to refute or support these findings.

C. A. Lawton, MD

22 Lung Cancer

Selection Criteria for Lung-Cancer Screening

Tammemägi MC, Katki HA, Hocking WG, et al (Brock Univ, St. Catharines, Ontario, Canada; Natl Cancer Inst, Rockville, MD; Marshfield Clinic Res Foundation, WI; et al)

N Engl J Med 368:728-736, 2013

Background.—The National Lung Screening Trial (NLST) used risk factors for lung cancer (e.g., ≥30 pack-years of smoking and <15 years since quitting) as selection criteria for lungcancer screening. Use of an accurate model that incorporates additional risk factors to select persons for screening may identify more persons who have lung cancer or in whom lung cancer will develop.

Methods.—We modified the 2011 lung-cancer risk-prediction model from our Prostate, Lung, Colorectal, and Ovarian (PLCO) Cancer Screening Trial to ensure applicability to NLST data; risk was the probability of a diagnosis of lung cancer during the 6-year study period. We developed and validated the model ($PLCO_{M2012}$) with data from the 80,375 persons in the PLCO control and intervention groups who had ever smoked. Discrimination (area under the receiver-operating-characteristic curve [AUC]) and calibration were assessed. In the validation data set, 14,144 of 37,332 persons (37.9%) met NLST criteria. For comparison, 14,144 highest-risk persons were considered positive (eligible for screening) according to $PLCO_{M2012}$ criteria. We compared the accuracy of $PLCO_{M2012}$ criteria with NLST criteria to detect lung cancer. Cox models were used to evaluate whether the reduction in mortality among 53,202 persons undergoing low-dose computed tomographic screening in the NLST differed according to risk.

Results.—The AUC was 0.803 in the development data set and 0.797 in the validation data set. As compared with NLST criteria, $PLCO_{M2012}$ criteria had improved sensitivity (83.0% vs. 71.1%, $P < 0.001$) and positive predictive value (4.0% vs. 3.4%, $P = 0.01$), without loss of specificity (62.9% and. 62.7%, respectively; $P = 0.54$); 41.3% fewer lung cancers were missed. The NLST screening effect did not vary according to $PLCO_{M2012}$ risk ($P = 0.61$ for interaction).

Conclusions.—The use of the $PLCO_{M2012}$ model was more sensitive than the NLST criteria for lung-cancer detection.

▶ Lung cancer remains the top cancer killer for both men and women in the United States with more than 80 000 men and more than 70 000 women dying annually. Smoking is clearly the most significant carcinogen in the development of this dreaded disease. Sadly, it is both smokers and the people close to them who most commonly develop lung cancer, the latter via secondhand smoke. Even more concerning is the increase in incidence of lung cancer in nonsmokers, the cause of which is yet to be well understood.

Screening for such a deadly disease has become an important health care opportunity. Yet finding lung cancer early is not simple without the use of expensive screening tests such as thin-sliced computed tomography, and thus evaluating and subsequently developing good criteria to know which patients to screen is imperative. The report here is another attempt to focus screening for lung cancer beyond the simple question of smoking history and timing. These authors have developed a tool that appears to more efficiently identify patients at high risk for lung cancer development and for whom lung cancer screening may be both cost-effective and lifesaving.

C. A. Lawton, MD

Results of Initial Low-Dose Computed Tomographic Screening for Lung Cancer

The National Lung Screening Trial Research Team (Univ of Minnesota School of Public Health, Minneapolis; Dartmouth–Hitchcock Med Ctr, Lebanon, NH; Univ of California at Los Angeles; et al)

N Engl J Med 368:1980-1991, 2013

Background.—Lung cancer is the largest contributor to mortality from cancer. The National Lung Screening Trial (NLST) showed that screening with low-dose helical computed tomography (CT) rather than with chest radiography reduced mortality from lung cancer. We describe the screening, diagnosis, and limited treatment results from the initial round of screening in the NLST to inform and improve lung-cancer–screening programs.

Methods.—At 33 U.S. centers, from August 2002 through April 2004, we enrolled asymptomatic participants, 55 to 74 years of age, with a history of at least 30 pack-years of smoking. The participants were randomly assigned to undergo annual screening, with the use of either low-dose CT or chest radiography, for 3 years. Nodules or other suspicious findings were classified as positive results. This article reports findings from the initial screening examination.

Results.—A total of 53,439 eligible participants were randomly assigned to a study group (26,715 to low-dose CT and 26,724 to chest radiography); 26,309 participants (98.5%) and 26,035 (97.4%), respectively, underwent screening. A total of 7191 participants (27.3%) in the low-dose CT group and 2387 (9.2%) in the radiography group had a positive screening result; in the respective groups, 6369 participants (90.4%) and 2176 (92.7%) had at least one follow-up diagnostic procedure, including imaging in 5717 (81.1%) and 2010 (85.6%) and surgery in 297 (4.2%) and 121 (5.2%). Lung cancer was diagnosed in 292 participants (1.1%) in the low-dose CT group versus 190 (0.7%) in the radiography group (stage 1 in 158 vs. 70 participants and stage IIB to IV in 120 vs. 112). Sensitivity and specificity were 93.8% and 73.4% for low-dose CT and 73.5% and 91.3% for chest radiography, respectively.

Conclusions.—The NLST initial screening results are consistent with the existing literature on screening by means of low-dose CT and chest radiography, suggesting that a reduction in mortality from lung cancer is achievable at U.S. screening centers that have staff experienced in chest CT. (Funded by the National Cancer Institute; NLST ClinicalTrials.gov number, NCT00047385.)

▶ Lung cancer kills more Americans annually than any other malignancy. Thus, efforts to screen for early lesions (which are often curable) are laudable. The challenge is that simple and inexpensive chest x-rays are not cost-effective for mass screening; the tumors found by this modality are often not curable because they are too large and may have already metastasized to regional lymph nodes or beyond.

Computed tomography (CT) of the chest is the obvious screening tool that could be used to find very early tumors. Yet cost is an issue here as is radiation exposure, and we are still left wondering which Americans should be considered for such screening.

The data reported here from the National Lung Screening Trial Research Team looked at screening for lung cancer in adults who are heavy smokers with annual chest x-ray vs low dose CT over 3 years. The low-dose CT group diagnosed more lung cancers compared with the chest x-ray cohort, suggesting that low-dose CT of the chest be applied as a screening tool. Yet two questions remain. First, what is the optimal group of patients (regarding age and smoking history) to which we should apply this screening technique? Second, what is the cost of such screening when applied to the appropriate population?

C. A. Lawton, MD

50-Year Trends in Smoking-Related Mortality in the United States

Thun MJ, Carter BD, Feskanich D, et al (American Cancer Society, Atlanta, GA; Brigham and Women's Hosp, Boston, MA; et al)

N Engl J Med 368:351-364, 2013

Background.—The disease risks from cigarette smoking increased in the United States over most of the 20th century, first among male smokers and later among female smokers. Whether these risks have continued to increase during the past 20 years is unclear.

Methods.—We measured temporal trends in mortality across three time periods (1959–1965, 1982–1988, and 2000–2010), comparing absolute and relative risks according to sex and self-reported smoking status in two historical cohort studies and in five pooled contemporary cohort studies, among participants who became 55 years of age or older during follow-up.

Results.—For women who were current smokers, as compared with women who had never smoked, the relative risks of death from lung cancer were 2.73, 12.65, and 25.66 in the 1960s, 1980s, and contemporary cohorts, respectively; corresponding relative risks for male current smokers, as compared with men who had never smoked, were 12.22, 23.81, and 24.97. In the contemporary cohorts, male and female current smokers also had similar relative risks for death from chronic obstructive pulmonary disease (COPD) (25.61 for men and 22.35 for women), ischemic heart disease (2.50 for men and 2.86 for women), any type of stroke (1.92 for men and 2.10 for women), and all causes combined (2.80 for men and 2.76 for women). Mortality from COPD among male smokers continued to increase in the contemporary cohorts in nearly all the age groups represented in the study and within each stratum of duration and intensity of smoking. Among men 55 to 74 years of age and women 60 to 74 years of age, all-cause mortality was at least three times as high among current smokers as among those who had never smoked. Smoking cessation at any age dramatically reduced death rates.

Conclusions.—The risk of death from cigarette smoking continues to increase among women and the increased risks are now nearly identical for men and women, as compared with persons who have never smoked. Among men, the risks associated with smoking have plateaued at the high levels seen in the 1980s, except for a continuing, unexplained increase in mortality from COPD.

▶ Smoking remains a huge health care problem in the United States and around the globe. The health risks incurred by smoking are monumental, with cancer representing only part of the overall problem—but clearly a significant part. So, as oncologists, it behooves all of us to work to decrease smoking not only in our patients but in the communities where we work and live.

Thus, having a sense of the actual mortality related to smoking is helpful to arm ourselves with data to support our message of smoking cessation. This data set provides just the type of information we need to get our antismoking message across.

Especially important to note in this data set is the impact of smoking-related illnesses and mortality on women. Sadly, many women, like their male counterparts, have taken up smoking, and equally sad is the fact that this has resulted in an increased risk of death for women that is now almost identical to that of men.

It is absolutely imperative that we as oncologists get the message to our patients and their families as well as our colleagues that smoking is extremely dangerous in terms of cancer risk, heart disease, lung disease, and beyond. We have to be advocates for smoking-cessation programs for our current smokers. In addition, we need to support educational programs for children and young adults who will be tempted to start this life-shortening habit.

C. A. Lawton, MD

23 Supportive Care

Palliative care always

Ramchandran K, Von Roenn JH (Stanford Hosp and Clinics, CA)
Oncology (Williston Park) 27:13-26, 2013

Palliative cancer care is the integration into oncologic care of therapies that address the issues that cause physical and psychosocial suffering for the patient and family. Effective provision of palliative cancer care requires an interdisciplinary team that can provide care in all settings (home, inpatient, and outpatient). There is clear evidence for improved outcomes in multiple domains-symptoms, quality of end-of-life care, provider satisfaction, cost of care-with the integration of palliative care into cancer care. As a result, there are now guideline-based recommendations for incorporating palliative care into cancer care. Unfortunately there continue to be barriers to effective integration; these include gaps in education and research, and a cultural stigma that equates palliative care with end-of-life care. These barriers will need to be addressed in order to achieve seamless palliative care integration across the continuum of cancer care for all patients and their families.

▶ Palliative care for cancer patients has often been equated to "end-of-life care," yet its correct use should span the time from oncologic diagnosis through treatment and survivorship as well as end of life. Several studies have shown actual improvement in survival for cancer patients who have had early intervention with palliative care. Yet the stigma of "we are just giving up" seems to stick to the palliative care of option, as inappropriate as that may be.

This article is an excellent update on the current status of the role of palliative care for cancer patients. It outlines very clearly which cancer patients should be considered for palliative care using the National Comprehensive Cancer Network guidelines and other indicators. It also helps oncologists understand who provides quality palliative care. It presents a clear case for palliative care to be multidisciplinary to address all aspects of the cancer patient's needs from physical and emotional to social and spiritual, and beyond. Finally the article addresses the issue of barriers to incorporating palliative care into quality oncologic care within the United States. The good news is that quality palliative care can actually help to reduce overall health care costs, which is a clear need given our current health care financial challenges.

C. A. Lawton, MD

Why Is Spiritual Care Infrequent at the End of Life? Spiritual Care Perceptions Among Patients, Nurses, and Physicians and the Role of Training

Balboni MJ, Sullivan A, Amobi A, et al (Harvard Med School, Boston, MA; Harvard School of Public Health, Boston, MA; et al)

J Clin Oncol 31:461-467, 2013

Purpose.—To determine factors contributing to the infrequent provision of spiritual care (SC) by nurses and physicians caring for patients at the end of life (EOL).

Patients and Methods.—This is a survey-based, multisite study conducted from March 2006 through January 2009. All eligible patients with advanced cancer receiving palliative radiation therapy and oncology physician and nurses at four Boston academic centers were approached for study participation; 75 patients (response rate = 73%) and 339 nurses and physicians (response rate = 63%) participated. The survey assessed practical and operational dimensions of SC, including eight SC examples. Outcomes assessed five factors hypothesized to contribute to SC infrequency.

Results.—Most patients with advanced cancer had never received any form of spiritual care from their oncology nurses or physicians (87% and 94%, respectively; *P* for difference = .043). Majorities of patients indicated that SC is an important component of cancer care from nurses and physicians (86% and 87%, respectively; *P* =.1). Most nurses and physicians thought that SC should at least occasionally be provided (87% and 80%, respectively; *P* =.16). Majorities of patients, nurses, and physicians endorsed the appropriateness of eight examples of SC (averages, 78%, 93%, and 87%, respectively; *P* =.01). In adjusted analyses, the strongest predictor of SC provision by nurses and physicians was reception of SC training (odds ratio [OR] = 11.20, 95% CI, 1.24 to 101; and OR = 7.22, 95% CI, 1.91 to 27.30, respectively). Most nurses and physicians had not received SC training (88% and 86%, respectively; *P* =.83).

Conclusion.—Patients, nurses, and physicians view SC as an important, appropriate, and beneficial component of EOL care. SC infrequency may be primarily due to lack of training, suggesting that SC training is critical to meeting national EOL care guidelines.

► The role of palliative care and the benefit of such is becoming more and more evident with randomized trials showing a clear advantage to its use. Palliative care is helpful not only in terms of quality of life but in quantity of life as well. Palliative care is and needs to be multidisciplinary with obvious issues such as pain control as just one part of the whole picture. Another aspect of quality palliative care includes the addressing of spirituality and religion. This aspect of a patient's life has been studied and found to be a significant issue for patients, especially those with advanced disease such as end-stage cancer. Addressing spirituality has been shown to improve these patients quality of life. Yet these data, although reinforcing the desire of patients and their caregivers to have spirituality addressed, show that in fact it is not happening routinely. The next obvious question is why not? Certainly our lack of education is an issue, and one that should be relatively easy to solve. Incorporation of training in spiritual care should be done for all oncologists and their oncologic team to help address this significant need for our patients who are facing end of life secondary to their malignancy.

C. A. Lawton, MD

Clinical Ascertainment of Health Outcomes Among Adults Treated for Childhood Cancer

Hudson MM, Ness KK, Gurney JG, et al (St Jude Children's Res Hosp and the Univ of Tennessee College of Medicine, Memphis; et al)

JAMA 309:2371-2381, 2013

Importance.—Adult survivors of childhood cancer are known to be at risk for treatment-related adverse health outcomes. A large population of survivors has not been evaluated using a comprehensive systematic clinical assessment to determine the prevalence of chronic health conditions.

Objective.—To determine the prevalence of adverse health outcomes and the proportion associated with treatment-related exposures in a large cohort of adult survivors of childhood cancer.

Design, Setting, and Participants.—Presence of health outcomes was ascertained using systematic exposure–based medical assessments among 1713 adult (median age, 32 [range, 18-60] years) survivors of childhood cancer (median time from diagnosis, 25 [range, 10-47] years) enrolled in the St Jude Lifetime Cohort Study since October 1, 2007, and undergoing follow-up through October 31, 2012.

Main Outcomes and Measures.—Age-specific cumulative prevalence of adverse outcomes by organ system.

Results.—Using clinical criteria, the crude prevalence of adverse health outcomes was highest for pulmonary (abnormal pulmonary function, 65.2% [95% CI, 60.4%- 69.8%]), auditory (hearing loss, 62.1% [95% CI, 55.8%-68.2%]), endocrine or reproductive (any endocrine condition, such as hypothalamic-pituitary axis disorders and male germ cell dysfunction, 62.0% [95% CI, 59.5%-64.6%]), cardiac (any cardiac condition, such as heart valve disorders, 56.4% [95% CI, 53.5%-59.2%]), and neurocognitive (neurocognitive impairment, 48.0% [95% CI, 44.9%-51.0%]) function, whereas abnormalities involving hepatic (liver dysfunction, 13.0% [95% CI, 10.8%- 15.3%]), skeletal (osteoporosis, 9.6% [95% CI, 8.0%-11.5%]), renal (kidney dysfunction, 5.0% [95% CI, 4.0%-6.3%]), and hematopoietic (abnormal blood cell counts, 3.0% [95% CI, 2.1%-3.9%]) function were less common. Among survivors at risk for adverse outcomes following specific cancer treatment modalities, the estimated cumulative prevalence at age 50 years was 21.6% (95% CI, 19.3%-23.9%) for cardiomyopathy, 83.5% (95% CI, 80.2%-86.8%) for heart valve disorder, 81.3% (95% CI, 77.6%-85.0%) for pulmonary dysfunction, 76.8% (95% CI, 73.6%-80.0%) for pituitary dysfunction, 86.5%

(95% CI, 82.3%-90.7%) for hearing loss, 31.9% (95% CI, 28.0%-35.8%) for primary ovarian failure, 31.1% (95% CI, 27.3%-34.9%) for Leydig cell failure, and 40.9% (95% CI, 32.0%-49.8%) for breast cancer. At age 45 years, the estimated cumulative prevalence of any chronic health condition was 95.5% (95% CI, 94.8%-98.6%) and 80.5% (95% CI, 73.0%-86.6%) for a serious/ disabling or life-threatening chronic condition.

Conclusions and Relevance.—Among adult survivors of childhood cancer, the prevalence of adverse health outcomes was high, and a systematic risk-based medical assessment identified a substantial number of previously undiagnosed problems that are more prevalent in an older population. These findings underscore the importance of ongoing health monitoring for adults who survive childhood cancer.

▶ Curing a childhood cancer is nothing short of fantastic for both patients and their families. Often those cures are a result of a multidisciplinary approach of surgery, chemotherapy, and/or radiation. Each of these modalities comes with their own toxicities. When combined as is often done in childhood malignancies, those toxicities can be magnified. Thus, evaluating the late toxicities resulting from these treatments is important to try to mitigate them as much as possible and to help prepare patients and their families for potential long-term effects.

The data presented here by the St Jude Lifetime Cohort Study looked at a large cohort of adult survivors of childhood cancers. Their results show that survivorship comes at a real price in terms of late toxicities. Lung capacity compromised, hearing loss, endocrine disorders, male germ cell dysfunction, and cardiac issues lead the long list of toxicities found. These data are important for oncologists to digest and comprehend to inform patients receiving treatment for childhood malignancies and their families. It is also critical for oncologists to note these data to help guide survivorship recommendations. Finally, it is critical for oncologists to know these data to try to improve the lives of survivors by changing our treatments through research so that the incidence of these late problems can decrease.

C. A. Lawton, MD

Randomized Phase III Trial of ABVD Versus Stanford V With or Without Radiation Therapy in Locally Extensive and Advanced-Stage Hodgkin Lymphoma: An Intergroup Study Coordinated by the Eastern Cooperative Oncology Group (E2496)

Gordon LI, Hong F, Fisher RI, et al (Northwestern Univ Feinberg School of Medicine and Robert H. Lurie Comprehensive Cancer Ctr, Chicago, IL; Dana-Farber Cancer Inst, Boston, MA; Univ of Rochester James P. Wilmot Cancer Ctr, NY; et al)

J Clin Oncol 31:684-691, 2013

Purpose.—Although ABVD (doxorubicin, bleomycin, vinblastine, and dacarbazine) has been established as the standard of care in patients with advanced Hodgkin lymphoma, newer regimens have been investigated, which have appeared superior in early phase II studies. Our aim was to determine if failure-free survival was superior in patients treated with the Stanford V regimen compared with ABVD.

Patients and Methods.—The Eastern Cooperative Oncology Group, along with the Cancer and Leukemia Group B, the Southwest Oncology Group, and the Canadian NCIC Clinical Trials Group, conducted this randomized phase III trial in patients with advanced Hodgkin lymphoma. Stratification factors included extent of disease (localized *v* extensive) and International Prognostic Factors Project Score (0 to 2 *v* 3 to 7). The primary end point was failure-free survival (FFS), defined as the time from random assignment to progression, relapse, or death, whichever occurred first. Overall survival, a secondary end point, was measured from random assignment to death as a result of any cause. This design provided 87% power to detect a 33% reduction in FFS hazard rate, or a difference in 5-year FFS of 64% versus 74% at two-sided .05 significance level.

Results.—There was no significant difference in the overall response rate between the two arms, with complete remission and clinical complete remission rates of 73% for ABVD and 69% for Stanford V. At a median follow-up of 6.4 years, there was no difference in FFS: 74% for ABVD and 71% for Stanford V at 5 years ($P = .32$).

Conclusion.—ABVD remains the standard of care for patients with advanced Hodgkin lymphoma.

▶ Hodgkin's disease has a fascinating history. Before the advent of the modern chemotherapy era, radiation therapy was the mainstay of treatment for virtually all patients. For patients with stage III disease, the volume and doses of radiation therapy required for "cure" resulted in significant and sometimes fatal complications, both acute and late. So the essential replacement of wide field radiation therapy by combination chemotherapy such as the "MOPP" regimen seemed to be a huge step forward—both in terms of disease control but also toxicity.

Advances within the multiagent chemotherapy arena also occurred with the advent of newer combinations of drugs such that the MOPP regimen was replaced by ABVD, which has been the standard for years. Yet ABVD has its own set of acute and late toxicities such that many institutions such as Stanford worked on the development of other regimens to try to keep the excellent control rates and yet decrease toxicities. In the end, the only way to ensure that any new regimen is equal or better or worse than ABVD (our current standard) is to run a trial such as was done here. These results confirm that ABVD remains the standard in North America. However, this does not mean that investigators should give up. ABVD works (with radiation for bulky sites), but given its toxicities, we need to continue to work to find equally effective and less toxic regimens.

C. A. Lawton, MD

Single-Fraction Radiotherapy Versus Multifraction Radiotherapy for Palliation of Painful Vertebral Bone Metastases—Equivalent Efficacy, Less Toxicity, More Convenient: A Subset Analysis of Radiation Therapy Oncology Group Trial 97-14

Howell DD, James JL, Hartsell WF, et al (Univ of Michigan Med School, Ann Arbor; Radiation Therapy Oncology Group Statistical Ctr, Philadelphia, PA; Advocate Good Shepherd Hosp, Barrington, IL; et al)
Cancer 119:888-896, 2013

Background.—The Radiation Therapy Oncology Group (RTOG) trial 97-14 revealed no difference between radiation delivered for painful bone metastases at a dose of 8 gray (Gy) in 1 fraction (single-fraction radiotherapy [SFRT]) and 30 Gy in 10 fractions (multifraction radiotherapy [MFRT]) in pain relief or narcotic use 3 months after randomization. SFRT for painful vertebral bone metastases (PVBM) has not been well accepted, possibly because of concerns about efficacy and toxicity. In the current study, the authors evaluated the subset of patients that was treated specifically for patients with PVBM.

Methods.—PVBM included the cervical, thoracic, and/or lumbar spine regions. Among patients with PVBM, differences in retreatment rates and in pain relief, narcotic use, and toxicity 3 months after randomization were evaluated.

Results.—Of 909 eligible patients, 235 (26%) had PVBM. Patients with and without PVBM differed in terms of the percentage of men (55% vs 47%, respectively; $P = .03$) and the proportion of patients with multiple painful sites (57% vs 38%, respectively; $P < .01$). Among those with PVBM, more patients who received MFRT had multiple sites treated (65% vs 49% for MFRT vs SFRT, respectively; $P = .02$). There were no statistically significant treatment differences in terms of pain relief (62% vs 70% for MFRT vs SFRT, respectively; $P = .59$) or freedom from narcotic use (24% vs 27%, respectively; $P = .76$) at 3 months. Significant differences in acute grade 2 through 4 toxicity (20% vs 10% for MFRT vs SFRT, respectively; $P = .01$) and acute grade 2 through 4 gastrointestinal toxicity (14% vs 6%, respectively; $P = .01$) were observed at 3 months, with lower toxicities seen in the patients treated with SFRT. Late toxicity was rare. No myelopathy was recorded. SFRT produced higher 3-year retreatment rates (5% vs 15%; $P = .01$).

Conclusions.—Results for the subset of patients with PVBM in the RTOG 94-17 randomized controlled trial were comparable to those for the entire population. SFRT produced less acute toxicity and a higher rate of retreatment than MFRT. SFRT and MFRT resulted in comparable pain relief and narcotic use at 3 months.

▶ The role of palliative care in general for cancer patients is a critical one with the overarching goal of increasing quality of life. Improving quality of life through palliative care has also been shown to correlate with increased quantity of life. Radiotherapy has played a critical role in palliative care for decades. The most common use of palliative radiation therapy is the treatment of painful bony metastasis.

Historically, palliative radiation for painful bony metastasis was given as a fractionated course of >10 fraction. Several trials have looked at the efficacy and potential toxicity of shorter courses of radiation including the option of a single fraction. It is obvious from a patient's perspective that a single-fraction approach would be the most convenient and, therefore, the more desired, radiation approach. However, radiation oncologists have had concerns regarding whether a single fraction of approximately 8 Gy would be efficacious and whether it would lead to potential increases in toxicities. One of the greatest fears for the radiation oncologist was concern about spinal cord injury in treating vertebral bony metastasis. So these data, which directly assess those concerns, is timely and helpful. It is clear from this analysis that 8 Gy as a palliative approach for vertebral bony metastasis is both safe and effective and as such should be seriously considered by all radiation oncologists when faced with a patient who needs such treatment. There are always extenuating situations in which this single-fraction approach may not be the best, such as a large soft-tissue component associated with the bony metastasis. In general, however, the single-fraction approach should be at the fore of the radiation oncologist's mind when considering palliative radiation therapy for vertebral bony metastasis. These data and others like them are the reason that short fractionation courses for palliative radiotherapy of bony metastasis was 1 of the 5 choosing-wisely items chosen by the American Society for Radiation Oncology in 2013. It shows that radiation oncologists do understand that for palliation, both efficacy and convenience for the patient need to be taken into consideration.

C. A. Lawton, MD

24 Cancer Screening

Body CT Scanning in Young Adults: Examination Indications, Patient Outcomes, and Risk of Radiation-induced Cancer

Zondervan RL, Hahn PF, Sadow CA, et al (Massachusetts General Hosp, Boston; et al)

Radiology 267:460-469, 2013

Purpose.—To quantify patient outcome and predicted cancer risk from body computed tomography (CT) in young adults and identify common indications for the imaging examination.

Materials and Methods.—This retrospective multicenter study was HIPAA compliant and approved by the institutional review boards of three institutions, with waiver of informed consent. The Research Patient Data Registry containing patient medical and billing records of three university-affiliated hospitals in a single metropolitan area was queried for patients 18–35 years old with a social security record who underwent chest or abdominopelvic CT from 2003 to 2007. Patients were analyzed according to body part imaged and scanning frequency. Mortality status and follow-up interval were recorded. The Biologic Effects of Ionizing Radiation VII method was used to calculate expected cancer incidence and death. Examination indication was determined with associated ICD-9 diagnostic code; 95% confidence intervals for percentages were calculated, and the binomial test was used to compare the difference between percentages.

Results.—In 21 945 patients, 16 851 chest and 24 112 abdominopelvic CT scans were obtained. During the average 5.5-year (± 0.1 [standard deviation]) follow-up, 7.1% (575 of 8057) of chest CT patients and 3.9% (546 of 13 888) of abdominal CT patients had died. In comparison, the predicted risk of dying from CT-induced cancer was 0.1% (five of 8057, $P < .01$) and 0.1% (eight of 12 472, $P < .01$), respectively. The most common examination indications were cancer and trauma for chest CT and abdominal pain, trauma, and cancer for abdominopelvic CT. Among patients without a cancer diagnosis in whom only one or two scans were obtained, mortality and predicted risk of radiation-induced cancer death were 3.6% (215 of 5914) and 0.05% (three of 5914, $P < .01$) for chest CT and 1.9% (219 of 11 291) and 0.1% (six of 11 291, $P < .01$) for abdominopelvic CT.

Conclusion.—Among young adults undergoing body CT, risk of death from underlying morbidity is more than an order of magnitude greater than death from long-term radiation-induced cancer.

▶ There is no question that patients should never be exposed unnecessarily to radiation of any sort. If we could pick a group of patients for which this is especially important, it would be children. The younger the age at the time of exposure to ionizing radiation the higher the incidence of potential cancers because the patients are likely to live longer than older patients with similar exposures.

For patients who need x-ray tests due to medical conditions, both patients and their physicians are left wondering what the risk of secondary cancers might be to balance that risk with the medical need for the examination. These authors have tried to quantitate that risk looking at both computed tomography (CT) of the chest as well as CT of the abdomen and pelvis in patients ages 18 to 35. The good news is that among these young adults, risk of death from their underlying medical conditions was much higher than the risk of death from long-term radiation-induced cancers. The only challenge to these conclusions relates to the follow-up in the study. Average follow-up was 5.5 years, which is short when one thinks about radiation-induced solid tumors, which may take a decade or more to develop. It will be interesting to look at these data once the average follow-up is closer to 10 years.

C. A. Lawton, MD

Risk of Ischemic Heart Disease in Women after Radiotherapy for Breast Cancer

Darby SC, Ewertz M, McGale P, et al (Univ of Oxford, UK; Univ of Southern Denmark, Odense, Denmark; et al)

N Engl J Med 368:987-998, 2013

Background.—Radiotherapy for breast cancer often involves some incidental exposure of the heart to ionizing radiation. The effect of this exposure on the subsequent risk of ischemic heart disease is uncertain.

Methods.—We conducted a population-based case–control study of major coronary events (i.e., myocardial infarction, coronary revascularization, or death from ischemic heart disease) in 2168 women who underwent radiotherapy for breast cancer between 1958 and 2001 in Sweden and Denmark; the study included 963 women with major coronary events and 1205 controls. Individual patient information was obtained from hospital records. For each woman, the mean radiation doses to the whole heart and to the left anterior descending coronary artery were estimated from her radiotherapy chart.

Results.—The overall average of the mean doses to the whole heart was 4.9 Gy (range, 0.03 to 27.72). Rates of major coronary events increased linearly with the mean dose to the heart by 7.4% per gray (95% confidence interval, 2.9 to 14.5; $P < 0.001$), with no apparent threshold. The increase started within the first 5 years after radiotherapy and continued into the third decade after radiotherapy. The proportional increase in the rate of major coronary events per gray was similar in women with and women without cardiac risk factors at the time of radiotherapy.

Conclusions.—Exposure of the heart to ionizing radiation during radiotherapy for breast cancer increases the subsequent rate of ischemic heart disease. The increase is proportional to the mean dose to the heart, begins within a few years after exposure, and continues for at least 20 years. Women with preexisting cardiac risk factors have greater absolute increases in risk from radiotherapy than other women. (Funded by Cancer Research UK and others.)

▶ Breast conservation in the form of lumpectomy and postoperative irradiation has become the gold standard for the management of most localized breast cancer patients. Multiple randomized trials have looked at this treatment versus mastectomy, and each has shown equivalence (at a minimum) to the disfiguring surgery of mastectomy.

It has also been well documented that, especially with older radiation techniques, collateral damage can occur within the lungs, and for left-sided breast cancers, within the heart. So it should come as no surprise that the data published by Darby and colleagues looking at breast cancer patients treated with radiation from 1958 through 2001 in Sweden and Denmark has produced evidence of cardiac toxicity. The good news is that with newer radiation techniques, such as prone positioning, the dose to the heart even in patients with left-sided breast cancers can be minimized significantly. These data should not cause women to avoid breast conservation with lumpectomy and radiation but should stimulate a conversation between the patient and her radiation oncologist as to how the heart can be maximally protected. In addition, it should push the radiation oncologist to continue to be vigilant in protecting the heart and other organs, such as the lungs, during breast radiation.

C. A. Lawton, MD

PART FOUR

KIDNEY, WATER, AND ELECTROLYTES

RENEE GARRICK, MD

Introduction

Mitigation of Progression and Consequences of Chronic Kidney Disease

Research this year has again focused on novel interventions that may help to mitigate the progression of CKD. Along these lines, the data from the KEEP investigators deserve our attention. The KEEP findings reviewed here demonstrated that something as straightforward and risk-free as reiterative educational programs may improve patient outcomes. For example, compared to matched control patients, those receiving CKD education had a greater likelihood of choosing home peritoneal dialysis, of receiving a transplant, of being placed on a transplant wait-list, and of preemptive placement of a permanent vascular access. The next several articles focus on the effect of protein calorie malnutrition in patients with CKD and demonstrate that these patients are at risk early on for protein energy wasting, which can have deleterious effects on both renal outcomes and on overall morbidity and mortality. The consensus statement from the International Society of Renal Nutrition and Metabolism provides an excellent framework for the discussion. The statement notes that although observational trials demonstrate that improvement in nutritional biomarkers is associated with enhanced survival, the impact of nutritional modifications on outcomes will best be directly established by randomized trials, and we eagerly await such studies. These data are further amplified by the remarkable studies by Silverwood and colleagues drawn from the British birth registry. That study began in 1946 in England, Scotland, and Wales, and the patients have been followed since enrollment. The registry data are quite interesting. The findings reviewed here highlight that low birth weight increases the lifetime risk of renal disease, and this risk seemed to be heightened by the later development of obesity. These findings suggest that low birth weight patients should be monitored closely and that attention to later-life obesity might mitigate the risk of later renal insufficiency. Other factors studied this year that may modify disease progression include salt restriction, exercise, and B/P management. McMahon and colleagues offer the first double-blind randomized controlled data to support the concept that dietary salt restriction may impact cardiovascular outcomes and CKD progression. The potential benefit of improved adherence to antihypertensive regimens and exercise and lifestyle intervention were the topic of papers by Roy and Howden and colleagues. Adherence to antihypertensive regimens was linked with risk reduction in ESRD, and exercise and lifestyle intervention were demonstrated to improve body composition, diastolic dysfunction, and cardio respiratory fitness. Whether these sorts of interventions will improve long-term mortality will require further study, but collectively the data suggest that life quality is improved.

Acute Kidney Injury

Multiple studies have identified acute kidney injury as an independent risk factor for death, and attention continues to focus on the deleterious long-term effects of a single episode of acute intrinsic kidney injury. Stads and colleagues performed a retrospective cohort study of patients with acute kidney injury severe enough to necessitate continuous renal replacement therapy during their hospital stay. They found that most patients still had impaired renal function at discharge and that the degree of renal dysfunction was closely associated with reduced patient and renal survival. Chawla and colleagues demonstrated co-morbid cardiovascular effects of acute kidney injury. Using patients from the Veterans Affairs database with the discharge diagnosis of acute myocardial infarction, they demonstrated that patients with acute kidney injury and acute kidney injury together with a myocardial infarction fared worse than patients with a myocardial infarction alone. These data have obvious clinical and prognostic significance. The linkage between renal disease and altered outcomes after cardiac surgery was the topic of separate studies by Arthur (for the SAKInet investigators) and Coca (for the TRIBE-AKI investigators) and colleagues. Arthur evaluated urinary biomarkers in patients with early-stage acute kidney injury following cardiac surgery. They demonstrated that a combination of interleukin-18 (IL-18) and kidney injury molecule 1 (KIM-1) result in improved identification of patients at risk for progressive acute kidney injury or death. Coca and colleagues evaluated the long-term predictive value of urinary acute kidney injury biomarkers following cardiac surgery. They demonstrated that IL-18 and KIM-1 measured on postoperative days 1–3 provided additional prognostic information regarding three-year mortality in patients with and without clinically apparent acute kidney injury. This latter finding suggests that biomarkers are likely more sensitive than the serum creatinine in detecting subtle, but clinically significant, acute kidney injury. This is reminiscent of the situation between the serum troponin I levels vs the EKG changes in patients with myocardial injury. The data from Wilson and colleagues demonstrates that the decisions, benefits, and timing of the initiation of dialysis in the setting of AKI is not necessarily a simple one. They evaluated patients with AKI without a clear clinical indication for emergency dialysis. Using a time-varying propensity score, they matched not-yet-dialyzed patients to each dialyzed patient and found that the initiation of dialysis was associated with improved survival when initiated at a higher creatinine level ($\geq$3.8 mg/dl) and was associated with a higher mortality when initiated in patients with a lower serum creatinine. The corollary of this finding is that patients in whom the creatinine is higher (over 3.8 mg/dl) fare better if dialysis is initiated rather than withheld.

The final two entries focus our attention on adverse drug events and acute kidney injury. The data from the single-center observational study by Cox and colleagues are quite worrisome. Among other findings, they demonstrated that patients with acute kidney injury (minimum rise in the creatinine of 0.5 mg/dL) commonly received nephrotoxic medications despite the diagnosis of acute kidney injury. The concluding selection by Gandhi reminds us that the co-administration of calcium channel blockers and clarithromycin has been linked to acute kidney injury serious enough to require hospitalization. This is especially true among older adults.

Clinical Nephrology

The first several selections cause us to rethink several previously held clinical axioms. First, the presence of urinary eosinophils, even at a 5% cutoff level rather than the usual 1% cutoff level typically used, is not generally useful in distinguishing acute interstitial nephritis from acute tubular necrosis or other kidney diseases. Second, renal artery stenting for atherosclerotic renal artery stenosis is not superior to medical therapy with regard to all-cause mortality and cardiovascular or renal outcomes, although there was a slight (2.3 mmHg) improvement in systolic blood pressure among the stent group. Third, among patients with diabetic nephropathy (albumin/creatinine ratio of at least 300 mg and eGFR of 32-89.9 mls/min/1.73 m^2), combined ACEi (lisinopril) and ABR (losartan), therapy was associated with increased risk of adverse events, which necessitated early discontinuation of the VA NEPHRON-D trial. And lastly, despite the findings of many observational studies, Mendelian randomization analysis failed to demonstrate any causal association between uric acid levels and ischemic heart disease or blood-pressure. The study did, however, support a causal effect between body mass index, uric acid levels, and hyperuricemia, suggesting that the BMI is a cofounder in observational associations. Having dealt with those troublesome issues, the selections next turn to a prospective trial drawn from the MESA data performed in community-living individuals without known cardiovascular disease, which demonstrated that an abnormal urinary albumin to creatinine ratio is strongly associated with cardiovascular disease events in persons with a low body weight. This association is driven primarily by the urine albumin concentration rather than by the loss of muscle mass and any subsequent decrease in the urinary creatinine concentration. The next selection by Rein and colleagues evaluated a consecutive cohort of patients who underwent coronary angiography for established or suspected coronary artery disease. The data demonstrate that a 5 ml/min/1.73 m^2 decrease in eGFR independently conferred a 60% increase in mortality risk. This finding represents a new independent predictive-risk marker for death and vascular events following coronary angiography. The last three selections all focus on renal stone disease. New information is presented regarding the safety and efficacy of febuxostat for the treatment of high uric acid excretion in patients at risk for calcium stone disease, the potential ability of the DASH diet to serve as an alternative to low-oxalate diets the prevention of calcium oxalate stone formation, and an update demonstrating that sugar-sweetened soda and punch are associated with a higher risk of stone formation as compared to other beverages such as coffee, tea, and orange juice.

Chronic Kidney Disease

When addressing any clinical problem, it is good to know the magnitude of the incidence within the population at risk. Using a Markov Monte Carlo model stimulation, Grams and colleagues estimated that the lifetime risk of developing CKD Stage IIIa (eGFR <60 mls/min/1.73 m^2) to ESRD is approximately 59%, and the lifetime risk of ESRD is approximately 3.6%, with a higher risk in blacks than whites, especially black women (7.8% risk of ESRD). These data demonstrate the importance of primary prevention and risk mitigation. Along the same lines, the data from Posada-Ayala are quite fascinating. These investigators used advanced chromatography and mass spectrometry to compare the urine metabolic signature in patients with CKD to normal controls. The investigators were able to demonstrate a pattern of urinary electrolytes that clearly differentiates patients with CKD. This proof-of-principle study may ultimately help clinicians identify and monitor patients at greatest risk for CKD and CKD progression. The next group of studies focuses on hypertension control among patients with CKD. The data of Tanner and colleagues demonstrate that apparent treatment-resistant hypertension is quite common among patients with CKD. The data from the Blood Pressure Lowering Treatment Trialists Collaboration demonstrate that, among patients with moderate reductions in eGFR (<60 mls/min/1.73 m^2), blood-pressure control reduces the risk of cardiovascular events, and there is little evidence to indicate that any particular class of drugs is superior to another for achieving this aim.

The next selection focuses on the management of atrial fibrillation, which occurs with increased frequency in patients with chronic kidney disease. The management and risk stratification of bleeding vs stroke prevention in this population remains quite complex. Data from the observational prospective multicenter SWEDEHEART study demonstrate that among patients with CKD and myocardial infarction with atrial fibrillation warfarin treatment can reduce the one-year risk of composite adverse cerebro- and cardiovascular outcomes without demonstrating an unacceptably high risk of bleeding. Before generalizing these findings, it should be noted that the monitoring and INR-control of these patients is tighter than that typically achieved in outpatient settings in the US, and only a relatively small number of patients had advanced CKD. The final selection again focuses our attention on patient safety in the setting of CKD. Ginsberg and colleagues demonstrate that adverse safety events are quite common and varied in this population and that, because of their frequency, more extensive data are needed to identify those patients at greatest risk for adverse events.

Dialysis and Transplantation

One of the themes in the renal literature this year has been the role of malnutrition and protein energy wasting in patients with CKD and ESRD. The study by Jia and colleagues demonstrates that low-serum IGF-I levels are associated with changes in body composition and with markers of bone and mineral metabolism. Moreover, reduced levels of IGF-1 predict increased mortality risk in incident dialysis patients.

The next two selections help demonstrate the breadth of the nutritional problem in patients with end-stage renal disease on dialysis. den Hoedt and colleagues demonstrate that despite compliant, guideline-based dialysis care, all inflammatory and nutritional parameters worsened over time among the dialysis population. In addition, the data from Park and colleagues demonstrates that race does not modify the association between a BMI and muscle mass and improved survival. Taken together, the data suggest that much more prospective, evidence-driven information is needed to help establish the most appropriate approach to nutritional supplementation in this high-risk population. The next paper by Park continues the observation of the U-shaped association between changes in blood pressure and all-cause mortality in patients on hemodialysis. In this study, the authors demonstrate that a modest decline in blood pressure after hemodialysis is acceptable, whereas any fall greater than 30 mm Hg, or any dialysis-associated increase in systolic blood pressure is associated with an increase in mortality. It is important for internists to be aware of these data and to work closely with the nephrologist to avoid excessive and potentially contradictory manipulations of antihypertensive agents on the day of dialysis treatment. The last two articles focus on cognitive dysfunction and safety in patients on dialysis. The data from Shaffi and colleagues suggest that 25 hydroxy vitamin D deficiency may contribute to the impaired cognitive function, which occurs among patients with CKD and ESRD. The final ESRD selection is the first demonstration that accidental falls are common in patients on peritoneal dialysis. The mean fall rate was 1.7 falls/patient year, and every successive fall was associated with a 1.62 fold higher mortality rate, which was not necessarily linked to the fall itself but likely to other co-morbidities, such as increased frailty. The data are important and establish that peritoneal as well as hemodialysis patients are at increased risk for falls and the associated mortality risk.

The last two selections turn our attention to transplantation donation. Together they demonstrate that organ donation is generally safe with regard to both overall donor health and future long-term renal function. It is important to note that though the absolute risk is small, the patients in the Norwegian donor study did have an increased risk of the ESRD (302 cases/million), which might have been related to either hereditary or immunologic factors. Thus, while these data likely should not deter living donation to a loved one, it is important for donors to be carefully screened, fully informed, and have appropriate long-term follow-up.

Renee Garrick, MD

25 Mitigation and Modulation of the Progression of Kidney Disease

Educational programs improve the preparation for dialysis and survival of patients with chronic kidney disease

Kurella Tamura M, on behalf of the KEEP Investigators (VA Palo Alto Health Care System, CA)

Kidney Int 85:686-692, 2014

Preparation for end-stage renal disease (ESRD) is widely acknowledged to be suboptimal in the United States. We sought to determine whether participation in a kidney disease screening and education program resulted in improved ESRD preparation and survival in 595 adults who developed ESRD after participating in the National Kidney Foundation Kidney Early Evaluation Program (KEEP), a community-based screening and education program. Non-KEEP patients were selected from a national ESRD registry and matched to KEEP participants based on demographic and clinical characteristics. The main outcomes were pre-ESRD nephrologist care, placement of permanent vascular access, use of peritoneal dialysis, pre-emptive transplant wait listing, transplantation, and mortality after ESRD. Participation in KEEP was associated with significantly higher rates of pre-ESRD nephrologist care (76.0% vs. 69.3%), peritoneal dialysis (10.3% vs. 6.4%), pre-emptive transplant wait listing (24.2% vs. 17.1%), and transplantation (9.7% vs. 6.4%) but not with higher rates of permanent vascular access (23.4% vs. 20.1%). Participation in KEEP was associated with a lower risk for mortality (hazard ratio 0.80), but this was not statistically significant after adjusting for ESRD preparation. Thus, participation in a voluntary community kidney disease screening and education program was associated with higher rates of ESRD preparation and survival.

▶ The Kidney Early Evaluation Program (KEEP) is a multicenter, community-based screening and education program that was initiated in 2000 and designed to identify individuals at increased risk of kidney disease. Individuals aged 18 years and older with hypertension or diabetes, or those having a first-degree relative with the same diagnoses, were encouraged to follow-up and participate in ongoing educational programs. The current study compared matched KEEP participants who developed end-stage renal disease (ESRD) between June 2005 and December 2010 to non-KEEP patients drawn from the United States Renal Data System. Patients were matched for clinical and demographic characteristics. Patients who participated in KEEP had significantly higher rates of pre-ESRD care by a nephrologist, higher rates of transplantation, and were more likely to receive home peritoneal dialysis. Most interesting was that KEEP participants had a longer survival following the initiation of dialysis, and this was associated with better preparation for ESRD. One limitation of the study is that patients who enrolled in the KEEP program were self-selected and, therefore, may have been more highly motivated and engaged in their own health care compared with the matched control population. Alternatively, KEEP participation itself may have simply been more effective in motivating patients to become more active participants in their own care. Because KEEP is an observational study by design, it is not possible to definitively establish a causal relationship between participation and ESRD preparation. However, the investigators did use propensity score matching to identify patients with similar clinical characteristics, and the findings are in keeping with other trials which of demonstrated that pre-ESRD education can improve ESRD outcomes and mortality.[1] There is much to be learned from the KEEP trial. For example, a better understanding of the cultural specificity and the optimal timing of "teaching interventions" may increase the favorable impact of any educational initiatives. The overall concept that repetitive access to, and engagement in, early kidney disease education can have a favorable impact on clinical outcomes suggests that ongoing widespread kidney educational programs could be of great clinical utility. In this study, participation in KEEP was associated with an approximately 5.4% absolute reduction in ESRD mortality over a median of 1.6 years, which translates into the prevention of one ESRD death for every 18 patients who participate. Given the obvious safety profile of participation in KEEP, it is hard to think of another clinical intervention with this degree of upside.

R. Garrick, MD

Reference

1. Manns BJ, Taub K, Vanderstraeten C, et al. The impact of education on chronic kidney disease patients' plans to initiate dialysis with self-care dialysis: a randomized trial. *Kidney Int.* 2005;68:1777-1783.

Prevention and treatment of protein energy wasting in chronic kidney disease patients: a consensus statement by the International Society of Renal Nutrition and Metabolism

Ikizler TA, Cano NJ, Franch H, et al (Vanderbilt Univ Med Ctr, North Nashville TN; CHU Clermont-Ferrand, France; Emory Univ, Atlanta, GA; et al)
Kidney Int 84:1096-1107, 2013

Protein energy wasting (PEW) is common in patients with chronic kidney disease (CKD) and is associated with adverse clinical outcomes, especially

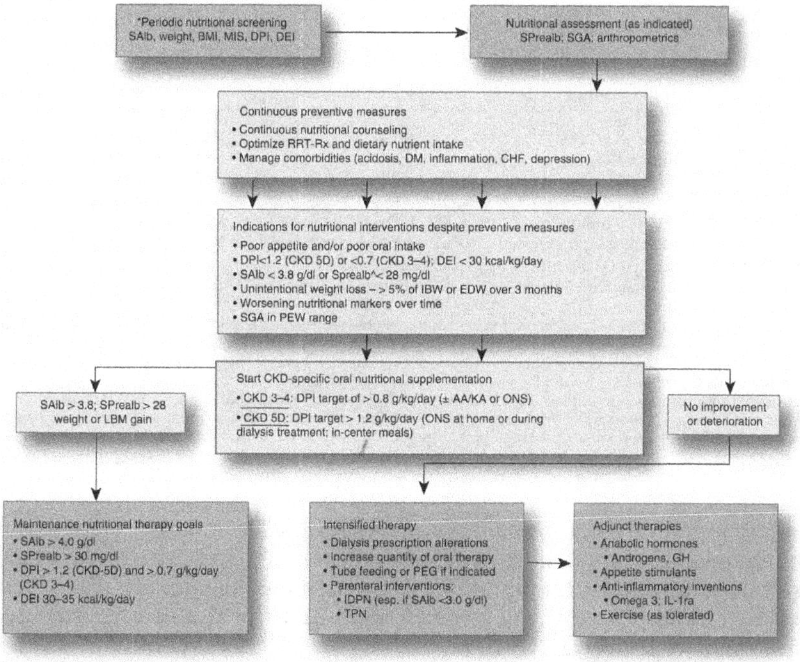

FIGURE 2.—Proposed algorithm for nutritional management and support in patients with chronic kidney disease. *Minimum every 3 months, monthly screening recommended. ^Only for ESRD patients without residual renal function. AA/KA, amino acid/keto acid; BMI, body mass index; CHF, congestive heart failure; CKD, chronic kidney disease; DEI, dietary energy intake; DM, diabetes mellitus; DPI, dietary protein intake; EDW, estimated dry weight; GH, growth hormone; IBW, ideal body weight; IDPN, intradialytic parenteral nutrition; IL-1ra, interleukin-1 receptor antagonist; LBM, lean body mass; MIS, malnutrition–inflammation score; ONS, oral nutritional supplement; PEG, percutaneous endoscopic gastrostomy; PEW, protein energy wasting; RRT-Rx, renal replacement therapy prescription; SAlb, serum albumin (measured by bromocresol green); SGA, subjective global assessment; SPrealb, serum prealbumin; TPN, total parenteral nutrition. (Reprinted with permission from Macmillan Publishers Ltd: Kidney International. Ikizler TA, Cano NJ, Franch H, et al. Prevention and treatment of protein energy wasting in chronic kidney disease patients: a consensus statement by the International Society of Renal Nutrition and Metabolism. *Kidney Int*. 2013;84:1096-1107, Copyright 2013, with permission from International Society of Nephrology.)

in individuals receiving maintenance dialysis therapy. A multitude of factors can affect the nutritional and metabolic status of CKD patients requiring a combination of therapeutic maneuvers to prevent or reverse protein and energy depletion. These include optimizing dietary nutrient intake, appropriate treatment of metabolic disturbances such as metabolic acidosis, systemic inflammation, and hormonal deficiencies, and prescribing optimized dialytic regimens. In patients where oral dietary intake from regular meals cannot maintain adequate nutritional status, nutritional supplementation, administered orally, enterally, or parenterally, is shown to be effective in replenishing protein and energy stores. In clinical practice, the advantages of oral nutritional supplements include proven efficacy, safety, and compliance. Anabolic strategies such as anabolic steroids, growth hormone, and exercise, in combination with nutritional supplementation or alone, have been shown to improve protein stores and

TABLE 1.—Recommended Minimum Protein, Energy, and Mineral Intakes for Chronic Kidney Disease (CKD) and Maintenance Dialysis Patients

	Nondialysis CKD	Hemodialysis	Peritoneal dialysis
Protein	0.6–0.8 g/kg/day Illness 1.0 g/kg	>1.2 g/kg/day	>1.2 g/kg/day Peritonitis >1.5 g/kg
Energy	30–35[a] kcal/kg/day	30–35[a] kcal/kg/day	30–35[a] kcal/kg/day including kcal from dialysate
Sodium	80–100 mmol/day	80–100 mmol/day	80–100 mmol/day
Potassium	<1 mmol/kg if elevated	<1 mmol/kg if elevated	Not usually an issue
Phosphorus	800–1000 mg and binders if elevated	800–1000 mg and binders if elevated	800–1000 mg and binders if elevated

Greater than 50% of high biological value protein (that is, complete protein sources, containing the full spectrum of essential amino acids) is recommended.

[a]Based on physical activity level. In sedentary elderly adults, recommended energy intake is 30 kcal/kg/day. All recommendations are based on ideal body weight. Regular follow-up supports compliance.

Reprinted with permission from Macmillan Publishers Ltd: Kidney International. Ikizler TA, Cano NJ, Franch H, et al. Prevention and treatment of protein energy wasting in chronic kidney disease patients: a consensus statement by the International Society of Renal Nutrition and Metabolism. Kidney Int. 2013;84:1096-1107. Copyright 2013.

represent potential additional approaches for the treatment of PEW. Appetite stimulants, anti-inflammatory interventions, and newer anabolic agents are emerging as novel therapies. While numerous epidemiological data suggest that an improvement in biomarkers of nutritional status is associated with improved survival, there are no large randomized clinical trials that have tested the effectiveness of nutritional interventions on mortality and morbidity (Fig 2, Table 1).

▶ This article represents a consensus statement from the International Society of Renal Nutrition and Metabolism regarding nutrition and renal disease. Studies have suggested that protein calorie protein energy wasting (PEW) adversely affects the outcomes of both chronic kidney disease and dialysis patients.[1-3] Several factors contribute to PEW in renal disease, including the accumulation of uremic toxins; the presence of comorbid conditions such as depression cardiovascular disease and diabetes; increased catabolism associated with dialysis; and a host of metabolic derangement including hyperparathyroidism, metabolic acidosis, and alterations in gonadal and pituitary hormones. PEW, in turn, can lead to infection, worsening cardiovascular function and wasting and increasing frailty. As outlined in Table 1, compared with the general population, among patients with renal dysfunction, the basal requirements needed to maintain appropriate protein-calorie and mineral balance are unique. In addition, in patients with CKD, the strategies needed to maintain appropriate protein balance can be challenging. For example, high-protein foods are usually high in phosphorus, so overzealous restriction of phosphate may increase the risk for PEW. However, injudicious phosphate intake can lead to hyperphosphatemia and other attendant secondary complications. Deleterious effects of metabolic acidosis, the potentially protective effect of a high fruit and fiber diet, and the need to adjust calorie intake for the more sedentary lifestyle of patients with advanced kidney disease all require consideration. In addition, the frequency and type of renal replacement therapy have an impact on metabolic balance and nutritional needs. Careful nutritional strategies are required to balance these dietary needs, and the consensus statement provides an algorithm for the nutritional management of these patients (Fig 2). In addition, the complexity of the dietary prescription highlights the need and value of education and early nutritional counseling.

R. Garrick, MD

References

1. Ikizler TA, Hakim RM. Nutrition in end-stage renal disease. *Kidney Int.* 1996;50: 343-357.
2. Kopple JD. Effect of nutrition on morbidity and mortality in maintenance dialysis patients. *Am J Kidney Dis.* 1994;24:1002-1009.
3. Fouque D, Kalantar-Zadeh K, Kopple J, et al. A proposed nomenclature and diagnostic criteria for protein-energy wasting in acute and chronic kidney disease. *Kidney Int.* 2008;73:391-398.

Low birth weight, later renal function, and the roles of adulthood blood pressure, diabetes, and obesity in a British birth cohort

Silverwood RJ, Pierce M, Hardy R, et al (London School of Hygiene and Tropical Medicine, UK; Univ College London, UK; et al)

Kidney Int 84:1262-1270, 2013

Low birth weight has been shown to be associated with later renal function, but it is unclear to what extent this is explained by other established kidney disease risk factors. Here we investigate the roles of diabetes, hypertension, and obesity using data from the Medical Research Council National Survey of Health and Development, a socially stratified sample of 5362 children born in March 1946 in England, Scotland, and Wales, and followed since. The birth weight of 2192 study members with complete data was related to three markers of renal function at age 60-64 (estimated glomerular filtration rate (eGFR) calculated using cystatin C (eGFRcys), eGFR calculated using creatinine and cystatin C (eGFRcr-cys), and the urine albumin—creatinine ratio) using linear regression. Each 1 kg lower birth weight was associated with a 2.25 ml/min per 1.73 m^2 (95% confidence interval 0.80—3.71) lower eGFRcys and a 2.13 ml/min per 1.73 m^2 (0.69—3.58) lower eGFRcr-cys. There was no evidence of an association with urine albumin-creatinine ratio. These associations with eGFR were not confounded by socioeconomic position and were not explained by diabetes or hypertension, but there was some evidence that they were stronger in study members who were overweight in adulthood. Thus, our findings highlight the role of lower birth weight in renal disease and suggest that in those born with lower birth weight particular emphasis should be placed on avoiding becoming overweight (Table 5).

▶ This is quite a fascinating data set. Drawn from the Medical Research Council National Survey of Health and Development, a diverse population of 5362 individuals born in March 1946 in England, Scotland, and Wales were followed up for the subsequent 60 to 64 years. The data here represent a subpopulation

TABLE 5.—Linear Regression Models for a 1-kg Increase in Birth Weight by Overweight Status at the Age of 36 Years

Outcome	Overweight at Age 36 Years	N	Coeff	95% CI	P^a
Cystatin C–based eGFR	No	1076	1.79	0.17 to 3.41	0.03
(ml/min per 1.73 m^2)	Yes	495	3.14	0.47 to 5.82	0.02
Creatinine and cystatin C–based	No	979	1.03	−0.59 to 2.65	0.21
eGFR (ml/min per 1.73 m^2)	Yes	445	4.03	1.34 to 6.71	0.003
Log-urine albumin–creatinine	No	1088	0.017	−0.062 to 0.096	0.68
ratio (mg/mmol)	Yes	504	−0.042	−0.192 to 0.108	0.58

Abbreviations: CI, confidence interval; Coeff, coefficient; eGFR, estimated glomerular filtration rate; HbA1c, glycated hemoglobin.

Restricted to study members nonmissing for childhood and adulthood socioeconomic status, self-reported diabetes by the age of 60–64 years, on diabetes treatment at the age of 60–64 years, HbA1c at the age of 60–64 years, midlife systolic blood pressure trajectory, on hypertension treatment at the age of 60–64 years, and systolic blood pressure at the age of 60–64 years.

Models adjusted for sex, age at renal function measurement, childhood and adulthood socioeconomic position, self-reported diabetes by the age of 60–64 years, on diabetes treatment at the age of 60–64 years, HbA1c at the age of 60–64 years, midlife systolic blood pressure trajectory, on hypertension treatment at the age of 60–64 years, systolic blood pressure at the age of 60–64 years, and diastolic blood pressure at the age of 60–64 years.

Wald test for effect modification by overweight status at the age of 36 years: $P = 0.08$ for cystatin C–based eGFR; $P = 0.01$ for creatinine and cystatin C–based eGFR; $P = 0.31$ for log-urine albumin–creatinine ratio.

[a]Likelihood ratio test.

of approximately 2200 individuals in whom complete data regarding birth weight and renal function are available. Prior investigations have suggested that low birth weight may be a harbinger of future kidney disease at middle age and beyond.[1] Theoretically, this could be because of a reduced nephron number and glomerular hyperfiltration. Along these lines, several investigations have linked low birth weight to the later development of hypertension and type 2 diabetes, both of which are risk factors for the later development of kidney disease.[2-6] In addition, a growing body of evidence suggests that obesity in adult life increases the risk of kidney disease.[7,8] The investigators sought to determine the effect of birth weight on later-life renal function and whether adult obesity modifies this relationship.

A particular strength of this study is that the prospective data were collected for 60 to 64 years using standardized protocols and, as such, the investigators were able to use statistical modeling to adjust for multiple potential confounders. The data show that lower birth weight is strongly associated with a lower estimated glomerular filtration rate (eGFR) (measured by formulas based on both creatinine and cystatin C) more than 60 years later. Interestingly, low birth weight did not strongly associate with the urine albumin/creatinine ratio. This effect was not influenced by socioeconomic position, diabetes, or systolic blood pressure. Compared with patients who were of normal weight, among individuals who were overweight by the age of 36, there was a much stronger association between lower birth weight and lower eGFR (Table 5). These longitudinal data are rich and quite interesting. They teach us that individuals of low birth weight should be monitored for factors that can augment their risk of renal disease. This is especially true for early-onset obesity, which appears to increase the rate of loss of renal function among those with low birth weight.

R. Garrick, MD

References

1. White SL, Perkovic V, Cass A, et al. Is low birth weight an antecedent of CKD in later life? A systematic review of observational studies. *Am J Kidney Dis.* 2009;54: 248-261.
2. Huxley RR, Shiell AW, Law CM. The role of size at birth and postnatal catch-up growth in determining systolic blood pressure: a systematic review of the literature. *J Hypertens.* 2000;18:815-831.
3. Mu M, Wang SF, Sheng J, et al. Birth weight and subsequent blood pressure: a meta-analysis. *Arch Cardiovasc Dis.* 2012;105:99-113.
4. Whincup PH, Kaye SJ, Owen CG, et al. Birth weight and risk of type 2 diabetes: a systematic review. *JAMA.* 2008;300:2886-2897.
5. Hsu CY, McCulloch CE, Darbinian J, Go AS, Iribarren C. Elevated blood pressure and risk of end-stage renal disease in subjects without baseline kidney disease. *Arch Intern Med.* 2005;165:923-928.
6. National Kidney Foundation. KDOQI clinical practice guideline for diabetes and CKD: 2012 update. *Am J Kidney Dis.* 2012;60:850-886.
7. Wang Y, Chen X, Song Y, Caballero B, Cheskin LJ. Association between obesity and kidney disease: a systematic review and meta-analysis. *Kidney Int.* 2008;73: 19-33.
8. Silverwood RJ, Pierce M, Thomas C, et al. Association between younger age when first overweight and increased risk for CKD. *J Am Soc Nephrol.* 2013;24:813-821.

A Randomized Trial of Dietary Sodium Restriction in CKD

McMahon EJ, Bauer JD, Hawley CM, et al (Princess Alexandra Hosp, Brisbane, Australia; Univ of Queensland, Brisbane Australia)
J Am Soc Nephrol 24:2096-2103, 2013

There is a paucity of quality evidence regarding the effects of sodium restriction in patients with CKD, particularly in patients with pre-end stage CKD, where controlling modifiable risk factors may be especially important for delaying CKD progression and cardiovascular events. We conducted a double-blind placebo-controlled randomized crossover trial assessing the effects of high versus low sodium intake on ambulatory BP, 24-hour protein and albumin excretion, fluid status (body composition monitor), renin and aldosterone levels, and arterial stiffness (pulse wave velocity and augmentation index) in 20 adult patients with hypertensive stage 3–4 CKD as phase 1 of the LowSALT CKD study. Overall, salt restriction resulted in statistically significant and clinically important reductions in BP (mean reduction of systolic/diastolic BP, 10/4 mm Hg; 95% confidence interval, 5 to 15 /1 to 6 mm Hg), extracellular fluid volume, albuminuria, and proteinuria in patients with moderate-to-severe CKD. The magnitude of change was more pronounced than the magnitude reported in patients without CKD, suggesting that patients with CKD are particularly salt sensitive. Although studies with longer intervention times and larger sample sizes are needed to confirm these benefits, this study indicates that sodium restriction should be emphasized in the management of patients with CKD as a means to reduce cardiovascular risk and risk for CKD progression.

▶ A few prior studies have suggested that patients with end-stage renal disease[1] and chronic kidney disease (CKD)[2] can benefit from dietary sodium restriction. The LOW SALT CKD STUDY is a double-blind, placebo-controlled, randomized, controlled crossover study aimed at evaluating the effects of dietary sodium restriction on various parameters of CKD progression. After a 1-week run-in period of low-sodium intake and dietary counseling, patients with stage 3 or stage 4 CKD (estimated glomerular filtration rate < 30 mL/min/1.73 m^2), with systolic blood pressure 130 to 169 mm Hg and diastolic blood pressure greater than 70 mm Hg were randomly assigned to either the low-salt group (60–80 mmol/d diet) or high-salt group (120 mmol/day Na tablet plus the low-sodium diet intake). After a 2-week interval, the patients underwent a 1-week washout and then switched groups. The study duration was 6 weeks. Several renal indicators were analyzed, and, as shown in Fig 4 of the original article, the mean urinary protein/creatinine ratio was lower in the low salt group, extracellular fluid volume decreased by approximately 0.8 L, and the mean reductions in systolic and diastolic blood pressures were approximately 10 and 4 mm Hg, respectively. As expected, plasma renin and aldosterone were higher in the low-salt phase.

A longer-term trial is needed to determine if these salutatory effects will be sustained over time. Nonetheless, the results of this well-designed trial suggest that patients with CKD are quite susceptible to the effects of dietary sodium. As such, their findings suggest that current patients may benefit from dietary salt restriction while we await the results of longer-term studies.

M. S. Shenoy, MD

References

1. Fine A, Fontaine B, Ma M. Commonly prescribed salt intake in continuous ambulatory peritoneal dialysis patients is too restrictive: results of a double-blind crossover study. *J Am Soc Nephrol.* 1997;8:1311-1314.
2. Vogt L, Waanders F, Boomsma F, de Zeeuw D, Navis G. Effects of dietary sodium and hydrochlorothiazide on the antiproteinuric efficacy of losartan. *J Am Soc Nephrol.* 2008;19:999-1007.

Adherence to antihypertensive agents improves risk reduction of end-stage renal disease

Roy L, White-Guay B, Dorais M, et al (Université de Montréal, Québec, Canada; et al)
Kidney Int 84:570-577, 2013

Uncontrolled hypertension is associated with an increased risk of end-stage renal disease (ESRD). Intensified blood pressure control may slow progression of chronic kidney disease; however, the impact of antihypertensive agent adherence on the prevention of ESRD has never been evaluated.

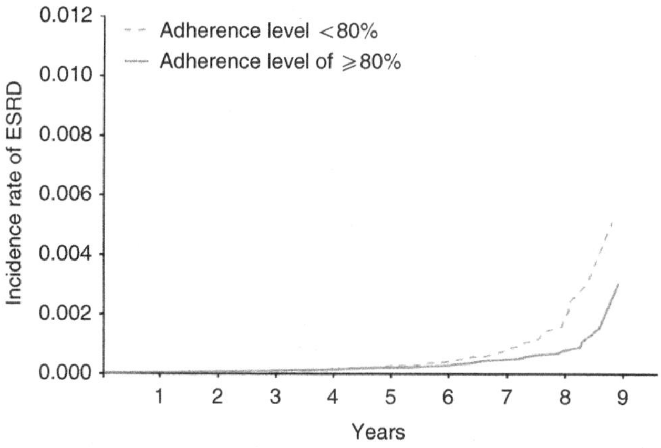

FIGURE 2.—Cumulative incidence rate of end-stage renal disease (ESRD) among high adherence level compared with the low level of adherence of antihypertensive (AH) agents over time in years. (Reprinted with permission from Macmillan Publishers Ltd: Kidney International. Roy L, White-Guay B, Dorais M, et al. Adherence to antihypertensive agents improves risk reduction of end-stage renal disease. *Kidney Int.* 2013;84:570-577, Copyright 2013, with permission from International Society of Nephrology.)

Here we assessed the impact of antihypertensive agent adherence on the risk of ESRD in 185,476 patients in the RAMQ databases age 45 to 85 and newly diagnosed/treated for hypertension between 1999 and 2007. A case cohort study design was used to assess the risk of and multivariate Cox proportional models were used to estimate the adjusted hazard ratio of ESRD. Adherence level was reported as a medication possession ratio. Mean patient age was 63 years, 42.2% male, 14.0% diabetic, 30.3% dyslipidemic, and mean follow-up was 5.1 years. A high adherence level of 80% or more to antihypertensive agent(s) compared to a lower one was related to a risk reduction of ESRD (hazard ratio 0.67; 95% confidence intervals 0.54—0.83). Sensitivity analysis revealed that the effect is mainly in those without chronic kidney disease. Risk factors for ESRD were male, diabetes, peripheral artery disease, chronic heart failure, gout, previous chronic kidney disease, and use of more than one agent. Thus, our study suggests that a better adherence to antihypertensive agents is related to a risk reduction of ESRD and this adherence needs to be improved to optimize benefits (Fig 2).

▶ There are many reasons for poorly controlled blood pressure, including nonadherence to antihypertensive agents. An estimated 50% of hypertensive patients do not adhere to the prescribed medications, and adherence declines after 6 months, especially among patients with newly diagnosed disease.[1-3] The impact of therapeutic adherence on the prevention of progression to end-stage renal disease (ESRD) has never been evaluated.

The authors examined this question in 185 476 patients between the ages of 45 to 85 in the Régie de l'assurance maladie du Québec (RAMQ) and Med-Echo databases, which are 2 large public health insurance databases in Canada. The patients were newly diagnosed (defined as receiving no antihypertensive drugs in the prior 2 years), and patients with known cases of secondary hypertension were excluded. Treatment with several medications was included, but α-blockers, vasodilators, and sympatholytics were excluded, as these drugs are rarely indicated as first-line treatments for essential hypertension, but rather, are often used for unrelated indications. Patients were followed up from 1 year to 9.5 years with a mean follow-up of 5.1 years.

As shown in Fig 2, after 5 years, an adherence rate of greater than 80% was associated with a 33% reduction in the incidence of ESRD. The impact of high adherence on the progression to ESRD was significant in patients without underlying kidney injury (Fig 3 in the original article). Additional subgroup analysis found that the benefit of therapeutic adherence was similar for patients older and younger than 65, suggesting that, at least in terms of blood pressure control, it's never too late to begin.

Like any cohort study based on administrative data, the study does have limitations. For example, it's possible that the development of worsening renal function influenced patients' adherence to their therapeutic regimen. Additionally, the data cannot be adjusted for clinical severity or, alternatively, for healthy user bias, and administrative data are always potentially hampered by faulty documentation. However, the study also has many strengths. It was very well designed, it was free of population bias, only incident users of antihypertensive medications were included, adherence was carefully defined, and the validity of the statistical modeling was established by showing that other high-adherence medications were not associated with a change in the cumulative incidence of ESRD.

These novel data are quite interesting. The effects of aggressive adherence appear to take years to achieve, and both patients and practitioners need to appreciate that reward requires patience. However, these data suggest that the rewards are clinically quite significant, and reducing the incidence of ESRD may be strong motivation for improved compliance.

A. Kapoor, MD

References

1. Park J, Campese V. Clinical characteristics of resistant hypertension: the importance of compliance and the role of diagnostic evaluation in delineating pathogenesis. *J Clin Hypertens (Greenwich)*. 2007;9:7-12.
2. Jackson KC 2nd, Sheng X, Nelson RE, Keskinaslan A, Brixner DI. Adherence with multiple-combination antihypertensive pharmacotherapies in a US managed care database. *Clin Ther.* 2008;30:1558-1563.
3. Burnier M. Medication adherence and persistence as the cornerstone of effective antihypertensive therapy. *Am J Hypertens.* 2006;19:1190-1196.

Effects of Exercise and Lifestyle Intervention on Cardiovascular Function in CKD

Howden EJ, Leano R, Petchey W, et al (Univ of Queensland, Australia; et al)
Clin J Am Soc Nephrol 8:1494-1501, 2013

Background and Objectives.—CKD is associated with poor cardiorespiratory fitness (CRF). This predefined substudy determined the effect of exercise training and lifestyle intervention on CRF and explored the effect on cardiovascular risk factors and cardiac and vascular function.

Design, Setting, Participants, & Measurements.—Between February 2008 and March 2010, 90 patients with stage 3–4 CKD were screened with an exercise stress echocardiogram before enrollment. Patients ($n = 83$) were randomized to standard care (control) or lifestyle intervention. The lifestyle intervention included multidisciplinary care (CKD clinic), a lifestyle program, and aerobic and resistance exercise training for 12 months. CRF (peak $\dot{V}o_2$), left ventricular function, arterial stiffness, anthropometric, and biochemical data were collected at baseline and 12 months.

Results.—Ten percent of randomized patients had subclinical myocardial ischemia at screening and completed the study without incident. There was no baseline difference among 72 patients who completed follow-up (36 in the lifestyle intervention group and 36 in the control group). The intervention increased peak $\dot{V}o_2$ (2.8 ± 0.7 ml/kg per minute versus −0.3 ± 0.9 ml/kg per minute; $P = 0.004$). There was small weight loss (−1.8 ± 4.2 kg versus 0.7 ± 3.7 kg; $P = 0.02$) but no change in BP or lipids. Diastolic function improved (increased e' of 0.75 ± 1.16 cm/s versus −0.47 ± 1.0 cm/s; $P = 0.001$) but systolic function was well preserved and did not change. The change in arterial elastance was attenuated (0.11 ± 0.76 mmHg/ml versus 0.76 ± 0.96 mmHg/ml; $P = 0.01$). Δ peak $\dot{V}o_2$ was associated with group allocation and improved body composition.

Conclusions.—Exercise training and lifestyle intervention in patients with CKD produces improvements in CRF, body composition, and diastolic function.

► Nephrologists continue to search for ways to slow the progression and deleterious clinical effects chronic kidney disease (CKD). As detailed by Howard and colleagues,[1] few well-controlled studies have been completed regarding the effects of lifestyle modification on the systemic effects of CKD. The current study is important because it is the first to demonstrate in a well-defined population that lifestyle intervention can improve cardiorespiratory fitness, cardiac function, and overall body composition. To achieve such gains from simple dietary modification and exercise training seems like a wish come true. Patients enrolled were age 18 to 75 years, with an estimated glomerular filtration rate between 25 and 60 mL/min/1.73 m^2 and 1 or more cardiovascular risk factors including hypertension, hyperlipidemia, poorly controlled diabetes, or obesity. Baseline demographics between the control and intervention group were similar. Exercise training included 150 minutes of moderate-intensity exercise per week, and after 8 weeks of supervised training, patients were encouraged to continue training at home. Compliance was carefully tracked via repetitive e-mails and calls. Lifestyle modification included 4 weeks of group counseling by dietitians and psychologists.

Although systolic and diastolic blood pressure did not improve, as shown in Fig 2 of the original article, lifestyle intervention was associated with improved cardiorespiratory fitness. Serum creatinine was not affected, but body mass index improved significantly.

Will these exercise-induced improvements in cardiac function translate into an improved quality of life or into a reduction in cardiac comorbidity? Those outcomes can only be definitively determine over time, but these results are encouraging, and it seems reasonable for us to share them with our patients and to advocate for these interventions.

M. S. Shenoy, MD

Reference

1. Howden EJ, Fassett RG, Isbel NM, Coombes JS. Exercise training in chronic kidney disease patients. *Sports Med.* 2012;42:473-488.

26 Acute Kidney Injury

Impaired Kidney Function at Hospital Discharge and Long-Term Renal and Overall Survival in Patients Who Received CRRT

Stads S, Fortrie G, van Bommel J, et al (Erasmus Med Ctr, Rotterdam, The Netherlands)

Clin J Am Soc Nephrol 8:1284-1291, 2013

Background and Objectives.—Critically ill patients with AKI necessitating renal replacement therapy (RRT) have high in-hospital mortality, and survivors are at risk for kidney dysfunction at hospital discharge. The objective was to evaluate the association between impaired kidney function at hospital discharge with long-term renal and overall survival.

Design, Setting, Participants, & Measurements.—Degree of kidney dysfunction in relation to long-term effects on renal survival and patient mortality was investigated in a retrospective cohort study of 1220 adults admitted to an intensive care unit who received continuous RRT between 1994 and 2010.

Results.—After hospital discharge, median follow-up of survivors (n=475) was 8.5 years (range, 1–17 years); overall mortality rate was 75%. Only 170 (35%) patients were discharged with an estimated GFR (eGFR) >60 ml/min per 1.73 m^2. Multivariate proportional hazards regression analysis demonstrated that age, nonsurgical type of admission, preexisting kidney disease, malignancy, and eGFR of 29–15 ml/min per 1.73 m^2 (hazard ratio [HR], 1.62; 95% confidence interval [CI], 1.01 to 2.58) and eGFR <15 ml/min per 1.73 m^2 (HR, 1.93; 95% CI, 1.23 to 3.02) at discharge were independent predictors of increased mortality. Renal survival was significantly associated with degree of kidney dysfunction at discharge. An eGFR of 29–15 ml/min per 1.73 m^2 (HR, 26.26; 95% CI, 5.59 to 123.40) and <15 ml/min per 1.73 m^2 (HR, 172.28; 95% CI, 37.72 to 786.75) were independent risk factors for initiation of long-term RRT.

Conclusions.—Most critically ill patients surviving AKI necessitating RRT have impaired kidney function at hospital discharge. An eGFR <30 ml/min per 1.73 m^2 is a strong risk factor for decreased long-term survival and poor renal survival.

► The concept that even a reversible episode of acute kidney injury (AKI) is associated with the development of chronic kidney disease (CKD) and increased mortality and risk has been gaining acceptance.[1] This, coupled with recent data (also reviewed here) that an episode of AKI increases cardiovascular risk,[2] shows the importance of better understanding the risk factors and outcomes of AKI. To accomplish this, the authors studied 470 postdischarge AKI intensive care unit patients for median follow-up of 8.5 years. The patient population studied was very typical of that seen in general clinical medicine. Pre-existing kidney disease was known in about 20% of patients, whereas 48% were known to have normal renal function at the time of admission. Patients were admitted for a variety of medical and surgical conditions, including sepsis, and had the typical array of underlying comorbid conditions, such as diabetes, malignancy, cardiovascular disease, and hypertension.

About a third of all patients who recovered from an episode of AKI necessitating dialysis were discharged with an estimated glomerular filtration rate (eGFR) less than 30 mL/min/1.73 m^2. There was a significant difference in patients' long-term survival depending on the severity of their renal dysfunction at the time of discharge, and multivariate proportional hazards analysis (Table 3 in the original article) found that pre-existing CKD (compared with normal renal function), and an eGFR of less than 30 mL/min/1.73 m^2 at discharge were risk factors for poor renal survival. One limitation of the study is that eGFR was used to estimate renal function, and because patients in the ICU may actually have lost muscle mass, it is possible that renal function was actually somewhat worse at the time of discharge. However, this would not negate the clinical significance of their observations. On balance, the findings show that ICU patients with an episode of AKI requiring dialysis are at risk for both worsening renal function and increased mortality in the years that follow. Clinically, the data suggest that these patients deserve close postdischarge follow-up. Although additional studies will be necessary to determine whether long-term outcome can be altered, these patients are certainly appropriate candidates for interventions, such as blood pressure control and dietary modification, that may ameliorate disease progression.

R. Garrick, MD

References

1. Bucaloiu ID, Kirchner HL, Norfolk ER, Hartle JE 2nd, Perkins RM. Increased risk of death and de novo chronic kidney disease following reversible acute kidney injury. *Kidney Int.* 2012;81:477-485.
2. Chawla LS, Amdur RL, Shaw AD, Faselis C, Palant CE, Kimmel PL. Association between AKI and long-term renal and cardiovascular outcomes in united states veterans. *Clin J Am Soc Nephrol.* 2014;9:448-456.

Association between AKI and Long-Term Renal and Cardiovascular Outcomes in United States Veterans

Chawla LS, Amdur RL, Shaw AD, et al (Veterans Affairs Med Ctr, Washington, DC; Duke Univ Med Ctr, Durham, NC; et al)
Clin J Am Soc Nephrol 9:448-456, 2014

Background and Objectives.—AKI is associated with major adverse kidney events (MAKE): death, new dialysis, and worsened renal function. CKD (arising from worsened renal function) is associated with a higher risk of major adverse cardiac events (MACE): myocardial infarction

(MI), stroke, and heart failure. Therefore, the study hypothesis was that veterans who develop AKI during hospitalization for an MI would be at higher risk of subsequent MACE and MAKE.

Design, Setting, Participants, & Measurements.—Patients in the Veterans Affairs (VA) database who had a discharge diagnosis with International Classification of Diseases, Ninth Revision, code of 584.xx (AKI) or 410.xx (MI) and were admitted to a VA facility from October 1999 through December 2005 were selected for analysis. Three groups of patients were created on the basis of the index admission diagnosis and serum creatinine values: AKI, MI, or MI with AKI. Patients with mean baseline estimated GFR < 45 ml/min per 1.73 m^2 were excluded. The primary outcomes assessed were mortality, MAKE, and MACE during the study period (maximum of 6 years). The combination of MAKE and MACE—major adverse renocardiovascular events (MARCE)—was also assessed.

Results.—A total of 36,980 patients were available for analysis. Mean age ± SD was 66.8 ± 11.4 years. The most deaths occurred in the MI + AKI group (57.5%), and the fewest (32.3%) occurred in patients with an uncomplicated MI admission. In both the unadjusted and adjusted time-to-event analyses, patients with AKI and AKI + MI had worse MARCE outcomes than those who had MI alone (adjusted hazard ratios, 1.37 [95% confidence interval, 1.32 to 1.42] and 1.92 [1.86 to 1.99], respectively).

Conclusions.—Veterans who develop AKI in the setting of MI have worse long-term outcomes than those with AKI or MI alone. Veterans with AKI alone have worse outcomes than those diagnosed with an MI in the absence of AKI.

► As the incidence of acute kidney injury (AKI) has increased and follow-up has improved, it has become quite apparent that it is anything but a benign event.[1,2] Additionally, certain concomitant comorbid conditions appear to uniquely influence a patient's long-term prognosis. This fact is highlighted in a retrospective observational study by Chawla and colleagues of approximately 37 000 veterans drawn from the Veterans Affair database. The authors hypothesized that patients who have AKI in the setting of a cardiac event may be at higher risk for both adverse cardiac (subsequent stroke, myocardial infarction [MI], or congestive heart failure [CHF]) and renal (end-stage renal disease, a 25% decline in estimated glomerular filtration rate, or death) outcomes. In addition, the combination of adverse renal and cardiovascular events (major adverse renocardiovascular events [MARCE]—a composite of each of these events), which is often used as a composite endpoint in clinical trials, was also assessed. The analysis was performed by identifying a group of patients with a primary diagnosis of MI with stable renal function; a second group with a primary diagnosis of AKI, identified by an increase in serum creatinine; and a third group with a primary diagnosis of MI together with an increase in serum creatinine level (AKI + MI).

Fig 3 in the original article shows the outcomes across the diagnostic groups. Interestingly, although the risk of cardiovascular events in the AKI group is lower than that in the MI alone, it remains substantial and suggests that an episode of AKI is associated with long-term cardiovascular events. In addition, patients with (MI + AKI) have twice the adjusted mortality risk of patients with MI alone. This finding is similar to that of prior cohort studies.[3] Patients with MI + AKI were almost twice as likely to be admitted with CHF as were patients with MI alone, and MI + AKI increases the incidence of major adverse kidney events. The authors note that together the data indicate a "bidirectional" deleterious effect. What is the clinical significance of this finding? After the myocardial event, patients receive counseling, begin exercise programs, and are placed on several cardiac-related medications in an effort to reduce cardiac risk. However, the same is not true for patients who suffered an episode of AKI. Observational studies such as this, despite the inherent limitations of retrospective, administrative database analyses, indicate the clear need for prospective controlled outcome trials aimed at identifying potential risk factors and interventions to improve the outcomes (especially the renal and cardiovascular outcomes) of patients who have suffered an episode of AKI.

R. Garrick, MD

References

1. Waikar SS, Curhan GC, Wald R, McCarthy EP, Chertow GM. Declining mortality in patients with acute renal failure, 1988 to 2002. *J Am Soc Nephrol.* 2006;17: 1143-1150.
2. Xue JL, Daniels F, Star RA, et al. Incidence and mortality of acute renal failure in Medicare beneficiaries, 1992 to 2001. *J Am Soc Nephrol.* 2006;17:1135-1142.
3. James MT, Ghali WA, Knudtson ML, et al. Alberta Provincial Project for Outcome Assessment in Coronary Heart Disease (APPROACH) Investigators. Associations between acute kidney injury and cardiovascular and renal outcomes after coronary angiography. *Circulation.* 2011;123:409-416.

Evaluation of 32 urine biomarkers to predict the progression of acute kidney injury after cardiac surgery

Arthur JM, for the SAKInet Investigators (Ralph H Johnson VA Med Ctr, Charleston, SC; et al)
Kidney Int 85:431-438, 2014

Biomarkers for acute kidney injury (AKI) have been used to predict the progression of AKI, but a systematic comparison of the prognostic ability of each biomarker alone or in combination has not been performed. In order to assess this, we measured the concentration of 32 candidate biomarkers in the urine of 95 patients with AKIN stage 1 after cardiac surgery. Urine markers were divided into eight groups based on the putative pathophysiological mechanism they reflect. We then compared the ability of the markers alone or in combination to predict the primary outcome of worsening AKI or death (23 patients) and the secondary outcome of AKIN stage 3 or death (13 patients). IL-18 was the best predictor of both outcomes (AUC of 0.74 and 0.89). L-FABP (AUC of 0.67 and 0.85), NGAL (AUC of 0.72 and 0.83), and KIM-1 (AUC of 0.73 and 0.81) were also good predictors. Correlation between most of the markers was generally related to

TABLE 4.—Biomarker Test Operating and Performance Characteristics for Combinations

	AUC	95% CI	MSE	Probability Threshold	T+, *N* (%)	PPV (D+|T+), *N* (%)	Sens (T+|D+), *N* (%)
AKIN 2/3 or death							
IL-18 +percentage of change in creatinine	0.80	(0.67, 0.89)	0.134	0.30	23 (24)	14 (61)	14 (61)
IL-8 +percentage of change in creatinine	0.81	(0.68, 0.89)	0.138	0.30	24 (25)	14 (58)	14 (61)
NGAL +percentage of change in creatinine	0.82	(0.70, 0.90)	0.139	0.28	27 (28)	15 (56)	15 (65)
AKIN 3 or death							
Cystatin C +percentage of change in creatinine	0.88	(0.70, 0.96)	0.067	0.13	26 (27)	10 (38)	10 (77)
KIM-1+IL-18	0.93	(0.80, 0.98)	0.069	0.31	16 (17)	10 (63)	10 (77)
NGAL +percentage of change in creatinine	0.89	(0.72, 0.96)	0.071	0.13	24 (25)	10 (42)	10 (77)
IL-18 +percentage of change in creatinine	0.93	(0.79, 0.98)	0.074	0.17	17 (18)	11 (65)	11 (85)

Abbreviations: AKIN, Acute Kidney Injury Network; AUC, area under the curve; CI, confidence interval; D+|T+, disease positive given test positive; IL, interleukin; KIM-1, kidney injury molecule-1; MSE, mean squared error; NGAL, neutrophil gelatinase–associated lipocalin; PPV, positive predictive value; Sens, sensitivity; T+, test positive; T+|D+, test positive given disease positive.

their predictive ability, but KIM-1 had a relatively weak correlation with other markers. The combination of IL-18 and KIM-1 had a very good predictive value with an AUC of 0.93 to predict AKIN 3 or death. Thus, a combination of IL-18 and KIM-1 would result in improved identification of high-risk patients for enrollment in clinical trials (Table 4).

▶ Ongoing attention has focused on the ability of biomarkers to predict the development of renal injury. Previous biomarker studies have focused largely on either predicting the development of acute kidney injury (AKI)[1,2] or on predicting any degree of worsening of AKI,[3,4] rather than on predicting the ultimate severity of the AKI. One previous biomarker study,[5] involving a small number of patients, demonstrated that neutrophil gelatinase-associated lipocalin (NGAL) might be useful for predicting the progression of an episode of AKI. The current large-scale prospective trial simultaneously compared the power of multiple biomarkers to predict AKI progression and included 95 subjects with early evidence of AKI after cardiac surgery. Detailed clinical information on each patient was available, and using carefully defined criteria for AKI progression, the authors evaluated whether a panel of 32 biomarkers alone or in combination could accurately predict progression of kidney injury or death.

The data are quite interesting. The authors demonstrated that some of the proteins they believed would be mechanistically similar actually failed to cluster together based on measurement of bioactivity and clinical outcomes. They found that the combination of markers including interleukin-18 and kidney injury molecule 1 (KIM-1) best predicted the progression to more severe levels of renal injury and death (Table 4). Although these results are not yet applicable to daily clinical medicine, it seems likely that will evolve quickly. In the meantime, we are reminded that AKI studies focusing on the benefit of therapeutic interventions are most robust when the population at risk for progression is first well defined. These results suggest that biomarkers may allow us to better define just such a population.

R. Garrick, MD

References

1. Han WK, Wagener G, Zhu Y, Wang S, Lee HT. Urinary biomarkers in the early detection of acute kidney injury after cardiac surgery. *Clin J Am Soc Nephrol.* 2009;4:873-882.
2. Katagiri D, Doi K, Honda K, et al. Combination of two urinary biomarkers predicts acute kidney injury after adult cardiac surgery. *Ann Thorac Surg.* 2012;93:577-583.
3. Hall IE, Coca SG, Perazella MA, et al. Risk of poor outcomes with novel and traditional biomarkers at clinical AKI diagnosis. *Clin J Am Soc Nephrol.* 2011;6:2740-2749.
4. Koyner JL, Garg AX, Coca SG, et al. Biomarkers predict progression of acute kidney injury after cardiac surgery. *J Am Soc Nephrol.* 2012;23:905-914.
5. Koyner JL, Vaidya VS, Bennett MR, et al. Urinary biomarkers in the clinical prognosis and early detection of acute kidney injury. *Clin J Am Soc Nephrol.* 2010;5:2154-2165.

Urinary biomarkers of AKI and mortality 3 years after cardiac surgery

Coca SG, TRIBE-AKI Consortium (Yale Univ School of Medicine, New Haven, CT; Western Univ, London, Ontario, Canada; et al)

J Am Soc Nephrol 25:1063-1071, 2014

Urinary biomarkers of AKI provide prognostic value for in-hospital outcomes, but little is known about their association with longer-term mortality after surgery. We sought to assess the association between kidney injury biomarkers and all-cause mortality in an international, multicenter, prospective long-term follow-up study from six clinical centers in the United States and Canada composed of 1199 adults who underwent cardiac surgery between 2007 and 2009 and were enrolled in the Translational Research in Biomarker Endpoints in AKI cohort. On postoperative days 1-3, we measured the following five urinary biomarkers: neutrophil gelatinase-associated lipocalin, IL-18, kidney injury molecule-1 (KIM-1), liver fatty acid binding protein, and albumin. During a median follow-up of 3.0 years (interquartile range, 2.2-3.6 years), 139 participants died (55 deaths per 1000 person-years). Among patients with clinical AKI, the highest tertiles of peak urinary neutrophil gelatinase-associated lipocalin, IL-18, KIM-1, liver fatty acid binding protein, and albumin associated independently with a 2.0- to 3.2-fold increased risk for mortality compared with the lowest tertiles. In patients without clinical AKI, the highest tertiles of peak IL-18 and KIM-1 also associated independently with long-term mortality (adjusted hazard ratios [95% confidence intervals] of 1.2 [1.0 to 1.5] and 1.8 [1.4 to 2.3] for IL-18 and KIM-1, respectively), and yielded continuous net reclassification improvements of 0.26 and 0.37, respectively, for the prediction of 3-year mortality. In conclusion, urinary biomarkers of kidney injury, particularly IL-18 and KIM-1, in the immediate postoperative period provide additional prognostic information for 3-year mortality risk in patients with and without clinical AKI.

▶ We included this study because it is the largest (and perhaps only) clinical study to date to assess whether urinary biomarkers can predict of long-term outcome. The TRIBE-AKI consortium is a multicenter, multinational trial that has evaluated acute kidney injury (AKI) in the setting of cardiac surgery. The current study evaluated the predictive value of 5 urinary biomarkers collected from approximately 1200 patients 1 to 3 days after cardiac surgery.

Patients were followed for the subsequent 3 years, and mortality events were collected and verified by review of vital records and databases. Patients who died were more likely to have a history of reduced estimated glomerular filtration rate, microalbuminuria, congestive heart failure, combined coronary artery bypass graft (CABG) and valve surgery, and longer perfusion cross-clamp times; were more likely to require postoperative ventilator support for more than 48 hours; and had longer intensive care unit and hospital stays. Fig 2 in the original article shows the adjusted survival curves and peak urinary biomarker levels stratified by AKI, in which AKI was defined as an increase in serum creatinine of $\geq$0.3 mg/dL or $\geq$50% from baseline preoperative levels.

Higher peak urinary biomarker levels were consistently associated with an increased relative risk of mortality in those with clinical AKI. In patients without AKI kidney injury molecule-1 (KIM-1) and interleukin (IL)-18 were independently associated with increased mortality risk. Urinary liver-type fatty acid-binding protein was inversely associated with mortality. The associations were strongest when the absolute value of the peak postoperative concentration was compared with the first postoperative value and was minimally confounded by perioperative factors known to influence mortality. Interesting, KIM-1 and IL-18 were independently associated with mortality even in patients without clinically apparent AKI.

These results are specific to patients who had cardiac surgery and cannot be generalized to other clinical settings. In addition, a statistical limitation was that multiple biomarkers were compared, which raises the chance of statistical interaction, and the data were not specifically corrected for this possibility. However, these issues aside, the data are the first of their kind and are quite interesting. They suggest that for both patients with and without prior clinically apparent AKI, urinary biomarkers can provide unique prognostic mortality information that is independent from other clinical data. If indeed the changes in biomarkers only reflect renal injury, then the data also raise the possibility that subclinical AKI after cardiac surgery may alter the long-term prognosis. This warrants further evaluation.

R. Garrick, MD

Dialysis versus Nondialysis in Patients with AKI: A Propensity-Matched Cohort Study

Wilson FP, Yang W, Machado CA, et al (Perelman School of Medicine at the Univ of Pennsylvania, Philadelphia; et al)
Clin J Am Soc Nephrol 9:673-681, 2014

Background and Objectives.—The benefit of the initiation of dialysis for AKI may differ depending on patient factors, but, because of a lack of robust evidence, the decision to initiate dialysis for AKI remains subjective in many cases. Prior studies examining dialysis initiation for AKI have examined outcomes of dialyzed patients compared with other dialyzed patients with different characteristics. Without an adequate nondialyzed control group, these studies cannot provide information on the benefit of dialysis initiation. To determine which patients would benefit from initiation of dialysis for AKI, a propensity-matched cohort study was performed among a large population of patients with severe AKI.

Design, Setting, Participants, & Measurements.—Adults admitted to one of three acute care hospitals within the University of Pennsylvania Health System from January 1, 2004, to August 31, 2010, who subsequently developed severe AKI were included (n = 6119). Of these, 602 received dialysis. Demographic, clinical, and laboratory variables were used to generate a time-varying propensity score representing the daily probability of initiation of dialysis for AKI. Not-yet-dialyzed patients were matched to each dialyzed patient according to day of AKI and propensity score. Proportional hazards analysis was used to compare time to all-cause mortality among dialyzed versus nondialyzed patients across a spectrum of prespecified variables.

Results.—After propensity score matching, covariates were well balanced between the groups, and the overall hazard ratio for death in dialyzed versus nondialyzed patients was 1.01 (95% confidence interval, 0.85 to 1.21; $P = 0.89$). Serum creatinine concentration modified the association between dialysis and survival, with a 20% (95% confidence interval, 9% to 30%) greater survival benefit from dialysis for each 1-mg/dl increase in serum creatinine concentration ($P = 0.001$). This finding persisted after adjustment for markers of disease severity. Dialysis initiation was associated with more benefit than harm at a creatinine concentration $\geq$ 3.8 mg/dl.

Conclusions.—Dialysis was associated with increased survival when initiated in patients with AKI who have a more elevated creatinine level but was associated with increased mortality when initiated in patients with lower creatinine concentrations.

▶ This is a very interesting study. Multiple factors influence nephrologists' decisions as to when to initiate dialysis in the setting of acute kidney injury (AKI). Often, dialysis is initiated because of oliguria, or a reduction in urine output relative to the obligate intake. In the nonoliguria setting, nephrologists may not be involved in the care of the patient early on and are only consulted when others have concluded that dialysis may be indicated.

The dialysis procedure itself can be associated hypotension, and other untoward effects, which can delay renal recovery,[1] and although several risk models exist, a more rigorous evidence-based approach to the initiation of dialysis would be welcome.

Patients were drawn from a single hospital system over a 6-year period, and 6199 patients with well-defined acute kidney injury and resolution (greater than 50% increase in serum creatinine or absolute increase of 0.3 mg/dL within 48 hours; with resolution defined as improvement of creatinine to within 10% of baseline) were evaluated. Using propensity matching based on clinical, laboratory, and patient factors, the authors created a time-varying propensity score of the probability of dialysis being initiated each day from the onset of AKI through day 14. On the day of initiation of dialysis, the dialyzed patients were matched to yet nondialyzed patients with the same duration of AKI. Primary outcome was time to all-cause mortality, and variables were assessed using rigorous statistical methodology. Of the full cohort of patients with AKI, 602 received dialytic therapy, and the median follow-up was 263 days. Utilizing this carefully matched cohort, the investigators evaluated the effect of several clinical variables, including patient demographics, urine output, parenteral and enteral nutrition, serum chemistries, and comorbid conditions (Fig 2 in the original article). The propensity analysis showed that initiating dialysis in patients with the serum creatinine $\geq$3.8 mg/dL was associated with a survival benefit compared with initiating dialysis at a lower creatinine level. As the authors indicate, the observed survival benefit may reflect a reduced muscle mass and overall frailty in patients with a lower creatinine level and superior muscle mass and nutritional status in patients with a higher creatinine level. Those possibilities cannot be determined from these data. In addition, data regarding fluid balance were not available to the authors, so the confounding effect of volume overload on the serum creatinine concentration could not be assessed. However, with these limitations in mind, the findings caution us that early intervention is not definitively linked to better outcomes and may help both guide our clinical decisions and provide groundwork for future outcome investigations.

R. Garrick, MD

Reference

1. Palevsky PM, Baldwin I, Davenport A, Goldstein S, Paganini E. Renal replacement therapy and the kidney: Minimizing the impact of renal replacement therapy on recovery of acute renal failure. *Curr Opin Crit Care.* 2005;11:548-554.

Adverse Drug Events during AKI and Its Recovery

Cox ZL, McCoy AB, Matheny ME, et al (Vanderbilt Univ Med Ctr, Nashville, TN; Vanderbilt Univ School of Medicine, Nashville, TN)
Clin J Am Soc Nephrol 8:1070-1078, 2013

Background and Objectives.—The impact of AKI on adverse drug events and therapeutic failures and the medication errors leading to these events have not been well described.

Design, setting, Participants, & Measurements.—A single-center observational study of 396 hospitalized patients with a minimum 0.5 mg/dl change in serum creatinine who were prescribed a nephrotoxic or renally eliminated medication was conducted. The population was stratified into two groups by the direction of their initial serum creatinine change: AKI and AKI recovery. Adverse drug events, potential adverse drug events, therapeutic failures, and potential therapeutic failures for 148 drugs and 46 outcomes were retrospectively measured. Events were classified for preventability and severity by expert adjudication. Multivariable analysis identified medication classes predisposing AKI patients to adverse drug events.

Results.—Forty-three percent of patients experienced a potential adverse drug event, adverse drug event, therapeutic failure, or potential therapeutic failure; 66% of study events were preventable. Failure to adjust for kidney function (63%) and use of nephrotoxic medications during AKI (28%) were the most common potential adverse drug events. Worsening AKI and hypotension were the most common preventable adverse drug events. Most adverse drug events were considered serious (63%) or life-threatening (31%), with one fatal adverse drug event. Among AKI patients, administration of angiotensin-converting enzyme inhibitors/angiotensin receptor blockers, antibiotics, and antithrombotics was most

TABLE 3.—Description of Potential Adverse Drug Events and Adverse Drug Events

Event	Incidence *n* (%)
pADE ($n = 93$)	
Contraindicated use for >24 hours	26 (28)
No dose adjustment for >24 hours	15 (16)
No interval adjustment for >24 hours	44 (47)
Ineffective at low creatinine clearance	2 (2)
No drug level monitoring	5 (5)
No creatinine monitoring	3 (3)
Other	6 (6)
Laboratory-only ADE ($n = 21$)	
Hyperkalemia	2 (10)
Supratherapeutic drug levels	19 (90)
Vancomycin	18
Tobramycin	1
ADE ($n = 52$)	
Hypotension	11 (21)
QT prolongation	2 (4)
Cognitive changes/somnolence	4 (8)
Delirium	1 (2)
Extrapyramidal symptoms	1 (2)
Oversedation	6 (11)
Rash	1 (2)
Major bleed	1 (2)
Minor bleed	5 (10)
Worsening AKI	24 (46)
Crystalurea	1 (2)
Respiratory depression	2 (4)
Hemodialysis	3 (6)
Colitis	1 (2)
Death	1 (2)

Subcategory numbers and percentages may exceed the total *n* or 100%, because one event could be composed of multiple adverse drug events (ADEs) or potential ADEs (pADEs). Supplemental Table 2 has definitions of each ADE and laboratoryonly ADE.

Reprinted from Cox ZL, McCoy AB, Matheny ME, et al. Adverse Drug Events during AKI and Its Recovery. Clin J Am Soc Nephrol. 2013;8:1070-1078. Copyright 2013, by the American Society of Nephrology.

strongly associated with the development of an adverse drug event or potential adverse drug event.

Conclusions.—Adverse drug events and potential therapeutic failures are common and frequently severe in patients with AKI exposed to nephrotoxic or renally eliminated medications (Table 3).

▶ Cox and colleagues are to be commended. This carefully defined and executed observational study was done to evaluate medication use and the risk of related adverse drug events in patients with acute kidney injury (AKI). Because there is no standard reference or consensus guiding drug utilization in individuals with concurrent AKI, the authors carefully defined their "at-risk group" and impaneled a committee of nephrologists, internists, and pharmacists, to perform chart reviews and identify both adverse drug events (ADEs), preventable adverse drug events (pADEs), and potential and actual therapeutic failures (pTFs;TFs) among hospitalized patients with either AKI (creatinine increase of 0.5 mg/dL) or during recovery from AKI. As expected, the patients had several underlying clinical conditions, including cancer, cerebrovascular disease, congestive heart failure, diabetes, and peripheral vascular disease, and individuals were excluded if they had undergone transplantation or were receiving chronic dialysis or palliative care. The results deserve our attention. Forty-three percent of the 396 patients at this single-center study experience a pTF, TF, ADE, or pADE. Patients with the most severe AKI were the most at risk for an ADE or pADE, and strikingly among the whole population studied, 66% of events were preventable. Antibiotics was the most frequently identified drug class associated with both potential and observed adverse drug events followed by nonsteroidal anti-inflammatory drugs, antivirals, and angiotensin-converting enzyme inhibitors, and angiotensin II receptor blockers. As shown in Table 3, a broad range of adverse events occurred, and 63% were considered either serious or life threatening (31%). Because the authors identified AKI-related adverse events from a prespecified list of ADEs, other events, as well as preadmission and post discharge events remain unrecognized. In addition, because causality could not be definitively substantiated, medications discontinued more than one day before the episode of AKI were excluded. Thus, the numbers of events may have actually been higher than detected. The data strongly indicate that drug selection and dosing among patients with and recovering from AKI require close and active monitoring.

R. Garrick, MD

Calcium-Channel Blocker–Clarithromycin Drug Interactions and Acute Kidney Injury

Gandhi S, Fleet JL, Bailey DG, et al (Western Univ, London, Ontario, Canada; Lawson Health Res Inst, London, Ontario, Canada, et al)
JAMA 310:2544-2553, 2013

Importance.—Calcium-channel blockers are metabolized by the cytochrome P450 3A4 (CYP3A4; EC 1.14.13.97) enzyme. Blood concentrations of these drugs may rise to harmful levels when CYP3A4 activity is inhibited. Clarithromycin is an inhibitor of CYP3A4 and azithromycin is not, which makes comparisons between these 2 macrolide antibiotics useful in assessing clinically important drug interactions.

Objective.—To characterize the risk of acute adverse events following coprescription of clarithromycin compared with azithromycin in older adults taking a calcium-channel blocker.

Design, Setting, and Participants.—Population-based retrospective cohort study in Ontario, Canada, from 2003 through 2012 of older adults (mean age, 76 years) who were newly coprescribed clarithromycin (n = 96 226) or azithromycin (n = 94 083) while taking a calcium-channel blocker (amlodipine, felodipine, nifedipine, diltiazem, or verapamil).

Main Outcomes and Measures.—Hospitalization with acute kidney injury (primary outcome) and hospitalization with hypotension and all-cause mortality (secondary outcomes examined separately). Outcomes were assessed within 30 days of a new coprescription.

Results.—There were no differences in measured baseline characteristics between the clarithromycin and azithromycin groups. Amlodipine was the most commonly prescribed calcium-channel blocker (more than 50% of patients). Coprescribing clarithromycin vs azithromycin with a calcium-channel blocker was associated with a higher risk of hospitalization with acute kidney injury (420 patients of 96 226 taking clarithromycin [0.44%] vs 208 patients of 94 083 taking azithromycin [0.22%]; absolute risk increase, 0.22% [95% CI, 0.16%-0.27%]; odds ratio [OR], 1.98 [95% CI, 1.68-2.34]). In a subgroup analysis, the risk was highest with dihydropyridines, particularly nifedipine (OR, 5.33 [95% CI, 3.39-8.38]; absolute risk increase, 0.63% [95% CI, 0.49%-0.78%]). Coprescription with clarithromycin was also associated with a higher risk of hospitalization with hypotension (111 patients of 96 226 taking clarithromycin [0.12%] vs 68 patients of 94 083 taking azithromycin [0.07%]; absolute risk increase, 0.04% [95% CI, 0.02%-0.07%]; OR, 1.60 [95% CI, 1.18-2.16]) and all-cause mortality (984 patients of 96 226 taking clarithromycin [1.02%] vs 555 patients of 94 083 taking azithromycin [0.59%]; absolute risk increase, 0.43% [95% CI, 0.35%-0.51%]; OR, 1.74 [95% CI, 1.57-1.93]).

Conclusions and Relevance.—Among older adults taking a calcium-channel blocker, concurrent use of clarithromycin compared with azithromycin was associated with a small but statistically significant greater 30-day risk of hospitalization with acute kidney injury. These findings support current safety warnings regarding concurrent use of CYP3A4 inhibitors and calcium-channel blockers.

▶ Clarithromycin, unlike azithromycin, is a clinically important inhibitor of cytochrome P453A4, the enzyme that metabolizes various classes of medications, including statins and calcium-channel blockers. Previous research[1,2] has shown that antibiotics and other agents can substantially increase blood concentrations of calcium channel blockers (by as much as 500%) and result in significant hypotension. In an effort to gauge the frequency and types of serious adverse drug-drug—related events, the authors conducted a population-based retrospective study of older adults in Ontario who were prescribed the 2 drugs together. Investigators identified 96 226 adults (mean age > 76), recently prescribed clarithromycin and 94 083 patients who were prescribed azithromycin while taking a calcium channel blocker (amlodipine, felodipine, nifedipine, diltiazem, or verapamil). For patients taking a calcium channel blocker, the absolute risk of hospitalization for acute kidney injury (AKI) was small but statistically higher in patients also taking clarithromycin than in those also taking azithromycin (420 of 96 226 or 0.44% vs 208 of 94 083 or 0.22%; odds ratio [OR], 1.98). Patient's co-prescribed clarithromycin also had a higher risk of all-cause mortality (OR, 1.74), and hospitalization for hypotension (111 of 96 226 [0.12%] vs 68/94 083 [0.07%]; OR, 1.60). It is presumed that hemodynamic instability contributed to the AKI. A subgroup analysis showed that dihydropyridines, particularly nifedipine, is associated with a higher risk of interaction with OR of 5.33. The study has many strengths: it is large, the population is well defined, appropriate comparator groups were included, and the outcomes were clearly predefined and demonstrated. Retrospective database studies are always limited by the potential for inaccuracies within the coded administrative data sets, and it is possible that the absolute risk increase may have actually been underestimated. This is the first large population-based study to assess AKI associated with the combined use of a calcium channel blocker and clarithromycin. The data demonstrate that this combination is frequently prescribed. Clarithromycin is mainly eliminated by the kidneys, and the data demonstrate that, surprisingly, the dosage is rarely appropriately adjusted for the prevalent renal function. Drug-drug interactions are usually underrecognized by prescribers, the use of built-in interaction recognition software and mobile applications may help mitigate this risk.

S. Chugh, MD

References

1. Westphal JF. Macrolide-induced clinically relevant drug interactions with cytochrome P-450A (CYP) 3A4: an update focused on clarithromycin, azithromycin and dirithromycin. *Br J Clin Pharmacol.* 2000;50:285-295.
2. Patel AM, Shariff S, Bailey DG, et al. Statin toxicity from macrolide antibiotic coprescription: a population-based cohort study. *Ann Intern Med.* 2013;158: 869-876.

27 Clinical Nephrology

Utility of Urine Eosinophils in the Diagnosis of Acute Interstitial Nephritis

Muriithi AK, Nasr SH, Leung N (Mayo Clinic, Rochester, MN)

Clin J Am Soc Nephrol 8:1857-1862, 2013

Background and Objectives.—Urine eosinophils (UEs) have been shown to correlate with acute interstitial nephritis (AIN) but the four largest series that investigated the test characteristics did not use kidney biopsy as the gold standard.

Design, Setting, Participants, & Measurements.—This is a retrospective study of adult patients with biopsy-proven diagnoses and UE tests performed from 1994 to 2011. UEs were tested using Hansel's stain. Both 1% and 5% UE cutoffs were compared.

Results.—This study identified 566 patients with both a UE test and a native kidney biopsy performed within a week of each other. Of these patients, 322 were men and the mean age was 59 years. There were 467 patients with pyuria, defined as at least one white cell per high-power field. There were 91 patients with AIN (80% was drug induced). A variety of kidney diseases had UEs. Using a 1% UE cutoff, the comparison of all patients with AIN to those with all other diagnoses showed 30.8% sensitivity and 68.2% specificity, giving positive and negative likelihood ratios of 0.97 and 1.01, respectively. Given this study's 16% prevalence of AIN, the positive and negative predictive values were 15.6% and 83.7%, respectively. At the 5% UE cutoff, sensitivity declined, but specificity improved. The presence of pyuria improved the sensitivity somewhat, with a decrease in specificity. UEs were no better at distinguishing AIN from acute tubular necrosis compared with other kidney diseases.

Conclusions.—UEs were found in a variety of kidney diseases besides AIN. At the commonly used 1% UE cutoff, the test does not shift pretest probability of AIN in any direction. Even at a 5% cutoff, UEs performed poorly in distinguishing AIN from acute tubular necrosis or other kidney diseases.

▶ The presence of urinary eosinophils is often considered to be a useful marker for diagnosis of acute interstitial nephritis (AIN). The sensitivity and specificity of this finding has typically been linked with clinical correlates rather than with a renal biopsy, which would permit a definitive diagnosis.[1-3] Thus, this study offers a unique evaluation of the clinical utility of eosinophiluria. The authors identified 566 patients with eosinophils identified in the urinalysis by Hansel's stain in patients who had undergone renal biopsy. As shown in Fig 2 of the original article, several inflammatory and noninflammatory diagnoses were associated with urinary eosinophils. The authors further evaluated whether the presence of pyuria or increasing the number of urinary eosinophils from 1% to 5% would change the sensitivity or specificity of the finding. When these were evaluated in patients in whom the diagnostic decision tree, as is often the case, was acute tubular necrosis (ATN) versus acute interstitial nephritis, the absence of urinary eosinophils did not secure the diagnosis.

When comparing drug-induced acute interstitial nephritis with all other (non-ATN) diagnoses in patients with pyuria at a cutoff level of 5% eosinophils, the negative predictive value was 89.6%.

One caveat is that patients undergoing biopsy likely represent a somewhat preselected population, as only patients in which the diagnosis of AIN is uncertain were likely to have received a biopsy. However, the clinically uncertain scenario is often the exact setting in which the diagnostic aphorism of urinary eosinophils equating with AIN is applied. Thus, the study has direct clinical applicability, as it cautions us that relying on the presence or absence of urinary eosinophils, especially when trying to distinguish ATN from AIN, can lead to incorrect diagnostic conclusions. In addition, the findings suggest the presence of urinary eosinophils alone offer inadequate diagnostic information and would not, alone, warrant the initiation of steroid therapy.

R. Garrick, MD

References

1. Corwin HL, Korbet SM, Schwartz MM. Clinical correlates of eosinophiluria. *Arch Intern Med.* 1985;45:1097-1099.
2. Corwin HL, Bray RA, Haber MH. The detection and interpretation of urinary eosinophils. *Arch Pathol Lab Med.* 1989;113:1256-1258.
3. Ruffing KA, Hoppes P, Blend D, Cugino A, Jarjoura D, Whittier FC. Eosinophils in urine revisited. *Clin Nephrol.* 1994;41:163-166.

Stenting and Medical Therapy for Atherosclerotic Renal-Artery Stenosis

Cooper CJ, for the CORAL Investigators (Univ of Toledo, OH; et al)

N Engl J Med 370:13-22, 2014

Background.—Atherosclerotic renal-artery stenosis is a common problem in the elderly. Despite two randomized trials that did not show a benefit of renal-artery stenting with respect to kidney function, the usefulness of stenting for the prevention of major adverse renal and cardiovascular events is uncertain.

Methods.—We randomly assigned 947 participants who had atherosclerotic renal-artery stenosis and either systolic hypertension while taking two or more antihypertensive drugs or chronic kidney disease to medical therapy plus renal-artery stenting or medical therapy alone. Participants were followed for the occurrence of adverse cardiovascular and renal events (a composite end point of death from cardiovascular or renal causes, myocardial infarction, stroke, hospitalization for congestive heart failure, progressive renal insufficiency, or the need for renal-replacement therapy).

Results.—Over a median follow-up period of 43 months (interquartile range, 31 to 55), the rate of the primary composite end point did not differ significantly between participants who underwent stenting in addition to receiving medical therapy and those who received medical therapy alone (35.1% and 35.8%, respectively; hazard ratio with stenting, 0.94; 95% confidence interval [CI], 0.76 to 1.17; $P = 0.58$). There were also no significant differences between the treatment groups in the rates of the individual components of the primary end point or in all-cause mortality. During follow-up, there was a consistent modest difference in systolic blood pressure favoring the stent group (−2.3 mm Hg; 95% CI, −4.4 to −0.2; $P = 0.03$).

Conclusions.—Renal-artery stenting did not confer a significant benefit with respect to the prevention of clinical events when added to comprehensive, multifactorial medical therapy in people with atherosclerotic renal-artery stenosis and hypertension or chronic kidney disease. (Funded by the National Heart, Lung and Blood Institute and others; ClinicalTrials.gov number, NCT00081731.)

▶ The benefit of arterial stenting in patients with renal-artery stenosis is uncertain. Previous studies[1,2] failed to show significant improvement in renal or cardiovascular outcomes. However, a concern regarding earlier studies was that patient enrollment was not limited to patients with severe/significant renal artery disease. The current CORAL trial was designed to compare the effects of stenting together with medical therapy versus medical therapy alone on cardiovascular and renal outcomes in patients with severe or potentially clinically significant renal artery stenosis. Stenosis was defined angiographically as a narrowing of at least 80% but less than 100% of the arterial diameter or of at least 60% but less than 80% along with a systolic pressure gradient of at least 20 mm Hg. Clinically patients with severe stenosis were defined as having systolic hypertension on 2 or more antihypertensives or normotensive patients with renal artery stenosis and chronic kidney disease (CKD; estimated glomerular filtration rate < 60 mL/min/1.73 m^2). After 43 months of follow-up, the primary outcomes between groups were similar (Table 2 in the original article).

There are a few important caveats. First, the antihypertensive treatment regimen and goals were completely proscriptive and standardized (angiotensin II receptor blockers with or without hydrochlorothiazide, amlodipine, and atorvastatin; B/P target goal 140/80 or if CKD/diabetes present 130/80 mm Hg). Second, patients in whom a positive response was unlikely (advanced CKD with serum creatinine > 4 mg/dL, kidneys under 7 cm, and lesions not amenable to treatment with a single stent) were excluded from the trial. Third, it is important to be aware that this study focused on renal-artery stenosis linked to atherosclerotic disease and excluded fibromuscular dysplasia, a lesion that is often responsive to arterial intervention and stenting. The CORAL study results are important and, together with the prior studies, offer strong, evidence-based guidance that renal-artery stenting is not superior to well-designed and implemented medical management for the prevention of clinical events in patients with either hypertension or CKD and atherosclerotic renal-artery stenosis.

R. Garrick, MD

References

1. ASTRAL Investigators, Wheatley K, Ives N, Gray R, et al. Revascularization versus medical therapy for renal-artery stenosis. *N Engl J Med.* 2009;361:1953-1962.
2. Bax L, Woittiez AJ, Kouwenberg HJ, et al. Stent placement in patients with atherosclerotic renal artery stenosis and impaired renal function: a randomized trial. *Ann Intern Med.* 2009;150:840-848.

Combined Angiotensin Inhibition for the Treatment of Diabetic Nephropathy

Fried LF, for the VA NEPHRON-D Investigators (Univ of Pittsburgh School of Medicine, PA; et al)
N Engl J Med 369:1892-1903, 2013

Background.—Combination therapy with angiotensin-converting–enzyme (ACE) inhibitors and angiotensin-receptor blockers (ARBs) decreases proteinuria; however, its safety and effect on the progression of kidney disease are uncertain.

Methods.—We provided losartan (at a dose of 100 mg per day) to patients with type 2 diabetes, a urinary albumin-to-creatinine ratio (with albumin measured in milligrams and creatinine measured in grams) of at least 300, and an estimated glomerular filtration rate (GFR) of 30.0 to 89.9 ml per minute per 1.73 m^2 of body-surface area and then randomly assigned them to receive lisinopril (at a dose of 10 to 40 mg per day) or placebo. The primary end point was the first occurrence of a change in the estimated GFR (a decline of ≥30 ml per minute per 1.73 m^2 if the initial estimated GFR was ≥60 ml per minute per 1.73 m^2 or a decline of ≥50% if the initial estimated GFR was <60 ml per minute per 1.73 m^2), end-stage renal disease (ESRD), or death. The secondary renal end point was the first occurrence of a decline in the estimated GFR or ESRD. Safety outcomes included mortality, hyperkalemia, and acute kidney injury.

Results.—The study was stopped early owing to safety concerns. Among 1448 randomly assigned patients with a median follow-up of 2.2 years, there were 152 primary endpoint events in the monotherapy group and 132 in the combination-therapy group (hazard ratio with combination therapy, 0.88; 95% confidence interval [CI], 0.70 to 1.12; $P = 0.30$). A trend toward a benefit from combination therapy with respect to the secondary end point (hazard ratio, 0.78; 95% CI, 0.58 to 1.05; $P = 0.10$) decreased with time ($P = 0.02$ for nonproportionality). There was no benefit with respect to mortality (hazard ratio for death, 1.04; 95% CI, 0.73 to 1.49; $P = 0.75$) or cardiovascular events. Combination therapy increased the risk of hyperkalemia (6.3 events per 100 person-years, vs. 2.6 events per 100 person-years with monotherapy; $P < 0.001$)

and acute kidney injury (12.2 vs. 6.7 events per 100 person-years, $P < 0.001$).

Conclusions.—Combination therapy with an ACE inhibitor and an ARB was associated with an increased risk of adverse events among patients with diabetic nephropathy. (Funded by the Cooperative Studies Program of the Department of Veterans Affairs Office of Research and Development; VA NEPHRON-D ClinicalTrials.gov number, NCT00555217.)

▶ The Ongoing Telmisartan Alone and in Combination with Ramipril Global Endpoint Trial (ON TARGET 1) demonstrated that in patients at increased cardiovascular risk, combined angiotensin converting enzyme inhibitor (ACEi) and angiotensin receptor blocker (ARB), therapy was associated with increased risk of hyperkalemia and acute kidney injury requiring dialysis compared with monotherapy.[1] The current study evaluated the efficacy of monotherapy versus combined ACEi and ARB therapy in reducing the rate of progression of diabetic nephropathy. If present, at the time of enrollment, ACEi and ARB therapy was discontinued, and patients were initially begun on losartan, which was increased from 50 to 100 mg per day provided that the serum potassium remained less than 5.5 mmol/L and creatinine remained stable (< 30% increase from baseline). After 1 month of treatment, patients were randomized to receive either lisinopril or placebo. The randomization was stratified based on underlying estimated glomerular filtration rate, the magnitude of proteinuria, and the use or nonuse of combination ACEi and ARB therapy at the time of enrollment.

Lisinopril was titrated from 10 mg to 40 mg/day provided that the potassium and creatinine remained stable (under 5.5 mm/L and < 30% increase in creatinine). This carefully designed study revealed that diabetics with residual proteinuria on full-dose ARB monotherapy are faced with an increased the risk of hyperkalemia and/or acute kidney injury (Fig 2 in the original article) if ACEi therapy is added on to attempt to lower the proteinuria with the hope of slowing disease progression.

The risk events necessitated study termination (mean patient follow-up 2.2 years), so it is impossible to know whether a subpopulation might have experienced any long-term benefit on disease progression with combined therapy. Overall, the data are important and again demonstrate the critical need for carefully controlled, prospective randomized trials that use hard, clinically relevant end points (acute kidney injury, hyperkalemia), rather than surrogate markers (proteinuria), to define efficacy.

R. Garrick, MD

Reference

1. Mann JF, Schmieder RE, McQueen M, et al. Renal outcomes with telmisartan, ramipril, or both, in people at high vascular risk (the ONTARGET study): a multicentre, randomised, double-blind, controlled trial. *Lancet.* 2008;372:547-553.

Association of plasma uric acid with ischaemic heart disease and blood pressure: mendelian randomisation analysis of two large cohorts

Palmer TM, Nordestgaard BG, Benn M, et al (Univ of Warwick, UK; Copenhagen Univ Hosp, Denmark; et al)

BMJ 347:f4262, 2013

Objectives.—To assess the associations between both uric acid levels and hyperuricaemia, with ischaemic heart disease and blood pressure, and to explore the potentially confounding role of body mass index.

Design.—Mendelian randomisation analysis, using variation at specific genes (*SLC2A9* (rs7442295) as an instrument for uric acid; and *FTO* (rs9939609), *MC4R* (rs17782313), and *TMEM18* (rs6548238) for body mass index).

Setting.—Two large, prospective cohort studies in Denmark.

Participants.—We measured levels of uric acid and related covariables in 58 072 participants from the Copenhagen General Population Study and 10 602 from the Copenhagen City Heart Study, comprising 4890 and 2282 cases of ischaemic heart disease, respectively.

Main Outcome.—Blood pressure and prospectively assessed ischaemic heart disease.

Results.—Estimates confirmed known observational associations between plasma uric acid and hyperuricaemia with risk of ischaemic heart disease and diastolic and systolic blood pressure. However, when using genotypic instruments for uric acid and hyperuricaemia, we saw no evidence for causal associations between uric acid, ischaemic heart disease, and blood pressure. We used genetic instruments to investigate body mass index as a potentially confounding factor in observational associations, and saw a causal effect on uric acid levels. Every four unit increase of body mass index saw a rise in uric acid of 0.03 mmol/L (95% confidence interval 0.02 to 0.04), and an increase in risk of hyperuricaemia of 7.5% (3.9% to 11.1%).

Conclusion.—By contrast with observational findings, there is no strong evidence for causal associations between uric acid and ischaemic heart disease or blood pressure. However, evidence supports a causal effect between body mass index and uric acid level and hyperuricaemia. This finding strongly suggests body mass index as a confounder in observational associations, and suggests a role for elevated body mass index or obesity in the development of uric acid related conditions.

▶ Uric acid is an antioxidant that in humans and other large primates is poorly metabolized due to a nonfunctional gene for urate oxidase.[1] It has even been hypothesized that this genetic anomaly may confer a selective advantage because of urate's antioxidant effects on the cardiovascular system.[2] It is a seeming paradox, therefore, that hyperuricemia has been positively correlated with increased risks of cardiovascular disease,[3] although no causal connection has ever been convincingly found. It has been hypothesized that the apparently higher incidence of cardiovascular diseases in patients with hyperuricemia can be explained by unmeasured confounders and by reverse causality, whereby the existence of subclinical or preclinical vascular disease somehow raises uric acid levels as a possibly protective mechanism.

Using data from prospective cohort studies, Palmer et al tried to uncover a causal connection using Mendelian genetic analysis of 2 genetic loci. They looked at a gene polymorphism of SLC2A9, which robustly associates with hyperuricemia and is able to divide the population into those likely to be hyperuricemic and those who are not, regardless of the existence of vascular disease and reverse causality. Similarly, polymorphisms of MC4R were used as markers for body mass index.

They evaluated more than 68 000 participants from 2 Danish prospective cohort studies, which included more than 7000 patients with ischemic heart disease. Their analysis confirmed well-described associations between uric acid levels and both ischemic heart disease and hypertension. An increase in uric acid of one standard deviation was associated with an adjusted hazard ratio (AHR) for ischemic heart disease of 1.21 and the categorical presence of hyperuricemia was associated with AHR of 1.41. A similar pattern of findings was reported for the relationship of uric acid to both systolic and diastolic hypertension. They found no significant causal relationship but were able to show that body mass index, which has been found to have both associative and causal relationships with ischemic heart disease and blood pressure, was found to be nearly linearly associated with the degree of hyperuricemia. This confounding association likely accounts for the strong association between hyperuricemia and both ischemic heart disease and hypertension.

These data suggest that hyperuricemia is a marker for increased body mass but is not directly responsible for the negative cardiovascular outcomes from ischemic heart disease and hypertension. This observation, combined with the fact that uric acid is a potent antioxidant, might suggest that treatment of hyperuricemia may be me more harmful than helpful. This is a question that still awaits a prospective trial.

M. Klein, MD

References

1. Wu XW, Muzny DM, Lee CC, Caskey CT. Two independent mutational events in the loss of urate oxidase during hominoid evolution. *J Mol Evol.* 1992;34:78-84.
2. Ames BN, Cathcart R, Schwiers E, Hochstein P. Uric acid provides an antioxidant defense in humans against oxidant- and radical-caused aging and cancer: a hypothesis. *Proc Natl Acad Sci U S A.* 1981;78:6858-6862.
3. Niskanen LK, Laaksonen DE, Nyyssönen K, et al. Uric acid level as a risk factor for cardiovascular and all-cause mortality in middle-aged men: a prospective cohort study. *Arch Intern Med.* 2004;164:1546-1551.

Influence of Urine Creatinine Concentrations on the Relation of Albumin-Creatinine Ratio With Cardiovascular Disease Events: The Multi-Ethnic Study of Atherosclerosis (MESA)

Carter CE, Katz R, Kramer H, et al (Univ of California San Diego; Univ of Washington, Seattle; Loyola Med Ctr, Maywood, IL; et al)

Am J Kidney Dis 62:722-729, 2013

Background.—Higher urine albumin-creatinine ratio (ACR) is associated with cardiovascular disease (CVD) events, an association that is stronger than that between spot urine albumin on its own and CVD. Urine creatinine excretion is correlated with muscle mass, and low muscle mass also is associated with CVD. Whether low urine creatinine concentration in the denominator of the ACR contributes to the association of ACR with CVD is uncertain.

Study Design.—Prospective cohort study.

Setting & Participants.—6,770 community-living individuals without CVD.

Predictors.—Spot urine albumin concentration, the reciprocal of the urine creatinine concentration (1/UCr), and ACR.

Outcome.—Incident CVD events.

Results.—During a mean of 7.1 years of follow-up, 281 CVD events occurred. Geometric mean values for spot urine creatinine concentration, urine albumin concentration, and ACR were 95 ± 2 (SD) mg/dL, 0.7 ± 3.7 mg/dL, and 7.0 ± 3.1 mg/g. Urine creatinine concentration was lower in older, female, and low-weight individuals. Adjusted HRs per 2-fold higher increment in each urinary measure with CVD events were similar (1/UCr: 1.07 [95% CI, 0.94-1.22]; urine albumin concentration: 1.08 [95% CI, 1.01-1.14]; and ACR: 1.11 [95% CI, 1.04-1.18]). ACR ≥10 mg/g was associated more strongly with CVD events in individuals with low weight (HR for lowest vs highest tertile: 4.34 vs 1.97; *P* for interaction = 0.006). Low weight also modified the association of urine albumin concentration with CVD (*P* for interaction = 0.06), but 1/UCr did not (*P* for interaction = 0.9).

Limitations.—We lacked 24-hour urine data.

Conclusions.—Although ACR is associated more strongly with CVD events in persons with low body weight, this association is not driven by differences in spot urine creatinine concentration. Overall, the associations of ACR with CVD events appear to be driven primarily by urine albumin concentration and less by urine creatinine concentration.

▶ Using a well-defined Multiethnic Study of Atherosclerosis (MESA) population,[1] Carter and colleagues[2] found in patients without known underlying cardiovascular disease that a urinary albumin-to-creatinine ratio (ACR) of 10 mg/g or greater predicted the likelihood of a cardiovascular disease event. This association persisted across age, sex, race/ethnicity, diabetes, hypertension, or chronic kidney disease status. Of note was that patients with an ACR ≥ 10 mg/g who were in the lowest weight tertile had the highest incidence of cardiovascular disease. Analysis found that this was related to an increase in urine albumin excretion rather than a reduction in creatinine excretion. The authors speculated that this may indicate the presence of subclinical disease burden or perhaps underlying vascular inflammation. These data, which are based on an older, multiethnic population, together with the PREVEND 2 (Prevention of Renal and Vascular End-Stage Disease) trial, which was based in Europe, suggest that this simple urinary study can be used to define patients at the greatest risk for cardiovascular disease development.

R. Garrick, MD

References

1. Bild DE, Bluemke DA, Burke GL, et al. Multi-Ethnic Study of Atherosclerosis: objectives and design. *Am J Epidemiol.* 2002;156:871-881.
2. Carter CE, Gansevoort RT, Scheven L, et al. Influence of urine creatinine on the relationship between the albumin-to-creatinine ratio and cardiovascular events. *Clin J Am Soc Nephrol.* 2012;7:595-603.

Usefulness of Serial Decline of Kidney Function to Predict Mortality and Cardiovascular Events in Patients Undergoing Coronary Angiography

Rein P, Saely CH, Vonbank A, et al (Vorarlberg Inst for Vascular Investigation and Treatment, Feldkirch, Austria)

Am J Cardiol 113:215-221, 2014

Chronic kidney disease increases cardiovascular risk and all-cause mortality. However, data on the predictive power of dynamic changes in kidney function are sparse. The aim of this research was to assess the predictive power of serial changes in kidney function on mortality and cardiovascular risk. Estimated glomerular filtration rate (eGFR) was calculated using the Chronic Kidney Disease Epidemiology Collaboration equation at baseline and at follow-up in a high-risk population of 619 consecutive patients who underwent coronary angiography. The population was stratified into 3 groups with respect to decreases in eGFR: stable kidney function (no decrease in eGFR) versus a mild decline (decrease in eGFR > 0 but <4 ml/min/1.73 m^2 per year) and a rapid decline in kidney function (decrease in eGFR ≥4 ml/min/1.73 m^2 per year). Mortality and nonfatal cardiovascular events were recorded over 4 years. Baseline coronary angiography revealed significant coronary stenoses (≥50%) in 368 patients (60%). Survival and event-free survival were significantly lower in patients with rapid decreases in eGFR compared with those with mild decreases ($P < 0.001$ and $P = 0.012$, respectively) and stable kidney function ($P < 0.001$ and $P = 0.004$, respectively). After multivariate adjustment in Cox regression analyses, the continuous variable decline in kidney function significantly predicted death (standardized adjusted hazard ratio 1.32, 95% confidence interval 1.03 to 1.70, $P = 0.032$) and the incidence of the composite end point death and nonfatal vascular events (hazard ratio 1.20, 95% confidence interval 1.01 to 1.43, $P = 0.038$). A 5 ml/min/1.73 m^2 decrease in eGFR independently conferred a 60% increase in

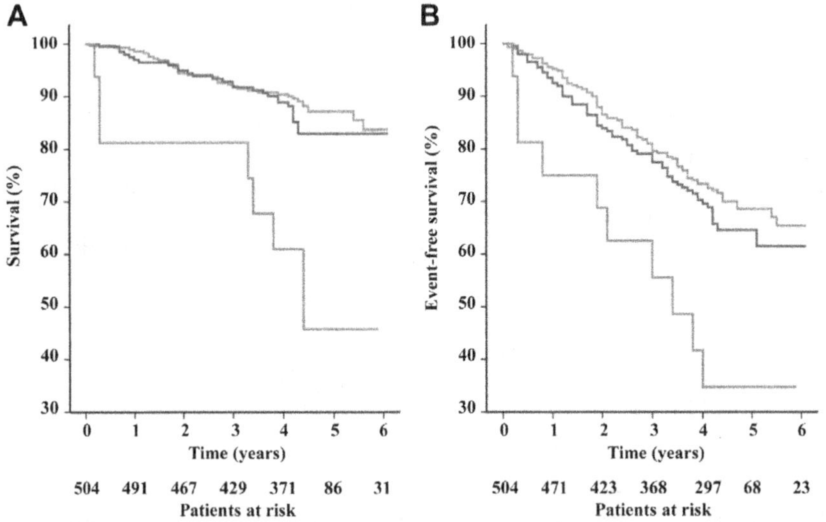

FIGURE 2.—Total mortality (*A*) and event-free survival (*B*) in patients with stable kidney function (*green line*) and those with mild (*blue line*) and rapid (*red line*) declines in kidney function in patients with coronary artery disease. For interpretation of the references to color in this figure legend, the reader is referred to web version of this article. For Interpretation of the references to color in this figure legend, the reader is referred to web version of this article. (Reprinted from the American Journal of Cardiology. Rein P, Saely CH, Vonbank A, et al. Usefulness of serial decline of kidney function to predict mortality and cardiovascular events in patients undergoing coronary angiography. *Am J Cardiol.* 2014;113:215-221, Copyright 2014, with permission from Elsevier.)

mortality risk ($P = 0.032$). In conclusion, a rapid decline in kidney function is a powerful and independent new risk marker for death and vascular events (Fig 2).

▶ Chronic kidney disease itself is a risk for all-cause mortality. Previous studies have found that both the rate of decline of renal function and the variability of glomerular filtration rate (GFR) are associated with an increased risk of mortality.[1,2] These important findings show for the first time that when tracked over several years, a decrease in estimated GFR (eGFR) independently predicts death and predicts that vascular disease will occur over the approximate ensuing 4 years. The data are particularly interesting because they emanate from a well-defined risk cohort in which angiographic characterization was performed on all patients at baseline and in which cardiovascular status and renal function were serially monitored. In addition, the hazard model was adjusted for cardiovascular risk and events; the presence of significant coronary stenosis at baseline; underlying diseases; habits such as smoking, diabetes, obesity, hypercholesterolemia, hypertension; and the use of angiotensin-converting-enzyme inhibitors, angiotensin II receptor blockers, and statins. The renal function/cardiac association was independent of baseline renal function and of angiographically demonstrated baseline coronary artery disease. Fig 2 shows the effect of a rapid decline in renal function on overall mortality and event-free survival in patients with underlying coronary artery disease. A similar eGFR effect stratification was found in the aggregate cohort as well. Overall, a 5-mL/min/1.73 m^2/y decrease in eGFR predicted a 60% increased risk of mortality. This interesting analysis suggests that, in this type of high-risk population, the rate of the decline of eGFR represents a built-in biomarker for mortality and for clinically relevant progression of atherothrombotic disease.

R. Garrick, MD

References

1. Al-Aly Z, Zeringue A, Fu J, et al. Rate of kidney function decline associates with mortality. *J Am Soc Nephrol*. 2010;21:1961-1969.
2. Al-Aly Z, Balasubramanian S, McDonald JR, Scherrer JF, O'Hare AM. Greater variability in kidney function is associated with an increased risk of death. *Kidney Int*. 2012;82:1208-1214.

Randomized Controlled Trial of Febuxostat Versus Allopurinol or Placebo in Individuals with Higher Urinary Uric Acid Excretion and Calcium Stones

Goldfarb DS, MacDonald PA, Gunawardhana L, et al (New York Univ Langone Med Ctr; Global Med Affairs, Deerfield, IL; Takeda Global Res & Development Ctr, Inc, Deerfield, IL; et al)

Clin J Am Soc Nephrol 8:1960-1967, 2013

Background and Objectives.—Higher urinary uric acid excretion is a suspected risk factor for calcium oxalate stone formation. Febuxostat, a xanthine oxidoreductase inhibitor, is effective in lowering serum urate concentration and urinary uric acid excretion in healthy volunteers and people with gout. This work studied whether febuxostat, compared with allopurinol and placebo, would reduce 24-hour urinary uric acid excretion and prevent stone growth or new stone formation.

Design, Setting, Participants, & Measurements.—In this 6-month, double-blind, multicenter, randomized controlled trial, hyperuricosuric participants with a recent history of calcium stones and one or more radio-opaque calcium stone ≥ 3 mm (as seen by multidetector computed tomography) received daily febuxostat at 80 mg, allopurinol at 300 mg, or placebo. The primary end point was percent change from baseline to month 6 in 24-hour urinary uric acid. Secondary end points included percent change from baseline to month 6 in size of index stone and change from baseline in the mean number of stones and 24-hour creatinine clearance.

Results.—Of 99 enrolled participants, 86 participants completed the study. Febuxostat led to significantly greater reduction in 24-hour urinary uric acid (−58.6%) than either allopurinol (−36.4%; $P = 0.003$) or placebo (−12.7%; $P < 0.001$). Percent change from baseline in the size of the largest calcium stone was not different with febuxostat compared with allopurinol or placebo. There was no change in stone size, stone number, or renal function. No new safety concerns were noted for either drug.

Conclusions.—Febuxostat (80 mg) lowered 24-hour urinary uric acid significantly more than allopurinol (300 mg) in stone formers with higher urinary uric acid excretion after 6 months of treatment. There was no change in stone size or number over the 6-month period.

▶ Nearly one-third of calcium stone formers have hyperuricosuria.[1,2] Febuxostat, a xanthine oxidoreductase inhibitor may be effective in the prevention of calcium stones. This study is the first randomized, multicentered, controlled trial comparing the efficacy of febuxostat with that of allopurinol in recurrent uric acid stone formers with high levels of urinary uric acid excretion. The study duration was 6 months and compared full-dose (80 mg) febuxostat with 300 mg allopurinol. The febuxostat lowered urinary uric acid more effectively than did allopurinol (Fig 2 in the original article) There was no change in the size or number of stones, suggesting that stone growth did not occur, although the study may have not have been long enough to detect a physical change in stone appearance. More than half of the patients complained of adverse events, and the most significant event was acute nephrolithiasis requiring hospitalization in a patient receiving placebo. Three participants prematurely discontinued treatment because of side effects: 1 subject in the placebo group (musculoskeletal pain) and 2 participants in the febuxostat group (1 participant with viral hepatitis and increased blood CPK levels and 1 patient on febuxostat with nausea, vomiting, and renal colic). This short-term trial indicates that febuxostat can safety reduced uric acid excretion in stone formers to a greater extent than 300 mg allopurinol. Longer-term studies will be needed to assess its effect on stone formation and growth.

M. Brogan, MD

References

1. Arowojolu O, Goldfarb DS. Treatment of calcium nephrolithiasis in the patient with hyperuricosuria. *J Nephrol.* 2014 [Epub ahead of print].
2. Ettinger B. Does hyperuricosuria play a role in calcium oxalate lithiasis? *J Urol.* 1989;141:738-741.

Urinary Lithogenic Risk Profile in Recurrent Stone Formers With Hyperoxaluria: A Randomized Controlled Trial Comparing DASH (Dietary Approaches to Stop Hypertension)-Style and Low-Oxalate Diets

Noori N, Honarkar E, Goldfarb DS, et al (Shahid Beheshti Univ of Med Sciences, Tehran, Iran; New York Harbor VA Healthcare System; et al)

Am J Kidney Dis 63:456-463, 2014

Background.—Patients with nephrolithiasis and hyperoxaluria generally are advised to follow a low-oxalate diet. However, most people do not eat isolated nutrients, but meals consisting of a variety of foods with complex combinations of nutrients. A more rational approach to nephrolithiasis prevention would be to base dietary advice on the cumulative effects of foods and different dietary patterns rather than single nutrients.

Study Design.—Randomized controlled trial.

Setting & Participants.—Recurrent stone formers with hyperoxaluria (urine oxalate > 40 mg/d).

Intervention.—The intervention group was asked to follow a calorie-controlled Dietary Approaches to Stop Hypertension (DASH)-style diet (a diet high in fruit, vegetables, whole grains, and low-fat dairy products and low in saturated fat, total fat, cholesterol, refined grains, sweets, and meat), whereas the control group was prescribed a low-oxalate diet. Study length was 8 weeks.

Outcomes.—Primary: change in urinary calcium oxalate supersaturation.

Secondary.—Changes in 24-hour urinary composition.

Results.—57 participants were randomly assigned (DASH group, 29; low-oxalate group, 28). 41 participants completed the trial (DASH group, 21; low-oxalate group, 20). As-treated analysis showed a trend for urinary oxalate excretion to increase in the DASH versus the low-oxalate group (point estimate of difference, 9.0 mg/d; 95% CI, −1.1 to 19.1 mg/d; $P = 0.08$). However, there was a trend for calcium oxalate supersaturation to decrease in the DASH versus the low-oxalate group (point estimate of difference, −1.24; 95% CI, −2.80 to 0.32; $P = 0.08$) in association with an increase in magnesium and citrate excretion and urine pH in the DASH versus low-oxalate group.

Limitations.—Limited sample size, as-treated analysis, nonsignificant results.

Conclusions.—The DASH diet might be an effective alternative to the low-oxalate diet in reducing calcium oxalate supersaturation and should be studied more.

▶ Dietary habits are believed to contribute to the incidence of kidney stones.[1-3] As such, dietary intake represents a potentially modifiable risk factor for stone formation. This is the first head-to-head controlled trial of the Dietary Approaches to Stop Hypertension (DASH) diet versus a low-oxalate diet for the metabolic control of oxalate stones.

The DASH-style diet was chosen to assess the effects of a presumably more satisfying and sustainable multinutrient diet versus the alternative approach of controlling a single nutrient.

The results showed that despite an increase in the urinary oxalate, calcium-oxalate supersaturation decreased on the 24-hour urine sample. This change in saturation may have been caused by an increased urine volume and other factors related to dietary intake, such as urine pH, that may favorably influence the molar concentration of oxalate.

The strength of the study was the randomization and close follow-up of the patients. Weaknesses of the trial are that the results may not be readily generalized, only single ethnicity was studied, and the lithogenic risk profile was assessed on a single urine test at the end of follow-up.

A concern was that, by dietary recall, calcium intake on a low-oxalate diet was lower than would be chronically advisable. Other dietary modifications, such as a low salt, low protein diet and vegetarian diets have each been utilized to reduce stone risk. The DASH diet may represent a novel approach to reduce the risk of oxalate stone formation.

M. Brogan, MD

References

1. Trinchieri A. A rapid food screener ranks potential renal acid load of renal stone formers similarly to a diet history questionnaire. *Urolithiasis*. 2013;41:3-7.
2. Borghi L, Schianchi T, Meschi T, et al. Comparison of two diets for the prevention of recurrent stones in idiopathic hypercalciuria. *N Engl J Med*. 2002;346:77-84.
3. Heilberg IP, 'Goldfarb DS. Optimum Nutrition for Kidney Stone Disease. *Adv Chronic Kidney Dis*. 2013;20:165-174.

Soda and Other Beverages and the Risk of Kidney Stones

Ferraro PM, Taylor EN, Gambaro G, et al (Catholic Univ of the Sacred Heart, Rome, Italy; Brigham and Women's Hosp, Boston, MA)
Clin J Am Soc Nephrol 8:1389-1395, 2013

Background and Objectives.—Not all fluids may be equally beneficial for reducing the risk of kidney stones. In particular, it is not clear whether sugar and artificially sweetened soda increase the risk.

Design, Setting, Participants, & Measurements.—We prospectively analyzed the association between intake of several types of beverages and incidence of kidney stones in three large ongoing cohort studies. Information on consumption of beverages and development of kidney stones was collected by validated questionnaires.

Results.—The analysis involved 194,095 participants; over a median follow-up of more than 8 years, 4462 incident cases occurred. There was a 23% higher risk of developing kidney stones in the highest category of consumption of sugar-sweetened cola compared with the lowest category (P for trend = 0.02) and a 33% higher risk of developing kidney stones for sugar-sweetened noncola (P for trend = 0.003); there was a marginally significant higher risk of developing kidney stones for artificially sweetened noncola (P for trend = 0.05). Also, there was an 18% higher risk for punch (P for trend = 0.04) and lower risks of 26% for caffeinated coffee (P for trend <0.001), 16% for decaffeinated coffee (P for trend = 0.01), 11%for tea (P for trend = 0.02), 31%−33%for wine (P for trend <0.005), 41% for beer (P for trend <0.001), and 12% for orange juice (P for trend = 0.004).

Conclusions.—Consumption of sugar-sweetened soda and punch is associated with a higher risk of stone formation, whereas consumption of coffee, tea, beer, wine, and orange juice is associated with a lower risk.

▶ A diet low in salt and animal protein are typically recommended to patients with stone disease. A high fluid intake is also advisable, but the types of fluid are often not specified. Ferraro and colleagues evaluated the influence of beverage consumption on the incidence of stone formation in large cohort patients with a follow-up time of up to 13 years. The numbers of patients enrolled and the length of follow-up make these data both interesting and clinically useful.

Most clinicians tell patients to drink water to prevent stones. It is good to know that both caffeinated and, less so, decaffeinated coffee and tea can also reduce stones, and wine (red and white) and beer can be safely consumed, at least with regard to stone formation.

A new finding was that sugary punch was found to increase stone formation. The daily consumption of sugar-sweetened colas and noncolas increased stone formation compared with artificially sweetened sodas. This finding differs from those found with analyses of other cohorts.[1,2] These findings may be due to the effects of fructose on stone formation, which are believed to be mediated by fructose-induced increases in urinary calcium oxalate and uric acid excretion.[3,4]

Conversely, beverages such as orange juice may reduce stone formation because their high citrate content offsets the effects of the high fructose content. Interestingly, the current study did not confirm a significant increase in stone formation via intake of apple and grapefruit juice.[1,2] The authors postulate that this may be due to differences in sample size and length of follow-up.

Diet is a modifiable risk factor in the treatment of stones. Practitioners and stone-forming patients should find the results of this large cohort-based study both interesting and clinically applicable.

R. Garrick, MD

References

1. Curhan GC, Willett WC, Rimm EB, Spiegelman D, Stampfer MJ. Prospective study of beverage use and the risk of kidney stones. *Am J Epidemiol.* 1996;143: 240-247.
2. Curhan GC, Willett WC, Speizer FE, Stampfer MJ. Beverage use and risk for kidney stones in women. *Ann Intern Med.* 1998;128:534-540.
3. Nguyen NU, Dumoulin G, Henriet MT, Regnard J. Increase in urinary calcium and oxalate after fructose infusion. *Horm Metab Res.* 1995;27:155-158.
4. Fox IH, Kelley WN. Studies on the mechanism of fructose-induced hyperuricemia in man. *Metabolism.* 1972;21:713-721.

28 Chronic Kidney Disease

Lifetime Incidence of CKD Stages 3–5 in the United States

Grams ME, Chow EKH, Segev DL, et al (Johns Hopkins Univ School of Medicine, Baltimore, MD; Johns Hopkins Univ Bloomberg School of Public Health, Baltimore, MD)

Am J Kidney Dis 62:245-252, 2013

Background.—Lifetime risk estimates of chronic kidney disease (CKD) can motivate preventative behaviors at the individual level and forecast disease burden and health care utilization at the population level.

Study Design.—Markov Monte Carlo model simulation study.

Setting & Population.—Current U.S. black and white population.

Model, Perspective, & Timeframe.—Markov models simulating kidney disease development, using an individual perspective and lifetime horizon.

Outcomes.—Age-, sex- and race-specific residual lifetime risks of CKD stages 3a+ (eGFR<60 ml/min/1.73 m^2), 3b+ (eGFR<45 ml/min/1.73 m^2), and 4+ (eGFR<30 ml/min/1.73 m^2), and end stage renal disease (ESRD).

Measurements.—State transition probabilities of developing CKD and of dying prior to its development were modeled using: 1) mortality rates from National Vital Statistics Report, 2) mortality risk estimates from a 2-million person meta-analysis, and 3) CKD prevalence from National Health and Nutrition Examination Surveys. Incidence, prevalence, and mortality related to ESRD were supplied by the US Renal Disease System.

Results.—At birth, the overall lifetime risks of CKD stages 3a+, 3b+, 4+, and ESRD were 59.1%, 33.6%, 11.5%, and 3.6%, respectively. Women experienced greater CKD risk yet lower ESRD risk than men; blacks of both sexes had markedly higher CKD stage 4+ and ESRD risk (lifetime risks for white men, white women, black men, and black women, respectively: 53.6%, 64.9%, 51.8%, and 63.6% [CKD stage 3a+]; 29.0%, 36.7%, 33.7%, and 40.2% [CKD stage 3b+]; 9.3%, 11.4%, 15.8%, and 18.5% [CKD stage 4+]; and 3.3%, 2.2%, 8.5%, and 7.8% [ESRD]). Risk of CKD increased with age, with approximately one-half of CKD stage 3a+ cases developing after 70 years of age.

Limitations.—CKD incidence estimates were modeled from prevalence in the U.S. population.

Conclusions.—In the U.S., the lifetime risk of developing CKD stage 3a+ is high, underscoring the importance of primary prevention and effective therapy to reduce CKD-related morbidity and mortality.

▶ Chronic kidney disease (CKD) is rising in prevalence, increasingly expensive, and associated with a high degree of morbidity and mortality; reduced renal function is now a well-accepted risk factor for all-cause mortality. Grams and colleagues used a variety of vital databases and Markov models to better estimate the future population burden end-stage renal disease (ESRD) among Americans. Investigators applied the CKD-EPI (Chronic Kidney Disease Epidemiology Collaboration) creatinine [2009] equation to derive estimated glomerular filtration rate (eGFR) and defined CKD stage 3a (CKD3a) as eGFR < 60 mL/min/1.73 m^2; CKD3b as eGFR < 45 mL/min/1.73 m^2; CKD4 as (eGFR < 30 mL/min/1.73 m^2), and ESRD (chronic kidney failure treated by dialysis or transplantation).

Fig 2 in the original article demonstrates the cumulative incidence of the various stages of CKD over lifetime stratified by race and sex. The statistical evaluation demonstrates that 63.8% (135.8 million people), in the current US white and black population either have (7.2%) or are expected to develop (56.6%) CKD stage 3a during their lifetime. Similarly, a projected 26.1 million either have or are expected to develop CKD4. A 40-year-old is more likely to develop CKD than either coronary disease or invasive cancer, and a 55-year-old has a greater risk of developing CKD than diabetes. The risk of CKD continues to dramatically increase with age, with approximately half the incident cases occurring after age 70.

The magnitude of these numbers causes us to reflect on the new American College of Physicians recommendations against screening for CKD.[1] Those recommendations would seem to contradict the magnitude of the lifetime risk of CKD/ESRD and its related effects on morbidity (cardiovascular disease, bone disease, cognitive dysfunction, protein energy wasting) and mortality.

Perhaps this apparent inconsistency lies in the distinction between the word screening and the concept of early detection of those at risk. Thus, the American College of Physicians recommends against screening for asymptomatic adults (early CKD is almost always asymptomatic) without risk factors for CKD; those factors include diabetes, older age, obesity, family history of CKD (especially among Native Americans, African Americans, and Hispanics), and hypertension. They also recommend the use of angiotensin converting enzyme (ACE) inhibitors and angiotensin II receptor blockers (ARBs) in hypertensive patients with CKD1–3 (and suggest those with diabetes or proteinuria are likely receiving an ACE inhibitors/ARB) and the use of statin therapy. These interventions, of course, would require measuring the serum creatinine, blood pressure, and urinary protein spillage to detect those at risk.

Thus, it would seem that the College guidelines must be interpreted carefully and actually apply to fairly small numbers of individuals, especially when judged against those at risk for CKD/ESRD.

R. Garrick, MD

Reference

1. Qaseem A, Hopkins RH Jr, Sweet DE, Starkey M, Shekelle P. Screening, monitoring, and treatment of stage 1–3 chronic kidney disease: a clinical practice guideline from the American College of Physicians. *Ann Intern Med.* 2013;159: 835-847.

Identification of a urine metabolomic signature in patients with advanced-stage chronic kidney disease

Posada-Ayala M, Zubiri I, Martin-Lorenzo M, et al (IIS-Fundacion Jimenez Diaz, Madrid, Spain; et al)

Kidney Int 85:103-111, 2014

The prevalence of chronic kidney disease (CKD) is increasing and frequently progresses to end-stage renal disease. There is an urgent demand to discover novel markers of disease that allow monitoring disease progression and, eventually, response to treatment. To identify such markers, and as a proof of principle, we determined if a metabolite signature corresponding to CKD can be found in urine. In the discovery stage, we analyzed the urine metabolome by NMR of 15 patients with CKD and compared that with the metabolome of 15 healthy individuals and found a classification pattern clearly indicative of CKD. A validation cohort of urine samples from an additional 16 patients with CKD and 15 controls was then analyzed by (Selected Reaction Monitoring) liquid chromatography-triple quadrupole mass spectrometry and indicated that a group of seven urinary metabolites differed between CKD and non-CKD urine samples. This profile consisted of 5-oxoproline, glutamate, guanidoacetate, α-phenylacetylglutamine, taurine, citrate, and trimethylamine N-oxide. Thus, we identified a panel of urine metabolites differentially present in urine that may help identify and monitor patients with CKD.

▶ We included this study because it is very forward-looking. For many years clinicians have struggled to find ways to identify patients with chronic kidney disease (CKD; with or without underlying comorbidities such as diabetes, proteinuria, hypertension, and cardiovascular disease) and to predict who will progress to more severe levels of renal dysfunction or end-stage renal disease (ESRD).[1-3]

Despite much progress, the tools in our armamentarium such as serum creatinine, cystatin C, protein/creatinine ratios, and selected biomarkers have remained somewhat blunt. The current study identified and validated a urine metabolomic signature to help identify and monitor patients with CKD. A metabolome is the downstream change in the genome, transcriptome, and proteome that reflects the real-time processes occurring in an organism. The proteome contains approximately 10 million proteins, whereas the metabolites of an organism are measured in the thousands and are, therefore, considerably less complex.[4] A major advantage of this applied technology is the absence of any preselection of candidate metabolites to be investigated, and as such, preselection bias is eliminated.

The investigators used nuclear magnetic resonance (NMR) to identify candidate metabolites initially. The results were then validated by using SRM (liquid chromatography–mass spectrometry) urinary assays which were carried out in both healthy controls and patients with known CKD. Through this discovery and validation process as shown in Fig 4 of the original article, a small array of candidate metabolites was identified.

Of interest is that the changes in the metabolomic signature have some concordance with metabolic changes that are known to occur during the progression of chronic kidney injury. For example, glutamate metabolism is linked to ammoniagenesis and the required daily excretion of acids. The changes noted may represent changes in renal production of ammonia in concert with changes in estimated glomerular filtration rate and renal mass, with glutamate levels increasing during earlier stages of CKD to compensate for metabolic acidosis and then falling in later stages of CKD due to reduced renal mass and a concomitant reduction in cellular function. Future studies will be needed to test the metabolomic signature in larger populations and to determine if the metabolomic signature can be used to predict progression in a wide array of patients.

R. Garrick, MD

References

1. Peralta CA, Shlipak MG, Judd S, et al. Detection of chronic kidney disease with creatinine, cystatin C, and urine albumin-to-creatinine ratio and association with progression to end-stage renal disease and mortality. *JAMA*. 2011;305: 1545-1552.
2. Fassett RG, Venuthurupalli SK, Gobe GC, Coombes JS, Cooper MA, Hoy WE. Biomarkers in chronic kidney disease: a review. *Kidney Int*. 2011;80:806-821.
3. Jardine MJ, Hata J, Woodward M, et al; ADVANCED Collaborative Group. Prediction of kidney-related outcomes in patients with type 2 diabetes. *Am J Kidney Dis*. 2012;60:770-778.
4. van der Kloet FM, Tempels FW, Ismail N, et al. Discovery of early-stage biomarkers for diabetic kidney disease using ms-based metabolomics (FinnDiane study). *Metabolomics*. 2012;8:109-119.

Prevalence of Apparent Treatment-Resistant Hypertension among Individuals with CKD

Tanner RM, Calhoun DA, Bell EK, et al (Univ of Alabama, Birmingham)
Clin J Am Soc Nephrol 8:1583-1590, 2013

Background and Objectives.—Apparent treatment-resistant hypertension is defined as systolic/diastolic BP ≥ 140/90 mmHg with concurrent use of three or more antihypertensive medication classes or use of four or more antihypertensive medication classes regardless of BP level.

Design, Setting, Participants, & Measurements.—The prevalence of apparent treatment-resistant hypertension among Reasons for Geographic and Racial Differences in Stroke study participants treated for hypertension (n = 10,700) was determined by level of estimated GFR and albumin-to-creatinine ratio, and correlates of apparent treatment-resistant hypertension among those participants with CKD were evaluated. CKD was defined as an albumin-to-creatinine ratio ≥ 30 mg/g or estimated GFR <60 ml/min per 1.73 m^2.

Results.—The prevalence of apparent treatment-resistant hypertension was 15.8%, 24.9%, and 33.4% for those participants with estimated GFR ≥60, 45–59, and <45 ml/min per 1.73 m^2, respectively, and 12.1%, 20.8%, 27.7%, and 48.3% for albumin-to-creatinine ratio <10, 10–29, 30–299, and ≥300 mg/g, respectively. The multivariable adjusted prevalence ratios (95% confidence intervals) for apparent treatment-resistant hypertension were 1.25 (1.11 to 1.41) and 1.20 (1.04 to 1.37) for estimated GFR levels of 45–59 and <45 ml/min per 1.73 m^2, respectively, versus ≥60 ml/min per 1.73 m^2 and 1.54 (1.39 to 1.71), 1.76 (1.57 to 1.97), and 2.44 (2.12 to 2.81) for albumin-to-creatinine ratio levels of 10–29, 30–299, and ≥300 mg/g, respectively, versus albumin-to-creatinine ratio <10 mg/g. After multivariable adjustment, men, black race, larger waist circumference, diabetes, history of myocardial infarction or stroke, statin use, and lower estimated GFR and higher albumin-to-creatinine ratio levels were associated with apparent treatment-resistant hypertension among individuals with CKD.

Conclusions.—This study highlights the high prevalence of apparent treatment-resistant hypertension among individuals with CKD.

▶ The control of hypertension in patients with chronic kidney disease (CKD) can be quite frustrating. Treatment-resistant hypertension (TRH) is typically defined as blood pressure ≥140/90 mm Hg on medications from ≥3 antihypertensive classes or while taking a total of ≥4 medications. To better understand the demographics and risk factors of resistant hypertension in this population, Tanner and colleagues used the REGARDS[1] study population, which was comprised of more than 30 000 African-American and white US adults ≥45 years of age. From this population, they culled approximately 15 000 non–end-stage renal disease patients with hypertension and blood pressure controlled with at least one class of antihypertensive medications and who had available information regarding renal function, urinary protein spillage, and medication compliance (based on total bottle review). Treatment-resistant hypertension was carefully defined; blood pressure was obtained by trained technicians; and full behavioral, medical, and socioeconomic histories were available. The prevalence of TRH was increased among patients with either CKD or an increased albumin/creatinine ratio (ACR). As shown in Fig 3 of the original article, within each estimated glomerular filtration rate (eGFR) level, the prevalence of TRH was increased at higher ACR levels. As shown, the prevalence of TRH among patients with CKD and albuminuria approaches almost 60%. This certainly helps explain why blood pressure control among this at- risk population is so clinically challenging. After full demographic adjustment, the population most associated with TRH was obese, diabetic, African-American men on statins, with an eGFR less than 45 mL/min/1.73 m^2 and increased ACR.

A strength of this study is that it was done on a well-defined, carefully monitored population. Although the cross-sectional design makes it impossible to determine whether TRH was primary or secondary to the CKD, the significance of the observation remains clinically relevant. Their results help define the phenotype of patients most at risk for treatment-resistant hypertension and can help us more carefully direct our attention and resources.

R. Garrick, MD

Reference

1. Howard VJ, Cushman M, Pulley L. The reasons for geographic and racial differences in stroke study: objectives and design. *Neuroepidemiology.* 2005;25: 135-143.

Blood pressure lowering and major cardiovascular events in people with and without chronic kidney disease: meta-analysis of randomised controlled trials

Blood Pressure Lowering Treatment Trialists' Collaboration (Univ of Sydney, New South Wales, Australia)

BMJ 347:f5680, 2013

Objective.—To define the cardiovascular effects of lowering blood pressure in people with chronic kidney disease.

Design.—Collaborative prospective meta-analysis of randomised trials.

Data Sources and Eligibility.—Participating randomised trials of drugs to lower blood pressure compared with placebo or each other or that compare different blood pressure targets, with at least 1000 patient years of follow-up per arm.

Main Outcome Measures.—Major cardiovascular events (stroke, myocardial infarction, heart failure, or cardiovascular death) in composite and individually and all cause death.

Participants.—26 trials (152 290 participants), including 30 295 individuals with reduced estimated glomerular filtration rate (eGFR), which was defined as eGFR <60 mL/min/1.73 m^2.

Data Extraction.—Individual participant data were available for 23 trials, with summary data from another three. Meta-analysis according to baseline kidney function was performed. Pooled hazard ratios per 5 mm Hg lower blood pressure were estimated with a random effects model.

Results.—Compared with placebo, blood pressure lowering regimens reduced the risk of major cardiovascular events by about a sixth per 5 mm Hg reduction in systolic blood pressure in individuals with (hazard ratio 0.83, 95% confidence interval 0.76 to 0.90) and without reduced eGFR (0.83, 0.79 to 0.88), with no evidence for any difference in effect ($P = 1.00$ for homogeneity). The results were similar irrespective of whether blood pressure was reduced by regimens based on angiotensin converting enzyme inhibitors, calcium antagonists, or diuretics/β blockers. There was no evidence that the effects of different drug classes on major cardiovascular events varied between patients with different eGFR (all $P > 0.60$ for homogeneity).

Conclusions.—Blood pressure lowering is an effective strategy for preventing cardiovascular events among people with moderately reduced eGFR. There is little evidence from these overviews to support the preferential choice of particular drug classes for the prevention of cardiovascular events in chronic kidney disease.

▶ The Blood Pressure Lowering Treatment Trialists Collaboration[1] was created to conduct prospectively defined overviews of randomized trials to establish the effect of blood pressure-lowering agents on cardiovascular morbidity and mortality. This study evaluated 26 trials with 152 000 participants, including approximately 30 000 patients within estimated glomerular filtration rate (eGFR) of less than 60 mL/min/1.73 m^2. Individual data were available from 23 trials. This large, carefully controlled, meta-analysis looked at 6 prespecified outcomes. The main outcome was major cardiovascular events comprising stroke, coronary heart disease, heart failure, and cardiovascular death. Blood pressure treatment comparisons were also prespecified in the original protocol of the Trialists' Collaboration and included broad-controlled trials comparing active treatment groups with placebo groups. Separate overviews were done for various blood pressure regimens such as ACEi, calcium antagonist-based regimens, β blockers, and diuretics. In addition, the target range of blood pressure control (more intensive vs less intensive control), was also compared. The eGFR was estimated from standard formula, and proteinuria was based on the urine albumin excretion rate of greater than 300 mg/d or urinary protein dipstick of greater than +1.

This multistudy analysis based on more than 150 000 participants shows cardiovascular benefits of blood pressure control in patients with stage 1 through 3 chronic kidney disease (eGFR > 30 mL/min/1.73 m^2). This cardiovascular protection occurred regardless of the regimen used. One caveat is that few participants had documented proteinuria and, therefore, the data cannot be completely generalized to all classes of renal injury. However, the data strongly support the concept of blood-pressure lowering per se, rather than the particular class of drug used, is clearly associated with lower cardiovascular risk during the early stages of chronic kidney disease. Although these findings may not be readily generalized to patients with more advanced kidney disease or those with hypertension along with more significant proteinuria, they can help guide medication selection, especially in patients with early CKD who are at risk for cardiovascular disease.

R. Garrick, MD

Reference

1. Protocol for prospective collaborative overviews of major randomized trials of blood-pressure-lowering treatments. World Health Organization-International Society of Hypertension Blood Pressure Lowering Treatment Trialists' Collaboration. *J Hypertens.* 1998;16:127-137.

Warfarin, Kidney Dysfunction, and Outcomes Following Acute Myocardial Infarction in Patients With Atrial Fibrillation

Carrero JJ, Evans M, Szummer K, et al (Karolinska Institutet, Stockholm, Sweden; et al)

JAMA 311:919-928, 2014

Importance.—Conflicting evidence exists regarding the association between warfarin treatment, death, and ischemic stroke incidence in patients with advanced chronic kidney disease (CKD) and atrial fibrillation.

Objective.—To study outcomes associated with warfarin treatment in relation to kidney function among patients with established cardiovascular disease and atrial fibrillation.

Design, Setting, and Participants.—Observational, prospective, multicenter cohort study from the Swedish Web-System for Enhancement and Development of Evidence-Based Care in Heart Disease Evaluated According to Recommended Therapies (SWEDEHEART) registry (2003-2010), which includes all Swedish hospitals that provide care for acute cardiac diseases. Participants included consecutive survivors of an acute myocardial infarction (MI) with atrial fibrillation and known serum creatinine (N = 24 317), including 21.8% who were prescribed warfarin at discharge. Chronic kidney disease stages were classified according to estimated glomerular filtration rate (eGFR).

Main Outcomes and Measures.—(1) Composite end point analysis of death, readmission due to MI, or ischemic stroke; (2) bleeding (composite of readmission due to hemorrhagic stroke, gastrointestinal bleeding, bleeding causing anemia, and others); or (3) the aggregate of these 2 outcomes within 1 year from discharge date.

Results.—A total of 5292 patients (21.8%) were treated with warfarin at discharge, and 51.7%had manifest CKD (eGFR <60 mL/min/1.73 m^2 [$eGFR_{<60}$]). Compared with no warfarin use, warfarin was associated with a lower risk of the first composite outcome (n = 9002 events) in each CKD stratum for event rates per 100 person-years: $eGFR_{>60}$ event rate, 28.0 for warfarin vs 36.1 for no warfarin; adjusted hazard ratio (HR), 0.73 (95% CI, 0.65 to 0.81); $eGFR_{>30\text{-}60}$: event rate, 48.5 for warfarin vs 63.8 for no warfarin; HR, 0.73 (95% CI, 0.66 to 0.80); $eGFR_{>15\text{-}30}$: event rate, 84.3 for warfarin vs 110.1 for no warfarin; HR, 0.84 (95% CI, 0.70-1.02); $eGFR_{\leq 15}$: event rate, 83.2 for warfarin vs 128.3 for no warfarin; HR, 0.57 (95% CI, 0.37-0.86). The risk of bleeding (n = 1202 events) was not significantly higher in patients treated with warfarin in any CKD stratum for event rates per 100 person-years: $eGFR_{>60}$ event rate, 5.0 for warfarin vs 4.8 for no warfarin; HR, 1.10 (95% CI, 0.86-1.41); $eGFR_{>30\text{-}60}$ event rate, 6.8 for warfarin vs 6.3 for no warfarin; HR, 1.04 (95% CI, 0.81-1.33); $eGFR_{>15\text{-}30}$ event rate, 9.3 for warfarin vs 10.4 for no warfarin; HR, 0.82 (95% CI, 0.48-1.39); $eGFR_{\leq 15}$ event rate, 9.1 for warfarin vs 13.5 for no warfarin; HR, 0.52 (95% CI, 0.16-1.65). Warfarin use in each CKD stratum was associated with lower hazards of the aggregate outcome (n = 9592 events) for event rates per 100 person-years: $eGFR_{>60}$ event rate, 32.1 for warfarin vs 40.0 for no warfarin; HR, 0.76 (95% CI, 0.69-0.84); $eGFR_{>30\text{-}60}$ event rate, 53.6 for warfarin vs 69.0 for no warfarin; HR, 0.75 (95% CI, 0.68-0.82); $eGFR_{>15\text{-}30}$ event rate, 90.2 for warfarin vs 117.7 for no warfarin; HR, 0.82 (95% CI, 0.68-0.99); $eGFR_{\leq 15}$ event rate, 86.2 for warfarin vs 138.2 for no warfarin; HR, 0.55 (95% CI, 0.37-0.83).

Conclusions and Relevance.—Warfarin treatment was associated with a lower 1-year risk for the composite outcome of death, MI, and ischemic stroke without a higher risk of bleeding in consecutive acute MI patients with atrial fibrillation. This association was not related to the severity of concurrent CKD.

▶ Confusion in the decision tree regarding the use of warfarin in individuals with atrial fibrillation and underlying chronic kidney disease continues.[1-4] Patients with chronic kidney disease are at increased risk of stroke; however, they are also at increased risk of bleeding. The breakpoint for this dynamic paradigm has remained unclear. A large database study such as the Danish registry study found that in patients with chronic kidney disease, warfarin alone decreased the risk of stroke but increased the risk of bleeding. In contrast, aspirin increased the risk of bleeding without reducing the risk of stroke in this same population cohort.[5] That study classified patients as normal renal function, chronic kidney disease (CKD), and end-stage renal disease on dialysis and used diagnostic treatment codes to determine the presence of renal dysfunction. The current observational, prospective study by Carrero and colleagues may help tilt our decision in certain scenarios. Using the evidence-based SWEDEHEART registry, data were gathered on almost 5300 patients who suffered an acute myocardial infarction (MI), complicated by atrial fibrillation. The database included more than 5000 patients, almost 22% of which were treated with warfarin at discharge, and about 52% had chronic kidney disease (estimated glomerular filtration rate [eGFR] < 60 mL/min/1.73 m^2). Warfarin therapy was associated with a lower 1-year risk for the composite outcome of death, MI, or ischemic stroke, and, unlike the Danish study, the risk of bleeding was not statistically increased. Of interest was the finding that the risk of bleeding did not increase across the spectrum of CKD, and stroke protection was observed even among patients with eGFR of less than 30 mL/min. Two important details must be noted. The first is that International Normalized Ratio (INR) data are not available, and although the authors note INR control in Scandinavian countries tends to be very good[6]; nonetheless, the degree of anticoagulation remains uncertain. The second is that the numbers of patients with severe (eGFR < 15 mL/min/1.73 m^2), was quite small. Thus, without further data, we should be careful to avoid quickly generalizing these data to all populations with CKD. However, they can help guide therapy for patients with even fairly advanced CKD and atrial fibrillation associated with a myocardial infarction.

R. Garrick, MD

References

1. Chan KE, Lazarus JM, Thadhani R, Hakim RM. Anticoagulant and antiplatelet usage associates with mortality among hemodialysis patients. *J Am Soc Nephrol.* 2009;20:872-881.
2. Chan KE, Lazarus JM, Thadhani R, Hakim RM. Warfarin use associates with increased risk for stroke in hemodialysis patients with atrial fibrillation. *J Am Soc Nephrol.* 2009;20:2223-2233.
3. Winkelmayer WC, Liu J, Setoguchi S, Choudhry NK. Effectiveness and safety of warfarin initiation in older hemodialysis patients with incident atrial fibrillation. *Clin J Am Soc Nephrol.* 2011;6:2662-2668.
4. Olesen JB, Lip GY, Kamper AL, et al. Stroke and bleeding in atrial fibrillation with chronic kidney disease. *N Engl J Med.* 2012;367:625-635.
5. Herzog CA, Asinger RW, Berger AK, et al. Cardiovascular disease in chronic kidney disease. A clinical update from Kidney Disease: Improving Global Outcomes (KDIGO). *Kidney Int.* 2011;80:572-586.
6. Wieloch M, Sjalander A, Frykman V, Rosenqvist M, Eriksson N, Svensson PJ. Anticoagulation control in Sweden: reports of time in therapeutic range, major bleeding, and thrombo-embolic complications from the national quality registry AuriculA. *Eur Heart J.* 2011;32:2282-2289.

Patient-Reported and Actionable Safety Events in CKD

Ginsberg JS, Zhan M, Diamantidis CJ, et al (Univ of Maryland, Baltimore)
J Am Soc Nephrol 2014 [Epub ahead of print]

Patients with CKD are at high risk for adverse safety events because of the complexity of their care and impaired renal function. Using data from our observational study of predialysis patients with CKD enrolled in the Safe Kidney Care study, we estimated the baseline frequency of adverse safety events and determined to what extent these events co-occur. We examined patient-reported adverse safety incidents (class I) and actionable safety findings (class II), conditioned on participant use of drugs that might cause such an event, and we used association analysis as a data-mining technique to identify co-occurrences of these events. Of 267 participants, 185 (69.3%) had at least one class I or II event, 102 (38.2%) had more than one event, and 48 (18.0%) had at least one event from both classes. The adjusted conditional rates of class I and class II events ranged from 2.9 to 57.6 per 100 patients and from 2.2 to 8.3 per 100 patients, respectively. The most common conditional class I and II events were patient-reported hypoglycemia and hyperkalemia (serum potassium >5.5 mEq/L), respectively. Reporting of hypoglycemia (in patients with diabetes) and falling or severe dizziness (in patients without diabetes) were most frequently paired with other adverse safety events. We conclude that adverse safety events are common and varied in CKD, with frequent association between disparate events. Further work is needed to define the CKD "safety phenotype" and identify patients at highest risk for adverse safety events.

▶ Prior studies have established that the risk of medication events and errors is increased in patients with underlying chronic kidney disease.[1,2] The potential for direct patient harm and for exacerbation of underlying conditions, including worsening of renal function, is self-evident. To better estimate the baseline frequency of adverse safety events and to determine if particular risk factors increase the likelihood of such events, the authors evaluated patients with chronic kidney disease enrolled in the Safe Kidney Care study. Two categories of adverse safety events were evaluated. Patient-reported adverse safety incidences (class I) were determined from a baseline self-reported safety event questionnaire. As part of this questionnaire, patients reported whether they had experienced hypoglycemia or hyperkalemia requiring intervention during the prior 12 months. Class 2 events were defined as potentially hazardous abnormalities of baseline laboratory and vital sign parameters associated with concomitant treatment with a drug known to cause such disturbances. The investigators also examined which class 1 and class 2 events were associated with other events within and between the classes. This was done using the statistical process of association analysis to examine the interrelationship between various safety findings. The results, as shown in Fig 1 in the original article, indicate that both class I and class II events are common and that almost 40% of patients had more than one event.

The data analysis used, although complex, allows for some unique observations regarding the potential linking of safety events. For example, among diabetics, an episode of hypoglycemia was frequently paired with other adverse safety events. This is a very novel way of trying to tease out complex interrelationships among safety events and could lead to more precise interventions which, in turn, could reduce both risk and harm.

R. Garrick, MD

References

1. Seliger SL, Zhan M, Hsu VD, Walker LD, Fink JC. Chronic kidney disease adversely influences patient safety. *J Am Soc Nephrol.* 2008;19:2414-2419.
2. Chapin E, Zhan M, Hsu VD, Seliger SL, Walker LD, Fink JC. Adverse safety events in chronic kidney disease: The frequency of "multiple hits". *Clin J Am Soc Nephrol.* 2010;5:95-101.

29 Dialysis and Transplantation

IGF-1 and Survival in ESRD

Jia T, Gama Axelsson T, Heimbürger O, et al (Karolinska Institutet, Stockholm, Sweden)

Clin J Am Soc Nephrol 9:120-127, 2014

Background and Objectives.—IGF-1 deficiency links to malnutrition in CKD patients; however, it is not clear to what extent it associates with survival among these patients.

Design, Setting, Participants, & Measurements.—Serum IGF-1 and other biochemical, clinical (subjective global assessment), and densitometric (dual energy x-ray absorptiometry) markers of nutritional status and mineral and bone metabolism were measured in a cohort of 365 Swedish clinically stable CKD stage 5 patients (median age of 53 years) initiating dialysis between 1994 and 2009; in 207 patients, measurements were also taken after 1 year of dialysis. Deaths were registered during a median follow-up of 5 years. Associations of mortality with baseline IGF-1 and changes of IGF-1 after 1 year of dialysis were evaluated by Cox models.

Results.—At baseline, IGF-1 concentrations associated negatively with age, diabetes mellitus, cardiovascular disease, poor nutritional status, IL-6, and osteoprotegerin and positively with body fat mass, bone mineral density, serum phosphate, calcium, and fibroblast growth factor-23. At 1 year, IGF-1 had increased by 33%. In multivariate regression, low age, diabetes mellitus, and high serum phosphate and calcium associated with IGF-1 at baseline, and in a mixed model, these factors, together with high fat body mass, associated with changes of IGF-1 during the first 1 year of dialysis. Adjusting for calendar year of inclusion, age, sex, diabetes mellitus, cardiovascular disease, IL-6, and poor nutritional status, a 1 SD higher level of IGF-1 at baseline associated with lower mortality risk (hazard ratio, 0.57; 95%confidence interval, 0.32 to 0.98). Persistently low or decreasing IGF-1 levels during the first 1 year on dialysis predicted worse survival (adjusted hazard ratio, 2.19; 95% confidence interval, 1.06 to 4.50).

Conclusion.—In incident dialysis patients, low serum IGF-1 associates with body composition and markers of mineral and bone metabolism, and it predicts increased mortality risk.

▶ Protein energy wasting and malnutrition are of concern in patients with end-stage renal disease and have become the subject of intense study. A prior cross-sectional study[1] on prevalent hemodialysis patients found an inverse association between insulin-like growth factor 1 (IGF-I) levels and all cause mortality. The current study is a post-hoc analysis of cross-sectional and longitudinal follow-up data drawn from 365 incident patients with advanced chronic kidney disease (CKD) who were enrolled at the initiation of dialysis. In addition, a subgroup of patients had further samples collected 1 year after the initiation of dialysis.[2] Mortality was registered during a median follow-up of 5 years. As shown in Fig 2 of the original article, both baseline and decreasing levels of IGF-I are markers of increased risk of mortality in incident hemodialysis patients.

This is a novel finding and is especially significant because the IGF-I data were independent of pre-existing known risk factors such as age, cardiovascular disease, diabetes, inflammation, or known protein energy wasting. In addition, the IGF-I levels were stratified between hemodialysis (where it tracked with mortality) and peritoneal dialysis (where it did not), suggesting that these 2 dialysis modalities may have differential effects on either nutritional biomarkers or possibly clinically relevant nutritional outcomes. With regard to the biological mechanism behind this finding, IGF-I has linkages to protein metabolism, glucose and lipid metabolism, and bone growth, and of interest is that changes in IGF-I concentrations also were appropriately directionally associated with other metabolic factors such as interleukin-6 levels, diabetes, cardiovascular disease, and markers of bone metabolism including FGF-23 and osteoprotegerin. Observational data can never prove causality. However, these unique findings show that IGF-I levels associate with markers of body composition and bone and mineral metabolism and are a strong independent marker of mortality risk in patients with advanced kidney disease

R. Garrick, MD

References

1. Qureshi AR, Alvestrand A, Divino-Filho JC, et al. Inflammation, malnutrition, and cardiac disease as predictors of mortality in hemodialysis patients. *J Am Soc Nephrol.* 2002;13:S28-S36.
2. Stenvinkel P, Heimbürger O, Paultre F, et al. Strong association between malnutrition, inflammation, and atherosclerosis in chronic renal failure. *Kidney Int.* 1999; 55:1899-1911.

Clinical Predictors of Decline in Nutritional Parameters over Time in ESRD

den Hoedt CH, for the CONTRAST Investigators (Maasstad Hosp, Rotterdam, The Netherlands; et al)

Clin J Am Soc Nephrol 9:318-325, 2014

Background and Objectives.—Inflammation and malnutrition are important features in patients with ESRD; however, data on changes in these parameters over time are scarce. This study aimed to gain insight into changes over time in serum albumin, body mass index, high-sensitivity C-reactive protein, and IL-6 in patients with ESRD and aimed to identify clinical risk factors for deterioration of these parameters.

Design, Setting, Participants, & Measurements.—Data were analyzed from the Convective Transport Study, a randomized controlled trial conducted from June 2004 to January 2011, in which 714 patients with chronic ESRD were randomized to either online hemodiafiltration or low-flux hemodialysis. Albumin and body mass index were measured up to 6 years and predialysis C-reactive protein and IL-6 were measured up to 3 years in a subset of 405 participants. Rates of change in these parameters over time were estimated across strata of predefined risk factors with linear mixed-effects models.

Results.—Albumin and body mass index decreased and C-reactive protein and IL-6 increased over time. For every incremental year of age at baseline, the yearly excess decline in albumin was 0.003 g/dl (−0.004 to −0.002; $P < 0.001$) and the excess decline in body mass index was 0.02 kg/m^2 per year (−0.02 to −0.01; $P < 0.001$). In patients with diabetes mellitus, there was a yearly excess decline of 0.05 g/dl in albumin (−0.09 to −0.02; $P = 0.002$). Compared with women, men had an excess decline of 0.03 g/dl per year in albumin (−0.06 to −0.001; $P = 0.05$) and an excess increase of 11.6% per year in IL-6 (0.63%−23.6%; $P = 0.04$).

Conclusions.—Despite guideline-based care, all inflammatory and nutritional parameters worsened over time. The deterioration of some of these parameters was more pronounced in men, older patients, and patients with diabetes mellitus. Special focus on the nutritional status of at-risk patients by individualizing medical care might improve their prognosis.

▶ The mortality rate in patients with end-stage renal disease (ESRD) is considerably higher than that in the general population, and inflammation and nutritional status[1] are believed to be predictors of ESRD mortality. This study is unique because it provides longitudinal data regarding changes in nutritional biomarkers in ESRD patients. Patients were drawn from the Convective Transport Study (CONTRAST) and were followed up over a 7-year period using guideline-based care. This multinational trial evaluated the effects of different types of hemodialysis and found that the modality, per se, did not influence the rate of change in albumin and minimally affected various markers of inflammation (interleukin [IL]-6 and C-reactive protein). In the current subpopulation, the annual decline in albumin was 0.08 g/dL, and this varied inversely with the change in C-reactive protein and IL-6. The decline was greatest in patients older than 66 years and in diabetics and men. The decrease in body mass index was also higher in older patients and was more marked in those with cardiovascular disease. IL-6 and C-reactive protein, both increased over time, and their rate of change was similar and not influenced by age, diabetes, or underlying cardiovascular disease.

The results are noteworthy. They suggest that nutritional and inflammatory markers deteriorate over time in patients with ESRD despite the provision of what is currently believed to be adequate evidence-based dialysis care and nutritional support. This trend is more pronounced in older patients, in men, and in patients with underlying diabetes and cardiovascular disease.

One clear implication of their findings is that, at least with regard to nutritional parameters, adherence to current standard-of-care guidelines cannot be used as a surrogate marked for the prediction of improved clinical outcomes. Whether additional interventions, such as other lifestyle modifications, would alter these results will require additional study. The findings reinforce the need for prospective, controlled trials to determine the most efficacious treatments for patients with dialysis-dependent renal failure.

S. Shenoy, MD

Reference

1. Tripepi G, Mallamaci F, Zoccali C. Inflammation markers, adhesion molecules, and all-cause and cardiovascular mortality in patients with ESRD: Searching for the best risk marker by multivariate modeling. *J Am Soc Nephrol.* 2005;16:S83-S88.

Mortality Predictability of Body Size and Muscle Mass Surrogates in Asian vs White and African American Hemodialysis Patients

Park J, Jin DC, Molnar MZ, et al (Univ of California Irvine, Orange; et al)
Mayo Clin Proc 88:479-486, 2013

Objective.—To determine whether the association of body size and muscle mass with survival among patients undergoing long-term hemodialysis (HD) is consistent across race, especially in East Asian vs white and African American patients.

Patients and Methods.—Using data from 20,818 patients from South Korea who underwent HD from February 1, 2001, to June 30, 2009, and 20,000 matched patients from the United States (10,000 whites and 10,000 African Americans) who underwent HD from July 1, 2001, to June 30, 2006, we compared mortality associations of baseline body mass index (BMI) and serum creatinine level as likely surrogates of obesity and muscle mass across the 3 races.

Results.—In Korean HD patients, higher BMI together with higher serum creatinine levels were associated with greater survival, as previously reported from US and European studies. In the matched cohort (10,000 patients from each of the 3 races), mortality risks were lower across higher BMI and serum creatinine levels, and these associations were similar in all 3 races (reference groups: patients with BMI >25.0 kg/m^2 or serum creatinine >12 mg/dL in each race). White, African American, and Korean patients with BMI levels of 18.5 kg/m^2 or less (underweight) had 78%, 79%, and 57% higher mortality risk, respectively, and white, African American, and Korean patients with serum creatinine levels of 6.0 mg/dL or less had 108%, 87%, and 78% higher mortality, respectively.

Conclusion.—This study shows that race does not modify the association of higher body size and muscle mass with greater survival in HD patients. Given the consistency of the obesity paradox, which may be related to a mitigated effect of protein-energy wasting on mortality irrespective of racial disparities, nutritional support to improve survival should be tested in HD patients of all races.

▶ Prior studies have found that obesity (as measured by the body mass index [BMI]) may offer a survival advantage in patients undergoing dialysis for chronic kidney disease.[1,2] Similarly, increased serum creatinine level is believed to be a marker of muscle mass and has also been associated with improved outcomes. It has been thought likely that protein energy wasting (PEW), with a reduction of muscle and body mass contributes to this apparent paradox. Most of the data have been generated on whites and African-Americans. Park and colleagues extended these observations by studying matched nonconcurrent dialysis cohorts from the United States, (African-Americans and whites) and South Korea. As shown in Fig 2 of the original article, similar to African-Americans, white and Korean hemodialysis patients with high BMIs and serum creatinine levels had improved rates of survival compared with patients with BMI levels of less than 18.5 kg/m^2 or creatinine levels of ≤6 mg/dL. Thus, among hemodialysis patients, the improved survival associated with higher BMI and muscle mass is not modified by race. The study is a retrospective observational study and, therefore, data on other markers of muscle mass were unavailable, and control for confounding factors was limited. In addition, residual renal function was not measured and, if present, could have contributed to a lower serum creatinine. However, residual function would typically reduce mortality risk and, therefore, would have attenuated their findings. Although this retrospective study does have limitations, it is strengthened by its size and lends support to the concept that undernutrition and protein energy wasting may add to the mortality risk of end-stage renal disease.

R. Garrick, MD

References

1. Kalantar-Zadeh K, Streja E, Molnar MZ, et al. Mortality prediction by surrogates of body composition: an examination of the obesity paradox in hemodialysis patients using composite ranking score analysis. *Am J Epidemiol.* 2012;175: 793-803.
2. Kalantar-Zadeh K, Streja E, Kovesdy CP, et al. The obesity paradox and mortality associated with surrogates of body size and muscle mass in patients receiving hemodialysis. *Mayo Clin Proc.* 2010;85:991-1001.

A comparative effectiveness research study of the change in blood pressure during hemodialysis treatment and survival

Park J, Rhee CM, Sim JJ, et al (Univ of California Irvine, Orange; Kaiser Permanente Med Ctr, Los Angeles, CA; et al)
Kidney Int 84:795-802, 2013

It is not clear to what extent changes in blood pressure (BP) during hemodialysis affect or predict survival. Studying comparative outcomes of BP changes during hemodialysis can have major clinical implications including the impact on management strategies in hemodialysis patients. Here we undertook a retrospective cohort study of 113,255 hemodialysis patients over a 5-year period to evaluate an association between change in BP during hemodialysis and mortality. The change in BP was defined as post-hemodialysis minus pre-hemodialysis BP, and mean of BP change values during the hemodialysis session was used as a mortality predictor. The patients' average age was 61 years old and consisted of 45% women, 32% African-Americans and 58% diabetics. Over a median follow-up of 2.2 years, a total of 53,461 (47.2%) all-cause and 21,548 (25.7%) cardiovascular deaths occurred. In a fully adjusted Cox regression model with restricted cubic splines, there was a U-shaped association between change in systolic BP and all-cause mortality. Post-dialytic drops in systolic BP between −30 and 0 mm Hg were associated with greater survival, but large decreases of systolic BP (more than −30 mm Hg) and any increase in systolic BP (over 0 mm Hg) were related to increased mortality. Peak survival was found at a change in systolic BP of −14 mm Hg. The U-shaped association was also found for cardiovascular mortality. Thus, modest declines in BP after hemodialysis are associated with the greatest survival, whereas any rise or large decline in BP is associated with worsened survival.

► We elected to include this article because the continuum of care of blood pressure (B/P) management in dialysis patients involves multiple practitioners in numerous settings. Studies have shown that the peridialysis B/P is not a good indicator of overall ambulatory B/P control,[1] which by itself means that many practitioners aside from the nephrologist will be engaged in B/P monitoring in this population. Earlier studies have suggested that both intradialytic hypertension and hypotension (typically defined as a 30–40 mm drop in B/P during the dialysis, eg, incoming volume expanded B/P of 165 mm Hg and end B/P of 120 mm Hg meets this criteria) are both associated with adverse short- and long-term cardiovascular outcomes.[2-4] The topic is further complicated by the demonstration that intradialytic B/P variability is associated with an increase in mortality in long-term dialysis patients.[5] Park and colleagues sought to use a large dialysis database to better define the extent to which the delta-change in the pre- and post-B/P affects survival. This retrospective analysis of 113 255 patients was conducted over a 5-year period with a median follow-up of 2.2 years. The data suggest that any delta increase between pre- and postdialysis systolic B/P is associated with higher mortality. A fall in pre- vs postdialysis B/P of greater than 30 mm Hg systolic and 15 mm Hg diastolic was also associated with an increase in mortality. The greatest survival was seen in patients who had the smallest change in pre- and postdialysis systolic statistics and diastolic pressures (−14 mm Hg and −6 mm Hg, respectively).

The details of the dialysis treatments were not available, and as such, it is unknown as to whether the patients were symptomatic, received fluid support for hypotension, or if ultrafiltration rates changed during the treatment in response to changes in blood pressure. Also, no data are available regarding the dialysis sodium gradient, and most of the patients were fairly new to dialysis and therefore may not have had their dry weight or B/P regimens fully established. However, despite these limitations, the study gives us much to consider. Many interventions may help improve the blood pressure stability in this population. Improved dietary salt intake, improved fluid balance, different antihypertensive regimens (perhaps guided by patient-specific physiologic parameters), longer dialysis treatments, and changes in ultrafiltration rates and profiles may all contribute to B/P stability. For the nonnephrologists, a key point is to help patients understand the unique importance of B/P control in the setting of hemodialysis where patients are exposed to repetitive (typically thrice weekly) dialysis, placing them at risk for rapid changes in sodium, volume, and B/P that are not otherwise experienced by patients with normal renal function. In addition, practitioners should be guiding patients with regard to those variables (such as salt and fluid intake) that are within individuals' control.

R. Garrick, MD

References

1. Agarwal R, Peixoto AJ, Santos SF, Zoccali C. Pre- and postdialysis blood pressures are imprecise estimates of interdialytic ambulatory blood pressure. *Clin J Am Soc Nephrol.* 2006;1:389-398.
2. McIntyre CW. Recurrent circulatory stress: the dark side of dialysis. *Semin Dial.* 2010;23:449-451.
3. Chen J, Gul A, Sarnak MJ. Management of intradialytic hypertension: the ongoing challenge. *Semin Dial.* 2006;19:141-145.
4. Inrig JK, Oddone EZ, Hasselblad V, et al. Association of intradialytic blood pressure changes with hospitalization and mortality rates in prevalent ESRD patients. *Kidney Int.* 2007;71:454-461.
5. Flythe JE, Inrig JK, Shafi T, et al. Association of intradialytic blood pressure variability with increased all-cause and cardiovascular mortality in patients treated with long-term hemodialysis. *Am J Kidney Dis.* 2013;61:966-974.

Low 25-Hydroxyvitamin D Levels and Cognitive Impairment in Hemodialysis Patients

Shaffi K, Tighiouart H, Scott T, et al (Tufts Med Ctr, Boston, MA)
Clin J Am Soc Nephrol 8:979-986, 2013

Background and Objectives.—25-hydroxyvitamin D (25[OH]D) deficiency and cognitive impairment are both prevalent in hemodialysis patients in the United States. This study tested the hypothesis that 25(OH)D deficiency may be associated with cognitive impairment because of its vasculoprotective, neuroprotective, and immune-modulatory properties.

Design, Setting, Participants, & Measurements.—This cross-sectional analysis involved 255 patients enrolled in the Dialysis and Cognition Study between 2004 and 2012. In linear regression models, 25(OH)D was the exposure variable; it was used first as a continuous variable and then stratified as deficient (<12 ng/ml), insufficient (12 to <20 ng/ml), and sufficient (≥20 ng/ml). Principal component analysis was used to obtain the memory and the executive function domains from the individual neurocognitive tests. Scores on individual tests as well as on the memory and executive function domains were the outcome variables. Multivariable models were adjusted for age, sex, race, education, and other potential confounding variables.

Results.—Mean serum 25(OH)D ± SD was 17.2 ± 7.4 ng/ml, with 14%, 55%, and 31% of patients in the deficient, insufficient, and sufficient groups, respectively. Patients in the deficient group were more likely to be women, African American, and diabetic and to have longer dialysis vintage. Higher 25(OH)D levels were independently associated with better performance on several tests of executive function (mean difference on component executive score, 0.16 [95% confidence interval, 0.04–0.28; $P = 0.01$] for each SD higher 25[OH]D). No association was seen with tests assessing memory.

Conclusions.—25(OH)D deficiency in hemodialysis patients is associated with worse cognitive function, particularly in domains that assess executive function.

▶ Cognitive impairment can have far-reaching consequences in patients with renal disease. Besides hampering patients' abilities to make informed decisions, it can limit their ability to comprehend complex medical information, including medication instructions, and can ultimately lead to increased morbidity and mortality. Traditional risk factors in patients with renal disease such as age, hypertension, hyperlipidemia, coronary artery disease, and peripheral vascular disease increase the risk for cerebrovascular dementia.[1,2] Recently, nontraditional risk factors, including vitamin D deficiency, have generated increased interest. The active form of vitamin D, 1,25 dihydroxy vitamin D3, has been found to have antioxidant, neuroprotective, and vasculoprotective properties. Its precursor hormone, 25 (OH)2 vitamin D3 is frequently reduced (insufficient) or low (deficient) in dialysis patients. To further evaluate the possible contributory role of vitamin D among dialysis patients, Shaffi and colleagues performed a cross-sectional study on 255 patients between 2004 and 2012. Patients were categorized based on vitamin D levels and underwent a battery of well-validated neurocognitive tests to evaluated executive and memory functions. The tests used are all standardized and have established age-, sex-, and education-matched normative scores.

Dialysis patients with deficient and insufficient vitamin D levels were found to have statistically significant lower levels of executive function than were vitamin D-sufficient patients. No significant difference was noticed in memory domain of neurocognitive tests.

Understandably, observational cross-sectional studies cannot prove causality, and it is possible that the vitamin D-deficient patients were simply more ill and debilitated, which, in turn, influenced their neurovascular or executive function test results. That is a legitimate concern, but, may we still gain insight from these intriguing data? Active 1, 25 Di-hydroxy vitamin D3 increases the activity of genes that are found to affect neuronal cell differentiation. Within the nervous system, most activated vitamin D is generated in vivo by the neuronal cells, rather than entering across the blood-brain barrier. Thus, the availability of intracellular precursor 25 hydroxy vitamin D is believed pivotal for the neuronal production of activated hormone. The current findings confirm that vitamin D deficiency is ubiquitous among dialysis patients. The authors postulate that this deficiency may lead to a reduction in intracellular activated 1,25 dihydroxy vitamin D3, which, in turn, may alter neuronal cellular function. Clinically, these cellular changes are then manifested by a loss of executive function. The authors previously found that the most common cognitive dysfunction in dialysis patients is a loss of executive function[2,3] and these findings provide a possible mechanism for this observation. As is the case with the general population, it is unclear whether dietary vitamin D supplementation will alter these neuronal processes in dialysis patients. Nonetheless, the findings are quite interesting and certainly open new opportunities for well-designed clinical studies and potential novel therapeutic intervention.

P. Vohra, MD

References

1. Kurella Tamura M, Yaffe K. Dementia and cognitive impairment in ESRD: diagnostic and therapeutic strategies. *Kidney Int.* 2011;79:14-22.
2. Weiner DE, Scott TM, Giang LM, et al. Cardiovascular disease and cognitive function in maintenance hemodialysis patients. *Am J Kidney Dis.* 2011;58:773-781.
3. Pereira AA, Weiner DE, Scott T, et al. Subcortical cognitive impairment in dialysis patients. *Hemodial Int.* 2007;11:309-314.

Accidental Falls and Risk of Mortality among Older Adults on Chronic Peritoneal Dialysis

Farragher J, Chiu E, Ulutas O, et al (Univ Health Network, Toronto, Ontario, Canada; et al)
Clin J Am Soc Nephrol 2014 [Epub ahead of print]

Background and Objectives.—More than 40% of elderly hemodialysis patients experience one or more accidental falls within a 1-year period. Such falls are associated with higher mortality. The objectives of this study were to assess whether falls are also common in elderly patients established on peritoneal dialysis and evaluate if patients with falls have a higher risk of mortality than patients who do not experience a fall.

Design, Setting, Participants, & Measurements.—Using a prospective cohort study design, patients ages ≥65 years on chronic peritoneal dialysis from April 2002 to April 2003 at the University Health Network were recruited. Patients were followed biweekly, and falls occurring within the first 15 months were recorded. Outcome data were collected until death, study end (July 31, 2012), transplantation, or transfer to another dialysis center.

Results.—Seventy-four of seventy-six potential patients were recruited, assessed at baseline, and followed biweekly for falls; 40 of 74 (54%) peritoneal dialysis patients experienced 89 falls (adjusted mean fall rate, 1.7 falls per patient-year; 95% confidence interval, 1.0 to 2.7). Patients with falls were more likely to have had previous falls, be more recently initiated onto dialysis, be men, be older, and have higher comorbidity. Twenty-eight patients died during the follow-up period. After adjustment for known risk factors, each successive fall was associated with a 1.62-fold higher mortality (hazard ratio, 1.62; 95% confidence interval, 1.29 to 2.02; $P < 0.001$).

Conclusions.—Accidental falls are common in the peritoneal dialysis population and often go unrecognized. Falls were associated with higher mortality risk. Because fall interventions are effective in other populations, screening peritoneal dialysis patients for falls may be a simple measure of clinical importance.

▶ Falls in older adults (aged ≥ 65 years) are a significant cause of morbidity and account for approximately 2-fold higher risk of death (after adjustment for known mortality risk factors) than patients who do not fall.[1] It is known from the study by Desmet et al that elderly patient on hemodialysis have an even higher risk of accidental falls (1.2—1.6 per person-year in hemodialysis population).[2] This was attributed to multiple factors including aging, multiple comorbidities, polypharmacy, muscular dysfunction, and rapid shifts in volume status occurring as a direct result of ultrafiltration associated with hemodialysis treatments. However, little was known in patients on peritoneal dialysis (PD) where less adverse events related to hemodynamic alterations are reported.[2,3]

This study is among the first prospective studies to examine the significance of accidental falls and their association with mortality among elderly individuals maintained on PD. The study recruited 74 patients on PD aged 65 years or older. Patients were followed biweekly for falls. More than half of the study sample (40 of 74) had at least 1 fall during the 1-year fall observation. Patients with falls were statistically more likely to have reported a fall in the previous 1 year. They were also nonstatistically more likely to be older with higher comorbidities and recently started on dialysis compared with those who had not fallen. Fall rates were similar to the rates reported in HD populations but almost 2 times the rates observed in large cohort studies of community-dwelling elderly populations. However, no relationship between fall risk and blood pressure was seen. When data were adjusted for known predictors of mortality, the number of fall events remained a significant predictor of death (hazard ratio 1.62). Prospective design, high rate of recruitment, and a close biweekly follow-up are the major strengths of this study, but the design may also have accounted for some errors. The number of falls could be higher because there is an observed relationship of falls with higher mortality, and patients who had a fall more than 1 year earlier or after the study were falsely classified as nonfallers, which may have underestimated the true association between falls and mortality.

Nonetheless, the data showed again that falls are among the major factors related to higher morbidity and mortality in elderly chronic kidney disease patients on renal replacement therapy. Randomized trials have demonstrated the effectiveness of a multidisciplinary approach to falls in individuals who are not dialysis patients.[4] This approach includes a review of medication, strength and gait testing with targeted training, assessment of the home environment, and measuring visual acuity. These strategies are likely to be effective in dialysis patients as well and could help reduce the morbidity associated with falls in this vulnerable population.

S. Chugh, MD

References

1. Centers for Disease Control and Prevention, National Center for Injury Prevention and Control. Web-based Injury Statistics Query and Reporting System (WISQARS). http://www.cdc.gov/injury/wisqars/. Accessed May 23, 2014.
2. Cook WL, Tomlinson G, Donaldson M, et al. Falls and fall-related injuries in older dialysis patients. *Clin J Am Soc Nephrol.* 2006;1:1197-1204.
3. Desmet C, Beguin C, Swine C; Jadoul MUniversité Catholique de Louvain Collaborative Group. Falls in hemodialysis patients: prospective study of incidence, risk factors, and complications. *Am J Kidney Dis.* 2005;45:148-153.
4. Close J, Ellis M, Hooper R, Glucksman E, Jackson S, Swift C. Prevention of falls in the elderly trial (PROFET): a randomised controlled trial. *Lancet.* 1999;353: 93-97.

Comorbidity Burden and Perioperative Complications for Living Kidney Donors in the United States

Schold JD, Goldfarb DA, Buccini LD, et al (Cleveland Clinic, OH; Case Western Reserve Univ, Cleveland, OH; et al)

Clin J Am Soc Nephrol 8:1773-1782, 2013

Background and Objectives.—Since 1998, 35% of kidney transplants in the United States have been derived from living donors. Research suggests minimal long-term health consequences after donation, but comprehensive studies are limited. The primary objective was to evaluate trends in comorbidity burden and complications among living donors.

Design, Setting, Participants, & Measurements.—The National Inpatient Sample (NIS) was used to identify donors from 1998 to 2010 (n = 69,117). Comorbid conditions, complications, and length of stay during hospitalization were evaluated. Outcomes among cohorts undergoing appendectomies, cholecystectomies and nephrectomy for nonmetastatic carcinoma were compared, and sample characteristics were validated with the Scientific Registry of Transplant Recipients (SRTR). Survey regression models were used to identify risk factors for outcomes.

Results.—The NIS captured 89% (69,117 of 77,702) of living donors in the United States. Donor characteristics were relatively concordant with those noted in SRTR (mean age, 40.1 versus 40.3 years [$P = 0.18$]; female donors, 59.0% versus 59.1% [$P = 0.13$]; white donors, 68.4% versus 69.8% [$P < 0.001$] for NIS versus SRTR). Incidence of perioperative complications was 7.9% and decreased from 1998 to 2010 (from 10.1% to 7.6%). Men (adjusted odds ratio [AOR], 1.37; 95% confidence interval [CI], 1.20 to 1.56) and donors with hypertension (AOR, 3.35; 95% CI, 2.24 to 5.01) were more likely to have perioperative complications. Median length of stay declined over time (from 3.7 days to 2.5 days), with longer length of stay associated with obesity, depression, hypertension, and pulmonary disorders. Presence of depression (AOR, 1.08;

95% CI, 1.04 to 1.12), hypothyroidism (AOR, 1.07; 95% CI, 1.04 to 1.11), hypertension (AOR, 1.38; 95% CI, 1.27 to 1.49), and obesity (AOR, 1.07; 95% CI, 1.03 to 1.11) increased over time. Complication rates and length of stay were similar for patients undergoing appendectomies and cholecystectomies but were less than those with nephrectomies for carcinoma.

Conclusions.—The NIS is a representative sample of living donors. Complications and length of stay after donation have declined over time, while presence of documented comorbid conditions has increased. Patients undergoing appendectomy and cholecystectomy have similar outcomes during hospitalization. Monitoring the health of living donors remains critically important.

▶ Living kidney donors provide a vital source of organs for those seeking to escape the burdens of dialysis. It is the physician's ethical responsibility to provide adequate information regarding the true risks of this procedure as part of the informed consent process. Long-term studies have suggested that there may be higher relative risks of hypertension, proteinuria, and maybe even end-stage renal disease[1,2] and mortality[3] after donation. However, the short-term surgical risks have not been well examined.

Schold et al set out to compare these surgical risks of kidney donation with the risks of other common abdominal surgeries. They used the National Inpatient Sample 3 to identify 69 117 donors over 12 years starting in 1998. They found that the incidence of perioperative complications was overall 7.9%, which incidentally showed steady improvement over the surveyed period. Subgroup evaluation found that men and those with hypertension were in a higher risk group for complications, as were African Americans and donors with no private pay insurance. Of note, the presence of preoperative donor hypertension as well as depression and hypothyroidism has increased steadily during the studied period. The types of complications varied, with the highest proportion being gastrointestinal (32%) and the lowest being cardiac (4%).

The investigators compared the short-term risks of donor nephrectomy, as well as length of stay (LOS), with the risks of other abdominal surgeries; specifically, cholecystectomy, appendectomy, and nephrectomy for carcinoma. All the procedures were associated with similar risk and LOS except nephrectomy for carcinoma, which had markedly higher complication rates and increased LOS. Over the study period, donor nephrectomy had the most pronounced improvement in risk profile, declining approximately 45% per year compared with around 18% to 25% for the other procedures. The mortality rate finding of 0.17% of living donors is high compared with that of prior studies and may represent errors in reliance on ICD9 coding for classification.

This study suggests that living donation presents similar short-term risks as cholecystectomy and appendectomy and that these risks have steadily improved over time. This study provides another meaningful piece of data that may help guide the process of informed consent in kidney donation.

M. Klein, MD, JD

References

1. Mjøen G, Hallan S, Hartmann A, et al. Long-term risks for kidney donors. *Kidney Int.* 2013 [Epub ahead of print].
2. Muzaale AD, Massie AB, Wang MC, et al. Risk of end-stage renal disease following live kidney donation. *JAMA.* 2014;311:579-586.
3. Healthcare Cost and Utilization Project. http://www.hcup-us.ahrq.gov/nisoverview.jsp. Accessed May 29, 2014.

Long-term risks for kidney donors

Mjøen G, Hallan S, Hartmann A, et al (Oslo Univ Hosp, Norway; St Olav Univ Hosp, Trondheim, Norway; et al)
Kidney Int 86:162-167, 2014

Previous studies have suggested that living kidney donors maintain long-term renal function and experience no increase in cardiovascular or all-cause mortality. However, most analyses have included control groups less healthy than the living donor population and have had relatively short follow-up periods. Here we compared long-term renal function and cardiovascular and all-cause mortality in living kidney donors compared with a control group of individuals who would have been eligible for donation. All-cause mortality, cardiovascular mortality, and end-stage renal disease (ESRD) was identified in 1901 individuals who donated a kidney during 1963 through 2007 with a median follow-up of 15.1 years. A control group of 32,621 potentially eligible kidney donors was selected, with a median follow-up of 24.9 years. Hazard ratio for all-cause death was significantly increased to 1.30 (95% confidence interval 1.11–1.52) for donors compared with controls. There was a significant corresponding increase in cardiovascular death to 1.40 (1.03–1.91), while the risk of ESRD was greatly and significantly increased to 11.38 (4.37–29.6). The overall incidence of ESRD among donors was 302 cases per million and might have been influenced by hereditary factors. Immunological renal disease was the cause of ESRD in the donors. Thus, kidney donors are at increased long-term risk for ESRD, cardiovascular, and all-cause mortality compared with a control group of non-donors who would have been eligible for donation.

▶ Living kidney donation requires major elective surgery, which subjects the voluntary donor to surgical hazards as well as to long-term clinical risks. Prior studies have been imperfect due to inadequate follow-up periods and poorly selected control groups. It behooves us as physicians to define more accurately the true long-term risks of elective kidney donation to more accurately counsel potential donors.

It is well accepted that unilateral nephrectomy in otherwise healthy individuals confers a increased risk of hypertension[1] and proteinuria[2] over the lifetime of the donor. Nevertheless, studies have not demonstrated that these risks significantly increase cardiovascular nor all-cause mortality. Mjoen et al present a sobering study, which demonstrates that if the follow-up is long enough and the control group is selected appropriately, a definite increased risk for mortality and end-stage renal disease (ESRD) in the donors can be detected.

They identified roughly 1900 kidney donors followed for a median of 15 years and compared them to nearly 33 000 healthy nondonor control subjects culled from the HUNT population survey[3] followed for a median of 25 years. Initially both groups had similar hazard ratios for mortality and ESRD, but after 10 years, they found an increased hazard ratio 1.48 for all-cause mortality, 1.5 for cardiovascular mortality, and 11.42 for development of ESRD. Although the absolute risk remained low at only 302 cases per million of ESRD compared with the risk in the unselected Norwegian population of 100 cases per million, the relative risk was increased more than 11-fold. For the absolute risks of all-cause and cardiovascular mortality, the differences were significant, although less dramatic between the 2 groups.

This study is well done. It included a control group of healthy individuals rather than the less healthy general population, a comparison that plagued prior studies and may have obscured otherwise prominent increased hazard ratios. In addition, the follow-up in this study was extremely long and well documented. Unfortunately, it was conducted at a single center, and all donors were Caucasian, confounding the generalization of these findings.

Nevertheless, this study may help interested donors make educated decisions regarding the risks to their own health. Despite the negative implications to the donors, this study should not significantly deter voluntary donation. A donor who is willing to accept a known surgical risk for the sake of a loved one would likely not be overly concerned about these small absolute risks in a remote future. Nonetheless, informed consent for donation should certainly include a discussion of these important data.

M. Klein, MD, JD

References

1. Boudville N, Prasad GV, Knoll G, et al. Donor Nephrectomy Outcomes Research (DONOR) Network. Meta-analysis: risk for hypertension in living kidney donors. *Ann Intern Med.* 2006;145:185-196.
2. Garg AX, Muirhead N, Knoll G, et al. Donor Nephrectomy Outcomes Research (DONOR) Network. Proteinuria and reduced kidney function in living kidney donors: a systematic review, meta-analysis, and meta-regression. *Kidney Int.* 2006;70:1801-1810.
3. Krokstad S, Langhammer A, Hveem K, et al. Cohort Profile: the HUNT Study, Norway. *Int J Epidemiol.* 2013;42:968-977.

30 Diabetes

Combined Angiotensin Inhibition for the Treatment of Diabetic Nephropathy

Fried LF, for the VA NEPHRON-D Investigators (Veterans Affairs (VA) Pittsburgh Healthcare System and Univ of Pittsburgh School of Medicine, PA; et al)

N Engl J Med 369:1892-1903, 2013

Background.—Combination therapy with angiotensin-converting–enzyme (ACE) inhibitors and angiotensin-receptor blockers (ARBs) decreases proteinuria; however, its safety and effect on the progression of kidney disease are uncertain.

Methods.—We provided losartan (at a dose of 100 mg per day) to patients with type 2 diabetes, a urinary albumin-to-creatinine ratio (with albumin measured in milligrams and creatinine measured in grams) of at least 300, and an estimated glomerular filtration rate (GFR) of 30.0 to 89.9 ml per minute per 1.73 m^2 of body-surface area and then randomly assigned them to receive lisinopril (at a dose of 10 to 40 mg per day) or placebo. The primary end point was the first occurrence of a change in the estimated GFR (a decline of ≥30 ml per minute per 1.73 m^2 if the initial estimated GFR was ≥60 ml per minute per 1.73 m^2 or a decline of ≥50% if the initial estimated GFR was <60 ml per minute per 1.73 m^2), end-stage renal disease (ESRD), or death. The secondary renal end point was the first occurrence of a decline in the estimated GFR or ESRD. Safety outcomes included mortality, hyperkalemia, and acute kidney injury.

Results.—The study was stopped early owing to safety concerns. Among 1448 randomly assigned patients with a median follow-up of 2.2 years, there were 152 primary end-point events in the monotherapy group and 132 in the combination-therapy group (hazard ratio with combination therapy, 0.88; 95% confidence interval [CI], 0.70 to 1.12; $P = 0.30$). A trend toward a benefit from combination therapy with respect to the secondary end point (hazard ratio, 0.78; 95% CI, 0.58 to 1.05; $P = 0.10$) decreased with time ($P = 0.02$ for nonproportionality). There was no benefit with respect to mortality (hazard ratio for death, 1.04; 95% CI, 0.73 to 1.49; $P = 0.75$) or cardiovascular events. Combination therapy increased the risk of hyperkalemia (6.3 events per 100 person-years, vs. 2.6 events per 100 person-years with monotherapy; $P < 0.001$) and acute kidney injury (12.2 vs. 6.7 events per 100 person-years, $P < 0.001$).

Conclusions.—Combination therapy with an ACE inhibitor and an ARB was associated with an increased risk of adverse events among patients with diabetic nephropathy. (Funded by the Cooperative Studies Program of the Department of Veterans Affairs Office of Research and Development; VA NEPHRON-D ClinicalTrials.gov number, NCT00555217.)

▶ Nephropathy leading to kidney insufficiency requiring dialysis is an often-observed complication of diabetes. To ameliorate this complication is a desirable goal. Proteinuria and the reduction of the glomerular filtration rate (GFR) are symptoms of nephropathy in which the degree of reduction in proteinuria correlates with the extent to which the decrease in GFR is slowed. Both blockers of the renin-angiotensin system, inhibitors of the angiotensin-converting enzyme (ACE inhibitors) and angiotensin-II-receptor blockers (ARBs), reduce proteinuria, and their combination results in a greater decrease in proteinuria than monotherapy with either an ACE inhibitor or ARB alone. The present study investigates whether the combination of an ACE inhibitor with ARB is more effective in slowing the progression of proteinuric diabetic nephropathy than therapy with an ACE inhibitor alone and whether this combination therapy is safe. This trial was stopped because of safety concerns, with acute kidney injury being the main serious adverse event. Hence the promise of the combination of 2 blockers of the renin-angiotensin system to effectively prevent end-stage renal disease in patients with proteinuric diabetic nephropathy was not fulfilled.

E. Oetjen, MD

Saxagliptin and Cardiovascular Outcomes in Patients with Type 2 Diabetes Mellitus

Scirica BM, for the SAVOR-TIMI 53 Steering Committee and Investigators (Brigham and Women's Hosp, Boston, MA; et al)
N Engl J Med 369:1317-1326, 2013

Background.—The cardiovascular safety and efficacy of many current antihyperglycemic agents, including saxagliptin, a dipeptidyl peptidase 4 (DPP-4) inhibitor, are unclear.

Methods.—We randomly assigned 16,492 patients with type 2 diabetes who had a history of, or were at risk for, cardiovascular events to receive saxagliptin or placebo and followed them for a median of 2.1 years. Physicians were permitted to adjust other medications, including antihyperglycemic agents. The primary end point was a composite of cardiovascular death, myocardial infarction, or ischemic stroke.

Results.—A primary end-point event occurred in 613 patients in the saxagliptin group and in 609 patients in the placebo group (7.3% and 7.2%, respectively, according to 2-year Kaplan–Meier estimates; hazard ratio with saxagliptin, 1.00; 95% confidence interval [CI], 0.89 to 1.12; $P = 0.99$ for superiority; $P < 0.001$ for noninferiority); the results were similar in the "on-treatment" analysis (hazard ratio, 1.03; 95% CI, 0.91 to 1.17). The major secondary end point of a composite of cardiovascular death, myocardial infarction, stroke, hospitalization for unstable angina, coronary revascularization, or heart failure occurred in 1059 patients in the saxagliptin group and in 1034 patients in the placebo group (12.8% and 12.4%, respectively, according to 2-year Kaplan–Meier estimates; hazard ratio, 1.02; 95% CI, 0.94 to 1.11; $P = 0.66$). More patients in the saxagliptin group than in the placebo group were hospitalized for heart failure (3.5% vs. 2.8%; hazard ratio, 1.27; 95% CI, 1.07 to 1.51; $P = 0.007$). Rates of adjudicated cases of acute and chronic pancreatitis were similar in the two groups (acute pancreatitis, 0.3% in the saxagliptin group and 0.2% in the placebo group; chronic pancreatitis, <0.1% and 0.1% in the two groups, respectively).

Conclusions.—DPP-4 inhibition with saxagliptin did not increase or decrease the rate of ischemic events, though the rate of hospitalization for heart failure was increased. Although saxagliptin improves glycemic control, other approaches are necessary to reduce cardiovascular risk in patients with diabetes. (Funded by AstraZeneca and Bristol-Myers Squibb; SAVOR-TIMI 53 ClinicalTrials.gov number, NCT01107886.)

▶ Since 2008, the Food and Drug Administration and the European Medicines Agency require a demonstration of cardiovascular safety for all new glucose-lowering therapies for their approval processes. In phase 2 and 3 studies, the dipeptidyl peptidase IV inhibitor saxagliptin improved glycemic control and reduced the risk of major cardiovascular events (Frederich R, Alexander JH, Fiedorek, 2010), but long-term data on the safety and efficacy of this drug in diabetic patients at risk for cardiovascular were still missing. In the present study, saxagliptin did not protect against cardiovascular events but increased the risk of hospitalization for heart failure and the risk of hypoglycemic events. These findings are disappointing, but in comparison to the UK Prospective Diabetes Study, the follow-up with a median of 2.1 years was rather short. Of note, cases of chronic or acute pancreatitis were similar in the saxagliptin and placebo groups.

E. Oetjen, MD

Linagliptin for patients aged 70 years or older with type 2 diabetes inadequately controlled with common antidiabetes treatments: a randomised, double-blind, placebo-controlled trial

Barnett AH, Huisman H, Jones R, et al (Heart of England NHS Foundation Trust, Birmingham, UK; Boehringer Ingelheim, Alkmaar, Netherlands; Boehringer Ingelheim, Bracknell, UK; et al)

Lancet 382:1413-1423, 2013

Background.—A substantial proportion of patients with type 2 diabetes are elderly (≥65 years) but this group has been largely excluded from clinical studies of glucose-lowering drugs. We aimed to assess the effectiveness of linagliptin, a dipeptidyl peptidase-4 inhibitor, in elderly patients with type 2 diabetes.

Methods.—In this randomised, double-blind, parallel-group, multinational phase 3 study, patients aged 70 years or older with type 2 diabetes, glycated haemoglobin A_{1c} (HbA_{1c}) of 7·0% or more, receiving metformin, sulfonylureas, or basal insulin, or combinations of these drugs, were randomised (by computer-generated randomisation sequence, concealed with a voice–response system, stratified by HbA_{1c} level [<8·5% *vs* ≥8·5%] and insulin use [yes *vs* no], block size four) in a 2:1 ratio to once-daily oral treatment with linagliptin 5 mg or matching placebo for 24 weeks. Investigators and participants were masked to assignment throughout the study. The primary endpoint was change in HbA_{1c} from baseline to week 24. This trial is registered with ClinicalTrials.gov, number NCT01084005.

Findings.—241 community-living outpatients were randomised (162 linagliptin, 79 placebo). Mean age was 74·9 years (SD 4·3). Mean HbA_{1c} was 7·8% (SD 0·8). At week 24, placebo-adjusted mean change in HbA_{1c} with linagliptin was −0·64% (95% CI −0·81 to −0·48, $p < 0{\cdot}0001$). Overall safety and tolerability were much the same between the linagliptin and placebo groups; 75·9% of patients in both groups had an adverse event (linagliptin n = 123, placebo n = 60). No deaths occurred. Serious adverse events occurred in 8·6% (14) of patients in the linagliptin group and 6·3% (five) patients in the placebo group; none were deemed related to study drug. Hypoglycaemia was the most common adverse event in both groups, but did not differ between groups (24·1% [39] in the linagliptin group, 16·5% [13] in the placebo group; odds ratio 1·58, 95% CI 0·78–3·78, $p = 0{\cdot}2083$).

Interpretation.—In elderly patients with type 2 diabetes linagliptin was efficacious in lowering glucose with a safety profile similar to placebo. These findings could inform treatment decisions for achieving individualised glycaemic goals with minimal risk in this important population of patients.

▶ Because of improved medical care, individuals with type 2 diabetes become older than ever. With increasing age, β-cell function further declines, which might result in inadequately controlled diabetes despite antidiabetic therapy. Elderly people have declined renal function, thereby prolonging the elimination of drugs or even aggravating adverse drug effects. However, in most clinical studies, people aged older than 65 years are excluded. The present study was specifically designed to investigate whether the dipeptidyl peptidase (DPP) IV inhibitor linagliptin was efficient in lowering blood glucose levels as an add on to existing antidiabetic therapy without causing undesired effects. To date, linagliptin is the only DPP IV inhibitor that is eliminated by the kidney only to a very small extent, making it suitable for use in elderly and in patients with impaired renal function without dose adjustment. The results of this study suggest that linagliptin, because of its favorable pharmacokinetic, could be used in elderly patients as well without increasing the risk of adverse drug effects.

E. Oetjen, MD

A small-molecule AdipoR agonist for type 2 diabetes and short life in obesity

Okada-Iwabu M, Yamauchi T, Iwabu M, et al (The Univ of Tokyo, Japan; et al)
Nature 503:493-499, 2013

Adiponectin secreted from adipocytes binds to adiponectin receptors AdipoR1 and AdipoR2, and exerts antidiabetic effects via activation of AMPK and PPAR-α pathways, respectively. Levels of adiponectin in plasma are reduced in obesity, which causes insulin resistance and type 2 diabetes. Thus, orally active small molecules that bind to and activate AdipoR1 and AdipoR2 could ameliorate obesity-related diseases such as type 2 diabetes. Here we report the identification of orally active synthetic small-molecule AdipoR agonists. One of these compounds, AdipoR agonist (AdipoRon), bound to both AdipoR1 and AdipoR2 *in vitro*. AdipoRon showed very similar effects to adiponectin in muscle and liver, such as activation of AMPK and PPAR-α pathways, and ameliorated insulin resistance and glucose intolerance in mice fed a high-fat diet, which was completely obliterated in AdipoR1 and AdipoR2 double-knockout mice. Moreover, AdipoRon ameliorated diabetes of genetically obese rodent model *db/db* mice, and prolonged the shortened lifespan of *db/db* mice on a high-fat diet. Thus, orally active AdipoR agonists such as AdipoRon are a promising therapeutic approach for the treatment of obesity-related diseases such as type 2 diabetes.

▶ Since the detection of adipose tissue as an endocrine-active organ, the function of the cytokines secreted from adipose tissue (ie, adipokines) has received much attention. With the finding that, by attenuating insulin resistance and glucose intolerance in mice, adiponectin exerts antidiabetic effects and that plasma adiponectin levels are reduced in obesity, insulin resistance, and type 2 diabetes, promoting adiponectin action has become a novel goal in the treatment of type 2 diabetes. This study by Okada-Iwabu et al addresses this goal. These authors have already described 2 adiponectin receptors that have slightly different functions and signal via activation of AMPK and peroxisome proliferator—activated receptor-α. They now describe 2 dual agonists for both adiponectin receptors. In an elegant experiment using mice deficient in these receptors, the authors confirm that these small molecules indeed act by binding to the adiponectin receptors. Thus, the panel of a potential novel antidiabetic is expanded by these agonists of the adiponectin receptors.

E. Oetjen, MD

Achievement of Goals in U.S. Diabetes Care, 1999–2010

Ali MK, Bullard KM, Saaddine JB, et al (Emory Univ, Atlanta, GA; et al)
N Engl J Med 368:1613-1624, 2013

Background.—Tracking national progress in diabetes care may aid in the evaluation of past efforts and identify residual gaps in care.

Methods.—We analyzed data for adults with self-reported diabetes from the National Health and Nutrition Examination Survey and the Behavioral Risk Factor Surveillance System to examine risk-factor control, preventive practices, and risk scores for coronary heart disease over the 1999–2010 period.

Results.—From 1999 through 2010, the weighted proportion of survey participants who met recommended goals for diabetes care increased, by 7.9 percentage points (95% confidence interval [CI], 0.8 to 15.0) for glycemic control (glycated hemoglobin level <7.0%), 9.4 percentage points (95% CI, 3.0 to 15.8) for individualized glycemic targets, 11.7 percentage points (95% CI, 5.7 to 17.7) for blood pressure (target, <130/80 mm Hg), and 20.8 percentage points (95% CI, 11.6 to 30.0) for lipid levels (target level of low-density lipoprotein [LDL] cholesterol, <100 mg per deciliter [2.6 mmol per liter]). Tobacco use did not change significantly, but the 10-year probability of coronary heart disease decreased by 2.8 to 3.7 percentage points. However, 33.4 to 48.7% of persons with diabetes still did not meet the targets for glycemic control, blood pressure, or LDL cholesterol level. Only 14.3% met the targets for all three of these measures and for tobacco use. Adherence to the recommendations for annual eye and dental examinations was unchanged, but annual lipid-level measurement and foot examination increased by 5.5 percentage points (95% CI, 1.6 to 9.4) and 6.8 percentage points (95% CI, 4.8 to 8.8), respectively. Annual vaccination for influenza and receipt of pneumococcal vaccination for participants 65 years of age or older rose by 4.5 percentage points (95% CI, 0.8 to 8.2) and 6.9 percentage points (95% CI, 3.4 to 10.4), respectively, and daily glucose monitoring increased by 12.7 percentage points (95% CI, 10.3 to 15.1).

Conclusions.—Although there were improvements in risk-factor control and adherence to preventive practices from 1999 to 2010, tobacco use remained high, and almost half of U.S. adults with diabetes did not meet the recommended goals for diabetes care.

▶ Obesity and diabetes are among the diseases showing the greatest increase worldwide and are reaching close to epidemic dimensions. Thus, the search for new antidiabetic therapies and efforts to improve antidiabetic therapy are important areas of research. The question remains of whether the goal of improved diabetes care is being achieved. These authors from the United States investigated this concern in a retrospective study, and the results are not encouraging. Despite a slight reduction in the 10-year probability of coronary heart disease, almost half of the adults with self-reported diabetes do not meet the recommended goals for diabetes care. Particularly, tobacco use remains high, and improvement of glycemic control (measured as HbA1c) is low. This study highlights the importance of diabetes care, putting the individual with diabetes into focus, and argues for improved individual diabetes care, control, and education.

E. Oetjen, MD

PART FIVE

PULMONARY DISEASE

JAMES A. BARKER, MD

Introduction

I continue to be amazed at the continued growth and enhancement of knowledge in Medicine and particularly in our field. Each year, we find new and exciting insights. Dr Sandra K. Willsie has provided two definitive articles on bronchial thermoplasty for asthma. The procedure works and is safe. But don't take my word for it; read the abstract and her thoughtful comments. Likewise, read the article by Amelink et al, "Severe adult-onset asthma: a distinct phenotype." They make a compelling argument that these asthmatics are different from those with mild to moderate manifestations. Many of us have thought this to be the case for years, but now there is evidence.

Dr Janet R. Mauer brings to light many new ideas and insights into COPD. For example, we know that COPD is actually an inflammatory disease and that cardiovascular mortality is increased in those with COPD. She has included articles that shed further light on these connections. The COPD Surveilllance data is also highly useful. Did you know that respiratory cause and specifically COPD cause admissions are decreasing this past decade? Three unique therapies are also discussed: macrolides, N-acetylcysteine, and statins. Each has promise, but also some pitfall. This is exciting!

Dr Lynn Tanoue has clearly outlined the new information and controversies in lung cancer. Current survival for all comers with new diagnosis of lung cancer is still horribly low at 16%. The death rate from lung cancer in women is beginning to drop for the first time, although lung cancer remains above breast cancer as mortality cause. She also points out the new development of the ACCP guidelines for lung cancer, so now we (pulmonologists and internists) have a single source to go to for up-to-date information on this important and devastating disease. Finally, the USPSTF guidelines have come out. Will all smokers or former smokers between ages 55 and 80 now be screened? Can we afford it? CMS is debating the issues as this goes to print.

Dr Christopher Spradley has again found some new and fascinating articles on interstitial lung disease, pleural diseases, and pulmonary hypertension. There is new molecular evidence to identify those with high risk and poor prognosis for IPF, for example. Did you know that the interstitial lung disease associated with collagen vascular disease was very treatable in comparison to idiopathic pulmonary fibrosis? See the enclosed articles and comments. I have been waiting years for an article on pleural plaques and Mesothelioma risk. Now we have one, and the findings are very helpful. Dr Maurer has also found some new and exciting articles on community-acquired pneumonia and on lung transplantation. For example, I always wanted to know what happens to those who are transplanted after lung volume reduction surgery. Now we can know!

Each year Dr Shirley Jones finds new and exciting articles on sleep disorders to share with us. This one is no exception. Dr Jones has included an important and definitive article on Servo ventilation vs Bipap for Complex Apnea. There are also some highly useful articles on ways to improve adherence to CPAP. Finally, there is a Critical Care section by Dr Jim Barker. This field continues to grow and expand. I have included some interesting articles and some seminal articles. Be sure to read about the latest in ECMO, and also be sure to read the latest on sepsis and septic shock from Dr Derek Angus and co-workers.

James A. Barker, MD, CPE, FACP, FCCP, FAASM

31 Asthma, Allergy, and Cystic Fibrosis

Bronchial thermoplasty: Long-term safety and effectiveness in patients with severe persistent asthma

Wechsler ME, for the Asthma Intervention Research 2 Trial Study Group (Natl Jewish Health, Denver, CO; et al)

J Allergy Clin Immunol 132:1295-1302.e3, 2013

Background.—Bronchial thermoplasty (BT) has previously been shown to improve asthma control out to 2 years in patients with severe persistent asthma.

Objective.—We sought to assess the effectiveness and safety of BT in asthmatic patients 5 years after therapy.

Methods.—BT-treated subjects from the Asthma Intervention Research 2 trial (ClinicalTrials.gov NCT01350414) were evaluated annually for 5 years to assess the long-term safety of BT and the durability of its treatment effect. Outcomes assessed after BT included severe exacerbations, adverse events, health care use, spirometric data, and high-resolution computed tomographic scans.

Results.—One hundred sixty-two (85.3%) of 190 BT-treated subjects from the Asthma Intervention Research 2 trial completed 5 years of follow-up. The proportion of subjects experiencing severe exacerbations and emergency department (ED) visits and the rates of events in each of years 1 to 5 remained low and were less than those observed in the 12 months before BT treatment (average 5-year reduction in proportions: 44% for exacerbations and 78% for ED visits). Respiratory adverse events and respiratory-related hospitalizations remained unchanged in years 2 through 5 compared with the first year after BT. Prebronchodilator FEV_1 values remained stable between years 1 and 5 after BT, despite a 18% reduction in average daily inhaled corticosteroid dose. High-resolution computed tomographic scans from baseline to 5 years after BT showed no structural abnormalities that could be attributed to BT.

Conclusions.—These data demonstrate the 5-year durability of the benefits of BT with regard to both asthma control (based on maintained reduction in severe exacerbations and ED visits for respiratory symptoms) and safety. BT has become an important addition to our treatment armamentarium and should be considered for patients with severe persistent

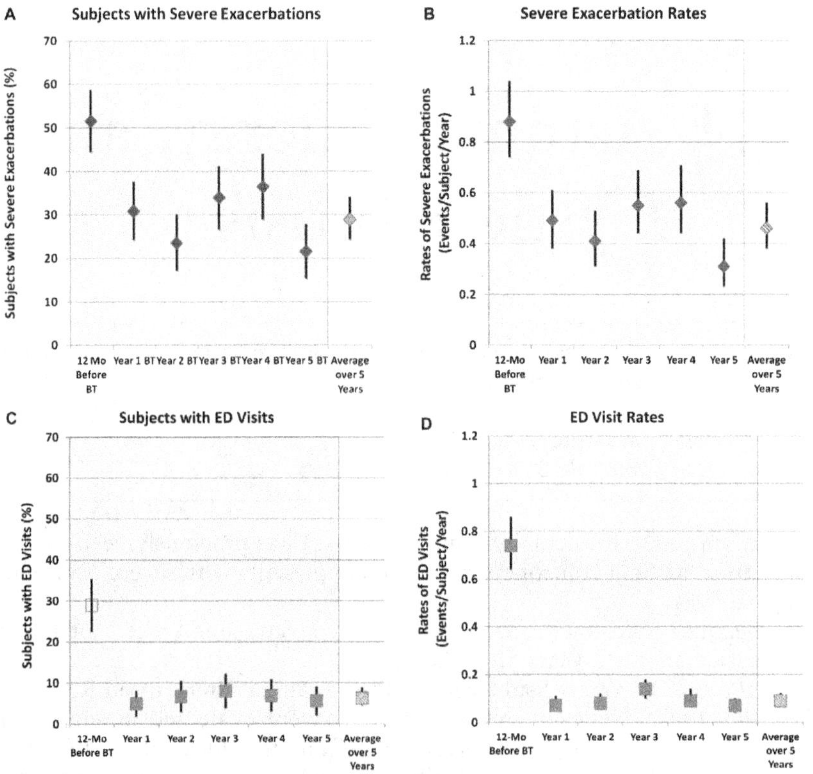

FIGURE 1.—Severe exacerbations and ED visits in the 5 years after BT. A, Proportion of subjects with severe exacerbations. B, Severe exacerbation rates. C, Proportion of subjects with ED visits for respiratory symptoms. D, ED visit rates. Values are point estimates with 95% upper and lower CIs. The 365-day period constituting year 1 began at 6 weeks after the last BT bronchoscopy. (Reprinted from The Journal of Allergy and Clinical Immunology. Wechsler ME, for the Asthma Intervention Research 2 Trial Study Group. Bronchial thermoplasty: long-term safety and effectiveness in patients with severe persistent asthma. *J Allergy Clin Immunol.* 2013;132:1295-1302.e3, Copyright, 2013, with permission from Elsevier.)

asthma who remain symptomatic despite taking inhaled corticosteroids and long-acting β_2-agonists (Figs 1 and 2, Table 1).

▶ What we've been waiting for: 5-year outcomes after bronchial thermoplasty (BTP) in severe persistent asthmatics! At baseline, 72% of subjects were taking a minimum of 2 maintenance medications (long-acting β_2 agonist [LABA] and high-dose inhaled corticosteroids [ICS]), whereas 28% of subjects required 3 maintenance medications. Although outcomes at 1 and 2 years have been published previously,[1-3] this report outlines baseline demographics (Table 1) and 5 years of annual follow-up after bronchial thermoplasty for 162 of 190 (85.3%) subjects with uncontrolled asthma (from the Asthma Intervention Research 2 trial). Fig 1 depicts results pre-BTP (pBTP) and annual follow-up for: percentage of subjects with severe exacerbations; rates of severe exacerbation (events per subject per year); percentage of subjects with emergency department

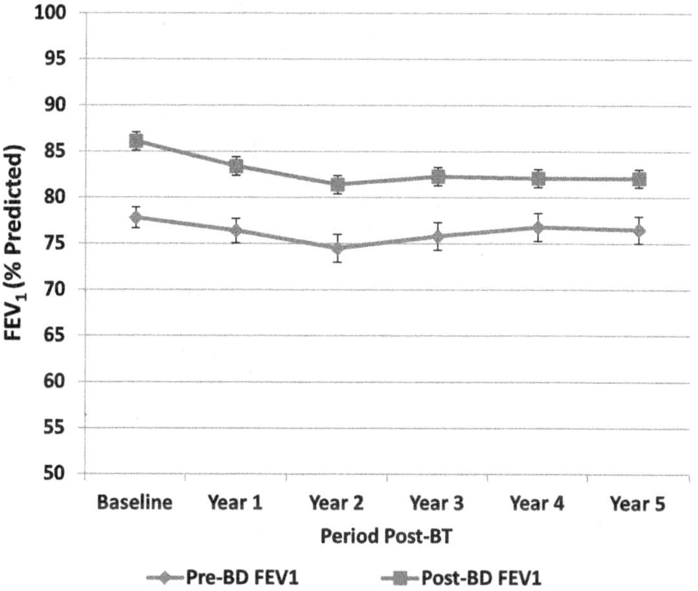

FIGURE 2.—Prebronchodilator and postbronchodilator FEV_1 over 5 years (percent predicted). Percent predicted prebronchodilator and postbronchodilator FEV_1 values (means ± SEMs) for subjects completing follow-up during each year. The percent predicted prebronchodilator FEV_1 values remained unchanged over the 5 years after BT. Postbronchodilator FEV_1 remained higher at all times; increase in percent predicted FEV_1 at baseline of 8.2% and at 5 years of 5.9%. *BD*, Bronchodilator. (Reprinted from The Journal of Allergy and Clinical Immunology. Wechsler ME, for the Asthma Intervention Research 2 Trial Study Group. Bronchial thermoplasty: long-term safety and effectiveness in patients with severe persistent asthma. *J Allergy Clin Immunol.* 2013;132:1295-1302.e3, Copyright 2013, with permission from Elsevier.)

(ED) visits; and ED visit rates (events per subject follow-up). Pre- and post-bronchodilator reactivity was monitored over the 5-year follow-up. For all of the above outcomes, statistically significant improvement was maintained over 5 years of annual follow-up showing essentially no change from pBTP (Fig 2). Overall, an 18% reduction was noted in ICS dose at 5 years, with 12% of subjects no longer taking ICS 5 years post-BPT, and 7% of subjects no longer taking ICS or LABA therapy. These data confirm the previously established safety profile for BTP reported at 2 years and support consideration of BTP for severe persistent symptomatic asthmatics on optimal therapy with ICS and LABA.

S. K. Willsie, DO, MA

References

1. Cox G, Thomson NC, Rubin AS, et al. Asthma control during the year after bronchial thermoplastsy. *N Engl J Med.* 2007;356:1327-1337.
2. Castro M, Rubin AS, Laviolette M, et al. Effectiveness and safety of bronchial thermoplasty in the treatment of severe asthma: a multicenter, randomized, double-blind, sham-controlled clinical trial. *Am J Respir Crit Care Med.* 2010; 181:116-124.
3. Castro M, Rubin A, Laviolette M, Hanania NA, Armstrong B, Cox G. Persistence of effectiveness of bronchial thermoplasty in patients with severe asthma. *Ann Allergy Asthma Immunol.* 2011;107:65-70.

TABLE 1.—Demographics and Clinical Characteristics

	All Subjects Undergoing BT at Baseline (n = 190)	Subjects Undergoing BT Completing 5-y Follow-up (n = 162)	Subjects Undergoing BT not Completing 5-y Follow-up (n = 28)
Age (y)	40.7 ± 11.9	41.5 ± 11.8	35.8 ± 11.3[§]
Sex	Male: 81 (42.6%) Female: 109 (57.4%)	Male: 68 (42.0%) Female: 94 (58.0%)	Male: 13 (46.4%) Female: 15 (63.6%)
Race			
White	151 (79.5%)	134 (82.7%)	17 (60.7%)
African American/black	19 (10.0%)	13 (8.0%)	6 (21.4%)
Hispanic	6 (3.2%)	4 (2.5%)	2 (7.1%)
Asian	4 (2.1%)	3 (1.9%)	1 (3.6%)
Other	10 (5.3%)	8 (4.9%)	2 (7.1%)
Weight (kg)	81.7 ± 18.4	81.4 ± 17.1	83.4 ± 24.6
ICS dose (μg)*	1960.7 ± 745.2	1958.9 ± 757.9	1900 ± 551.6
LABA dose (μg)[†]	116.8 ± 34.4	120.8 ± 47.7	108.9 ± 23.8
Symptom-free days (%)	16.4 ± 24.0	16.1 ± 24.1	18.4 ± 24.1
Asthma Control Questionnaire score	2.1 ± 0.87	2.1 ± 0.84	2.3 ± 1.02
AQLQ score	4.30 ± 1.17	4.32 ± 1.17	4.23 ± 1.16
ED visits for respiratory symptoms in prior 12 mo,[‡] no. of events (no. of subjects)	141 (55)	115 (47)	26 (8)
Hospitalizations for respiratory symptoms in prior 12 mo,[‡] no. of events (no. of subjects)	10 (8)	10 (8)	0 (0)
Seasonal allergies, no. (%)[‡]			
Yes	103 (54.5%)	85 (52.8%)	18 (64.3%)
No	86 (45.5%)	76 (47.2%)	10 (35.7%)
Lung function measures			
Prebronchodilator FEV_1	77.8 ± 15.65	77.8 ± 15.84	78.0 ± 14.75
Postbronchodilator FEV_1	86.1 ± 15.76	85.9 ± 15.83	87.1 ± 15.57
Morning PEF (L/min)	383.8 ± 104.3	380.9 ± 106.0	400.7 ± 93.8
Methacholine PC_{20} (mg/mL), geometric mean (range)	0.27 (0.22-0.34)	0.27 (0.21-0.35)	0.29 (0.15-0.54)

Values are means ± SDs, except when indicated otherwise.
PEF, Peak expiratory flow.
*Beclomethasone or equivalent.
[†]Salmeterol or equivalent.
[‡]Patient reported.
[§]$P = .019$ comparing subjects completing 5-year follow-up versus subjects not completing 5-year follow-up (*t* test).
Reprinted from The Journal of Allergy and Clinical Immunology. Wechsler ME, for the Asthma Intervention Research 2 Trial Study Group. Bronchial thermoplasty: long-term safety and effectiveness in patients with severe persistent asthma. J Allergy Clin Immunol. 2013;132:1295-1302.e3, Copyright, 2013, with permission from Elsevier.

Safety of bronchial thermoplasty in patients with severe refractory asthma

Pavord ID, for the Research in Severe Asthma Trial Study Group (Univ Hosps of Leicester NHS Trust, UK)
Ann Allergy Asthma Immunol 111:402-407, 2013

Background.—Patients with severe refractory asthma treated with bronchial thermoplasty (BT), a bronchoscopic procedure that improves asthma control by reducing excess airway smooth muscle, were followed up for 5 years to evaluate long-term safety of this procedure.

Objectives.—To assess long-term safety of BT for 5 years.

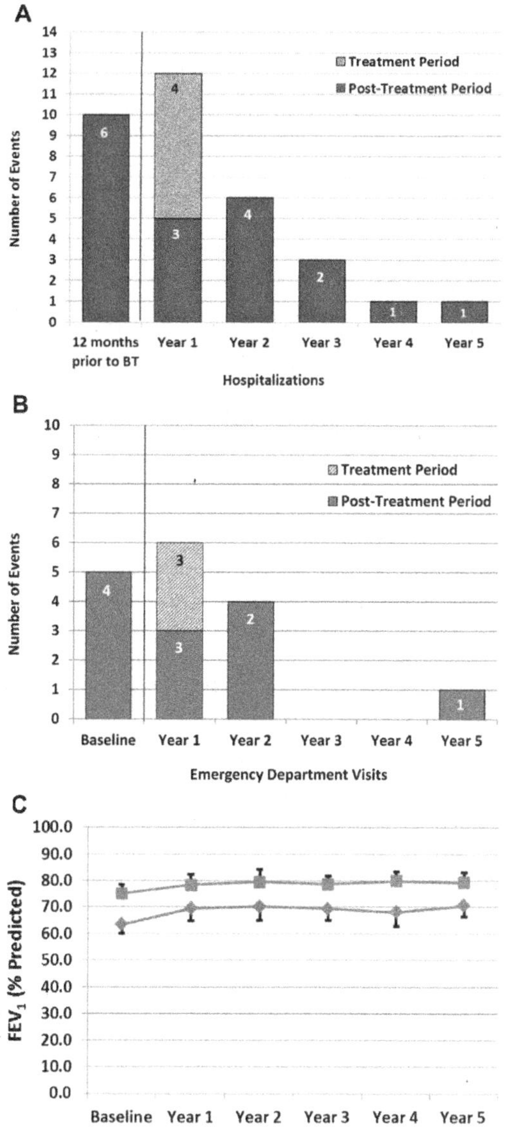

FIGURE 1.—Summary of health care utilization events. A, Hospitalizations for respiratory symptoms. B, Emergency department (ED) visits for respiratory symptoms. Bars represent number of events. Numbers within bars represent the number of patients contributing to the events. Year 1 data represent events occurring in the treatment period (day of first BT procedure until 6 weeks after the third BT procedure) and the posttreatment period (46-week period beginning 6 weeks after the last BT procedure to 12 months). $P = .16$ for the trend in the percentage of patients with hospitalizations for respiratory symptoms and $P = .22$ for the trend in the percentage of patients with ED visits for respiratory symptoms across years 1 to 5 (posttreatment period) using a repeated-measures logistic regression (generalized estimating equation), modeling the percentage of patients reporting an event. C, Prebronchodilator and postbronchodilator forced expiratory volume in 1 second (FEV_1) over time. Values represent mean (SEM) percent predicted prebronchodilator (◇) and postbronchodilator (□) FEV_1 values. (Reprinted from Annals of Allergy, Asthma and Immunology. Pavord ID, for the Research in Severe Asthma Trial Study Group. Safety of bronchial thermoplasty in patients with severe refractory asthma. *Ann Allergy Asthma Immunol.* 2013;111:402-407, Copyright 2013, with permission from American College of Allergy, Asthma & Immunology.)

TABLE 1.—Baseline Demographics and Clinical Characteristics

Parameter	Bronchial Thermoplasty (n = 14)
Age, mean (SD), y	38.6 (13.3)
Sex, No. (%)	
Male	6 (43)
Female	8 (57)
White race, No. (%)	14 (100)
Height, mean (SD), cm	165.8 (7.9)
Weight, mean (SD), kg	90.5 (19.5)
Inhaled corticosteroid dose, mean (SD), μg^a	1,179 (421)
LABA dose, mean (SD), μg^b	127 (62)
OCS dose, mean (SD), mg (n = 7)	15 (5.8)
Symptom-free days, mean (SD), %	5.6 (14.1)
Asthma Control Questionnaire score, mean (SD)	2.8 (1.0)
Asthma Quality of Life Questionnaire score, mean (SD)	4.1 (1.3)
Rescue medication use, mean (SD), No. of puffs per 7 days	60.1 (60.1)
Emergency department visits for respiratory symptoms in prior 12 months,[c]	5 (4)
No. of events (No. of patients)	
Hospitalizations for respiratory symptoms in prior 12 months,[c]	10 (6)
No. of events (No. of patients)	
Seasonal allergies (self-reported), No. (%)	10 (71)
Lung function measures	
Morning peak expiratory flow rate, mean (SD), L/min	370.0 (82.0)
Prebronchodilator FEV_1, mean (SD), % predicted	63.5 (12.5)
Postbronchodilator FEV_1, mean (SD), % predicted	75.2 (11.9)
Methacholine PC_{20}, geometric mean (range), mg/mL	0.24 (0.1-1.1)

Abbreviations: FEV_1, forced expiratory volume in 1 second; LABA, long-acting β_2-agonist; OCS, oral corticosteroid; PC_{20}, provocative concentration causing a 20% decrease in FEV_1.

[a]Fluticasone or equivalent.

[b]Salmeterol or equivalent.

[c]Patient reported.

Reprinted from Pavord ID, for the Research in Severe Asthma Trial Study Group. Safety of bronchial thermoplasty in patients with severe refractory asthma. Ann Allergy Asthma Immunol. 2013;111:402-407, Copyright 2014, with permission from American College of Annals of Allergy, Asthma & Immunology.

TABLE 2.—Adverse Events by Year

Year	Total No. of Events	Total No. (%) of Patients Reporting	No. of Events per Patient per Year
Year 1[a] (n = 14)	118	14 (100)	8.4
Year 2 (n = 14)	20	11 (78.6)	1.4
Year 3 (n = 14)	34	12 (85.7)	2.4
Year 4 (n = 12)	20	10 (83.3)	1.7
Year 5 (n = 12)	29	12 (100)	2.4

[a]Year 1 data (posttreatment period only; ie, the 46-week period beginning 6 weeks after the last bronchial thermoplasty procedure to 12 months) for 14 patients who enrolled in long-term follow-up trial. Adverse events solicited from patient during multiple office visits in year 1. In subsequent years, adverse events solicited only at annual follow-up visit.

Reprinted from Pavord ID, for the Research in Severe Asthma Trial Study Group. Safety of bronchial thermoplasty in patients with severe refractory asthma. Ann Allergy Asthma Immunol. 2013;111:402-407, Copyright 2014, with permission from American College of Annals of Allergy, Asthma & Immunology.

Methods.—Patients with asthma aged 18 to 65 years requiring high-dose inhaled corticosteroids (ICSs) (>750 μg/d of fluticasone propionate or equivalent) and long-acting β_2-agonists (LABAs) (at least 100 μg/d of salmeterol or equivalent), with or without oral prednisone (≤30 mg/d), leukotriene modifiers, theophylline, or other asthma controller medications were enrolled in the Research in Severe Asthma (RISA) Trial. Patients had a prebronchodilator forced expiratory volume in 1 second of 50% or more of predicted, demonstrated methacholine airway hyperresponsiveness, had uncontrolled symptoms despite taking maintenance medication, abstained from smoking for 1 year or greater, and had a smoking history of less than 10 pack-years.

Results.—Fourteen patients (of the 15 who received active treatment in the RISA Trial) participated in the long-term follow-up study for 5 years. The rate of respiratory adverse events (AEs per patient per year) was 1.4, 2.4, 1.7, and 2.4, respectively, in years 2 to 5 after BT. There was a decrease in hospitalizations and emergency department visits for respiratory symptoms in each of years 1, 2, 3, 4, and 5 compared with the year before BT treatment. Measures of lung function showed no deterioration for 5 years.

Conclusion.—Our findings suggest that BT is safe for 5 years after BT in patients with severe refractory asthma.

Trial Registration.—clinicaltrials.gov Identifier: NCT00401986 (Fig 1, Tables 1 and 2).

► This is a 5-year follow-up report of 14 subjects with severe persistent asthma (mean prebronchodilator forced expiratory volume in 1 second [FEV_1]: 63.5% with standard deviation [SD] of 12.5), who underwent bronchial thermoplasty (BT) in the Research in Severe Asthma (RISA) trial. Table 1 depicts baseline demographics and pre-BT dosing of long-acting β agonists (LABA) and inhaled corticosteroids (ICS) and Table 2 lists adverse events by year after BT. Fig 1 shows data from 12 months before BT through 5-year follow-up. As with the report of the Asthma Intervention Research 2 (AIR2) trial in which subjects with severe persistent asthma (mean prebronchodilator FEV_1 of 77.8%, SD 16.5) underwent BT,[1] pre- and postbronchodilator FEV_1 was maintained over 5 years in all subjects. The incidence of hospitalization and ED visits trended toward improvement but did not reach statistical significance. No significant change in asthma medication use was found over the monitoring period. Data from the RISA trial are additive to the AIR2 5-year outcome data concerning the safety of BT.[1]

S. K. Willsie, DO, MA

Reference

1. Wechsler ME, Laviolette M, Aalberto SR, et al. Bronchial thermoplasty: long-term safety and effectivenss in patients with severe persistent asthma. *J Allergy Clin Immunol.* 2013;132:1296-1302.

Severe adult-onset asthma: A distinct phenotype

Amelink M, de Groot JC, de Nijs SB, et al (Univ of Amsterdam, The Netherlands; Med Centre Leeuwarden, The Netherlands; et al)

J Allergy Clin Immunol 132:336-341, 2013

Background.—Some patients with adult-onset asthma have severe disease, whereas others have mild transient disease. It is currently unknown whether patients with severe adult-onset asthma represent a distinct clinical phenotype.

Objective.—We sought to investigate whether disease severity in patients with adult-onset asthma is associated with specific phenotypic characteristics.

Methods.—One hundred seventy-six patients with adult-onset asthma were recruited from 1 academic and 3 nonacademic outpatient clinics. Severe refractory asthma was defined according to international Innovative Medicines Initiative criteria, and mild-to-moderate persistent asthma was defined according to Global Initiative for Asthma criteria. Patients were characterized with respect to clinical, functional, and inflammatory

TABLE 1.—Symptoms, Medication Use, and Health Care Use

	Mild-to-Moderate Persistent Asthma (n = 98)	Severe Asthma (n = 78)	*P* Value
ACQ score*	1.17 (0.94)	1.91 (0.98)	<.001
AQLQ score*	5.4 (1.28)	4.8 (1.15)	.002
ICS dose (fluticasone equivalent)†	500 (250-500)	1000 (1000-1500)	<.001
OCS (%)	0	59	<.001
Anti-IgE (%)	0	11.5	.001
Exacerbations (%)			<.001
0	70	17	
1-2	18	32	
≥3	12	51	
Doctor's office visits (%)			<.001
0	14	0	
1-2	65	22	
≥3	21	78	
ED visits (%)			.04
0	90	75	
1-2	8	17	
≥3	2	8	
Hospitalizations (%)			.003
0	93	74	
1-2	5	22	
≥3	2	4	
ICU admissions (%)			.01
0	99	86	
1-2	1	10	
≥3	0	1	

Exacerbations, doctor's office visits, emergency department visits, and hospitalizations are defined as the number of events in the past 12 months. Intensive care unit admissions are the number of admissions ever to the intensive care unit.

ACQ, Asthma Control Questionnaire; *AQLQ*, Asthma Quality of Life Questionnaire; *ED*, emergency department; *ICS*, inhaled corticosteroids; *ICU*, intensive care unit; *OCS*, oral corticosteroids.

*Mean (SD).

†Median (first and third interquartiles).

TABLE 2.—Patients' Characteristics

	Mild-to-Moderate Persistent Asthma (N = 98)	Severe Asthma (n = 78)	*P* Value
Age (y)*	53.6 (11.4)	54.4 (9.8)	.6
Sex (% female)	59.2	61.5	.7
Age of onset (y)*	41.8 (13.8)	40.2 (11.9)	.4
Asthma duration (y)†	9 (3-18.5)	10 (5-21)	.07
White race (%)	82.7	87.2	.4
(Ex)smoker (%)	33.7	47.4	.08
Pack years smoked†	0 (0-4.5)	0 (0-7.6)	.3
Total IgE (kU/L)†	77.5 (26.3-277)	112 (51.7-325)	.1
Atopy (positive RAST result [%])	52	34.6	.02
IgE against *Aspergillus species* (%)	10	9	.7
Family history of atopy (%)	36.6	27.6	.2
Family history of asthma (%)	34.4	38.2	.6
BMI (kg/m^2)†	27.3 (24.5-29.9)	28.6 (24.8-31.6)	.2
Nasal polyposis (%)	26.5	53.8	<.001
History of NSAID sensitivity (%)	11.2	16.7	.4
SNOT score*	1.15 (0.76)	1.4 (0.86)	.02
Use of nasal corticosteroids (%)	45	74.4	<.001

NSAID, Nonsteroidal anti-inflammatory drug; *SNOT*, 22-item Sino-Nasal Outcome Test.
*Mean (SD).
†Median (first and third interquartiles).

TABLE 4.—Inflammatory Markers

	Mild-to-Moderate Persistent Asthma (n = 98)	Severe Asthma (n = 78)	*P* Value
Blood eosinophils (10^9/L)	0.18 (0.09-0.31)	0.25 (0.14-0.5)	.05
Blood neutrophils (10^9/L)	4 (3.1-4.9)	5.3 (3.9-6.8)	<.001
FENO (ppb)	27 (16-50)	38 (19-73)	.02
Sputum eosinophils (% [n = 110])	0.8 (0.1-7.1)	11.6 (1.5-33.4)	<.001
Sputum neutrophils (% [n = 110])	73.5 (46.7-84.9)	67.2 (37.9-83.2)	.9

Values are presented as medians (first and third interquartiles).

parameters. Unpaired *t* tests and χ^2 tests were used for group comparisons; both univariate and multivariate logistic regression were used to determine factors associated with disease severity.

Results.—Apart from the expected high symptom scores, poor quality of life, need for high-intensity treatment, low lung function, and high exacerbation rate, patients with severe adult-onset asthma were more often nonatopic (52% vs 34%, $P = .02$) and had more nasal symptoms and nasal polyposis (54% vs 27%, $P \leq .001$), higher exhaled nitric oxide levels (38 vs 27 ppb, $P = .02$) and blood neutrophil counts (5.3 vs 4.0 10^9/L, $P \leq .001$) and sputum eosinophilia (11.8% vs 0.8%, $P \leq .001$). Multiple logistic regression analysis showed that increased blood neutrophil (odds ratio, 10.9; $P = .002$) and sputum eosinophil (odds ratio, 1.5; $P = .005$) counts were independently associated with severe adult-onset disease.

Conclusion.—The majority of patients with severe adult-onset asthma are nonatopic and have persistent eosinophilic airway inflammation. This suggests that severe adult-onset asthma has a distinct underlying mechanism compared with milder disease (Tables 1, 2, and 4).

▶ This is an important investigation aimed at characterizing severe adult-onset asthma. A total of 176 subjects with adult-onset asthma were evaluated: 98 were characterized as mild-moderate asthmatics and 78 as severe asthmatics (forming the group upon which the study focused). More than 50% of the severe asthmatic population was receiving daily oral corticosteroids and greater than 10% were receiving anti-immunoglobulin E therapy. Tables 1 and 2 show that adult-onset severe asthmatics used higher-dose inhaled corticosteroids (ICS) ($P < .001$) and nasal corticosteroids ($P < .001$) than the mild-moderate asthmatics. Table 4 summarizes the results of inflammatory marker testing, which show that the adult-onset severe asthmatic is more likely to have peripheral neutrophilia and eosinophilia and sputum eosinophilia. They are more likely to be nonatopic and to have more nasal symptoms/nasal polyposis and higher exhaled nitric oxide levels. The investigators suggest that these data show the likelihood of a distinct phenotype, which may help to explain why adult-onset severe asthmatics often are seemingly less responsive to guideline-directed care. These data should lead to additional investigations surrounding the pathophysiology of this distinct phenotype with one result being the design of preventive steps to eliminate severe adult-onset asthma.

S. K. Willsie, DO, MA

Asthma During Pregnancy and Clinical Outcomes in Offspring: A National Cohort Study

Tegethoff M, Olsen J, Schaffner E, et al (Univ of Basel, Switzerland; Univ of California at Los Angeles)

Pediatrics 132:483-491, 2013

Background and Objective.—Maternal asthma is a common pregnancy complication, with adverse short-term effects for the offspring. The objective was to determine whether asthma during pregnancy is a risk factor of offspring diseases.

Methods.—We studied pregnant women from the Danish National Birth Cohort (births: 1996–2002; prospective data) giving birth to live singletons ($n = 66\,712$ mother-child pairs), with 4145 (6.2%) women suffering from asthma during pregnancy. We estimated the associations between asthma during pregnancy and offspring diseases (*International Classification of Diseases, 10th Revision* diagnoses from national registries), controlling for potential confounders and validating findings by secondary analyses.

Results.—Offspring median age at end of follow-up was 6.2 (3.6–8.9) years. Asthma was associated with an increased offspring risk of infectious and parasitic diseases (hazard ratio [HR] 1.34; 95% confidence interval [CI] 1.23–1.46), diseases of the nervous system (HR 1.43; CI

1.18–1.73), ear (HR 1.33; CI 1.19–1.48), respiratory system (HR 1.43; CI 1.34–1.52), and skin (HR 1.39; CI 1.20–1.60), and potentially (not confirmed in secondary analyses) of endocrine and metabolic disorders (HR 1.26; CI 1.02–1.55), diseases of the digestive system (HR 1.17; CI 1.04–1.32), and malformations (odds ratio 1.13; CI 1.01–1.26), but not of neoplasms, mental disorders, or diseases of the blood and immune system, circulatory system, musculoskeletal system, and genitourinary system.

Conclusions.—To the best of our knowledge, this is the first comprehensive study of the associations between asthma during pregnancy and a wide spectrum of offspring diseases. In line with previous data on selected outcomes, asthma during pregnancy may be a risk factor for numerous offspring diseases, suggesting that careful monitoring of women with asthma during pregnancy and their offspring is important.

▶ This study of more than 65 000 pregnant asthmatic-child pairs reports linkage between several diseases occurring in childhood, some not previously reported. Follow-up ended at a median age of 6.2 years (3.6–8.9 years), and the investigators reviewed data from the Danish National Birth Cohort (prospectively obtained data from 1996–2002). Table 2 in the original article lists the results of Cox regression models of offspring diseases associated with asthma during pregnancy. Adjusted odds ratios (OR) ranged from 0.85 for diseases of blood immune system to 1.51 for diseases of the respiratory system; diseases of the nervous system (1.51), diseases of the skin (1.43), infections and parasitic diseases (1.42), diseases of the ear (1.41), and mental disorders (1.35) were estimated to be associated with maternal asthma. There was no assessment of what in the asthmatic maternal condition led to these disorders (eg, medication effects, physiology). Further research is needed about possible genetic influences vs environment to fully understand the impact and potential for intervention to prevent disease development in the offspring of asthmatic women.

S. K. Willsie, DO, MA

Omalizumab: A review of its Use in Patients with Severe Persistent Allergic Asthma

McKeage K (Adis, North Shore, Auckland, New Zealand)
Drugs 73:1197-1212, 2013

Omalizumab (Xolair®) is a subcutaneously administered monoclonal antibody that targets circulating free IgE and prevents its interaction with the high-affinity IgE receptor (FCϵRI), thereby interrupting the allergic cascade. In the EU, the drug is approved as add-on therapy in adults, adolescents and children aged ≥ 6 years with severe persistent allergic asthma. In well designed clinical trials, add-on omalizumab significantly reduced the asthma exacerbation rate (primary endpoint) compared with placebo in adults, adolescents and children with severe persistent allergic asthma. Furthermore, add-on omalizumab reduced the need for inhaled corticosteroids in adults and adolescents, and improved asthma control and

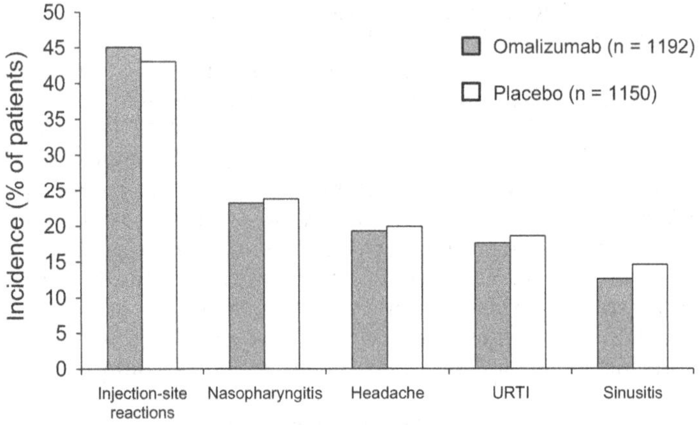

FIGURE 1.—Tolerability of add-on omalizumab in adults and adolescents with persistent allergic asthma. Results are from a review of data from several placebo-controlled trials of 16–32 weeks' duration, and include adverse events that occurred in >10 % of patients in either group [51]. Most patients had severe allergic asthma, but some studies were conducted in patients with moderate to severe disease. The omalizumab dose was based on body weight and pre-treatment total serum IgE levels. *URTI* upper respiratory tract infection. Editor's Note: Please refer to original journal article for full references. (Reprinted from McKeage K. Omalizumab: a review of its use in patients with severe persistent allergic asthma. *Drugs*. 2013;73:1197-1212, with permission from Springer International Publishing Switzerland, Copyright 2013, with permission from Adis Data Information BV.)

symptoms, and asthma-related quality of life in all age groups. The efficacy of omalizumab was also demonstrated in the real-world setting, with add-on therapy leading to reduced rates of hospitalizations, emergency room visits and unscheduled doctor's visits, as well as improvements in asthma symptom scores and the physician's overall assessment of treatment response. More data are needed to determine the optimum duration of treatment, and currently the duration is at the discretion of the treating physician. Omalizumab was generally well tolerated in clinical trials; the most common adverse event was transient injection-site reactions. In cost-utility analyses modelled over a life-time horizon, add-on omalizumab was cost effective compared with standard therapy, with incremental cost-effectiveness ratios falling within generally accepted willingness-to-pay thresholds. Thus, in difficult-to-treat patients with severe persistent allergic asthma, omalizumab provides a valuable treatment option (Fig 1).

▶ This is a comprehensive review of the use of omalizumab (subcutaneously administered recombinant DNA-derived humanized immunoglobulin E monoclonal antibody)[1] in the treatment of severe persistent allergic asthmatics. The author reviews several investigations evaluating the pharmacodynamics, pharmacokinetics, tolerability, and therapeutic uses and efficacy of omalizumab in severe persistent allergic asthma.[2] The most common adverse event attributable to omalizumab is transient injection-site reactions. Fig 1 depicts the tolerability of omalizumab vs placebo in adult and adolescent persistent allergic asthmatics. No significant differences between omalizumab vs placebo-related side effects were noted for injection site reactions, nasopharyngitis, headache, upper respiratory tract infections, and sinusitis. Omalizumab is indicated according to Global Initiative for Asthma Guidelines[3] for add-on use in patients with persistent allergic asthma that remains uncontrolled despite step 4 treatment (combinations of high-dose inhaled corticosteroids and other controller medications). Approved dosing, administration, and cost effectiveness is discussed.

S. K. Willsie, DO, MA

References

1. Soresi S, Togias A. Mechanisms of action of anti-immunoglobulin E therapy. *Allergy Asthma Proc.* 2006;27:S15-S23.
2. Corren J, Casale TB, Lanier B, Buhl R, Holgate S, Jimenez P. Safety and tolerability of omalizumab. *Clin Exp Allergy.* 2009;39:788-797.
3. Global Initiative for Asthma. *Global strategy for asthma management and prevention.* 2012. Updated, http://www.ginasthma.org/local/uploads/files/GINA_Report_2012Feb13.pdf. Accessed February 05, 2014.

Prescription fill patterns in underserved children with asthma receiving subspecialty care

Bollinger ME, Mudd KE, Boldt A, et al (Univ of Maryland, Baltimore)
Ann Allergy Asthma Immunol 111:185-189, 2013

Background.—Children with asthma receiving specialty care have been found to have improved asthma outcomes. However, these outcomes can be adversely affected by poor adherence with controller medications.

Objective.—To analyze pharmacy fill patterns as a measure of primary adherence in a group of underserved minority children receiving allergy subspecialty care.

Methods.—As part of a larger 18-month nebulizer use study in underserved children (ages 2-8 years) with persistent asthma, 53 children were recruited from an urban allergy practice. Pharmacy records were compared with prescribing records for all asthma medications.

Results.—Allergist controller prescriptions were written in 30-day quantities with refills and short-acting β-agonists (SABAs) with no refills. Only 49.1% of inhaled corticosteroid (ICS), 49.5% of combination ICS and long-acting β-agonist, and 64.5% of leukotriene modifier (LTM) initial and refill prescriptions were ever filled during the 18-month period. A mean of 5.1 refills (range, 0-14) for SABAs were obtained during 18 months, although only 1.28 SABA prescriptions were prescribed by the allergist. Mean times between first asthma prescription and actual filling were 30 days (range, 0-177 days) for ICSs, 26.6 days (range, 0-156 days) for LTMs, and 16.8 days (range, 0-139 days) for SABAs.

Conclusion.—Underserved children with asthma receiving allergy subspecialty care suboptimally filled controller prescriptions, yet filled abundant rescue medications from other prescribers. Limiting albuterol prescriptions to one canister without additional refills may provide an opportunity to monitor fill rates of both rescue and controller medications

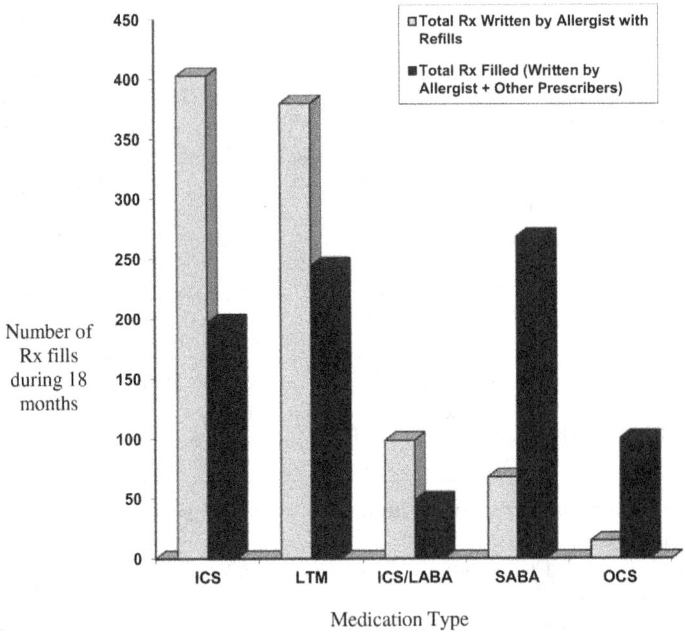

FIGURE 1.—Number of prescriptions written by an allergist (initial and refills) vs prescriptions filled in underserved children with asthma. (Reprinted from Annals of Allergy, Asthma and Immunology. Bollinger ME, Mudd KE, Boldt A, et al. Prescription fill patterns in underserved children with asthma receiving subspecialty care. *Ann Allergy Asthma Immunol*. 2013;111:185-189, Copyright 2014, with permission from American College of Allergy, Asthma & Immunology.)

and provide education to patients about appropriate use of medications to improve adherence (Fig 1).

▶ We prescribe guideline-directed care for our asthmatics and wonder why our patients' asthma is not improving! Underserved pediatric asthmatics receiving allergist subspecialty care were monitored over 18 months for prescription filling practices. Initial allergist-prescribed medications included a 30-day supply of controller medication (with refills) and 1 canister of short-acting β agonist (SABA) (no refill). Over the 18-month period of monitoring, patients refilled primarily the SABAs (mean 5.1 refills over 18 months, while allergists prescribed a mean of only 1.28 SABA refills). These data (Fig 1) indicate that the asthmatics are filling and refilling additional SABA prescriptions from nonsubspecialists. The increased filling/refilling of SABAs occurred in the face of less than 50% of controller prescriptions ever being filled or refilled and approximately 65% of leukotriene modifier prescriptions being filled or refilled. This clearly represents a need for better education of the parties caring for the asthmatics in the home as well as the referring providers (should coordinate care with specialists). Successful education and changed prescription-filling practices have great potential to improve control of asthma in children.

S. K. Willsie, DO, MA

32 Chronic Obstructive Pulmonary Disease

Cardiovascular Risk, Myocardial Injury, and Exacerbations of Chronic Obstructive Pulmonary Disease

Patel ARC, Kowlessar BS, Donaldson GC, et al (Univ College London, UK)

Am J Respir Crit Care Med 188:1091-1099, 2013

Rationale.—Patients with chronic obstructive pulmonary disease (COPD) have elevated cardiovascular risk, and myocardial injury is common during severe exacerbations. Little is known about the prevalence, magnitude, and underlying mechanisms of cardiovascular risk in community-treated exacerbations.

Objectives.—To investigate how COPD exacerbations and exacerbation frequency impact cardiovascular risk and myocardial injury, and whether this is related to airway infection and inflammation.

Methods.—We prospectively measured arterial stiffness (aortic pulse wave velocity [aPWV]) and cardiac biomarkers in 98 patients with stable COPD. Fifty-five patients had paired stable and exacerbation assessments, repeated at Days 3, 7, 14, and 35 during recovery. Airway infection was identified using polymerase chain reaction.

Measurements and Main Results.—COPD exacerbation frequency was related to stable-state arterial stiffness (rho = 0.209; $P = 0.040$). Frequent exacerbators had greater aPWV than infrequent exacerbators (mean ± SD aPWV, 11.4 ± 2.1 vs. 10.3 ± 2.0 ms^{-1}; $P = 0.025$). Arterial stiffness rose by an average of 1.2 ms^{-1} (11.1%) from stable state to exacerbation (n = 55) and fell slowly during recovery. In those with airway infection at exacerbation (n = 24) this rise was greater (1.4 ± 1.6 vs. 0.7 ± 1.3 ms^{-1}; $P = 0.048$); prolonged; and related to sputum IL-6 (rho = 0.753; $P < 0.001$). Increases in cardiac biomarkers at exacerbation were higher in those with ischemic heart disease (n = 12) than those without (n = 43) (mean ± SD increase in troponin T, 0.011 ± 0.009 vs. 0.003 ± 0.006 μg/L, $P = 0.003$; N-terminal pro-brain natriuretic peptide, 38.1 ± 37.7 vs. 5.9 ± 12.3 pg/ml, $P < 0.001$).

Conclusions.—Frequent COPD exacerbators have greater arterial stiffness than infrequent exacerbators. Arterial stiffness rises acutely during COPD exacerbations, particularly with airway infection. Increases in arterial stiffness are related to inflammation, and are slow to recover. Myocardial injury is common and clinically significant during COPD exacerbations, particularly in those with underlying ischemic heart disease.

▶ Chronic obstructive pulmonary disease (COPD) is now well recognized as a systemic inflammatory process that is often accompanied by other medical conditions. It remains the third leading cause of death worldwide, ranking behind ischemic cardiovascular and cerebrovascular disease. Smoking is frequently a common risk factor in all these processes; therefore, vasculopathy and other cardiac disease and obstructive lung disease often go hand in hand. In addition, several studies have documented that patients with COPD are at increased risk for cardiac events or increased mortality in various medical situations, particularly in the setting of COPD exacerbations. This study attempts to better quantify the risk of myocardial events in the peri-exacerbation period and begins to study the mechanisms that lie behind this risk, a first step to designing prevention measures. Several other studies were published in 2013 that further defined cardiac risks associated with comorbid COPD. Almassi et al[1] reported a large, randomized trial in which cardiac bypass graft surgery was performed either on-pump or off-pump in patients with comorbid COPD. The reason for the study was the known high risk of cardiac events in COPD patients undergoing cardiac surgery. In this study, patients who had surgery off pump had more complications at the time of surgery; however, long-term outcomes were not different between the 2 approaches. Gunter et al[2] reported a study of aortic valve replacement with or without bypass grafting in COPD patients. Of the 2379 patients reported, more than one-fifth had varying severities of COPD. COPD did not seem to impact the early perioperative mortality, but long-term survival (> 3 years) was worse across all levels of COPD, with severe disease carrying the worst odds ratio of 2.28. Stone et al[3] addressed the outcomes of patients undergoing abdominal aortic aneurysm (AAA) repair, both endovascular and open, who also had COPD. Smoking is a well-described risk factor for AAA, so it is not surprising that more than a third of patients coming for repair have a COPD diagnosis. Both types of repair were associated with higher in-hospital morbidity and mortality in oxygen-requiring COPD patients. Five-year survival was diminished in all levels of COPD; however, oxygen-dependency was an independent predictor of death.

Brenner et al[4] tried to assess the impact of COPD on survival in patients with systolic heart failure. They found, however, that it was very difficult to tell which patients had COPD because obstruction was variable in this population except when serial pulmonary functions were done in stable patients. Congestion was hard to separate from fixed obstruction except in patients shown to have hyperinflation. Only proven COPD was associated with increased mortality. Finally, Jensen et al[5] used the Copenhagen City Heart Study, a population-based study covering more than 35 years of follow-up, to define a relationship between resting heart rate and mortality in COPD patients. Higher resting heart rate was associated with reduced survival across all levels of COPD. The authors found that when resting heart rate was added to the Global Obstructive Lung Disease Guidelines, risk prediction was significantly enhanced. Resting heart rate levels can, in some cases, change survival predictions by years according to this study. Each of these studies provides some additional information about the impact of COPD as a comorbidity on management or survival. The better we understand these interactions, the easier it will be to treat our COPD patients.

J. R. Maurer, MD

References

1. Almassi GH, Shroyer AL, Collins JF, et al. Chronic obstructive pulmonary disease impact upon outcomes: the veterans affairs randomized on/off bypass trial. *Ann Thorac Surg*. 2013;96:1302-1309.
2. Gunter RL, Kilgo P, Guyton RA, et al. Impact of preoperative chronic lung disease on survival after surgical aortic valve replacement. *Ann Thorac Surg*. 2013;96: 1322-1328.
3. Stone DH, Goodney PP, Kalish J, et al. Vascular Study Group of New England. Severity of chronic obstructive pulmonary disease is associated with adverse outcomes in patients undergoing elective abdominal aortic aneurysm repair. *J Vasc Surg*. 2013;57:1531-1536.
4. Brenner S, Guder G, Berliner D, et al. Airway obstruction in systolic heart failure—COPD or congestion? *Int J Cardiol*. 2013;168:1910-1916.
5. Jensen MT, Marott JL, Lange P, et al. Resting heart rate is a predictor of mortality in COPD. *Eur Respir J*. 2013;42:341-349.

Chronic Pain and Pain Medication Use in Chronic Obstructive Pulmonary Disease: A Cross-Sectional Study

Roberts MH, Mapel DW, Hartry A, et al (Health Services Res Division, Albuquerque, NM; Health Economics & Outcomes Res, Malvern, PA)

Ann Am Thorac Soc 10:290-298, 2013

Rationale.—Pain is a common problem for patients with chronic obstructive pulmonary disease (COPD). However, pain is minimally discussed in COPD management guidelines.

Objectives.—The objective of this study was to describe chronic pain prevalence among patients with COPD compared with similar patients with other chronic diseases in a managed care population in the southwestern United States (age ≥ 40 yr).

Methods.—Using data for the period January 1, 2006 through December 31, 2010, patients with COPD were matched to two control subjects without COPD but with another chronic illness based on age, sex, insurance, and healthcare encounter type. Odds ratios (OR) for evidence of chronic pain were estimated using conditional logistic regression. Pulmonary function data for 200 randomly selected patients with COPD were abstracted.

Measurements and Main Results.—Retrospectively analyzed recurrent pain-related utilization (diagnoses and treatment) was considered evidence of chronic pain. The study sample comprised 7,952 patients with COPD (mean age, 69 yr; 42% male) and 15,904 patients with other chronic diseases (non-COPD). Patients with COPD compared with non-COPD patients had a higher percentage of chronic pain (59.8 vs. 51.7%; $P < 0.001$), chronic use of pain-related medications (41.2 vs. 31.5%; $P < 0.001$), and chronic use of short-acting (24.2 vs. 15.1%; $P < 0.001$) and long-acting opioids (4.4 vs.

1.9%; $P < 0.001$) compared with non-COPD patients. In conditional logistic regression models, adjusting for age, sex, Hispanic ethnicity, and comorbidities, patients with COPD had higher odds of chronic pain (OR, 1.56; 95% confidence interval [CI], 1.43–1.71), chronic use of pain-related medications (OR, 1.60; 95% CI, 1.46–1.74), and chronic use of short-acting or long-acting opioids (OR, 1.74; 95% CI, 1.57–1.92).

Conclusions.—Chronic pain and opioid use are prevalent among adults with COPD. This finding was not explained by the burden of comorbidity.

▶ Anxiety and depression have been shown to be prevalent in nearly half of all patients with chronic obstructive pulmonary disease (COPD) and significantly impact quality of life in that population. The increasing attention to these mood disorders has prompted numerous studies in the last few years so that patients are now routinely screened, and many get appropriate interventions. Pain, especially chronic pain, is much less often associated with COPD; most patients are not systematically assessed for pain. However, a few studies suggest that pain may be quite common in these patients and that, on average, they are more apt to be using more narcotics than age-matched controls.[1] Interestingly, there is virtually no discussion of pain assessment or approaches to treatment in COPD guidelines.[2] Pain can be a major factor in the development of anxiety and depression and in impaired quality of life. The risk for pain in these patients may be more related to the multiple comorbidities that are related to smoking, for example, cardiac disease and osteoporosis. The current cross-sectional study sought to better define the prevalence of pain, risk factors for pain, and the use of pain medications. In almost 8000 COPD patients, this study confirmed the high rates of pain when compared with almost 16 000 people with other chronic illnesses (Fig 1 in the original article). More COPD patients complained of pain and had higher use of narcotic pain medications as had been noted previously; the COPD patients range across the spectrum of airflow obstruction. The types of pain were primarily inflammatory and mechanical/compressive back pain. Adding pain into the mix with mood disorders undoubtedly reduces further the quality of life for COPD patients and may even impact survival. Very little is known about the best approaches to management of pain in this population, the risk factors, or preventive strategies.

This poorly studied and rarely discussed area deserves attention in clinical trials aimed at an overall better understanding and improved outcomes.

J. R. Maurer, MD

References

1. Blinderman CD, Homel P, Billings JA, Tennstedt S, Portenoy RK. Symptom distress and quality of life in patients with advanced chronic obstructive pulmonary disease. *J Pain Symptom Manage.* 2009;38:115-123.
2. Gold. Global strategy for the diagnosis, management, and prevention of copd, global initiative for chronic obstructive lung disease (GOLD). www.goldcopd.org. Accessed January 8, 2014.

COPD Surveillance—United States, 1999-2011

Ford ES, Croft JB, Mannino DM, et al (Ctrs for Disease Control and Prevention, Atlanta, GA; Univ of Kentucky College of Public Health, Lexington)
Chest 144:284-305, 2013

This report updates surveillance results for COPD in the United States. For 1999 to 2011, data from national data systems for adults aged ≥25 years were analyzed. In 2011, 6.5% of adults (approximately 13.7 million) reported having been diagnosed with COPD. From 1999 to 2011, the overall age-adjusted prevalence of having been diagnosed with COPD declined (P =.019). In 2010, there were 10.3 million (494.8 per 10,000) physician office visits, 1.5 million (72.0 per 10,000) ED visits, and 699,000 (32.2 per 10,000) hospital discharges for COPD. From 1999 to 2010, no significant overall trends were noted for physician office visits and ED visits; however, the age-adjusted hospital discharge rate for COPD declined significantly (P =.001). In 2010 there were 312,654 (11.2 per 1,000) Medicare hospital discharge claims submitted for COPD. Medicare claims (1999-2010) declined overall (P =.045), among men (P =.022) and among enrollees aged 65 to 74 years (P =.033). There were 133,575 deaths (63.1 per 100,000) from COPD in 2010. The overall age-adjusted death rate for COPD did not change during 1999 to 2010 (P =.163). Death rates (1999-2010) increased among adults aged 45 to 54 years (P < .001) and among American Indian/Alaska Natives (P =.008) but declined among those aged 55 to 64 years (P =.002) and 65 to 74 years (P < .001), Hispanics (P =.038), Asian/Pacific Islanders (P < .001), and men (P =.001). Geographic clustering of prevalence, Medicare hospitalizations, and deaths were observed. Declines in the age-adjusted prevalence, death rate in men, and hospitalizations for COPD since 1999 suggest progress in the prevention of COPD in the United States.

▶ In 2002 the Centers for Disease Control released its first chronic obstructive pulmonary disease (COPD) surveillance report. It was recognition of the increasing burden of this disease in the United States population and the cost of managing the disease. That report included disease prevalence, data about hospitalizations, outpatient visits, emergency room visits, and mortality. By 2008, chronic lower respiratory diseases, of which the principal component is COPD, became the third most common cause of death in the United States. This happened primarily because deaths from cerebrovascular disease, previously number 3, have continued a steady decline over a number of years.[1] In 2008, it was estimated that the direct economic cost of COPD and asthma was almost $54 billion per year including prescription medications (largest component at $20.4 billion); outpatient, emergency, and hospital stays; and home health care. The information presented in this report is expanded considerably. For the report, a large group of data sources were accessed. These included Behavioral Risk Factor Surveillance System (BRFSS), National Health Interview Survey, National Ambulatory Medical Care Survey, National Hospital Ambulatory Medical Care Survey, National Hospital Discharge Survey, death certificates from the National Vital Statistics

System, and Medicare Part A hospital claims administrative data. The primary message of the report is a slight decrease in death rate for men and a decrease in hospitalization rates in both men and women since 1999. Another 2013 study using Medicare data reported a decrease in respiratory hospitalizations from 58 to 44 per 100 person-years, while the prevalence of COPD in Medicare patients did not change; in addition, the rate of hospitalization for multiple COPD exacerbations also decreased.[2] These changes may be related to the ongoing decline in smoking in this country. Between 1965 and 2010, in both men and women, the number of smokers decreased by half—to 21.5% in men and 17.3% in women. Or it may be a combination of the decline in smoking, increased awareness of COPD, and better management. No matter what the cause, this is a glimmer of hope in the war against COPD.

J. R. Maurer, MD

References

1. Minino AM, Xu J, Kochanek KD. Division of Vital Statistics. Deaths: preliminary data for 2008. *Natl Vital Stat Rep*. 2010;59:1-52.
2. Baillargeon J, Wang Y, Kuo YF, Holmes HM, Sharma G. Temporal trends in hospitalization rates for older adults with chronic obstructive pulmonary disease. *Am J Med*. 2013;126:607-613.

A meta-analysis on the prophylactic use of macrolide antibiotics for the prevention of disease exacerbations in patients with Chronic Obstructive Pulmonary Disease

Donath E, Chaudhry A, Hernandez-Aya LF, et al (Univ of Miami Miller School of Medicine – Regional Campus, Atlantis, FL; Univ of Michigan School of Medicine, Ann Arbor; et al)

Respir Med 107:1385-1392, 2013

Introduction.—Macrolides are of unique interest in preventing COPD exacerbations because they possess a variety of antibacterial, antiviral and anti-inflammatory properties. Recent research has generated renewed interest in prophylactic macrolides to reduce the risk of COPD exacerbations. Little is known about how well these recent findings fit within the context of previous research on this subject. The purpose of this article is to evaluate, via exploratory meta-analysis, whether the overall consensus favors prophylactic macrolides for prevention of COPD exacerbations.

Methods.—EMBASE, Cochrane and Medline databases were searched for all relevant randomized controlled trials (RCTs). Six RCTs were identified. The primary endpoint was incidence of COPD exacerbations. Secondary endpoints including mortality, hospitalization rates, adverse events and likelihood of having at least one COPD exacerbation were also examined.

Results.—There was a 37% relative risk reduction (RR = 0.63, 95% CI: 0.45–0.87, *p* value = 0.005) in COPD exacerbations among patients taking macrolides compared to placebo. Furthermore, there was a 21% reduced risk of hospitalization (RR = 0.79, 95% CI: 0.69–0.90, *p*-value = 0.01) and 68% reduced risk of having at least one COPD exacerbation (RR = 0.34, 95% CI 0.21–0.54, *p*-value = 0.001) among patients taking macrolides versus placebo. There was also a trend toward decreased mortality and increased adverse events among patients taking macrolides but these were not statistically significant.

Conclusions.—Prophylactic macrolides are an effective approach for reducing incident COPD exacerbations. There were several limitations to this study including a lack of consistent adverse event reporting and some degree of clinical and statistical heterogeneity between studies.

▶ Macrolide antibiotics are unique among antibiotics because of their multiple types of activity. They are also antiviral and, particularly, immunomodulatory. These multiple actions have resulted in their use in a wide variety of circumstances, including the successful treatment of panbronchiolitis and prevention of cystic fibrosis exacerbations as well as reduction in development of bronchiolitis obliterans syndrome in lung transplant patients. It has also been used to prevent chronic obstructive pulmonary disease (COPD) exacerbations. Clinical trials have been conducted in each of these diseases, usually with success in reducing symptoms, preventing acute events, or generally improving patient quality of life. Probably the most cited trial in COPD was a multicenter study published in 2011. Albert et al[1] reported in a placebo-controlled trial that patients taking daily azithromycin had a longer period to first exacerbation; however, some hearing loss side effects were reported in this study. What remained unclear was the impact of potential development of microbial resistance patterns using a continuous prophylaxis regimen such as this. The meta-analysis presented here reviews the Albert et al[1] trial, but also 6 other randomized, controlled trials to assess consistency in findings. The authors found that all but one of the studies reported a reduction in COPD exacerbations when using prophylactic macrolides. However, this benefit is offset by adverse events. The one measure of adverse events that was relatively constant—and relatively common—across trials was discontinuation of the trial because of the adverse event. The authors found it difficult to capture the emergence of antibiotic resistance, although they note this is a worldwide concern. The evidence for reduction of acute exacerbations is compelling; however, the literal cost and the cost in adverse events and resistance are considerable. This argues for studies to assess different approaches in a robust, controlled way, such as intermittent administration or administration of lower doses of drug.

J. R. Maurer, MD

Reference

1. Albert R, Connett J, Bailey W, et al. Azithromycin for prevention of exacerbations of COPD. *N Engl J Med.* 2011;365:689-698.

High-Dose N-Acetylcysteine in Stable COPD: The 1-Year, Double-Blind, Randomized, Placebo-Controlled HIACE Study

Tse HN, Raiteri L, Wong KY, et al (Kwong Wah Hosp, Hong Kong, China; Wong Tai Sin Hosp, Hong Kong, China; Zambon Company SpA, Bresso, Italy)

Chest 144:106-118, 2013

Background.—The mucolytic and antioxidant effects of N-acetylcysteine (NAC) may have great value in COPD treatment. However, beneficial effects have not been confirmed in clinical studies, possibly due to insufficient NAC doses and/or inadequate outcome parameters used. The objective of this study was to investigate high-dose NAC plus usual therapy in Chinese patients with stable COPD.

Methods.—The 1-year HIACE (The Effect of High Dose N-acetylcysteine on Air Trapping and Airway Resistance of Chronic Obstructive Pulmonary Disease—a Double-blinded, Randomized, Placebo-controlled Trial) double-blind trial conducted in Kwong Wah Hospital, Hong Kong, randomized eligible patients aged 50 to 80 years with stable COPD to NAC 600 mg bid or placebo after 4-week run-in. Lung function parameters, symptoms, modified Medical Research Council (mMRC) dyspnea and St. George's Respiratory Questionnaire (SGRQ) scores, 6-min walking distance (6MWD), and exacerbation and admission rates were measured at baseline and every 16 weeks for 1 year.

Results.—Of 133 patients screened, 120 were eligible (93.2% men; mean age, 70.8 ± 0.74 years; %FEV_1 53.9 ± 2.0%). Baseline characteristics were similar in the two groups. At 1 year, there was a significant improvement in forced expiratory flow 25% to 75% ($P = .037$) and forced oscillation technique, a significant reduction in exacerbation frequency (0.96 times/y vs 1.71 times/y, $P = .019$), and a tendency toward reduction in admission rate (0.5 times/y vs 0.8 times/y, $P = .196$) with NAC vs placebo. There were no significant between-group differences in mMRC dypsnea score, SGRQ score, and 6MWD. No major adverse effects were reported.

Conclusion.—In this study, 1-year treatment with high-dose NAC resulted in significantly improved small airways function and decreased exacerbation frequency in patients with stable COPD.

Trial Registry.—ClinicalTrials.gov; No.: NCT01136239; URL: www.clinicaltrials.gov.

▶ N-acetyl cysteine (NAC) has for decades been considered a potential treatment in obstructive lung disease and other lung diseases. Not only is it a mucolytic, it also has antioxidant and anti-inflammatory properties. It scavenges reactive oxygen species and is a precursor of reduced glutathione. However, previous clinical trials assessing NAC treatment of chronic obstructive pulmonary disease (COPD) has been inconsistent. A Cochrane systematic review of 30 studies and a meta-analysis suggested a small, but inconsistent, benefit of NAC in reducing exacerbations[1,2]; however, the 3-year Bronchitis Randomized On NAC Cost-Utility Study (BRONCUS), which was a double-blinded randomized, controlled study, did not show either a reduction of exacerbations or an improvement in flow rates.[3] The Chinese investigators conducting the current study reasoned that the BRONCUS study may have been negative because (1) the dose of NAC used was too small or (2) no tool was used to measure small airway function and, therefore, measurements were not sensitive enough to actually detect the impact of the treatment. So they used more than twice the dose of NAC than BRONCUS investigators did, and they implemented 2 small airway measurements: forced expiratory flow 25 to 75 and forced external oscillation, which can detect airflow in the small airways. This was a relatively small study with a total of 120 patients and 58 in the NAC arm. Although the authors were able to show a significant difference in the rate of exacerbations and small airway function (barely), they were unable to show a difference in hospitalizations or other functional parameters. This leaves in question the clinical significance of the findings. Although intriguing, the use of NAC at this high dosage requires a larger, longer study to justify its place in COPD management.

J. R. Maurer, MD

References

1. Poole P, Black PN. Mucolytic agents for chronic bronchitis or chronic obstructive pulmonary disease. *Cochrane Database syst Rev.* 2010;(2):CD001287.
2. Grandjean EM, Berthet P, Ruffmann R, Leuenberger P. Efficacy of oral long-term N-acetylcysteine in chronic bronchopulmonary disease: a meta-analysis of published double-blind, placebo-controlled clinical trials. *Clin Ther.* 2000;22: 209-221.
3. Decramer M, Rutten-van Molken M, Dekhuijzen PN, et al. Effects of N-acetylcysteine on outcomes in chronic obstructive pulmonary disease (Bronchitis Randomized on NAC Cost-Utility Study, BRONCUS): a randomised placebo-controlled trial. *Lancet.* 2005;365:1552-1560.

Statin Use and Risk of COPD Exacerbation Requiring Hospitalization

Wang M-T, Lo Y-W, Tsai C-L, et al (School of Pharmacy, Taipei, Taiwan, Republic of China; Natl Defense Med Ctr, Taipei, Taiwan, Republic of China; et al)
Am J Med 126:598-606.e2, 2013

Background.—Despite recent studies that suggested statins' beneficial effects on chronic obstructive pulmonary disease (COPD) outcomes, the impact, if any, of statins on COPD exacerbations remains unclear. This study aimed to examine the association between statin use and risk of hospitalized COPD exacerbation, and to assess whether the association varied by statin initiation, dose, or duration of use.

Methods.—A retrospective nested case-control study among patients with COPD was conducted analyzing a nationwide health insurance claims database in Taiwan. Cases were subjects hospitalized for COPD exacerbations; each case was matched to 4 randomly selected controls on age, sex, cohort entry, and number of COPD-related outpatient visits by an incident-density sampling approach. Conditional logistic regressions were employed to quantify the COPD exacerbation risk associated with statin use.

Results.—The study cohort comprised 14,316 COPD patients, from which 1584 cases with COPD exacerbations and 5950 matched controls were identified. Any use of statins was associated with a 30% decreased risk of COPD exacerbation (95% confidence interval [CI], 0.56-0.88), and current use of statins was related to a greater reduced risk (adjusted odds ratio [OR] 0.60; 95% CI, 0.44-0.81). A dose-dependent reduced risk of COPD exacerbation by statins was observed (medium average daily dose: adjusted OR 0.60; 95% CI, 0.41-0.89; high daily dose: adjusted OR 0.33; 95% CI, 0.14-0.73). The reduced risk remained significant for either short or long duration of statin use.

Conclusions.—Statin use was associated with a reduced risk of COPD exacerbation, with a further risk reduction for statins prescribed more recently or at high doses.

▶ Several publications in the last 10 years purportedly showed a significant benefit of statins in reducing the rates of chronic obstructive pulmonary disease (COPD) exacerbations by as much as 40% and even have shown a substantial decreased mortality risk.[1,2] The proposed reasons for this impact are anti-inflammatory and immunomodulary effects, which have been identified both in human and in animal models.[3,4] In some cases, this seems to be a greater benefit than the commonly used inhaled medications that are recommended in major COPD management guidelines.[5] In the 2013 edition of the Global Initiative for Chronic Obstructive Lung Disease guidelines, one paragraph is devoted to immunomodulary drugs (not statins) and does not make any recommendations for their use.[5] Certainly, the lack of attention to statins cannot be because of adverse side effects or cost: Statins are one of the most widely used drugs for control of cholesterol in the world, and generic versions are much lower in cost than many of the pulmonary inhaled medications. The reasons that statins have not been incorporated into the armamentarium of COPD management are probably best stated by 1 of 2 systematic reviews that both came to the same general conclusion: "...the majority of published studies have inherent methodological limitations of retrospective studies and population-based analyses. There is a need for prospective interventional trials designed specifically to assess the impact of statins on clinically relevant outcomes in COPD."[6,7] The study abstracted here is not that definitive prospective study; it is a study based on information from a nationwide health insurance database of pharmacy and medical encounters. The authors were able to study more than 14 000 COPD patients during the period from January 2000 through December 2008. Again, there was a strong association between statin use and reduced exacerbations. But is this relationship causal? We continue to await that definitive prospective trial.

J. R. Maurer, MD

References

1. Blamoun AI, Batty GN, DeBari VA, Rashid AO, Sheikh M, Khan MA. Statins may reduce episodes of exacerbation and the requirement for intubation in patients with COPD: evidence from a retrospective cohort study. *Int J Clin Pract*. 2008; 62:1373-1378.

2. Mancini GB, Etminan M, Zhang B, Levesque LE, FitzGerald JM, Brophy JM. Reduction of morbidity and mortality by statins, angiotensin-converting enzyme inhibitors, and angiotensin receptor blockers in patients with chronic obstructive pulmonary disease. *J Am Coll Cardiol.* 2006;47:2554-2560.
3. Takahashi S, Nakamura H, Seki M, et al. Reversal of elastase-induced pulmonary emphysema and promotion of alveolar epithelial cell proliferation by simvastatin in mice. *Am J Physiol Lung Cell Mol Physiol.* 2008;294:L882-L890.
4. Arnaud C, Veillard NR, Mach F. Cholesterol-independent effects of statins in inflammation, immunomodulation and atherosclerosis. *Curr Drug Targets Cardiovasc Haematol Disord.* 2005;5:127-134.
5. Gold. Global strategy for the diagnosis, management, and prevention of COPD, global initiative for chronic obstructive lung disease (GOLD). www.goldcopd.org. Accessed January 8, 2014.
6. Dobler CC, Wong KK, Marks GB. Associations between statins and COPD: a systematic review. *BMC Pulm Med.* 2009;9:32.
7. Janda S, Park K, FitzGerald JM, Etminan M, Swiston J. Statins in COPD: a systematic review. *Chest.* 2009;136:734-743.

Predictors of Mortality in Hospitalized Adults with Acute Exacerbation of Chronic Obstructive Pulmonary Disease: A Systematic Review and Meta-analysis

Singanayagam A, Schembri S, Chalmers JD (St. Mary's Hosp, London, UK; Ninewells Hosp, Dundee, Scotland, UK)
Ann Am Thorac Soc 10:81-89, 2013

Rationale.—There is a need to identify clinically meaningful predictors of mortality following hospitalized COPD exacerbation.

Objectives.—The aim of this study was to systematically review the literature to identify clinically important factors that predict mortality after hospitalization for acute exacerbation of chronic obstructive pulmonary disease (COPD).

Methods.—Eligible studies considered adults admitted to hospital with COPD exacerbation. Two authors independently abstracted data. Odds ratios were then calculated by comparing the prevalence of each predictor in survivors versus nonsurvivors. For continuous variables, mean differences were pooled by the inverse of their variance, using a random effects model.

Measurements and Main Results.—There were 37 studies included (189,772 study subjects) with risk of death ranging from 3.6% for studies considering short-term mortality, 31.0% for long-term mortality (up to 2 yr after hospitalization), and 29.0% for studies that considered solely intensive care unit (ICU)–admitted study subjects. Twelve prognostic factors (age, male sex, low body mass index, cardiac failure, chronic renal failure, confusion, long-term oxygen therapy, lower limb edema, Global Initiative for Chronic Lung Disease criteria stage 4, cor pulmonale, acidemia, and elevated plasma troponin level) were significantly associated with increased short-term mortality. Nine prognostic factors (age, low body mass index, cardiac failure, diabetes mellitus, ischemic heart disease, malignancy, FEV_1, long-term oxygen therapy, and PaO_2 on admission) were significantly associated with long-term mortality. Three factors (age, low Glasgow Coma Scale score, and pH) were significantly associated with increased risk of mortality in ICU-admitted study subjects.

Conclusion.—Different factors correlate with mortality from COPD exacerbation in the short term, long term, and after ICU admission. These parameters may be useful to develop tools for prediction of outcome in clinical practice.

▶ Exacerbations are serious events in the life of a patient with chronic obstructive pulmonary disease (COPD). Not only might they presage an ongoing decline in lung function and worsening quality of life, but they also bring an increased risk of short-term and long-term mortality. Community-acquired pneumonia (CAP) is also a serious event, particularly in the life of an elderly patient also potentially with negative impacts on survival and postpneumonia morbidity. Unlike COPD exacerbations, however, tools have been developed that are used to predict, at the time of presentation of patients with CAP, the prognosis of that particular patient. Those tools not only provide information for the patient and the physician; they also help to determine the most appropriate approach to care. Pulmonary physicians have recently recognized the need to develop tools such as those that exist for CAP; however, before the tools can be designed, it is necessary to sort through existing evidence to determine if there is adequate information about risk factors in specific populations of COPD patients (for example, differing phenotypes) to develop useable tools. That was the purpose of this meta-analysis. The authors were successful in identifying from 37 studies, 12 short-term risk factors and 9 long-term risk factors. This is a great first step toward developing predictive tools. The next steps are harder, that is, to simplify the factors (eliminate those that add little, for example) to the extent they can be easily used by primary care and emergency department physicians and to properly weight the chosen factors to provide valuable prognostic and management guidance.

J. R. Maurer, MD

33 Community-Acquired Pneumonia

Functional Disability, Cognitive Impairment, and Depression After Hospitalization for Pneumonia

Davydow DS, Hough CL, Levine DA, et al (Univ of Washington, Seattle; Univ of Michigan, Ann Arbor)

Am J Med 126:615-624, 2013

Objective.—The study objective was to examine whether hospitalization for pneumonia is associated with functional decline, cognitive impairment, and depression, and to compare this impairment with that seen after known disabling conditions, such as myocardial infarction or stroke.

Methods.—We used data from a prospective cohort of 1434 adults aged more than 50 years who survived 1711 hospitalizations for pneumonia, myocardial infarction, or stroke drawn from the Health and Retirement Study (1998-2010). Main outcome measures included the number of Activities and Instrumental Activities of Daily Living requiring assistance and the presence of cognitive impairment and substantial depressive symptoms.

Results.—Hospitalization for pneumonia was associated with 1.01 new impairments in Activities and Instrumental Activities of Daily Living (95% confidence interval [CI], 0.71-1.32) among patients without baseline functional impairment and 0.99 new impairments in Activities and Instrumental Activities of Daily Living (95% CI, 0.57-1.41) among those with mild-to-moderate baseline limitations, as well as moderate-to-severe cognitive impairment (odds ratio, 2.46; 95% CI, 1.60-3.79) and substantial depressive symptoms (odds ratio, 1.63; 95% CI, 1.06-2.51). Patients without baseline functional impairment who survived pneumonia hospitalization had more subsequent impairments in Activities and Instrumental Activities of Daily Living than those who survived myocardial infarction hospitalization. There were no significant differences in subsequent moderate-to-severe cognitive impairment or substantial depressive symptoms between patients who survived myocardial infarction or stroke and those who survived pneumonia.

Conclusions.—Hospitalization for pneumonia in older adults is associated with subsequent functional and cognitive impairment. Improved pneumonia prevention and interventions to ameliorate adverse sequelae during and after hospitalization may improve outcomes.

▶ Hospitalizations for chronic conditions in elderly patients are often associated with an overall worsening of their baseline state—a lower level of physical functionality after discharge as well as possible cognitive decline. Community-acquired pneumonia (CAP), however, is typically considered a discrete illness that is treatable and usually resolves completely. However, it is unknown whether the insult of pneumonia transiently or permanently impacts the functional or mental baseline state of the elderly patient. This is an important question because pneumonia is extremely common in an aging population, and the health care system will need to plan for the impact of postpneumonia impairment if it is a common problem. The Davydow study is a longitudinal study that suggests that not only does such impairment occur, it may actually be worse than the declines observed after hospitalization for some chronic illnesses. In a second study published this year, Shah et al[1] showed that patients with even mild cognitive changes are more likely to develop pneumonia than patients without cognitive changes: patients with even mild cognitive changes often had accelerated changes after the pneumonia episode. With around 390 000 hospitalizations per year in older patients[2] and an anticipated near doubling of that number in around 25 years, it is very important to further study the postpneumonia status of elderly patients with an eye toward prevention and early intervention.

J. R. Maurer, MD

References

1. Shah FA, Pike F, Alvarez K, et al. Bidirectional relationship between cognitive function and pneumonia. *Am J Resp Crit Care Med.* 2013;188:586-592.
2. Thomas CP, Ryan M, Chapman JD, et al. Incidence and cost of pneumonia in medicare beneficiaries. *Chest.* 2012;142:973-981.

Readmission Following Hospitalization for Pneumonia: The Impact of Pneumonia Type and Its Implication for Hospitals

Shorr AF, Zilberberg MD, Reichley R, et al (Washington Hosp Ctr, DC; EviMed Research Group, LLC, Goshen, MA; Barnes-Jewish Hosp, St Louis, MO)

Clin Infect Dis 57:362-367, 2013

Background.—Readmission rates following discharge after pneumonia are thought to represent the quality of care. Factors associated with readmission, however, remain poorly described. It is unclear if readmission rates vary based on pneumonia type.

Methods.—We retrospectively identified adults admitted to an index hospital with non-nosocomial pneumonia (January through December 2010) and who survived to discharge. We only included patients with bacterial evidence of infection. Readmission in the 30 days following discharge to any of 9 hospitals comprising the index hospital's healthcare system served as the primary end point. We recorded demographics, severity of illness, comorbidities, and infection-related factors. We noted whether the patient had healthcare-associated pneumonia (HCAP) versus community-acquired pneumonia. We utilized logistic regression analysis to determine factors independently associated with readmission.

Results.—The cohort included 977 subjects; 78.9% survived to discharge. The readmission rate equaled 20%. Neither disease severity nor the rate of initially inappropriate antibiotic therapy correlated with readmission. Subjects with HCAP were 7.5 (95% confidence interval [CI], 3.6–15.7) times more likely to be readmitted. Four HCAP criteria were independently associated with readmission: admission from long-term care (adjusted odds ratio [AOR], 2.2 [95% CI, 1.4–3.4]); immunosuppression (AOR, 1.9 [95% CI, 1.3–2.9]); prior antibiotics (AOR, 1.7 [95% CI, 1.2–2.6]); and prior hospitalization (AOR, 1.7 [95% CI, 1.1–2.5]).

Conclusions.—Readmission for pneumonia is common but varies based on pneumonia type. The variables associated with readmission do not reflect factors that hospitals directly control. Use of one rule to guide payment that fails to account for HCAP and the HCAP criteria on readmission seems inappropriate.

▶ High rates of readmission for certain diseases such as pneumonia have been targeted by the Centers for Medicare and Medicaid Services (CMS) as areas for improvement. To try to reduce these rates, CMS supports improved transitions in care and has implemented reduced payments for hospitals that have excessive readmission rates for acute myocardial infarctions, congestive heart failure, and pneumonia. COPD exacerbations and arthroplasties will be added to the CMS excess readmission program in fiscal year 2015. One of the challenges for physicians and hospitals is that there are few studies that identify the specific risk factors for readmission. A better understanding of the patients most likely to require readmission could be valuable on 2 fronts: It could help the providers better prepare a posthospitalization environment for the patient (eg, home care, multiple calls or visits) and help CMS better risk-adjust for hospitals that have high-risk discharges. This study tries to identify these risks with a retrospective analysis. The authors note that studies from outside the United States identify a lower readmission rate than that seen in US hospitals and suggest that "healthcare system organization and structure may be an important contributor to readmission rates." That is likely true. Other systems often have a better care transition structure. A valuable addition to this analysis would be a prospective study in which specific interventions designed for the high-risk readmission patients identified here were implemented at discharge to ensure adequate care in the early postdischarge timeframe.

J. R. Maurer, MD

Inhaled corticosteroids in COPD and the risk of serious pneumonia

Suissa S, Patenaude V, Lapi F, et al (McGill Univ, Montreal, Québec, Canada)
Thorax 68:1029-1036, 2013

Background.—Inhaled corticosteroids (ICS) are known to increase the risk of pneumonia in patients with chronic obstructive pulmonary disease (COPD). It is unclear whether the risk of pneumonia varies for different inhaled agents, particularly fluticasone and budesonide, and increases with the dose and long-term duration of use.

Methods.—We formed a new-user cohort of patients with COPD treated during 1990–2005. Subjects were identified using the Quebec health insurance databases and followed through 2007 or until a serious pneumonia event, defined as a first hospitalisation for or death from pneumonia. A nested case–control analysis was used to estimate the rate ratio (RR) of serious pneumonia associated with current ICS use, adjusted for age, sex, respiratory disease severity and comorbidity.

Results.—The cohort included 163 514 patients, of which 20 344 had a serious pneumonia event during the 5.4 years of follow-up (incidence rate 2.4/100/year). Current use of ICS was associated with a 69% increase in the rate of serious pneumonia (RR 1.69; 95% CI 1.63 to 1.75). The risk was sustained with long-term use and declined gradually after stopping ICS use, disappearing after 6 months (RR 1.08; 95% CI 0.99 to 1.17). The rate of serious pneumonia was higher with fluticasone (RR 2.01; 95% CI 1.93 to 2.10), increasing with the daily dose, but was much lower with budesonide (RR 1.17; 95% CI 1.09 to 1.26).

Conclusions.—ICS use by patients with COPD increases the risk of serious pneumonia. The risk is particularly elevated and dose related with fluticasone. While residual confounding cannot be ruled out, the results are consistent with those from recent randomised trials.

► Several studies have suggested that inhaled corticosteroids are associated with an increased risk of bacterial pneumonia in chronic obstructive pulmonary disorder (COPD) patients. Two large multicenter clinical treatment trials, the TORCH (Toward a Revolution in COPD Health) trial and the INSPIRE (Investigating New Standards for Prophylaxis in Reduction of Exacerbations) trial studied inhaled corticosteroids as part of 1 of 2 treatment arms for COPD. TORCH was a trial comparing inhaled fluticasone/salmeterol with placebo and the primary endpoint was mortality.[1] A secondary endpoint was morbidity related to exacerbations. INSPIRE was a trial comparing tiotropium and fluticasone/salmeterol in terms of efficacy with respect to exacerbations.[2] However, in both these studies, an adverse event finding in the analysis was an excess number of pneumonias in patients in the study arms in which inhaled corticosteroids were used—even though in both cases the absolute numbers of pneumonias were small. Subsequent meta-analysis on multiple studies evaluating inhaled corticosteroids in COPD have found mixed results of the impact of inhaled corticosteroids.[3,4] It has been speculated that part of this inconsistency may be caused by a differential effect of various inhaled corticosteroids. In this study, the authors assessed the Quebec population database of COPD patients and confirmed that the population using inhaled corticosteroids had a higher rate of pneumonia, but probably more importantly, they found that fluticasone use created the highest risk and was dose-related, particularly compared with budesonide (the second most commonly used inhaled corticosteroid). This is consistent with both TORCH and INSPIRE in which the steroid used was fluticasone. Whether the difference between fluticasone and budesonide is real requires further evaluation. Of note, one of the meta-analyses found no increase in pneumonia with the use of inhaled corticosteroids evaluated budesonide, not fluticasone.[4] Fluticasone is generally considered a more potent drug and has a longer half-life, but its association with pneumonias may also be because it is used more often than budesonide in this population and possibly across a population of more severely ill patients.

J. R. Maurer, MD

References

1. Calverley PM, Anderson JA, Celli B, et al. Salmeterol and fluticasone propionate and survival in chronic obstructive pulmonary disease. *N Engl J Med.* 2007;356: 775-789.
2. Calverley PM, Stockley PA, Seemungal TA, et al. Reported pneumonia in patients with COPD: findings from the INSPIRE study. *Chest.* 2011;139:505-512.
3. Drummond MB, Dasenbrook EC, Pitz MW, Murphy DJ, Fan E. Inhaled corticosteroids in patients with stable chronic obstructive pulmonary disease: a systematic review and meta-analysis. *JAMA.* 2008;300:2407-2416.
4. Sin DD, Tashkin D, Zhang X, et al. Budesonide and the risk of pneumonia: a meta-analysis of individual patient data. *Lancet.* 2009;374:712-719.

34 Lung Transplantation

Lung Transplantation in Patients with Pretransplantation Donor-Specific Antibodies Detected by Luminex Assay

Brugière O, Suberbielle C, Thabut G, et al (Hôpital Bichat, Paris, France; et al)

Transplantation 95:761-765, 2013

Background.—New methods of solid-phase assays, such as Luminex assay, with high sensitivity in detecting anti–human leukocyte antigen (HLA) antibodies (Abs), have increased the proportion of sensitized candidates waiting for lung transplantation (LTx). However, how to apply these results clinically during graft allocation is debated: strict exclusion of candidates with Luminex-positive results can lead to lost opportunities for Tx. We retrospectively analyzed the clinical impact of pre-LTx Luminex-detected Abs on post-LTx outcomes for patients who underwent LTx before the availability of Luminex assay.

Methods.—We analyzed data for 56 successive patients who underwent LTx before 2008 and were considered to not have anti-HLA Abs by then-available methods of detection at the date of their LTx. Pre-LTx sera from these patients were retested by Luminex assay. Using log-rank test, freedom from bronchiolitis obliterans syndrome (BOS) and graft survival were compared between patients with and without pre-LTx Luminex-detected anti-HLA Abs classes I and II and donor-specific Abs (DSA) classes I and II.

Results.—Freedom from bronchiolitis obliterans syndrome was lower, and mortality was higher for patients with than those without pre-LTx Luminex-detected DSA class II ($P = 0.004$ and $P = 0.007$, respectively) but did not differ for patients with and without DSA class I or anti-HLA Abs class I or II.

Conclusions.—It suggests to avoid attributing graft with forbidden antigens to sensitized candidates with Luminex-detected DSA class II and to evaluate the role of specific posttransplantation protocols for LTx candidates who require emergency LTx.

▶ Preformed anti-human leukocyte (anti-HLA) antibodies in potential transplant recipients are a known risk for rejection and early mortality, particularly in renal transplantation. Patients with certain levels of antibodies are typically prematched against potential suitable donors to ensure compatibility or may be pretreated to remove antibodies. In recent years, the widespread availability of a much more sensitive assay for preformed antibodies, the Luminex assay, has shown that many—possibly as many as half of potential recipients—have some level of preformed anti-HLA antibodies. This has left many transplant centers with a perplexing question: How important are these antibodies in the outcomes of patients? Could they be responsible for some of the early graft dysfunction? What role, if any, do they contribute to long-term graft survival? And, if they do impact the graft, how important is that impact? This study starts to evaluate the potential impact of these antibodies, particularly on intermediate and later outcomes. These preliminary data suggest the antibodies impact outcomes; however, this retrospective study needs to be confirmed by a large, carefully designed prospective evaluation, as the outcome could have significant implications for donor and recipient matching.

J. R. Maurer, MD

35 Lung Cancer

Cancer Statistics, 2013
Siegel R, Naishadham D, Jemal A (American Cancer Society, Atlanta, GA)
CA Cancer J Clin 63:11-30, 2013

Each year, the American Cancer Society estimates the numbers of new cancer cases and deaths expected in the United States in the current year and compiles the most recent data on cancer incidence, mortality, and survival based on incidence data from the National Cancer Institute, the Centers for Disease Control and Prevention, and the North American Association of Central Cancer Registries and mortality data from the National Center for Health Statistics. A total of 1,660,290 new cancer

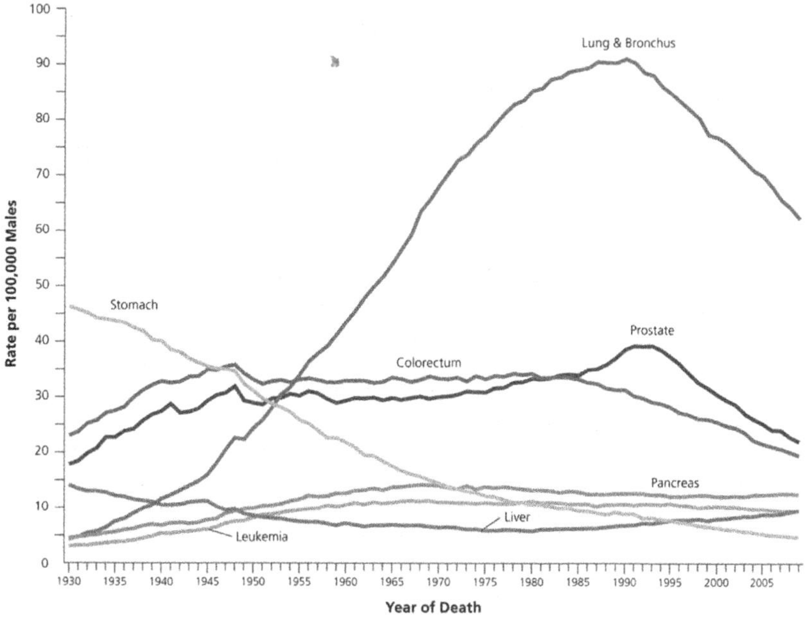

FIGURE 4.—Trends in Death Rates Among Males for Selected Cancers, United States, 1930 to 2009. Rates are age adjusted to the 2000 US standard population. Due to changes in International Classification of Diseases (ICD) coding, numerator information has changed over time. Rates for cancers of the lung and bronchus, colorectum, and liver are affected by these changes. (Reprinted from Siegel R, Naishadham D, Jemal A. Cancer statistics, 2013. *CA Cancer J Clin.* 2013;63:11-30, with permission from CA: A Cancer Journal for Clinicians and John Wiley and Sons, www.interscience.wiley.com.)

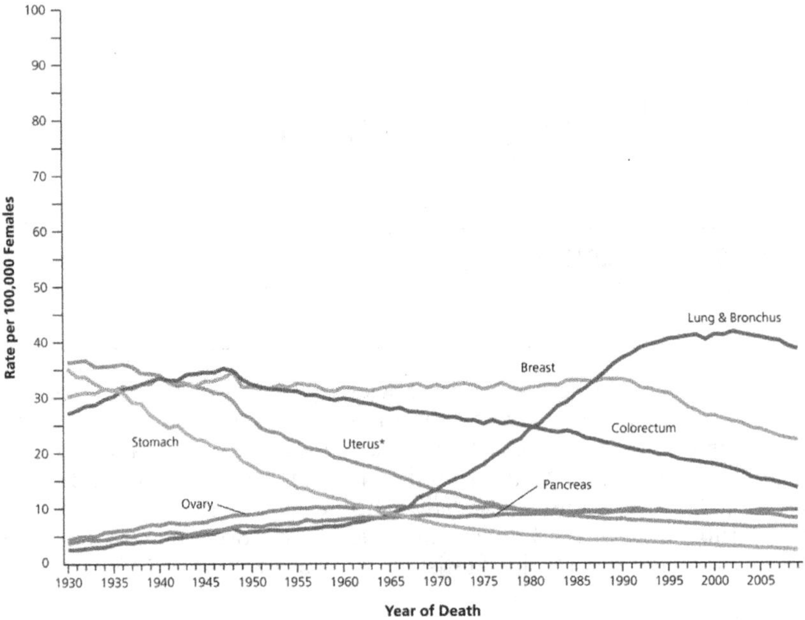

FIGURE 5.—Trends in Death Rates Among Females for Selected Cancers, United States, 1930 to 2009. Rates are age adjusted to the 2000 US standard population. Due to changes in International Classification of Diseases (ICD) coding, numerator information has changed over time. Rates for cancers of the uterus, ovary, lung and bronchus, and colorectum are affected by these changes. *Uterus includes uterine cervix and uterine corpus. (Reprinted from Siegel R, Naishadham D, Jemal A. Cancer statistics, 2013. *CA Cancer J Clin.* 2013;63:11-30, with permission from CA: A Cancer Journal for Clinicians and John Wiley and Sons, www.interscience.wiley.com.)

cases and 580,350 cancer deaths are projected to occur in the United States in 2013. During the most recent 5 years for which there are data (2005-2009), delay-adjusted cancer incidence rates declined slightly in men (by 0.6% per year) and were stable in women, while cancer death rates decreased by 1.8% per year in men and by 1.5% per year in women. Overall, cancer death rates have declined 20% from their peak in 1991 (215.1 per 100,000 population) to 2009 (173.1 per 100,000 population). Death rates continue to decline for all 4 major cancer sites (lung, colorectum, breast, and prostate). Over the past 10 years of data (2000-2009), the largest annual declines in death rates were for chronic myeloid leukemia (8.4%), cancers of the stomach (3.1%) and colorectum (3.0%), and non-Hodgkin lymphoma (3.0%). The reduction in overall cancer death rates since 1990 in men and 1991 in women translates to the avoidance of approximately 1.18 million deaths from cancer, with 152,900 of these deaths averted in 2009 alone. Further progress can be accelerated by applying existing cancer control knowledge across all segments of the

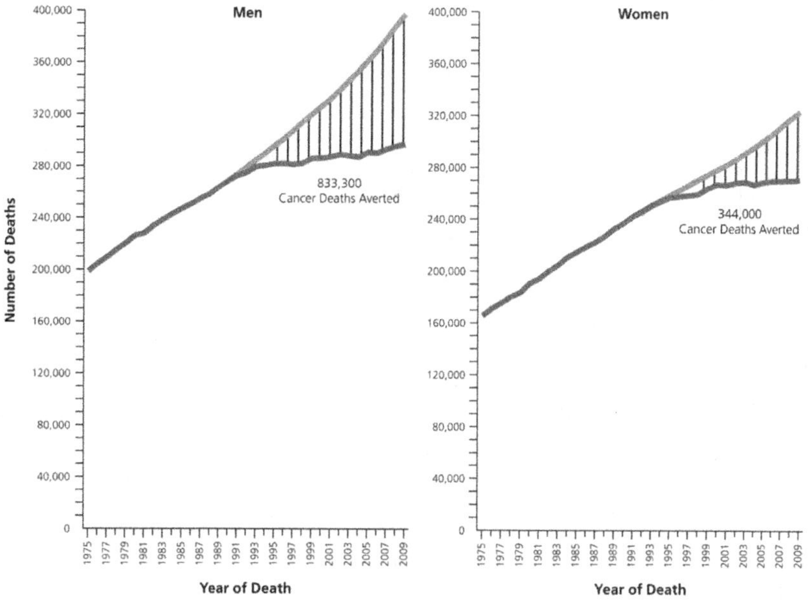

FIGURE 6.—Total Number of Cancer Deaths Averted From 1991 to 2009 in Men and From 1992 to 2009 in Women. The blue line represents the actual number of cancer deaths recorded in each year, and the red line represents the number of cancer deaths that would have been expected if cancer death rates had remained at their peak. For Interpretation of the references to color in this figure legend, the reader is referred to web version of this article. (Reprinted from Siegel R, Naishadham D, Jemal A. Cancer statistics, 2013. *CA Cancer J Clin.* 2013;63:11-30, with permission from CA: A Cancer Journal for Clinicians and John Wiley and Sons, www.interscience.wiley.com.)

population, with an emphasis on those groups in the lowest socioeconomic bracket and other underserved populations (Figs 4-6, Table 12).

▶ Lung cancer is the leading cause of cancer death in both men and women in the United States. In 2013, the American Cancer Society estimated that 87 260 men and 72 220 women died from lung cancer (total deaths 159 480). Lung cancer accounts for 28% of all male cancer deaths and 26% of all female cancer deaths. Although the mortality toll related to lung cancer still exceeds the next 3 leading causes of cancer death (breast, colorectal, and prostate cancers) combined, the good news is that these numbers in both sexes are less than in 2012. As can be seen in Fig 4, the lung cancer death rate in American men has been declining steadily since about 1990. Fig 5 shows that the lung cancer death rate curve in women is finally also bending downward. The 2 figures also point out that death from cancers in general are decreasing, with the total number of cancer deaths averted from 1991 to 2009 demonstrated in Fig 6.

Of all cancers, lung cancer has the largest variation in geographic distribution, which predominantly reflects the differences in smoking prevalence among states. Over the 5-year period from 2005 to 2009, age-adjusted lung cancer death rates in men and women in Kentucky were 128.2 and 55.5 per 100 000, respectively. In contrast, age-adjusted lung cancer death rates in men and women in Utah were 28.1 and 16.1 per 100 000, respectively. Table 12 shows

TABLE 12.—Trends in 5-Year Relative Survival Rates* (%) by Race and Year of Diagnosis, United States, 1975 to 2008

	All Races			White			African American		
	1975 TO 1977	1987 TO 1989	2002 TO 2008	1975 TO 1977	1987 TO 1989	2002 TO 2008	1975 TO 1977	1987 TO 1989	2002 TO 2008
All sites	49	56	68†	50	57	69†	39	43	60†
Brain & other nervous system	22	29	35†	22	28	34†	25	32	41†
Breast (female)	75	84	90†	76	85	92†	62	71	78†
Colon	51	61	65†	51	61	66†	45	53	55†
Esophagus	5	10	19†	6	11	21†	3	7	14†
Hodgkin lymphoma	72	79	87†	72	80	88†	70	72	83†
Kidney & renal pelvis	50	57	72†	50	57	72†	49	55	70†
Larynx	66	66	63†	67	67	65	59	56	51
Leukemia	34	43	58†	35	44	59†	33	35	51†
Liver & intrahepatic bile duct	3	5	16†	3	6	16†	2	3	11†
Lung & bronchus	12	13	17†	12	13	17†	11	11	14†
Melanoma of the skin	82	88	93†	82	88	93†	57‡	79‡	70‡
Myeloma	25	28	43†	25	27	43†	30	30	43†
Non-Hodgkin lymphoma	47	51	71†	47	52	72†	48	46	63†
Oral cavity & pharynx	53	54	65†	54	56	67†	36	34	45†
Ovary	36	38	43†	35	38	43†	42	34	36
Pancreas	2	4	6†	3	3	6†	2	6	5†
Prostate	68	83	100†	69	85	100†	61	72	98†
Rectum	48	58	68†	48	59	69†	45	52	61†
Stomach	15	20	28†	14	19	27†	16	19	28†
Testis	83	95	96†	83	96	97†	73‡,§	88‡	89
Thyroid	92	95	98†	92	94	98†	90	92	96†
Urinary bladder	73	79	80†	74	80	81†	50	63	62†
Uterine cervix	69	70	69	70	73	70	65	57	61
Uterine corpus	87	83	83†	88	84	85†	60	57	63

*Survival rates are adjusted for normal life expectancy and are based on cases diagnosed in the Surveillance, Epidemiology, and End Results (SEER) 9 areas from 1975 to 1977, 1987 to 1989, and 2002 to 2008 and followed through 2009.

†The difference in rates between 1975 to 1977 and 2002 to 2008 is statistically significant ($P < .05$).

‡The standard error of the survival rate is between 5 and 10 percentage points.

§Survival rate is for 1978 to 1980.

Reprinted from Siegel R, Naishadham D, Jemal A. Cancer statistics, 2013. CA Cancer J Clin. 2013;63:11-30, with permission from CA: A Cancer Journal for Clinicians and John Wiley and Sons, www.interscience.wiley.com.

that the overall 5-year survival rate for lung cancer now stands at 17%, which is dismal compared with all sites (overall 5-year survival rate, 68%), in particular compared with the other major causes of cancer death, including breast (5-year survival rate, 90%), colon (5-year survival rate, 65%), and prostate (5-year survival rate, 100%) cancers. Nonetheless, there has been improvement in lung cancer survival, largely related to reduction in tobacco use.[1] In contrast, decreases in death rates for prostate, colorectal, and breast cancers are generally attributed to improvements in early detection and treatment.[2-4] With much attention now focused on screening, we may over the coming years see a change in lung cancer mortality related to early detection for lung cancer as well.[5]

However, clear disparities in outcomes exist and need to be addressed, with African-Americans in particular showing lower 5-year survival rates overall and in lung cancer (5-year survival rate,14%) specifically. With cancer accounting for 23% of all deaths in the United States annually and the leading cause of death among both men and women age 40 to 79 years, much more work is still to be done in primary prevention, early detection, and improving treatment for advanced disease.

L. T. Tanoue, MD

References

1. Jemal A, Thun MJ, Ries LA, et al. Annual report to the nation on the status of cancer, 1975–2005, featuring trends in lung cancer, tobacco use, and tobacco control. *J Natl Cancer Inst.* 2008;100:1672-1694.
2. Berry DA, Cronin KA, Plevritis SK, et al. Effect of screening and adjuvant therapy on mortality from breast cancer. *N Engl J Med.* 2005;353:1784-1792.
3. Etzioni R, Tsodikov A, Mariotto A, et al. Quantifying the role of PSA screening in the US prostate cancer mortality decline. *Cancer Causes Control.* 2008;19:175-181.
4. Edwards BK, Ward E, Kohler BA, et al. Annual report to the nation on the status of cancer, 1975–2006, featuring colorectal cancer trends and impact of interventions (risk factors, screening, and treatment) to reduce future rates. *Cancer.* 2010; 116:544-573.
5. National Lung Screening Trial Research Team, Aberle DR, Adams AM, Berg CD, et al. Reduced lung-cancer mortality with low-dose computed tomographic screening. *N Engl J Med.* 2011;365:395-409.

Epidemic of Lung Cancer in Patients With HIV Infection

Winstone TA, Man SFP, Hull M, et al (Univ of British Columbia, Canada)
Chest 143:305-314, 2013

The survival of patients with HIV infection has improved dramatically over the past 20 years, largely owing to a significant reduction in opportunistic infections and AIDs-defining malignancies, such as lymphoma and Kaposi sarcoma. However, with improved survival, patients with HIV are experiencing morbidity and mortality from other (non-AIDs-defining) complications, such as solid organ malignancies. Of these, the leading cause of mortality in the HIV-infected population is lung cancer, accounting for nearly 30% of all cancer deaths and 10% of all non-HIV-related deaths. Importantly, the average age of onset of lung cancer in the HIV-infected population is 25 to 30 years earlier than that in the general population and at lower exposure to cigarette smoke. This article provides an overview of the epidemiology of lung cancer in the HIV-infected population and discusses some of the important risk factors and pathways that may enhance the risk of lung cancer in this population.

▶ The 2 most frequent AIDS-defining cancers are Kaposi sarcoma and non-Hodgkin's lymphoma. The incidence of both of these malignancies has decreased since the introduction of combination antiretroviral therapies. As in the general population, lung cancer is the most prevalent non–AIDS-defining cancer. Several features highlight why practitioners should be thinking about lung cancer in their patients with AIDS: (1) the risk of lung cancer is approximately 3-fold that of the general population, even with antiretroviral treatment; (2) the age at diagnosis is typically considerably younger than in the general population, on average between 38 and 57 years, and (3) the AIDS population as a group tends to display other characteristics and behaviors increasing the risk of lung cancer. Sixty percent to 80% of persons with HIV in the United States smoke.[1,2] They often have chronic pulmonary inflammation, primarily related to infections and smoking, and they are likely to have impaired immune surveillance, particularly when the CD4 count is low. As is seen in the general population, stage distribution is unfortunately weighted toward diagnosis of advanced disease; what follows inevitably is overall survival tends to be poor, as the stage of tumor is the predominant driver of prognosis.

Survival with HIV in the era of effective antiretroviral therapy has improved dramatically. As a consequence, the number of persons living with HIV and AIDS is growing. Given this, practitioners need to be aware of the increased risk of lung cancer, even in their younger AIDS patients, and should counsel their patients who smoke about the importance of quitting.

L. T. Tanoue, MD

References

1. Engels EA, Brock MV, Chen J, Hooker CM, Gillison M, Moore RD. Elevated incidence of lung cancer among HIV-infected individuals. *J Clin Oncol.* 2006;24: 1383-1388.
2. Giordano TP, Kramer JR. Does HIV infection independently increase the incidence of lung cancer? *Clin Infect Dis.* 2005;40:490-491.

Screening for Lung Cancer: U.S. Preventive Services Task Force Recommendation Statement

Moyer VA, on behalf of the U.S. Preventive Services Task Force (U.S. Preventive Services Task Force, Rockville, MD) *Ann Intern Med* 2013 [Epub ahead of print]

Description.—Update of the 2004 U.S. Preventive Services Task Force (USPSTF) recommendation on screening for lung cancer.

Methods.—The USPSTF reviewed the evidence on the efficacy of low-dose computed tomography, chest radiography, and sputum cytologic

TABLE.—Screening Scenarios From CISNET Models*

Screening Scenario†			Benefit			Harm‡			
Minimum Pack-Years at Screening, *n*	Minimum Age at Which to Begin Screening, *y*	Time Since Last Cigarette, *y*	Population Ever Screened, %	Lung Cancer Deaths Averted, %	Lung Cancer Deaths Averted, *n*	Total CT Screens, *n*	Radiation-Induced Lung Cancer Deaths, *n*	Overdiagnosis, %§	CT Screens per Lung Cancer Death Averted, *n*
40	60	25	13.0	11.0	410	171 924	17	11.2	437
40	55	25	13.9	12.3	458	221 606	20	11.1	506
30	60	25	18.8	13.3	495	253 095	21	11.9	534
30	**55**	**15**	**19.3**	**14.0**	**521**	**286 813**	**24**	**9.9**	**577**
20	60	25	24.8	15.4	573	327 024	25	9.8	597
30	55	25	20.4	15.8	588	342 880	25	10.0	609
20	55	25	27.4	17.9	664	455 381	31	10.4	719
10	55	25	36.0	19.4	721	561 744	35	9.5	819

CISNET = Cancer Intervention and Surveillance Modeling Network; CT = computed tomography.

*All scenarios model the results of following a cohort of 100 000 persons from age 45 to 90 y or until death from any cause, with a varying number of smokers and former smokers screened on the basis of smoking history, age, and years since stopping smoking. Bold text indicates the screening scenario with a reasonable balance of benefits and harms and that is recommended by the U.S. Preventive Services Task Force.

†In all scenarios, screening is continued through age 80 y.

‡Number of CT screenings is a measure of harm because it relates to the number of patients who will have risk for overdiagnosis and potential consequences from false-positive results.

§Percentage of screen-detected cancer that is overdiagnosis; that is, cancer that would not have been diagnosed in the patient's lifetime without screening.

Reprinted from Moyer VA, on behalf of the U.S. Preventive Services Task Force. Screening for Lung Cancer: U.S. Preventive Services Task Force Recommendation Statement. Ann Intern Med. Epub ahead of print. Copyright 2013, with permission from the American College of Physicians.

evaluation for lung cancer screening in asymptomatic persons who are at average or high risk for lung cancer (current or former smokers) and the benefits and harms of these screening tests and of surgical resection of early-stage non–small cell lung cancer. The USPSTF also commissioned modeling studies to provide information about the optimum age at which to begin and end screening, the optimum screening interval, and the relative benefits and harms of different screening strategies.

Population.—This recommendation applies to asymptomatic adults aged 55 to 80 years who have a 30 pack-year smoking history and currently smoke or have quit within the past 15 years.

Recommendation.—The USPSTF recommends annual screening for lung cancer with low-dose computed tomography in adults aged 55 to 80 years who have a 30 pack-year smoking history and currently smoke or have quit within the past 15 years. Screening should be discontinued once a person has not smoked for 15 years or develops a health problem that substantially limits life expectancy or the ability or willingness to have curative lung surgery. (B recommendation) (Table)

▶ The United States Preventive Services Task Force (USPSTF) finalized its updated recommendation on screening for lung cancer at the end of 2013. The new recommendation is as follows:

"The USPSTF recommends annual screening for lung cancer with low-dose computed tomography in adults aged 55 to 80 years who have a 30 pack-year smoking history and currently smoke or have quit within the past 15 years. Screening should be discontinued once a person has not smoked for 15 years or develops a health problem that substantially limits life expectancy or the ability or willingness to have curative lung surgery."

The recommendation was given a B grade, the definition of which is, "The USPSTF recommends the service. There is high certainty that the net benefit is moderate or there is moderate certainty that the net benefit is moderate to substantial." The USPSTF suggestion for practice is "Offer/provide this service." To inform this recommendation, the USPSTF performed a comprehensive systematic evidence review of all relevant screening trials, the largest and most compelling of which was the National Lung Screening Trial.[1] Additionally, modeling studies were performed by the Cancer Intervention and Surveillance Modeling Network (CISNET), which examined the harms and benefits relating to different screening scenarios.[2] CISNET considered scenarios with varying minimum pack-years of smoking, ages at beginning screening, and years since the last cigarette smoked. As is evident in the Table, the number of computed tomography screenings needing to be performed to avert one lung cancer death was lowest in the highest risk group, which had the most intense smoking history and was older at the age of screening initiation. This article also describes the guidelines of several of the major societies and institutions focusing on lung cancer, as these differ from each other as well as from the USPSTF in the specific recommendations relating to the intensity of smoking that would warrant screening, at what ages to start and stop screening, and whether to consider risk factors for lung cancer other than smoking.

The USPSTF recommendation is the most powerful endorsement of lung cancer screening to date. It now seems inevitable that insurance carriers, including Medicare, will cover the service. It is our responsibility to ensure that screening, as it is introduced into the community, is performed appropriately and safely to maximize benefit and minimize harm.

L. T. Tanoue, MD

References

1. National Lung Screening Trial Research Team, Aberle DR, Adams AM, Berg CD, et al. Reduced lung-cancer mortality with low-dose computed tomographic screening. *N Engl J Med.* 2011;365:395-409.
2. de Koning H, Meza R, Plevritis SK, et al. *Benefits and Harms of Computed Tomography Lung Cancer Screening Programs for High-Risk Populations.* AHRQ Publication No. 13–05196-EF-2. Rockville, MD: Agency for Healthcare Research and Quality; 2013.

Benefits and Harms of Computed Tomography Lung Cancer Screening Programs for High-Risk Populations

National Cancer Institute, Cancer Intervention and Surveillance Modeling Network, Lung Cancer Working Group (Erasmus MC, the Netherlands; Univ of Michigan, Ann Arbor; Stanford Univ, CA; et al) 2013

Background.—The National Lung Screening Trial (NLST) demonstrated that three annual computed tomography (CT) screenings reduced lung cancer-specific mortality by 20% compared with annual chest radiography screenings in a volunteer population of current and former smokers ages 55 to 74 years with at least 30 pack-years of cigarette smoking history and no more than 15 years since quitting for former smokers. To inform the updated U.S. Preventive Services Task Force recommendations on lung cancer screening, we assessed the benefits and harms of CT screening programs that varied by age, pack-year, and years since quitting criteria, as well as the frequency of screening.

Methods.—Five independent microsimulation models estimated the long-term harms and benefits of screening as experienced by the U.S. cohort born in 1950. The five models were calibrated to the NLST to predict lung cancer outcomes consistent with the trial's observations. These models were also then calibrated to the lung cancer screening portion of the Prostate, Lung, Colorectal, and Ovarian Cancer Screening Trial. We evaluated 576 scenarios with annual or less frequent screening of individuals between the ages of 45 and 85 years, for a range of minimum smoking exposure (measured in pack-years) and maximum time since quitting. Screening benefits are expressed in terms of the percentage of cancers detected at an early stage (stages I or II), percentage and absolute number of lung cancer deaths prevented, and life-years gained compared with a reference scenario with no screening. Screening harms are expressed as the number of CT screenings required (and percentage of the cohort ever screened), number of followup imaging examinations, and number of overdiagnosed lung cancers and radiation-related lung cancer deaths. We identified consensus strategies that the models identified as efficient, preventing the greatest number of lung cancer deaths for the screening examinations required. Counts and percentages reported are calculated as averages of outcomes from the five models, following a 100,000 person cohort from ages 45 to 90 years.

Results.—The models ranked strategies similarly and identified a consensus set of programs. We focus in this report on 26 efficient screening scenarios that start screening at age 50, 55, or 60 years and stop screening at age 80 or 85 years. Among these 26 programs, triennial screening reduced total lung cancer mortality in the cohort by 5% to 6% compared with biennial programs that reduced mortality by 7% to 10% and annual programs that reduced mortality by 11% to 21%. When we focused on annual programs that began screening at age 55 or 60 years, ended screening at age 80 years, and required between 200,000 to 600,000 screenings per 100,000 persons, a set of seven programs remained. We added a lower-intensity reference scenario, for a total of eight programs. These eight programs include a program similar to the NLST criteria except for the stopping age: starting annual screening at age 55 years, ending at age 80 years for ever-smokers with at least 30 pack-years, and no more than 15 years since quitting for former smokers. With this program, 19.3% of the cohort would be screened at least once, requiring 287,000 CT screenings per 100,000 persons, leading to 50% of lung cancers being detected at an early stage and a 14% lung cancer mortality reduction (about 520 lung cancer deaths averted per 100,000 population), resulting in about 5,500 life-years gained per 100,000 population. These benefits must be weighed against the following harms: 330,000 CT examinations per 100,000 persons (screenings and followup CT scans), an estimated 4% overdiagnosis rate (of all lung cancers in the cohort), and 0.8% of lung cancer deaths (24 per 100,000 population) related to radiation exposure (based on two models). Important tradeoffs between the eight programs are discussed.

Conclusions.—Our findings support a range of possible lung cancer screening programs, including annual lung cancer screening of individuals with at least 30 pack-years of smoking who are between the ages of 55 and 80 years, but cannot determine which tradeoff of harms and benefits is "best." Scenarios with an older starting age (60 years) but increased maximum years since quitting (from 15 to 25 years) offer different tradeoffs of benefits and harms (depending on the minimum pack-years). Extending eligibility to individuals with fewer pack-years—although still efficient—leads to additional benefits but more additional harms. Overdiagnosis remained limited for annual screening (Fig 3, Table 2).

▶ The current draft recommendation by the United States Preventive Services Task Force (USPSTF) now supports screening of high-risk individuals with low-dose computed tomography (CT).[1] This publication by de Koning and colleagues on behalf of the Cancer Intervention and Surveillance Modeling Network (CISNET) was prepared for the Agency for Healthcare Research and

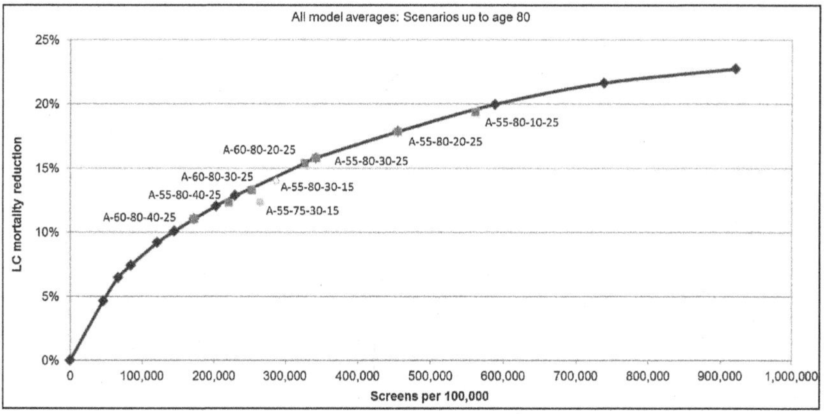

FIGURE 3.—Estimated lung cancer mortality reduction (Average of Five Models) from annual computed tomography screening in the 1950 birth cohort for programs with eligible ages of 55 to 80 years and different smoking eligibility cutoffs*. (Reprinted from de Koning HJ, Plevritis SK, ten Haaf K, et al. Benefits and harms of computed tomography lung cancer screening programs for high-risk populations. AHRQ Publication No. 13-05196-EF-2. Agency for Healthcare Research and Quality. Copyright 2013.)

Quality. It provides the important analysis leading to the change in the USPSTF recommendation.

Using individual de-identified data from the National Lung Screening Trial (NLST) and the lung cancer screening portion of the Prostate, Lung, Colorectal and Ovarian Cancer Screening Trial, the CISNET group developed 5 independent models estimating the benefits and long-term harms of screening as experienced by the US cohort born in 1950. All 5 models included dose-response information relating to cigarette exposure. Importantly, CISNET conducted the study with the intent of extrapolating the NLST findings to screening programs that could potentially be adopted in the general population. Twenty-six scenarios were examined, with variation in the ages of when screening would start (range, 45—60 years) and end (range, 75—85 years), the frequency of screening (annual, biennial, triennial), and eligibility based on minimum number of pack-years smoked (range, 10—40 pack-years) and maximum number of years since quitting (10—25 years). As outlined in Table 2, these scenarios then were applied to yield a series of outcome measurements, including lung cancer mortality reduction, CT screenings, life-years gained, and screenings per lung cancer death averted, with considerable variation in outcomes depending on the screening scenario. In Table 2, the NLST criteria are identified as A55-75-30-15. Expanding the NLST age criteria by 5 years (A55-80-30-15) or extending the beginning and stopping of screening by 5 years and extending the time since quitting to up to 25 years (A60-80-30-25), resulted in the same number of screenings leading to more lung cancer deaths averted than in the NLST. Table 2 also shows that extending the age of screening to 85 also achieves larger lung cancer mortality reductions but at the expense of a substantial increase in the number of screenings. The study group elected to focus on scenarios stopping screening at age 80 because of the increased risk of treatment in older individuals with heavy smoking histories and presumed higher comorbidities. Fig 3

TABLE 2.—Benefits of 26 Selected Efficient Screening Programs and the Screening Program Most Similar to NLST Eligibility Criteria (Average of Results From Five Models)

Scenario	Percentage Ever Screened	CT Screenings Per 100,000	Percentage of Cases Detected at an Early Stage*	Lung Cancer Mortality Reduction	Average Lung Cancer Deaths Averted Per 100,000**	Life-Years Gained Per 100,000	Life-Years Gained Per Death Averted	Relative Increase in Screenings Compared With Previous Scenario (%)	Relative Increase in Lung Cancer Deaths Averted Compared With Previous Scenario (%)	Screenings Per Life-Year Gained	Screenings Per Lung Cancer Death Averted	Number of Persons Needed to Screen (Ever) Per Lung Cancer Death Averted
Triennial Screening												
T-60-80-40-10	11.2%	45,685	42.0%	4.6%	172	1,823	10.6			25	265	65
T-60-85-40-10	11.3%	48,317	42.6%	5.1%	190	1,894	10.0			26	254	59
T-60-85-40-15	12.0%	55,316	43.3%	5.4%	201	2,000	10.0			28	275	60
T-60-85-40-25	13.0%	66,333	44.1%	6.0%	225	2,252	10.0			29	294	58
Biennial Screening												
B-60-80-40-10	11.2%	67,167	44.0%	6.5%	241	2,526	10.5			27	278	47
B-60-85-40-10	11.3%	69,662	44.3%	6.9%	256	2,665	10.4			26	272	44
B-60-85-40-15	12.0%	79,757	45.3%	7.4%	275	2,882	10.5			28	290	44
B-60-80-40-25	13.0%	90,337	45.5%	7.7%	286	3,017	10.6			30	315	45
B-60-85-40-25	13.0%	95,914	46.3%	8.4%	312	3,045	9.8			32	307	42
B-60-85-30-20	17.9%	127,046	47.5%	9.6%	358	3,451	9.6			37	354	50
Annual Screening												
A-60-80-40-25†	13.0%	171,924	48.1%	11.0%	410	4,211	10.3	ref	ref	41	419	32
A-60-85-40-25	13.0%	185,451	49.4%	12.1%	449	4,203	9.4			44	413	29
A-55-85-40-20	14.0%	220,505	50.0%	13.0%	485	4,811	9.9			46	454	29

A-55-80-40-25†	13.9%	221,606	49.2%	12.3%	458	4,777	10.4	29%	12%	46	483	30
A-60-80-30-25†	18.8%	253,095	50.4%	13.3%	495	4,940	10.0	14%	8%	51	511	38
A-55-75-30-15‡	19.2%	265,049	48.4%	12.3%	459	5,375	11.7			49	577	42
A-60-85-30-25	18.8%	271,152	52.1%	14.7%	547	5,322	9.7			51	495	34
A-50-85-40-25	14.6%	281,218	51.4%	14.6%	542	5,908	10.9			48	518	27
A-55-80-30-15†	19.3%	286,813	50.5%	14.0%	521	5,517	10.6	13%	5%	52	550	37
A-60-80-20-25†	24.8%	327,024	51.9%	15.4%	573	5,707	10.0	14%	10%	57	570	43
A-55-80-30-25†	20.4%	342,880	52.1%	15.8%	588	6,321	10.8	5%	3%	54	583	35
A-60-85-20-25	24.8%	348,894	53.7%	16.8%	624	5,934	9.5			59	559	40
A-55-80-20-25†	27.4%	455,381	53.9%	17.9%	664	7,092	10.7	33%	13%	64	685	41
A-55-85-20-25	27.4%	477,334	55.6%	19.1%	712	7,490	10.5			64	670	38
A-55-80-10-25†	36.0%	561,744	55.2%	19.4%	721	7,693	10.7	23%	9%	73	777	50
A-50-80-20-25	29.0%	588,516	55.2%	20.0%	743	8,530	11.5			69	792	39
A-50-85-20-25	29.0%	610,443	56.9%	21.2%	787	8,948	11.4			68	775	37

Note: All counts are cumulative, per a cohort of 100,000 persons age 45 years, followed until age 90 years. Radiation-related lung cancer deaths are not included in lung cancer deaths in Table 2 (see Table 3).

*Percentage of cases detected at an early stage in no screening scenario was 37.4%.

**Average lung cancer deaths in no screening scenario was 3,719 per 100,000 persons.

†Consensus efficient annual programs with a stopping age of 80 years and screening counts between 200,000 and 600,000, plus an 8th program (A60-80-40-25) with just under 200,000 screenings included as a reference program.

‡Denotes eligibility most similar to the NLST.

Reprinted from de Koning HJ, Plevritis SK, ten Haaf K, et al. Benefits and harms of computed tomography lung cancer screening programs for high-risk populations. AHRQ Publication No. 13-05196-EF-2. Agency for Healthcare Research and Quality. Copyright 2013.

graphically depicts the efficiency (lung cancer mortality reduction vs number of screens per 100 000) for multiple annual lung cancer screening scenarios. As would be anticipated, annual screening in an older population with more intense smoking was more efficient than screening a younger population with less smoking, but benefit was gained even in the latter groups, although at the price of considerably more screening interventions.

The take-home message is that, based on the CISNET modeling, a range of different screening scenarios are possible and arguably valid, with different balances of benefits and harms. The most efficient scenarios offer an efficiency of screening similar to that of the NLST. Extending screening to individuals who are younger or have fewer pack-years of smoking may still be beneficial and efficient but will lead to additional harms. The current USPSTF draft recommendation, which recommends screening for individuals ages 55 to 80, already extends the age of screening by 5 years more than the NLST and, at least in its current format, refrains from dictating the exact number of pack-years or the number of years since quitting. This leaves a fair amount of discretion in the hands of practitioners for whom this work by CISNET should provide some guidance.

L. T. Tanoue, MD

Reference

1. Screening for Lung Cancer: Draft Recommendation Statement. AHRQ Publication No. 13–05196-EF-3, 2013. (Accessed December 9, 2013)

50-Year Trends in Smoking-Related Mortality in the United States

Thun MJ, Carter BD, Feskanich D, et al (American Cancer Society, Atlanta, GA; Harvard Med School, Boston, MA; et al)
N Engl J Med 368:351-364, 2013

Background.—The disease risks from cigarette smoking increased in the United States over most of the 20th century, first among male smokers and later among female smokers. Whether these risks have continued to increase during the past 20 years is unclear.

Methods.—We measured temporal trends in mortality across three time periods (1959–1965, 1982–1988, and 2000–2010), comparing absolute and relative risks according to sex and self-reported smoking status in two historical cohort studies and in five pooled contemporary cohort studies, among participants who became 55 years of age or older during follow-up.

Results.—For women who were current smokers, as compared with women who had never smoked, the relative risks of death from lung cancer were 2.73, 12.65, and 25.66 in the 1960s, 1980s, and contemporary cohorts, respectively; corresponding relative risks for male current smokers, as compared with men who had never smoked, were 12.22, 23.81, and 24.97. In the contemporary cohorts, male and female current smokers also had similar relative risks for death from chronic obstructive pulmonary disease (COPD) (25.61 for men and 22.35 for women), ischemic heart disease (2.50 for men and 2.86 for women), any type of stroke (1.92 for men and 2.10 for women), and all causes combined (2.80 for men and 2.76 for women). Mortality from COPD among male smokers continued to increase in the contemporary cohorts in nearly all the age groups represented in the study and within each stratum of duration and intensity of smoking. Among men 55 to 74 years of age and women 60 to 74 years of age, all-cause mortality was at least three times as high among current smokers as among those who had never smoked. Smoking cessation at any age dramatically reduced death rates.

Conclusions.—The risk of death from cigarette smoking continues to increase among women and the increased risks are now nearly identical for men and women, as compared with persons who have never smoked. Among men, the risks associated with smoking have plateaued at the high levels seen in the 1980s, except for a continuing, unexplained increase in mortality from COPD.

▶ The first US Surgeon General's report on the health consequences of smoking issued in 1964 suggested that women were less likely than men to suffer from cigarette smoking.[1] The fallacy of that statement was, of course, related to the fact that in 1964 women had not been smoking long enough for those adverse health consequences to have yet become evident. In this report by Thun and colleagues, trends in mortality from 1959 to 2010 were examined in men and women, with specific reference to the influence of cigarette smoking. The authors highlight several points:

- The relative risks of death from the major cigarette-related diseases, including chronic obstructive pulmonary disease (COPD), ischemic heart disease, stroke, and all causes are now essentially equal for both sexes. This reflects the fact that smoking patterns among men and women have converged since the 1960s, when that first Surgeon General's report was published. As demonstrated in Fig 1 of the original article, the rate of death from lung cancer in men has plateaued, whereas in women it is still increasing, and the rate of COPD deaths has increased over time in both sexes.
- The rate of death for men 55 to 74 years and women 60 to 74 years is at least 3 times as high among current smokers compared with never smokers. This observation recapitulates the findings of the newly published US National Health Interview Survey[2] as well as the landmark British Doctors' Study.[3]
- The rate of death from COPD is increasing in both men and women smokers.
- Quitting smoking at any age decreases mortality for all the major smoking-related diseases. As demonstrated in Fig 2 of the original article, smoking cessation before the age of 40 results in a diminution of risk for lung cancer and COPD to nearly that of never smokers.

It is unfortunate that one of the few examples of gender equality resides in the recognition that the risks of the devastating consequences of smoking in women are now equal to those in men.

L. T. Tanoue, MD

References

1. US Public Health Service. *Smoking and health. Report of the Advisory committee to the Surgeon General for the Public Health Service.* Publication No. 1103. Washington, DC: US Department of Health, Education, and Welfare, Public Health Service; 1964.
2. Jha P, Ramasundarahettige C, Landsman V, et al. 21st-century hazards of smoking and benefits of cessation in the United States. *N Engl J Med.* 2013;368:341-350.
3. Doll R, Peto R, Wheatley K, Gray R, Sutherland I. Mortality in relation to smoking: 40 years' observations on male British doctors. *BMJ.* 1994;309:901-911.

21st-Century Hazards of Smoking and Benefits of Cessation in the United States

Jha P, Ramasundarahettige C, Landsman V, et al (Ctr for Global Health Res, Toronto, Canada; et al)
N Engl J Med 368:341-350, 2013

Background.—Extrapolation from studies in the 1980s suggests that smoking causes 25% of deaths among women and men 35 to 69 years of age in the United States. Nationally representative measurements of the current risks of smoking and the benefits of cessation at various ages are unavailable.

Methods.—We obtained smoking and smoking-cessation histories from 113,752 women and 88,496 men 25 years of age or older who were interviewed between 1997 and 2004 in the U.S. National Health Interview Survey and related these data to the causes of deaths that occurred by December 31, 2006 (8236 deaths in women and 7479 in men). Hazard ratios for death among current smokers, as compared with those who had never smoked, were adjusted for age, educational level, adiposity, and alcohol consumption.

Results.—For participants who were 25 to 79 years of age, the rate of death from any cause among current smokers was about three times that among those who had never smoked (hazard ratio for women, 3.0; 99% confidence interval [CI], 2.7 to 3.3; hazard ratio for men, 2.8; 99% CI, 2.4 to 3.1). Most of the excess mortality among smokers was due to neoplastic, vascular, respiratory, and other diseases that can be caused by smoking. The probability of surviving from 25 to 79 years of age was about twice as great in those who had never smoked as in current smokers (70% vs. 38% among women and 61% vs. 26% among men). Life expectancy was shortened by more than 10 years among the current smokers, as compared with those who had never smoked. Adults who had quit smoking at 25 to 34, 35 to 44, or 45 to 54 years of age gained about 10, 9, and 6 years of life, respectively, as compared with those who continued to smoke.

Conclusions.—Smokers lose at least one decade of life expectancy, as compared with those who have never smoked. Cessation before the age

TABLE 2.—Adjusted Hazard Ratios for Various Causes of Death among Current Smokers, as Compared with Those Who Never Smoked, among Women and Men 25 to 79 Years of Age*

Cause of Death	Women: Never Smoked (No. of Deaths)	Women: Current Smoker (No. of Deaths)	Women: Adjusted Hazard Ratio (99% CI)	Women: Deaths Attributable to Smoking among Smokers No. (%)	Men: Never Smoked (No. of Deaths)	Men: Current Smokers (No. of Deaths)	Men: Adjusted Hazard Ratio (99% CI)	Men: Deaths Attributable to Smoking among Smokers No. (%)
Lung cancer	61	267	17.8 (11.4–27.8)	252 (94)	44	348	14.6 (9.1–23.4)	324 (93)
Cancers other than lung cancer	544	258	1.7 (1.4–2.1)	106 (41)	280	317	2.2 (1.7–2.8)	173 (55)
All cancers	605	525	3.2 (2.6–3.9)	360 (69)	324	665	3.8 (3.1–4.8)	491 (74)
Ischemic heart disease	382	251	3.5 (2.7–4.6)	179 (72)	285	416	3.2 (2.5–4.1)	288 (69)
Stroke	150	88	3.2 (2.2–4.7)	60 (69)	74	66	1.7 (1.0–2.8)	27 (40)
Other vascular disease	252	137	3.1 (2.2–4.4)	93 (68)	141	161	2.1 (1.5–3.0)	84 (52)
All vascular diseases	784	476	3.2 (2.7–3.9)	328 (69)	500	643	2.6 (2.1–3.2)	395 (61)
Respiratory diseases	119	206	8.5 (6.1–11.8)	182 (88)	45	188	9.0 (5.6–14.4)	167 (89)
Other medical disorders not shown above	581	277	2.2 (1.7–2.8)	151 (55)	295	370	2.2 (1.7–2.9)	205 (55)
All medical disorders	2089	1484	3.0 (2.7–3.3)	986 (66)	1164	1866	2.9 (2.5–3.2)	1211 (65)
Accidents and injuries	101	95	3.9 (2.4–6.2)	0	119	164	2.1 (1.4–3.0)	0
All causes†	2190	1579	3.0 (2.7–3.3)	986 (62)	1283	2030	2.8 (2.4–3.1)	1211 (60)

*Hazard ratios were adjusted for age, educational level, alcohol consumption, and body-mass index.

†Deaths attributable to smoking were determined with the use of the hazard ratios for all medical causes of death. With the exclusion of the 199 women and 222 men who had quit smoking less than 5 years before their deaths and the exclusion of the 1795 women and 2184 men who reported a history of coronary heart disease, stroke, or cancer, the hazard ratios for all-cause mortality were 3.1 for women and 2.8 for men.

Reprinted from Jha P, Ramasundarahettige C, Landsman V, et al. 21st-Century Hazards of Smoking and Benefits of Cessation in the United States. N Engl J Med. 2013;368:341-350.

of 40 years reduces the risk of death associated with continued smoking by about 90% (Table 2).

▶ Smoking causes premature death. This indisputable fact is driven home by this study evaluating the impact of smoking and smoking cessation on mortality and survival in 113 752 women and 88 496 men, 25 years or older, who were interviewed as part of the United States National Health Interview Survey between 1997 and 2004. Table 2 shows the adjusted hazard ratios for causes of death among current smokers compared with never smokers. The adjusted hazard ratio for all causes of death in women was 3.0 (95% confidence interval [CI], 2.7–3.3) and in men was 2.8 (95% CI, 2.4–3.1). Simply put, these data indicate that the rate of death from any cause among current smokers was 3-fold that of people who never smoked. For lung cancer specifically, the adjusted hazard ratio for lung cancer in women was a staggering 17.8 (95% CI, 11.4–27.8) and in men was 14.6 (95% CI, 9.1–23.4).

Smoking cessation has predictable benefit with regard to improving survival. As was demonstrated in previous work by Peto and colleagues,[1] smoking cessation even into the sixth and seventh decades of life is associated with benefit, including reduction in lung cancer risk. Patients may be better able to understand the magnitude of benefit if it is expressed as years of life gained as opposed to probability of survival. As shown in Fig 3 of the original article, the younger one is at the time of smoking cessation, the more life years are gained. Smokers who quit at age 25 to 34 gain, on average, 10 years of life; smokers who quit at age 55 to 64 gain, on average, 4 years of life. It is important to note that there is still benefit even when smoking cessation comes at an older age, that is, it is never too late to quit!

L. T. Tanoue, MD

Reference

1. Peto R, Darby S, Deo H, Silcocks P, Whitley E, Doll R. Smoking, smoking cessation, and lung cancer in the UK since 1950: combination of national statistics with two case-control studies. *BMJ*. 2000;321:323-329.

Electronic cigarettes for smoking cessation: a randomised controlled trial

Bullen C, Howe C, Laugesen M, et al (The Univ of Auckland, New Zealand; Health New Zealand, Lyttelton, Christchurch; et al)

Lancet 382:1629-1637, 2013

Background.—Electronic cigarettes (e-cigarettes) can deliver nicotine and mitigate tobacco withdrawal and are used by many smokers to assist quit attempts. We investigated whether e-cigarettes are more effective than nicotine patches at helping smokers to quit.

Methods.—We did this pragmatic randomised-controlled superiority trial in Auckland, New Zealand, between Sept 6, 2011, and July 5, 2013. Adult (≥18 years) smokers wanting to quit were randomised (with computerised block randomisation, block size nine, stratified by ethnicity [Māori; Pacific; or non-Māori, non-Pacific], sex [men or women], and level of nicotine dependence [>5 or ≤5 Fagerström test for nicotine dependence]) in a 4:4:1 ratio to 16 mg nicotine e-cigarettes, nicotine patches (21 mg patch, one daily), or placebo e-cigarettes (no nicotine), from 1 week before until 12 weeks after quit day, with low intensity behavioural support via voluntary telephone counselling. The primary outcome was biochemically verified continuous abstinence at 6 months (exhaled breath carbon monoxide measurement <10 ppm). Primary analysis was by intention to treat. This trial is registered with the Australian New Zealand Clinical Trials Registry, number ACTRN12610000866000.

Findings.—657 people were randomised (289 to nicotine e-cigarettes, 295 to patches, and 73 to placebo e-cigarettes) and were included in the intention-to-treat analysis. At 6 months, verified abstinence was 7·3% (21 of 289) with nicotine e-cigarettes, 5·8% (17 of 295) with patches, and 4·1% (three of 73) with placebo e-cigarettes (risk difference for nicotine e-cigarette vs patches 1·51 [95% CI −2·49 to 5·51]; for nicotine e-cigarettes vs placebo e-cigarettes 3·16 [95% CI −2·29 to 8·61]). Achievement of abstinence was substantially lower than we anticipated for the power calculation, thus we had insufficient statistical power to conclude superiority of nicotine e-cigarettes to patches or to placebo e-cigarettes. We identified no significant differences in adverse events, with 137 events in the nicotine e-cigarettes group, 119 events in the patches group, and 36 events in the placebo e-cigarettes group. We noted no evidence of an association between adverse events and study product.

Interpretation.—E-cigarettes, with or without nicotine, were modestly effective at helping smokers to quit, with similar achievement of abstinence as with nicotine patches, and few adverse events. Uncertainty exists about the place of e-cigarettes in tobacco control, and more research is urgently needed to clearly establish their overall benefits and harms at both individual and population levels (Fig 2).

▶ Electronic cigarettes (e-cigarettes) appear to be increasingly used as aids to quit smoking. They are obvious alternatives to traditional tobacco cigarettes, but unless they are marketed as smoking cessation devices, regulation by the US Food and Drug Administration is not required. Little rigorous research exists about their effects on health other than as related to smoking cessation, and even for that there have been little data available. This study by Bullen and colleagues compared the effects of e-cigarettes containing nicotine, placebo e-cigarettes without nicotine, and nicotine patches on smoking cessation in subjects who were habitual smokers of at least one-half pack of cigarettes per day. The primary outcome was abstinence from traditional cigarettes. Fig 2 shows the main findings. The use of e-cigarettes containing nicotine for 13 weeks resulted in increased smoking abstinence at 6 months compared with placebo e-cigarettes or nicotine patches, but there was no statistical difference, and the relapse to smoking rates were high in all groups. The authors conclude that nicotine e-cigarettes were at least as effective as nicotine patches.

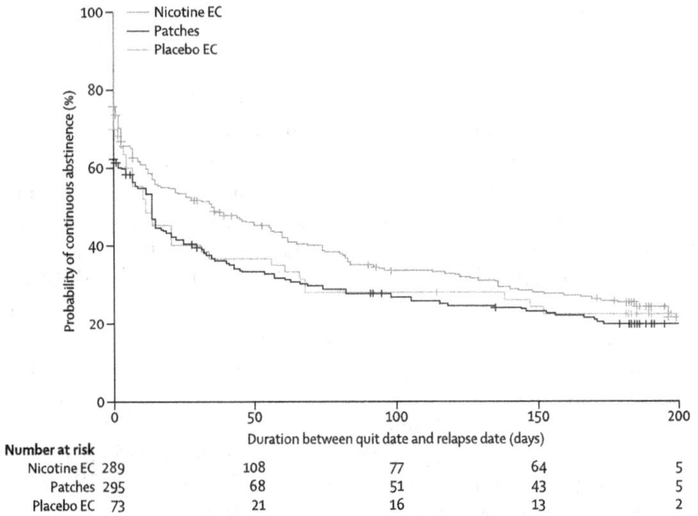

FIGURE 2.—Kaplan-Meier analysis of time to relapse. EC=e-cigarettes. (Reprinted from Bullen C, Howe C, Laugesen M, et al. Electronic cigarettes for smoking cessation: a randomised controlled trial. *Lancet*. 2013;382:1629-1637, Copyright 2013, with permission from Elsevier.)

The e-cigarette literature is full of controversy. The cartridges with which these devices are loaded vary in ingredients. Because they are not regulated, cartridge contents other than nicotine likely vary by manufacturer. Of concern, a number of potential harmful substances, including N-nitrosamines, polycyclic aromatic hydrocarbons, glycerin, and oils, have been identified in these devices, and a number of reports have documented adverse events related to their use.[1-3] It is also clear that some patients may decrease or eliminate traditional cigarette use but then become habitual e-cigarette smokers. It may take years for us to understand the health effects of substituting one smoking habit for another. Nonetheless, the consequences of cigarette smoking are very clear. Given the struggle to get the smoking rate of adult Americans below its current level of approximately 20%, it will be necessary to try to understand the short- and long-term risks as well as benefits of cigarette replacement therapies of all varieties.

L. T. Tanoue, MD

References

1. Avdalovic MV, Murin S. Electronic cigarettes: no such thing as a free lunch...Or puff. *Chest*. 2012;141:1371-1372.
2. Vardavas CI, Anagnostopoulos N, Kougias M, Evangelopoulou V, Connolly GN, Behrakis PK. Short-term pulmonary effects of using an electronic cigarette: impact on respiratory flow resistance, impedance, and exhaled nitric oxide. *Chest*. 2012; 141:1400-1406.
3. McCauley L, Markin C, Hosmer D. An unexpected consequence of electronic cigarette use. *Chest*. 2012;141:1110-1113.

36 Pleural, Interstitial Ling, and Pulmonary Vascular Disease

The Toll-like Receptor 3 L412F Polymorphism and Disease Progression in Idiopathic Pulmonary Fibrosis

O'Dwyer DN, Armstrong ME, Trujillo G, et al (Univ College Dublin, Belfield, Ireland; Univ of Michigan Med School, Ann Arbor; et al)

Am J Respir Crit Care Med 188:1442-1450, 2013

Rationale.—Idiopathic pulmonary fibrosis (IPF) is a fatal progressive interstitial pneumonia. The innate immune system provides a crucial function in the recognition of tissue injury and infection. Toll-like receptor 3 (TLR3) is an innate immune system receptor. We investigated the role of a functional *TLR3* single-nucleotide polymorphism in IPF.

Objectives.—To characterize the effects of the *TLR3* Leu412Phe polymorphism in primary pulmonary fibroblasts from patients with IPF and disease progression in two independent IPF patient cohorts. To investigate the role of TLR3 in a murine model of pulmonary fibrosis.

Methods.—TLR3-mediated cytokine, type 1 IFN, and fibroproliferative responses were examined in TLR3 wild-type (Leu/Leu), heterozygote (Leu/Phe), and homozygote (Phe/Phe) primary IPF pulmonary fibroblasts by ELISA, real-time polymerase chain reaction, and proliferation assays. A murine model of bleomycin-induced pulmonary fibrosis was used in TLR3 wild-type ($tlr3^{+/+}$) and TLR3 knockout mice ($tlr3^{-/-}$). A genotyping approach was used to investigate the role of the TLR3 L412F polymorphism in disease progression in IPF using survival analysis and longitudinal decline in FVC.

Measurements and Main Results.—Activation of TLR3 in primary lung fibroblasts from *TLR3* L412F-variant patients with IPF resulted in defective cytokine, type I IFN, and fibroproliferative responses. We demonstrate increased collagen and profibrotic cytokines in TLR3 knockout mice ($tlr3^{-/-}$) compared with wild-type mice ($tlr3^{+/+}$). *TLR3* L412F was also associated with a significantly greater risk of mortality and an accelerated decline in FVC in patients with IPF.

Conclusions.—This study reveals the crucial role of defective TLR3 function in promoting progressive IPF.

▶ In this compelling study by O'Dwyer et al published in the *Blue Journal*, the authors conduct a series of well-designed investigations to identify and elaborate on the role of the toll-like receptor 3 (TLR3) L412F polymorphism in rapid progression of idiopathic pulmonary fibrosis (IPF). The polymorphism has been shown to confer protection against age-related macular degeneration and is implicated in increased risk for cardiomyopathy after viral myocarditis.

The authors investigated 2 large cohorts of human subjects with IPF (the UK IPF cohort and subjects from the INSPIRE IPF trial) and a murine model for the polymorphism using a bleomycin-induced lung injury model.

The findings pose a strong case for the role of TLR3 L412F polymorphism in rapidly progressive IPF. These findings pave the way toward a better understanding of the pathogenesis of IPF. This polymorphism may also serve as a marker for patients with more aggressive disease and may eventually provide a therapeutic target for severe, rapidly progressive IPF.

C. D. Spradley, MD

Patients with Idiopathic Pulmonary Fibrosis with Antibodies to Heat Shock Protein 70 Have Poor Prognoses

Kahloon RA, Xue J, Bhargava A, et al (Univ of Pittsburgh, PA; et al)

Am J Respir Crit Care Med 187:768-775, 2013

Rationale.—Diverse autoantibodies are present in most patients with idiopathic pulmonary fibrosis (IPF). We hypothesized that specific autoantibodies may associate with IPF manifestations.

Objectives.—To identify clinically relevant, antigen-specific immune responses in patients with IPF.

Methods.—Autoantibodies were detected by immunoblots and ELISA. Intrapulmonary immune processes were evaluated by immunohistochemistry. Anti–heat shock protein 70 (HSP70) IgG was isolated from plasma by immunoaffinity. Flow cytometry was used for leukocyte functional studies.

Measurements and Main Results.—HSP70 was identified as a potential IPF autoantigen in discovery assays. Anti-HSP70 IgG autoantibodies were detected by immunoblots in 3% of 60 control subjects versus 25% of a cross-sectional IPF cohort (n = 122) ($P = 0.0004$), one-half the patients with IPF who died ($P = 0.008$), and 70% of those with acute exacerbations ($P = 0.0005$). Anti-HSP70 autoantibodies in patients with IPF were significantly associated with HLA allele biases, greater subsequent FVC reductions ($P = 0.0004$), and lesser 1-year survival (40 ± 10% vs. 80 ± 5%; hazard ratio = 4.2; 95% confidence interval, 2.0–8.6; $P < 0.0001$). HSP70 protein, antigen–antibody complexes, and complement were prevalent in IPF lungs. HSP70 protein was an autoantigen for IPF CD4 T cells, inducing lymphocyte proliferation ($P = 0.004$) and IL-4 production ($P = 0.01$). IPF anti-HSP70 autoantibodies activated monocytes ($P = 0.009$) and increased monocyte IL-8 production ($P = 0.049$). ELISA confirmed the association between anti-HSP70 autoreactivity and IPF outcome. Anti-HSP70 autoantibodies were also found in patients with other interstitial lung diseases but were not associated with their clinical progression.

Conclusions.—Patients with IPF with anti-HSP70 autoantibodies have more near-term lung function deterioration and mortality. These findings suggest antigen-specific immunoassays could provide useful clinical information in individual patients with IPF and may have implications for understanding IPF progression.

▶ Through diligent investigation and deductive reasoning, Kahloon et al identified heat shock protein 70 (HSP70) as a potential auto-antigen with prognostic value in idiopathic pulmonary fibrosis (IPF). The authors then showed CD4T cell activation and elaboration of IL 4 in IPF patients in response to HSP70. This was not observed in non-IPF controls. Anti-HSP70 autoantibodies were also found to activate monocytes and drive production of interleukin 8.

IPF patients with anti-HSP70 positivity were found to have more reduction in forced vital capacity, and survival was decreased. Anti-HSP70 was also present in two-thirds of patients presenting with acute exacerbations of IPF and 75% of those who showed exacerbation within 1 year. Mortality associated with exacerbation at 6 months was 100% in anti-HSP70 subjects verses 33% in autoantibody-negative patients. Mortality associated with anti-HSP70 was also assessed in a post-hoc analysis of nontransplanted patients, and the survival difference was apparent. Comparison of autoantibody positive and negative groups is provided in Fig 4 of the original article. In addition, a specific human leukocyte antigen class II allele, DRB1*11, was found to be protective, whereas DRB1*15 conferred risk of autoantibody positivity.

The authors also investigated another heat shock protein with similar weight and autoantigenicity in IPF and detected no meaningful clinical difference between antibody-positive and antibody-negative subjects.

The finding of a specific autoantibody that confers greater risk in IPF patients may prove helpful in prognostication and planning for transplantation. It may also pave the way for future targeted therapies in this disease, which currently evades effective treatment.

C. D. Spradley, MD

Morbidity and mortality in patients with usual interstitial pneumonia (UIP) pattern undergoing surgery for lung biopsy

Plönes T, Osei-Agyemang T, Elze M, et al (Univ Med Ctr Freiburg, Germany)
Respir Med 107:629-632, 2013

Background.—Previous studies revealed that surgical lung biopsy in usual interstitial pneumonia (UIP) patients is accompanied with higher morbidity and mortality. The aim of this retrospective analysis was to assess morbidity and mortality of patients with suspected UIP undergoing surgical lung biopsy.

Methods.—We conducted a retrospective study of 45 patients with suspected UIP pattern undergoing surgical biopsy for diffuse pulmonary infiltrates in our department. Data concerning medical history, histology, and survival status were extracted from the medical database of the University Medical Center Freiburg.

Results.—UIP was diagnosed by experienced pneumo-pathologists according to the criteria of American Thoracic Society/European Respiratory Society (ATS/ERS) consensus classification. Due to adhesions the surgeon decided in two patients to perform wedge resection via open surgery. In 43 patients lung biopsy was performed via Video-assisted thoracoscopy (VATS). No intraoperative complications were observed. Postoperative complications consisted of bradyarrhythmia ($n = 1$), gastrointestinal bleeding ($n = 1$), bacterial pneumonia ($n = 1$), candida pneumonia ($n = 1$) and acute exacerbation ($n = 1$). There was no 30-day mortality, but one patient was lost in follow-up and therefore censored. The intraoperative placed thoracic drain was removed at the first postoperative day in most cases (mean day of removal 1.9, ±2.6). The mean length of hospital stay was 8.1 days (±6.8).

Conclusions.—We conclude that surgical biopsy can be safely performed in patients with suspected UIP.

▶ In the era of computed tomography-based diagnosis, need for open lung biopsy in the evaluation of interstitial lung disease has declined. Still, it is occasionally necessary to make firm diagnoses and guide appropriate treatment. The decision to proceed with biopsy is often difficult to make because of studies that suggest mortality rates of 5.3% to 14%.

This retrospective review of 45 consecutive cases at a single German center by Plönes et al contradicts the findings of earlier studies. Although one patient was lost to follow-up, the remainder were alive at 30 days. There were no intraoperative complications. Postoperative complications, each occurring in 1 patient, were bradyarrhythmia, gastrointestinal bleeding, bacterial pneumonia, *Candida* pneumonia, and undefined adverse event. There was no need for reintubation or noninvasive ventilation. Chest drains were removed by the second postoperative day, and the mean length of stay was 8 days.

Based on American Society of Anesthesiology (ASA) class, the patients had a high severity of illness, and pulmonary function testing showed significant impairment. The retrospective nature of this study does leave the sample open to selection bias. Regardless, the authors have shown an impressive success rate obtaining a safe tissue diagnosis in a sick patient population.

C. D. Spradley, MD

Diagnosis and Treatment of Connective Tissue Disease-Associated Interstitial Lung Disease

Vij R, Strek ME (The Univ of Chicago, IL)

Chest 143:814-824, 2013

Interstitial lung disease (ILD) is one of the most serious pulmonary complications associated with connective tissue diseases (CTDs), resulting in significant morbidity and mortality. Although the various CTDs associated with ILD often are considered together because of their shared autoimmune nature, there are substantial differences in the clinical presentations and management of ILD in each specific CTD. This heterogeneity and the cross-disciplinary nature of care have complicated the conduct of prospective multicenter treatment trials and hindered our understanding of the development of ILD in patients with CTD. In this update, we present new information regarding the diagnosis and treatment of patients with ILD secondary to systemic sclerosis, rheumatoid arthritis, dermatomyositis and polymyositis, and Sjögren syndrome. We review information on risk factors for the development of ILD in the setting of CTD. Diagnostic criteria for CTD are presented as well as elements of the clinical evaluation that increase suspicion for CTD-ILD. We review the use of medications in the treatment of CTD-ILD. Although a large, randomized study has examined the impact of immunosuppressive therapy for ILD secondary to systemic sclerosis, additional studies are needed to determine optimal treatment strategies for each distinct form of CTD-ILD. Finally, we review new information regarding the subgroup of patients with ILD who meet some, but not all, diagnostic criteria for a CTD. A careful and systematic approach to diagnosis in patients with ILD may reveal an unrecognized CTD or evidence of autoimmunity in those previously believed to have idiopathic ILD (Tables 1 and 3).

▶ In this excellent, concise review of connective tissue disease—associated interstitial lung disease, Vij and Strek provide a helpful overview of diagnosis and treatment for these patients. The review focuses on systemic sclerosis, rheumatoid arthritis, dermatomyositis/polymyositis, and Sjögren's syndrome. A logical approach to evaluation is outlined in Table 1 and a summary of clinical pearls is provided in Table 3. Additionally, the authors provide an appendix that summarizes diagnostic criteria for the connective tissue diseases discussed.

The authors also discuss autoimmune-featured interstitial lung disease (AIF ILD), which Vij et al[1] described in an earlier paper in *CHEST* in 2011. These patients have autoimmune features but do not meet classic criteria for a firm diagnosis. These patients have a better prognosis if they present with an antinuclear antibody titer of ≥1:1280. This finding helps reinforce the underlying theme of this review, namely, that it is important to identify these patients because

TABLE 1.—Clinical Approach to Evaluating Patients With ILD for CTDs

Clinical Evaluation	Approach
Key elements of history	Presence of: Rashes Raynaud phenomenon Constitutional symptoms Arthralgias Sicca symptoms Dysphagia Proximal muscle weakness
Physical examination	Evaluate for: Rashes Mechanic's hands Gottron papules Sclerodactyly Digital ulcers Synovitis Oral ulcers Proximal muscle weakness
Laboratory	Antinuclear antibody Anti-double-stranded DNA Anti-ribonucleoprotein antibody Anti-Smith antibody Anti-Scl-70 Anti-Ro (SSA) Anti-La (SSB) Rheumatoid factor Anticyclic citrullinated peptide Anti-Jo-1 antibody Creatine kinase Aldolase Erythrocyte sedimentation rate C-reactive protein
Pulmonary function testing, 6-min walk test	Perform at diagnosis and for serial monitoring: Total lung capacity FVC DLCO 6-min walk distance and oxygen saturation
Radiographic	All patients should undergo HRCT scan NSIP pattern seen most often in CTD-ILD
Pathologic	Utility of surgical lung biopsy specimen in established CTD-ILD unclear Biopsy samples from upper, middle, and lower lung fields OP and cellular NSIP more likely to respond to immunosuppressive treatment

Anti-Jo-1 = antihistidyl transfer RNA synthetase; anti-Scl-70 = autoantibodies targeted against type I topoisomerase; CTD = connective tissue disease; DLCO = diffusing capacity of lung for carbon monoxide; HRCT = high-resolution CT; ILD = interstitial lung disease, NSIP = nonspecific interstitial pneumonia; OP = organizing pneumonia; SSA = Sjögren syndrome antigen A; SSB = Sjögren syndrome antigen B.

Reprinted from Vij R, Strek ME. Diagnosis and Treatment of Connective Tissue Disease-Associated Interstitial Lung Disease. Chest. 2013;143:814-824. © 2013, American College of Chest Physicians.

treatment options and prognoses differ between this population and those with idiopathic disease. Indeed, as a group they appear to have better outcomes.

C. D. Spradley, MD

TABLE 3.—Clinical Pearls for CTD-ILD

CTD	Diagnosis	Management
Systemic sclerosis	Esophageal dilation on HRCT scan increases clinical suspicion.	Esophageal dysfunction and gastroesophageal reflux are common. Annual screening for pulmonary hypertension is recommended by the WHO.
Rheumatoid arthritis	Consider drug-induced pneumonitis for new or worsening ILD.	Radiographic and histopathologic findings of UIP portend a worse prognosis. Tobacco cessation is strongly recommended.
Dermatomyositis and polymyositis	Myositis may be subtle and present after ILD. Myositis-associated and -specific antibodies aid in diagnosis.	Early treatment with prednisone and additional immunosuppressive agents may improve outcomes.
Sjögren syndrome	Cysts on HRCT scan increase clinical suspicion.	Severe ILD, with UIP on HRCT scan and pathology, has been reported. LIP may be less common than other histopathologic patterns.
Autoimmune-featured ILD	Comprehensive and systematic evaluation will identify these patients. Seen in patients with UIP on HRCT scan and pathology.	Patients with ANA titer ≥ 1:1,280 may have improved survival.

ANA = antinuclear antibody; LIP = lymphocytic interstitial pneumonia; UIP = usual interstitial pneumonia; WHO = World Health Organization. See Table 1 and 2 legends for expansion of other abbreviations.

Reprinted from Vij R, Strek ME. Diagnosis and Treatment of Connective Tissue Disease-Associated Interstitial Lung Disease. Chest. 2013;143:814-824. © 2013, American College of Chest Physicians.

Reference

1. Vij R, Noth I, Strek ME. Autoimmune-featured interstitial lung disease: a distinct entity. *Chest.* 2011;140:1292-1299.

Mycophenolate Mofetil Improves Lung Function in Connective Tissue Disease-associated Interstitial Lung Disease

Fischer A, Brown KK, Du Bois RM, et al (Natl Jewish Health, Denver, CO; Imperial College, London, UK)

J Rheumatol 40:640-646, 2013

Objective.—Small series suggest mycophenolate mofetil (MMF) is well tolerated and may be an effective therapy for connective tissue disease-associated interstitial lung disease (CTD-ILD). We examined the tolerability and longitudinal changes in pulmonary physiology in a large and diverse cohort of patients with CTD-ILD treated with MMF.

Methods.—We identified consecutive patients evaluated at our center between January 2008 and January 2011 and prescribed MMF for CTD-ILD. We assessed safety and tolerability of MMF and used longitudinal data analyses to examine changes in pulmonary physiology over time, before and after initiation of MMF.

Results.—We identified 125 subjects treated with MMF for a median 897 days. MMF was discontinued in 13 subjects. MMF was associated with significant improvements in estimated percentage of predicted forced vital capacity (FVC%) from MMF initiation to 52, 104, and 156 weeks (4.9% ± 1.9%, $p = 0.01$; 6.1% ± 1.8%, $p = 0.0008$; and 7.3% ± 2.6%, $p = 0.004$, respectively); and in estimated percentage predicted diffusing capacity (DLCO%) from MMF initiation to 52 and 104 weeks (6.3% ± 2.8%, $p = 0.02$; 7.1% ± 2.8%, $p = 0.01$). In the subgroup without usual interstitial pneumonia (UIP)-pattern injury, MMF significantly improved FVC% and DLCO%, and in the subgroup with UIP-pattern injury, MMF was associated with stability in FVC% and DLCO%.

Conclusion.—In a large diverse cohort of CTD-ILD, MMF was well tolerated and had a low rate of discontinuation. Treatment with MMF was associated with either stable or improved pulmonary physiology over a median 2.5 years of followup. MMF appears to be a promising therapy for the spectrum of CTD-ILD.

▶ In this study published in the *Journal of Rheumatology*, Fischer and colleagues present retrospective data describing a 4-year experience treating 125 patients with mycophenolate mofetil (MMF) for connective tissue disease–associated interstitial lung disease (CTD ILD). In the run up to the conclusion of the Scleroderma Lung Study II, the experience may give some early insight into the results.

The group describes average duration of treatment of almost 900 days and follows up with patients for 3 years. Drug was well tolerated and discontinued in only 10% of subjects. In 29%, MMF replaced cyclophosphamide, and in 15% it replaced azathioprine. Median daily prednisone dose decreased from 20 mg at initiation to 5 mg at 9 to 12 months (Fig 2 in the original article). Patients also showed a statistically significant improvement in forced vital capacity and diffusion capacity (Fig 3 in the original article).

As identified by the authors, the study suffers from its retrospective nature and the potential for referral bias. It is also not entirely clear how clinically significant the statistically significant improvements in lung function are. MMF appears to be an attractive option for the treatment of CTD ILD.

C. D. Spradley, MD

Pleural Plaques and the Risk of Pleural Mesothelioma

Pairon J-C, Laurent F, Rinaldo M, et al (Université Paris-Est Créteil, France; Centre cardiothoracique INSERM 1045, Bordeaux, France; Centre INSERM 897, Bordeaux, France; et al)
J Natl Cancer Inst 105:293-301, 2013

Background.—The association between pleural plaques and pleural mesothelioma remains controversial. The present study was designed to examine the association between pleural plaques on computed tomography (CT) scan and the risk of pleural mesothelioma in a follow-up study of asbestos-exposed workers.

Methods.—Retired or unemployed workers previously occupationally exposed to asbestos were invited to participate in a screening program for asbestos-related diseases, including CT scan, organized between October 2003 and December 2005 in four regions in France. Randomized, independent, double reading of CT scans by a panel of seven chest radiologists focused on benign asbestos-related abnormalities. A 7-year follow-up study was conducted in the 5287 male subjects for whom chest CT scan was available. Annual determination of the number of subjects eligible for free medical care because of pleural mesothelioma was carried out. Diagnosis certification was obtained from the French mesothelioma panel of pathologists. Survival regression based on the Cox model was used to estimate the risk of pleural mesothelioma associated with pleural plaques, with age as the main time variable and time-varying exposure variables, namely duration of exposure, time since first exposure, and cumulative exposure index to asbestos. All statistical tests were two-sided.

Results.—A total of 17 incident cases of pleural mesothelioma were diagnosed. A statistically significant association was observed between mesothelioma and pleural plaques (unadjusted hazard ratio (HR) = 8.9,

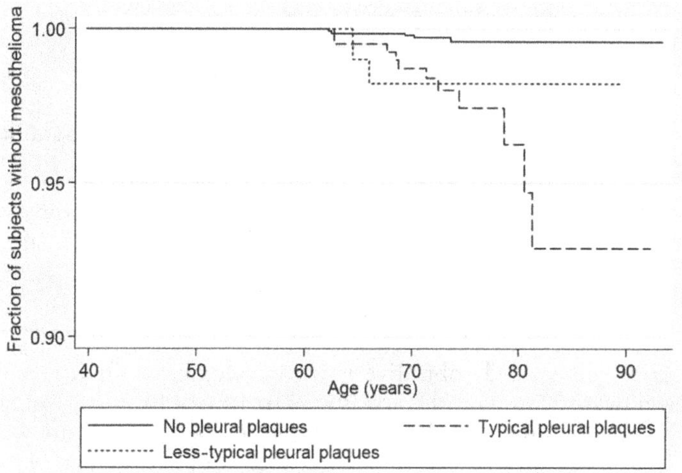

FIGURE 2.—Proportion of subjects without pleural mesothelioma at any given age according to the presence of pleural plaques on computed tomography (CT) scan (Kaplan–Meier survival curve, log-rank test $P < .0001$). N = 34 091 subject-years. At-risk subjects at different ages were as follows for the different groups: subjects with no plaques on CT scan: 1870 at 65 years, 1646 at 70 years, 353 at 75 years, 113 at 80 years, and 23 at 85 years; subjects with typical parietal or diaphragmatic pleural plaques on CT scan: 297 at 65 years, 353 at 70 years, 146 at 75 years, 63 at 80 years, and 22 at 85 years; subjects with other less typical plaques on CT scan: 108 at 65 years, 134 at 70 years, 43 at 75 years, 22 at 80 years, and 8 at 85 years. Parietal pleural plaques were considered to be typical when they were bilateral, thicker than 2 mm, and with an extent greater than 1 cm, regardless of whether they were calcified. (Reprinted from Pairon J-C, Laurent F, Rinaldo M, et al. Pleural plaques and the risk of pleural mesothelioma. *J Natl Cancer Inst.* 2013;105:293-301, by permission of Oxford University Press.)

95% confidence interval [CI] = 3.0 to 26.5; adjusted HR = 6.8, 95% CI = 2.2 to 21.4 after adjustment for time since first exposure and cumulative exposure index to asbestos).

Conclusion.—The presence of pleural plaques may be an independent risk factor for pleural mesothelioma (Fig 2).

▶ In this French study by Pairon et al, the investigators evaluated a large sample (5287 subjects) of men with prior occupational exposure to asbestos. The aim was to evaluate the relationship between presence of pleural plaques on computed tomography (CT) scan and risk for mesothelioma. Prior studies evaluating the link based on chest radiograph did not show a relationship.

The study relied on a cumulative exposure index based on duration and intensity of exposure, as quantitative fiber exposure data were not available. The study also censored female subjects.

In this study, the authors found an unadjusted hazard ratio of 8.9 for those exposed subjects with CT evidence of plaque verses those without. Patients with plaques had longer mean duration of exposure than patients without plaques. Fig 2, illustrating a fraction of subjects without mesothelioma, shows the statistically significant difference between the groups ($P < .0001$).

The study benefited from strong standards surrounding the definition of pleural plaques, double over-reading of scans with triple reading in the case of disagreement, and reliance on an expert panel of pathologists for confirmation of mesothelioma diagnosis in all but 3 of the 17 incident cases.

Based on this study, it does appear that pleural plaques are a marker for both increased exposure and increased risk of mesothelioma. These patients, therefore, will benefit from closer surveillance than exposed patients without evidence of pleural plaques on CT scan.

C. D. Spradley, MD

Surgical decortication as the first-line treatment for pleural empyema

Shin JA, Chang YS, Kim TH, et al (Yonsei Univ College of Medicine, Seoul, Korea)

J Thorac Cardiovasc Surg 145:933-939.e1, 2013

Objective.—The study objective was to evaluate the clinical outcomes of surgical decortication as the first line of treatment for pleural empyema.

Methods.—We analyzed the medical records of 111 patients who presented with empyema and were treated with simple drainage or surgical decortication as the first line of treatment at Gangnam Severance Hospital, a tertiary referral medical center in Seoul, Korea.

Results.—Of 111 patients with empyema, 27 underwent surgical decortication as the first intervention. Surgical decortication showed a better treatment success rate in all study subjects (96.3%, 26/27 patients) compared with simple drainage (58.3%, 49/84 patients; $P < .0001$ for method comparison). After propensity-scored matching, decortication resulted in a better outcome (95.0%, 19/20 patients) versus drainage (56.7%, 17/30 patients; $P = .003$). Surgical decortication as the first line of treatment for empyema was the best predictor of treatment success after adjustment for compounding factors (odds ratio, 14.529; 95% confidence interval, 1.715-123.074; $P = .014$).

Conclusions.—The first treatment choice for pleural empyema is a critical determinant of ultimate therapeutic success. After adjusting for confounding variables, surgical decortication is the optimal first treatment choice for advanced empyema (Fig 1).

▶ In this single-center, retrospective study published in *The Journal of Thoracic and Cardiovascular Surgery* by Shin and colleagues, the authors compare primary surgical therapy with decortication to simple pleural drainage for empyema.

The authors define empyema radiographically by septation on computed tomography scan and by appearance of gross puss or microbiologic positivity. The 2 groups studied differed in terms of Eastern Cooperative Oncology Group score, Charleston comorbidity index, and Acute Physiology and Chronic Health Evaluation (APACHE) II score with sicker patients being more common in the simple drainage group. Before propensity matching, body mass index ≥17, APACHE II score less than 20, mean blood pressure ≥60, and serum albumin ≥3.0 were predictors of superior outcome (Fig 1).

To correct for the difference, the authors used propensity matching. They excluded 61 of the original 111 patients and after matching, primary decortication remained the only significant predictor of success ($P = .003$). Treatment failure correlated with culture positivity after matching ($P < .001$).

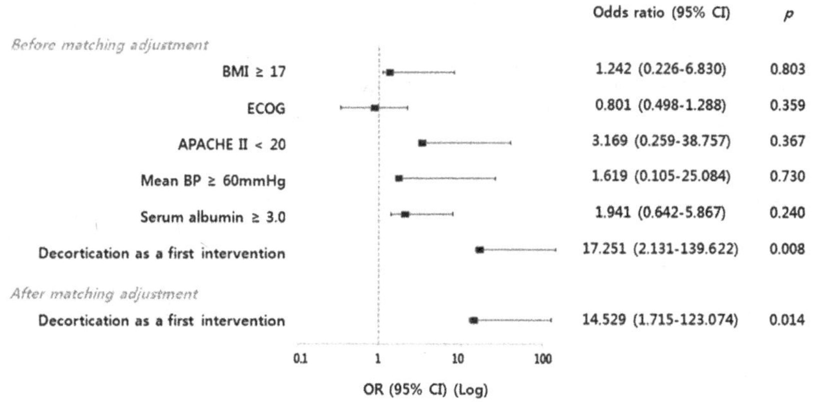

FIGURE 1.—Multivariate analysis of overall treatment success. Odds ratios (95% confidence intervals) of overall treatment success with BMI of 17 kg/m^2 or greater, ECOG score, APACHE II score less than 20, mean arterial pressure 60 mm Hg or greater, serum albumin 3.0 g/dL or greater, and decortications as a first treatment were analyzed using logistic regression in stepwise manner. After propensity-scored matching adjustment, decortication as a first intervention remained the most important predictive factor of a successful treatment outcome. *APACHE II*, Acute Physiology and Chronic Health Evaluation II; *BMI*, body mass index; *BP*, blood pressure; *CI*, confidence interval; *ECOG*, Eastern Cooperative Oncology Group; *OR*, odds ratio. (Reprinted from the Journal of Thoracic and Cardiovascular Surgery. Shin JA, Chang YS, Kim TH, et al. Surgical decortication as the first-line treatment for pleural empyema. *J Thorac Cardiovasc Surg*. 2013;145:933-939.e1, Copyright 2013, with permission from The American Association for Thoracic Surgery.)

Author-identified weaknesses of this study included the retrospective nature, the potential for selection bias (proven by the difference in the nonmatched populations), and the inclusion of tuberculous effusions with other forms of empyema.

Although this study does have flaws, as noted above, it supports the growing consensus that surgical intervention is the treatment of choice for loculated empyema.

C. D. Spradley, MD

Anticoagulation and Survival in Pulmonary Arterial Hypertension: Results From the Comparative, Prospective Registry of Newly Initiated Therapies for Pulmonary Hypertension (COMPERA)

Olsson KM, Delcroix M, Ghofrani HA, et al (Hannover Med School, Germany; Univ Hosps of Leuven, Germany; Univ of Giessen and Marburg Lung Ctr (UGMLC), Hannover, Germany; et al)

Circulation 129:57-65, 2014

Background.—For almost 30 years, anticoagulation has been recommended for patients with idiopathic pulmonary arterial hypertension (IPAH). Supporting evidence, however, is limited, and it is unclear whether this recommendation is still justified in the modern management era and whether it should be extended to patients with other forms of pulmonary arterial hypertension (PAH).

Methods and Results.—We analyzed data from Comparative, Prospective Registry of Newly Initiated Therapies for Pulmonary Hypertension (COMPERA), an ongoing European pulmonary hypertension registry. Survival rates of patients with IPAH and other forms of PAH were compared by the use of anticoagulation. The sample consisted of 1283 consecutively enrolled patients with newly diagnosed PAH. Anticoagulation was used in 66% of 800 patients with IPAH and in 43% of 483 patients with other forms of PAH. In patients with IPAH, there was a significantly better 3-year survival ($P = 0.006$) in patients on anticoagulation compared with patients who never received anticoagulation, albeit the patients in the anticoagulation group had more severe disease at baseline. The survival difference at 3 years remained statistically significant ($P = 0.017$) in a matched-pair analysis of n = 336 IPAH patients. The beneficial effect of anticoagulation on survival of IPAH patients was confirmed by Cox multivariable regression analysis (hazard ratio, 0.79; 95% confidence interval, 0.66-0.94). In contrast, the use of anticoagulants was not associated with a survival benefit in patients with other forms of PAH.

Conclusions.—The present data suggest that the use of anticoagulation is associated with a survival benefit in patients with IPAH, supporting current treatment recommendations. The evidence remains inconclusive for other forms of PAH.

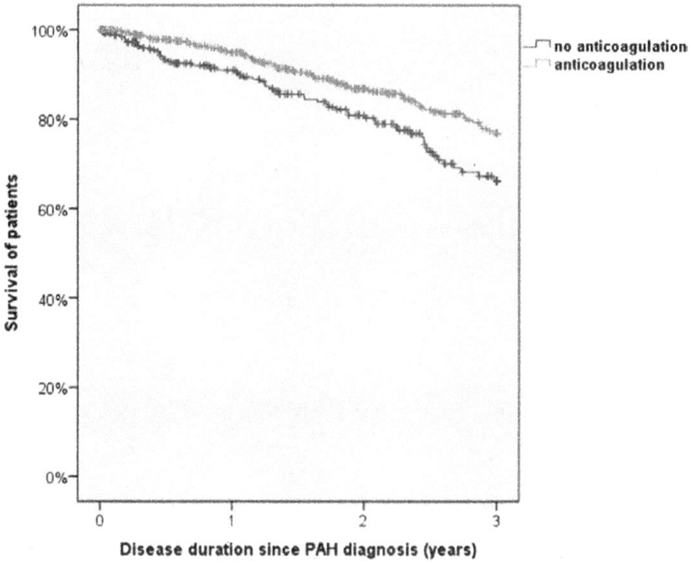

FIGURE 3.—Estimated survival of the idiopathic pulmonary arterial hypertension (IPAH) cohort in accordance with anticoagulation therapy. The numbers of patients at risk at baseline and after 1, 2, and 3 years were 528, 390, 247, and 155 in the anticoagulation group and 272, 180, 127, and 65 in the no anticoagulation group. The survival difference between both groups was statistically significant ($P = 0.006$). (Reprinted from Olsson KM, Delcroix M, Ghofrani HA, et al. Anticoagulation and survival in pulmonary arterial hypertension: results from the comparative, prospective registry of newly initiated therapies for pulmonary hypertension (COMPERA). *Circulation.* 2014;129:57-65, Copyright 2014, with permission from American Heart Association, Inc.)

Clinical Trial Registration.—URL: http://www.clinicaltrials.gov. Unique identifier: NCT01347216 (Figs 3 and 4).

▶ Hypercoagulability and in situ thrombosis of small pulmonary arteries is the hallmark of idiopathic pulmonary arterial hypertension (IPAH). This has led to the concept that therapeutic anticoagulation is beneficial in the management of this disease. Small observational studies have shown anticoagulants to be associated with better survival in patients with IPAH, but to date, there are no randomized clinical trials. The benefit of anticoagulation with other forms of pulmonary arterial hypertension (PAH) remains controversial. Accordingly, the aim of this study was to compare anticoagulation to no anticoagulation in a contemporary cohort of patients with IPAH and PAH from the noninterventional, prospective COMPERA registry. There were 800 patients in the IAPH cohort of which 528 (66%) received anticoagulants. Estimated survival probabilities by Kaplan-Meier at 1, 2, and 3 years in the anticoagulation group were 94.9%, 86.8%, and 76.9%, which was significantly greater than survival rates in the no anticoagulation group (90.9%, 80.9%, and 66.3%, respectively; $P = .006$; Fig 3). Match paired analysis of 336 IAPH demonstrated a statistically significant survival difference between both groups favoring patients in the anticoagulation group (survival rates at 1, 2, and 3 year of 93.9%, 88.2%, and 73.6%

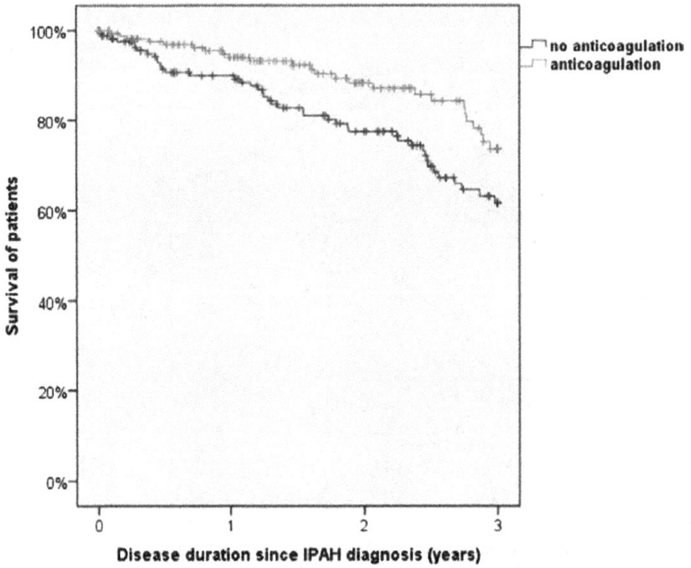

FIGURE 4.—Estimated survival of matched-pair idiopathic pulmonary arterial hypertension (IPAH) cohort. The numbers of patients at risk at baseline and after 1, 2, and 3 years were 168, 124, 76, and 46 in the anticoagulation group and 168, 120, 84, and 41 in the no anticoagulation group. The survival difference between both groups was statistically significant ($P = 0.017$). (Reprinted from Olsson KM, Delcroix M, Ghofrani HA, et al. Anticoagulation and survival in pulmonary arterial hypertension: results from the comparative, prospective registry of newly initiated therapies for pulmonary hypertension (COMPERA). *Circulation.* 2014;129:57-65, Copyright 2014, with permission from American Heart Association, Inc.)

in the anticoagulation group vs 89.9%, 77.5%, and 61.6% in the no anticoagulation group; $P = .017$; Fig 4). There were 483 patients with other forms of PAH of whom 210 (43%) received anticoagulants. Kaplan-Meier estimated survival rates at 1, 2, and 3 years were not statistically different between groups. In this study, patients with IPAH treated with anticoagulants had a survival benefit. Although groups were not entirely comparable in terms of severity of disease, a matched-paired analysis of a smaller cohort showed similar difference in survival. Although these data lend support to the use of anticoagulation in patients with IPAH, randomized, controlled trials are still needed. Despite a lack of supporting evidence and increased risk of bleeding, a surprising large number of patients with other forms of PAH were taking anticoagulants. Based on these data, the benefit of anticoagulation is inconclusive in this group.

T. Todoran, MD, MSc

37 Sleep Disorders

Randomized Controlled trial of Noninvasive Positive Pressure Ventilation (NPPV) Versus Servoventilation in Patients with CPAP-Induced Central Sleep Apnea (Complex Sleep Apnea)

Dellweg D, Kerl J, Hoehn E, et al (Kloster Grafschaft, Schmallenberg, Germany)

Sleep 36:1163-1171, 2013

Study Objectives.—To compare the treatment effect of noninvasive positive pressure ventilation (NPPV) and anticyclic servoventilation in patients with continuous positive airway pressure (CPAP)-induced central sleep apnea (complex sleep apnea).

Design.—Randomized controlled trial.

Setting.—Sleep center.

Patients.—Thirty patients who developed complex sleep apnea syndrome (CompSAS) during CPAP treatment.

Interventions.—NPPV or servoventilation.

Measurements and Results.—Patients were randomized to NPPV or servo-ventilation. Full polysomnography (PSG) was performed after 6 weeks. On CPAP prior to randomization, patients in the NPPV and servo-ventilator arm had comparable apnea-hypopnea indices (AHI, 28.6 ± 6.5 versus 27.7 ± 9.7 events/h (mean ± standard deviation [SD])), apnea indices (AI, 19 ± 5.6 versus 21.1 ± 8.6 events/h), central apnea indices (CAI, 16.7 ± 5.4 versus 18.2 ± 7.1 events/h), oxygen desaturation indices (ODI, 17.5 ± 13.1 versus 24.3 ± 11.9 events/h). During initial titration NPPV and servoventilation significantly improved the AHI (9.1 ± 4.3 versus 9 ± 6.4 events/h), AI (2 ± 3.1 versus 3.5 ± 4.5 events/h) CAI (2 ± 3.1 versus 2.5 ± 3.9 events/h) and ODI (10.1 ± 4.5 versus 8.9 ± 8.4 events/h) when compared to CPAP treatment (all $P < 0.05$). After 6 weeks we observed the following differences: AHI (16.5 ± 8 versus 7.4 ± 4.2 events/h, $P = 0.027$), AI (10.4 ± 5.9 versus 1.7 ± 1.9 events/h, $P = 0.001$), CAI (10.2 ± 5.1 versus 1.5 ± 1.7 events/h, $P < 0.0001$)) and ODI (21.1 ± 9.2 versus 4.8 ± 3.4 events/h, $P < 0.0001$) for NPPV and servoventilation, respectively. Other sleep parameters were unaffected by any form of treatment.

Conclusions.—After 6 weeks, servoventilation treated respiratory events more effectively than NPPV in patients with complex sleep apnea syndrome.

▶ The prevalence of complex sleep apnea is 15% of patients undergoing polysomnography at a large referral center. Clinical characteristics of patients with complex sleep apnea are similar to those with obstructive sleep apnea syndrome.[1] No reliable clinical markers are predictive of the appearance of complex sleep apnea.[2] Furthermore, there are no published guidelines on how to treat or who to treat. Complex sleep apnea is best thought of as a dynamic process with some individuals' apnea resolving and others in whom the complex apnea continues. Furthermore, Cassel et al reported the development of complex sleep apnea at 3-month follow-up in patients who had no evidence of it initially.[3] This finding only adds to the difficulty of treating this entity.

In this article, at 6 week follow-up those randomly assigned to noninvasive positive pressure ventilation (NPPV) had significantly higher apnea-hypopnea indices (AHI) than those receiving servoventilation. Central events represent the greatest number of respiratory events at follow-up, despite the fact that both groups had similar AHI on the titration night. It is unclear from this study why NPPV failed to control the complex sleep apnea at follow-up, but what I think we can glean from this study plus the existing literature is that this group of patients needs close follow-up because there are no clear predictors of the course for complex sleep apnea and that servoventilation appears to treat complex apnea more effectively over time compared with NPPV.

S. F. Jones, MD, FCCP, DABSM

References

1. Morgenthaler TI, Kagramanov V, Hanak V, Decker PA. Complex sleep apnea syndrome: is it a unique clinical syndrome? *Sleep*. 2006;36:1203-1209.
2. Kuźniar TJ, Morgenthaler TI. Treatment of complex sleep apnea syndrome. *Chest*. 2012;142:1049-1057.
3. Cassel W, Canisius S, Becker HF, et al. A prospective polysomnographic study on the evolution of complex sleep apnoea. *Eur Respir J*. 2011;38:329-337.

An Official American Thoracic Society Clinical Practice Guideline: Sleep Apnea, Sleepiness, and Driving Risk in Noncommercial Drivers: An Update of a 1994 Statement

Strohl KP, on behalf of the ATS Ad Hoc Committee on Sleep Apnea, Sleepiness, and Driving Risk in Noncommercial Drivers

Am J Respir Crit Care Med 187:1259-1266, 2013

Background.—Sleepiness may account for up to 20% of crashes on monotonous roads, especially highways. Obstructive sleep apnea (OSA) is the most common medical disorder that causes excessive daytime sleepiness, increasing the risk for drowsy driving two to three times. The purpose of these guidelines is to update the 1994 American Thoracic Society Statement that described the relationships among sleepiness, sleep apnea, and driving risk.

Methods.—A multidisciplinary panel was convened to develop evidence-based clinical practice guidelines for the management of sleepy driving due to OSA. Pragmatic systematic reviews were performed, and the Grading of Recommendations, Assessment, Development, and Evaluation approach was used to formulate and grade the recommendations. Critical outcomes included crash-related mortality and real crashes, whereas important outcomes included near-miss crashes and driving performance.

Results.—A strong recommendation was made for treatment of confirmed OSA with continuous positive airway pressure to reduce driving risk, rather than no treatment, which was supported by moderate-quality evidence. Weak recommendations were made for expeditious diagnostic evaluation and initiation of treatment and against the use of stimulant medications or empiric continuous positive airway pressure to reduce driving risk. The weak recommendations were supported by very low–quality evidence. Additional suggestions included routinely determining the driving risk, inquiring about additional causes of sleepiness, educating patients about the risks of excessive sleepiness, and encouraging clinicians to become familiar with relevant laws.

Discussion.—The recommendations presented in this guideline are based on the current evidence, and will require an update as new evidence and/or technologies becomes available.

▶ This is an update of the previous statement (which was last published in 1994!). A lot has happened since that time: litigations, drowsy driving laws passed in some states, and overall an increase in public awareness. So an update on this statement is timely (and overdue). The authors of the report are well-recognized experts in the field of sleep medicine and driving safety who have reviewed the available literature. Obstructive sleep apnea is associated with an increased risk of motor vehicle accidents. Furthermore, considering the possible number of near misses on the roadways today, it is important that our patients are aware of the public risk of drowsy driving and the importance of treatment and education. It is important that a timely evaluation and diagnostic testing is performed on high-risk individuals. There is emphasis on use of home sleep testing in the appropriate candidate. This, of course, would expedite diagnosis and management.

S. F. Jones, MD, FCCP, DABSM

Impact of Group Education on Continuous Positive Airway Pressure Adherence

Lettieri CJ, Walter RJ (Walter Reed Natl Military Med Ctr, Bethesda, MD)
J Clin Sleep Med 9:537-541, 2013

Study Objectives.—To compare the impact of a group educational program versus individual education on continuous positive airway pressure (CPAP) adherence.

Methods.—Post hoc assessment of a performance improvement initiative designed to improve clinic efficiency, access to care, and time to initiate therapy. Consecutive patients newly diagnosed with obstructive sleep apnea (OSA) initiating CPAP therapy participated in either an individual or group educational program. The content and information was similar in both strategies.

Results.—Of 2,116 included patients, 1,032 received education regarding OSA and CPAP through a group clinic, and 1,084 received individual education. Among the cohort, 76.6% were men, mean age 48.3 ± 9.2 years, mean body mass index 29.6 ± 4.6 kg/m^2, and mean apnea-hypopnea index was 33.3 ± 24.4 events/hour. Baseline characteristics were similar between groups. CPAP adherence was significantly greater in those participating in a group program than those receiving individual education. Specifically, CPAP was used for more nights (67.2% vs. 62.1%, $p = 0.02$) and more hours per night during nights used (4.3 ± 2.1 vs. 3.7 ± 2.8, $p = 0.03$). Further, fewer individuals discontinued therapy (10.6% vs. 14.5%, $p < 0.001$), more achieved regular use of CPAP (45.2%. vs. 40.6%, $p = 0.08$), and time to initiate therapy was shorter (13.2 ± 3.1 versus 24.6 ± 7.4 days, $p < 0.001$). Group education resulted in a 3- to 4-fold increase in the number of patients seen per unit time.

Conclusions.—A group educational program facilitated improved CPAP adherence. If confirmed by prospective randomized studies, group CPAP education may be an appropriate alternative to individual counseling, may improve acceptance of and adherence to therapy, and decrease time to treatment.

▶ I read this article with enthusiasm because I find the topic of continuous positive airway pressure (CPAP) adherence interesting and because I see the applicability in a busy clinical practice. In a practice with many referrals, we must find ways to be efficient and deliver outstanding service and, most importantly, provide excellent care for our patients. Of course, this all needs to be done early in the course of CPAP initiation, a time in which patterns of adherence (or not) emerge.

In this article, the authors evaluated adherence in patients who received education in an individual or group construct. By using group therapy, more patients could be seen in one time period compared, hence, improved efficiency. Subjects who received group education used their CPAP for more hours per night and a greater portion of nights than those who received individual attention. But alas! Although there is a statistically significant improvement in the adherence numbers, the mean hours of use and portion of nights used as a group are still less than ideal and fall below the CMS definition of compliance. Nevertheless, a positive note is that group therapy is feasible to use in the clinical setting with adherence rates that are better than those of individual education.

In my practice setting, we attempted a group education initiative for a short time. I think there were certain patients who found a group setting enjoyable, and for others it was not. By gaining a better understanding of the patient and medical-related factors, along with the technical challenges of CPAP adherence, we can adjust our methods of CPAP education and hopefully improve the current rates of treatment acceptance. I encourage you to read the article by Wickwire et al (also a selection in the Year Book).[1]

S. F. Jones, MD, FCCP, DABSM

Reference

1. Wickwire EM, Lettieri CJ, Cairns AA, Collop NA. Maximizing positive airway pressure adherence in adults. *Chest.* 2013;144:680-693.

Maximizing Positive Airway Pressure Adherence in Adults: A Common-Sense Approach

Wickwire EM, Lettieri CJ, Cairns AA, et al (Pulmonary Disease and Critical Care Associates, Columbia, MD; Uniformed Services Univ and Walter Reed Natl Military Med Ctr, Bethesda, MD; et al)

Chest 144:680-693, 2013

Positive airway pressure (PAP) therapy is considered the most efficacious treatment of obstructive sleep apnea (OSA), especially moderate to severe OSA, and remains the most commonly prescribed. Yet suboptimal adherence presents a challenge to sleep-medicine clinicians. The purpose of the current review is to highlight the efficacy of published interventions to improve PAP adherence and to suggest a patient-centered clinical approach to enhancing PAP usage.

▶ Nonadherence to continuous positive airway pressure (CPAP) is a common and daily problem clinicians see in practice. Although technologies continue to advance the field to make the prescribed pressure more acceptable, patient-related factors are important. We need to understand the multiple variables that make treatment so difficult for our patients, or otherwise we will continue to see rates of CPAP abandonment at 25%,[1] and long-term treatment adherence in less than 50% of patients.[2] This article nicely outlines patient, medical, and psychiatric disease-related factors and equipment-related issues associated with adherence. The available data on interventions that have been tried are reviewed. I think many of us focus on education, making it the center of our methods to promote adherence, but that alone is not enough. It is likely that we need to understand what inhibits our patients from CPAP use just as much as what is the best intervention. Individualization and interdisciplinary teams are important. There is a need for behavioral specialists on the team, and I think (and hope) that more sleep centers will incorporate such experts.

S. F. Jones, MD, FCCP, DABSM

References

1. van Zeller M, Severo M, Santos AC, Drummond M. 5-year APAP adherence in OSA patients—do first impressions matter? *Respir Med.* 2013;107: 2046-2052.
2. Weaver TE, Grunstein RR. Adherence to continuous positive airway pressure therapy: the challenge to effective treatment. *Proc Am Thorac Soc.* 2008;5: 173-178.

5-Years APAP adherence in OSA patients – Do first impressions matter?

van Zeller M, Severo M, Santos AC, et al (Centro Hospitalar de São João, Porto, Portugal; Univ of Porto Med School, Portugal)

Respir Med 107:2046-2052, 2013

Background.—Although continuous positive airway pressure (CPAP) is effective in treating obstructive sleep apnoea (OSA), inadequate adherence remains a major cause of treatment failure. This study aimed to determine long term adherence to auto adjusting-CPAP (APAP) and its influencing factors including the role of initial compliance.

Methods.—Eighty-eight male patients with newly diagnosed moderate/severe OSA were included. After initiation of APAP treatment, patients had periodic follow-up appointments at 2 weeks, 6 months and then annually for at least 5 years. Patient's compliance to therapy was assessed in each appointment and predictors to treatment abandonment and poor compliance were evaluated.

Results.—The studied population had a mean age of 53.8 years and mean apnoea–hypopnoea index of 52.71/h.

The mean time of follow-up was 5.2 (±1.6) years, during that time 22 (25%) patients abandoned APAP, those who maintained treatment had good compliance to it since 94% of them used it more than 4 h/day for at least 70% of days.

A significant negative association was found between age, % of days and mean time of APAP use on 12th day and 6th month and the risk of abandoning. APAP use lower than 33% and 57% of days at 12th day and 6th month, respectively had high specificity (~100%) to detect treatment abandonment.

Conclusions.—The majority of patients adheres to long term APAP treatment and has good compliance after 5-years of follow-up. Age and initial compliance (% days of use and mean hour/day) have the ability to predict future adherence, as soon as 12 days and 6 months after initiation.

▶ Although continuous positive airway pressure (CPAP) is first-line therapy for obstructive sleep apnea (OSA), adherence to therapy is difficult for many patients. It is estimated that up to 83% of patients use their CPAP machines less than 4 hours per night for less than 70% of nights.[1] While recognizing the association between OSA and cardiovascular morbidity and mortality, clinicians need to be able to identify early who is going to be nonadherent to therapy and consider alternative treatments for OSA or methods to improve adherence. Recognition should ideally occur before the patient abandons therapy with CPAP and is lost to follow-up.

The authors in this study performed 5-year longitudinal follow-up of 88 men with moderate to severe OSA. Subjects received an autotitrating PAP (APAP) machine and were followed up at regular intervals. Overall, 25% of the study subjects abandoned treatment. The first visit was at 12 days on average, and APAP use lower than 33% at the 12th day had a 100% specificity to detect treatment abandonment. There was also a negative relationship between age and risk of abandonment. Patients who report problems during the first night of APAP use the treatment less than those who do not.[2] If signs of abandonment are seen as early as 12th day, for how long should we continue to ask our patients to keep using PAP before we switch therapies or initiate an intervention strategy to promote adherence? What is the ideal strategy to improve adherence? That answer is not clear.

On a positive note, the treatment adherence in this study was high. Seventy percent of subjects still used PAP at 5 years, with 94% of patients using it for at least 4 hours per night on 70% of nights. Although this study did not find an association between apnea-hypopnea index and abandonment, the study included only patients with moderate to severe OSA. Disease severity has been found to be a weak but consistent factor to CPAP use.[3] For those who abandon therapy, the authors summarize that first impressions seem to last. I would agree with that.

S. F. Jones, MD, FCCP, DABSM

References

1. Weaver TE, Grunstein RR. Adherence to continuous positive airway pressure therapy: the challenge to effective treatment. *Proc Am Thorac Soc.* 2008;5:173-178.
2. Lewis KE, Seale L, Bartle IE, Watkins AJ, Ebden P. Early predictors of CPAP use for the treatment of obstructive sleep apnea. *Sleep.* 2004;27:134-138.
3. Sawyer AM, Gooneratne NS, Marcus CL, Ofer D, Richards KC, Weaver TE. A systematic review of CPAP adherence across age groups: clinical and empiric insights for developing CPAP adherence interventions. *Sleep Med Rev.* 2011;15:343-356.

38 Critical Care Medicine

Acute Respiratory Distress Syndrome After Spontaneous Intracerebral Hemorrhage

Elmer J, Hou P, Wilcox SR, et al (Univ of Pittsburgh Med Ctr, PA; Brigham and Women's Hosp, Boston, MA; Harvard Med School, Boston, MA; et al)

Crit Care Med 41:1992-2001, 2013

Objectives.—Acute respiratory distress syndrome develops commonly in critically ill patients in response to an injurious stimulus. The prevalence and risk factors for development of acute respiratory distress syndrome after spontaneous intracerebral hemorrhage have not been reported. We sought to determine the prevalence of acute respiratory distress syndrome after intracerebral hemorrhage, characterize risk factors for its development, and assess its impact on patient outcomes.

Design.—Retrospective cohort study at two academic centers.

Patients.—We included consecutive patients presenting from June 1, 2000, to November 1, 2010, with intracerebral hemorrhage requiring mechanical ventilation. We excluded patients with age less than 18 years, intracerebral hemorrhage secondary to trauma, tumor, ischemic stroke, or structural lesion; if they required intubation only during surgery; if they were admitted for comfort measures; or for a history of immunodeficiency.

Interventions.—None.

Measurements and Main Results.—Data were collected both prospectively as part of an ongoing cohort study and by retrospective chart review. Of 1,665 patients identified by database query, 697 met inclusion criteria. The prevalence of acute respiratory distress syndrome was 27%. In unadjusted analysis, high tidal volume ventilation was associated with an increased risk of acute respiratory distress syndrome (hazard ratio, 1.79 [95% CI, 1.13–2.83]), as were male sex, RBC and plasma transfusion, higher fluid balance, obesity, hypoxemia, acidosis, tobacco use, emergent hematoma evacuation, and vasopressor dependence. In multivariable modeling, high tidal volume ventilation was the strongest risk factor for acute respiratory distress syndrome development (hazard ratio, 1.74 [95% CI, 1.08–2.81]) and for inhospital mortality (hazard ratio, 2.52 [95% CI, 1.46–4.34]).

TABLE 2.—Multivariable Model of Risk Factors for Development of Acute Respiratory Distress Syndrome

Characteristic	Multivariable Hazard Ratio	*P*
Tidal volume >8 mL/kg	1.74 (1.08–2.81)	0.02
Male	1.70 (1.27–2.28)	0.02
Vasopressor dependence	1.70 (1.24–2.24)	0.001
Obesity	1.67 (1.25–2.24)	<0.001
Hypoxemia at presentation	1.59 (1.18–2.10)	<0.001
Packed RBC exposure (per unit)	1.20 (1.13–1.28)	<0.001
Fluid balance (per liter)	1.10 (1.02–1.18)	0.01
Fresh frozen plasma exposure (per unit)	1.04 (1.01–1.08)	0.03
Intracerebral hemorrhage volume		
<30 mL	Reference	
30 to <60 mL	0.81 (0.57–1.14)	0.23
60 to <90 mL	0.72 (0.47–1.11)	0.14
≥90 mL	0.41 (0.24–0.71)	0.001

Reprinted from Elmer J, Hou P, Wilcox SR, et al. Acute Respiratory Distress Syndrome After Spontaneous Intracerebral Hemorrhage. Crit Care Med. 2013;41:1992-2001.

Conclusions.—Development of acute respiratory distress syndrome is common after intubation for intracerebral hemorrhage. Modifiable risk factors, including high tidal volume ventilation, are associated with its development and in-patient mortality (Table 2).

▶ Neurogenic pulmonary edema is a relatively common form of noncardiogenic pulmonary edema. How often it progresses to acute respiratory distress syndrome (ARDS) has been heretofore unknown. Similarly, it has long been known that a significant number of patients with subarachnoid hemorrhage or intracerebral hemorrhage will develop ARDS, yet the precise incidence and risk factors have not been well elucidated before this study.

Twenty-seven percent, or roughly one-quarter of these patients, developed ARDS. And clearly that combination was associated with worse mortality. I was also surprised at the prevalence of male vs female patients. Likewise, the inverse relationship to age surprised me. Not discussed here but probably important is whether triple H therapy (hypervolemia, hypertension, and hypernatremia) was done, as this has also been previously associated with an increased ARDS rate in neurologically injured patients.

As in many other pathologic states associated with ARDS, these patients likely do have capillary leak phenomenon. This probably helps explain the high correlation with high tidal volume ventilation (eg, volutrauma is worse with volume overload) and with overall volume overload. Table 2 nicely identifies these risk factors.

Several of these factors could theoretically be altered by different care strategies.

J. A. Barker, MD, FACP, FCCP

Emerging Indications for Extracorporeal Membrane Oxygenation in Adults with Respiratory Failure

Abrams D, Brodie D (Columbia Univ College of Physicians and Surgeons/New York–Presbyterian Hosp)

Ann Am Thorac Soc 10:371-377, 2013

Recent advances in technology have spurred the increasing use of extracorporeal membrane oxygenation (ECMO) in patients with severe hypoxemic respiratory failure. However, this accounts for only a small percentage of patients with respiratory failure. We envision the application of ECMO in many other forms of respiratory failure in the coming years. Patients with less severe forms of acute respiratory distress syndrome, for instance, may benefit from enhanced lung-protective ventilation with the very low tidal

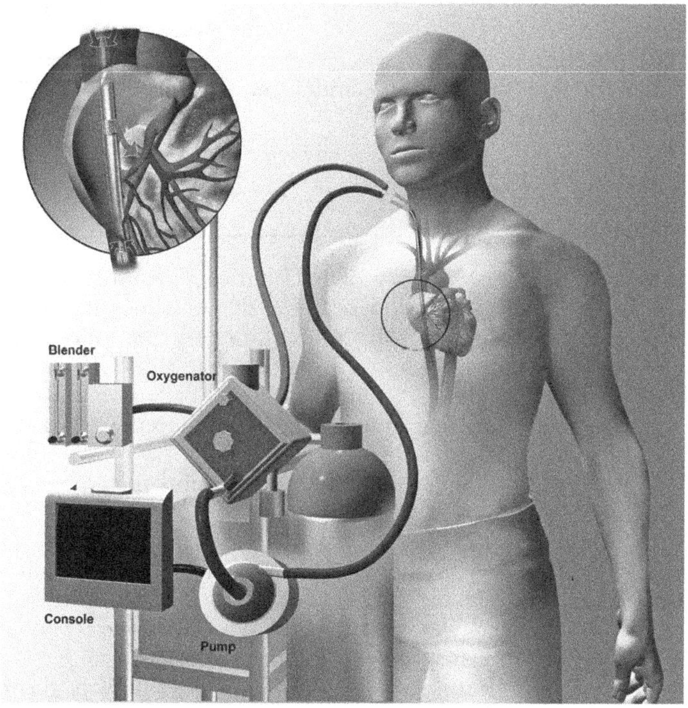

FIGURE 1.—Single-site approach to venovenous extracorporeal membrane oxygenation (ECMO) in the ambulatory patient. A dual-lumen cannula inserted in the internal jugular vein permits both the withdrawal of venous blood from the vena cavae and the reinfusion of oxygenated blood into the right atrium. Avoidance of femoral cannulation, in combination with more compact circuit components that can be easily mobilized, facilitates ambulation and physical rehabilitation in patients with respiratory failure requiring extracorporeal support. *Inset:* deoxygenated blood is withdrawn through ports positioned in both the superior and inferior vena cavae. The reinfusion port is oriented such that oxygenated blood is directed toward the tricuspid valve. Illustration used with permission from COACHsurgery.com and Columbia University. (Reprinted from Abrams D, Brodie D. Emerging indications for extracorporeal membrane oxygenation in adults with respiratory failure. *Ann Am Thorac Soc.* 2013;10:371-377, with permission from the American Thoracic Society.)

volumes made possible by direct carbon dioxide removal from the blood. For those in whom hypercapnia predominates, extracorporeal support will allow for the elimination of invasive mechanical ventilation in some cases. The potential benefits of ECMO may be further enhanced by improved techniques, which facilitate active mobilization. Although ECMO for these and other expanded applications is under active investigation, it has yet to be proven beneficial in these settings in rigorous controlled trials. Ultimately, with upcoming and future technological advances, there is the promise of true destination therapy, which could lead to a major paradigm shift in the management of respiratory failure (Fig 1).

▶ Extracorporeal membrane oxygenation (ECMO) is hitting mainstream in medical intensive care units now. These authors push the envelope on ECMO use. In other words, ECMO can be used for several types of respiratory failure. Newer setups (see Fig 1) enable ambulation and extubation.

J. A. Barker, MD, FACP, FCCP

Central or Peripheral Catheters for Initial Venous Access of ICU Patients: A Randomized Controlled Trial

Ricard J-D, Salomon L, Boyer A, et al (Hôpital Louis Mourier, Colombes, France; Hôpital Pellegrin–Tripode, Bordeaux, France; et al)

Crit Care Med 41:2108-2115, 2013

Objectives.—The vast majority of ICU patients require some form of venous access. There are no evidenced-based guidelines concerning the use of either central or peripheral venous catheters, despite very different complications. It remains unknown which to insert in ICU patients. We investigated the rate of catheter-related insertion or maintenance complications in two strategies: one favoring the central venous catheters and the other peripheral venous catheters.

Design.—Multicenter, controlled, parallel-group, open-label randomized trial.

Setting.—Three French ICUs.

Patients.—Adult ICU patients with equal central or peripheral venous access requirement.

Intervention.—Patients were randomized to receive central venous catheters or peripheral venous catheters as initial venous access.

Measurements and Results.—The primary endpoint was the rate of major catheter-related complications within 28 days. Secondary endpoints were the rate of minor catheter-related complications and a composite score-assessing staff utilization and time spent to manage catheter insertions. Analysis was intention to treat. We randomly assigned 135 patients to receive a central venous catheter and 128 patients to receive a peripheral venous catheter. Major catheter-related complications were greater in the peripheral venous catheter than in the central venous catheter group (133 vs 87, respectively, $p = 0.02$) although none of those was life threatening. Minor catheter-related complications were 201 with central venous catheters and 248 with peripheral venous catheters ($p = 0.06$). 46% (60/128) patients were managed throughout their ICU stay with peripheral venous catheters only. There were significantly more peripheral venous catheter-related complications per patient in patients managed solely with peripheral venous catheter than in patients that received peripheral venous catheter and at least one central venous catheter: 1.92 (121/63) versus 1.13 (226/200), $p < 0.005$. There was no difference in central venous catheter-related complications per patient between patients initially randomized to peripheral venous catheters but subsequently crossed-over to central venous catheter and patients randomized to the central venous catheter group. Kaplan–Meier estimates of survival probability did not differ between the two groups.

Conclusion.—In ICU patients with equal central or peripheral venous access requirement, central venous catheters should preferably be inserted: a strategy associated with less major complications.

▶ This is a very important study. The rate of peripherally inserted central catheter (PICC) lines in inpatients has increased phenomenally over the last decade. Yet, these lines are not actually safer than central lines, as shown very nicely by these French investigators. PICC lines still get infected if left in for several days, and they also carry a relatively high upper extremity venous thrombosis rate as well. This very well done study confirms these findings. PICC lines may also decrease viability of one upper extremity for dialysis access as well.

In addition, subclavian lines are much more comfortable for the awake and moving patient. Think twice about a PICC in an intensive care unit patient!

J. A. Barker, MD, FACP, FCCP

Removing nonessential central venous catheters: evaluation of a quality improvement intervention

Ilan R, Doan J, Cload B, et al (Queen's Univ, Kingston, Ontario, Canada; Royal Univ Hosp, Saskatoon, Saskatchewan, Canada; et al)

Can J Anesth 59:1102-1110, 2012

Introduction.—Nonessential central venous catheters (CVCs) should be removed promptly to prevent adverse events. Little is known about effective strategies to achieve this goal. The present study evaluates the effectiveness of a quality improvement (QI) initiative to remove nonessential CVCs in the intensive care unit (ICU).

Methods.—A prospective observational study was performed in two ICUs following a QI intervention that included a daily checklist, education, and reminders. During 28 consecutive days, all CVCs were identified and the presence of ongoing indications for CVC placement was recorded. The proportions of nonessential CVCs and CVC days were compared with pre-intervention proportions and between the participating units. Rates of

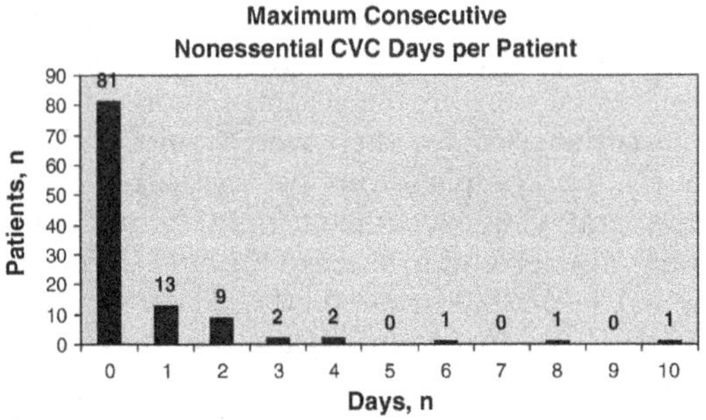

FIGURE 1.—Maximum consecutive nonessential CVC days per patient. CVC, central venous catheter. (With kind permission from Springer Science+Business Media. Ilan R, Doan J, Cload B, et al. Removing nonessential central venous catheters: evaluation of a quality improvement intervention. *Can J Anesth.* 2012;59:1102-1110.)

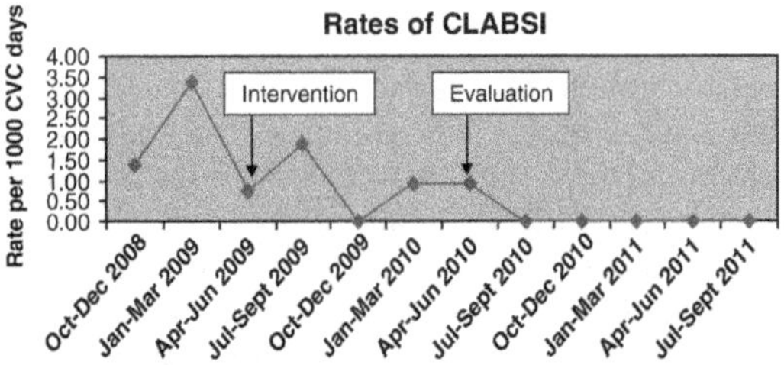

FIGURE 3.—CLABSI rates before, during and after the intervention. * CLABSI, central line associated bloodstream infection; CVC, central venous catheter. (With kind permission from Springer Science+Business Media. Ilan R, Doan J, Cload B, et al. Removing nonessential central venous catheters: evaluation of a quality improvement intervention. *Can J Anesth.* 2012;59:1102-1110.)

central line-associated bloodstream infections (CLABSI) were measured separately through Ontario's Critical Care Information System.

Results.—One hundred and ten patients and 159 CVCs were reviewed. Eighty-eight (11%) of 820 catheter days showed no apparent indication for CVC placement, and compared with the pre-intervention period, the proportion of patients with any number of nonessential CVC days decreased from 51% to 26% (relative risk 0.51; 95% confidence interval 0.34 to 0.74; $P < 0.001$). There was no significant difference in the proportion of nonessential catheter days between participating units. Reported rates of CLABSI decreased substantially during the intervention.

Discussion.—A checklist tool supported by a multifaceted QI intervention effectively ensured prompt removal of nonessential CVCs in two ICUs (Figs 1 and 3).

▶ The importance of diligent care for central lines has been previously proven by Pronovost et al.[1] One of the most important features of the central line care bundle devised by Pronovost was the prompt removal of lines that are no longer needed. It stands to reason that lines can't become infected or thrombose veins if they are no longer in the patient. Yet this part of the bundle is frequently overlooked. No doubt that venous access is truly the lifeline for the intensive care unit patient. Thus, it can also become the death knell.

These Canadian investigators show very nicely how quality improvement can yield real results. Fig 1 shows the rapid decrease in nonessential catheter days once the focus is placed on the issue. The important data are presented in Fig 3. Namely, the run chart shows the intervention followed by decrease in central line—associated infection rates culminating in multiple zero infection months.

It is simple! It works! Take it out when it isn't needed.

J. A. Barker, MD, FACP, FCCP

Reference

1. Pronovost P, Needham D, Berenholtz S, et al. An intervention to decrease catheter-related bloodstream infections in the ICU. *N Engl J Med.* 2006;355:2725-2732.

Severe Sepsis and Septic Shock

Angus DC, van der Poll T (Univ of Pittsburgh School of Medicine, PA; Univ of Amsterdam, The Netherlands)
N Engl J Med 369:840-851, 2013

Background.—The definition of sepsis has evolved over generations. Today, the view is that sepsis is a systemic inflammatory response to infection that can follow multiple infectious causes and does not require the presence of septicemia. Severe sepsis and sepsis are terms often used interchangeably to describe infection complicated by acute organ dysfunction. The current state of knowledge about severe sepsis and septic shock was outlined.

Incidence and Causes.—US data indicate that 2% of patients admitted to the hospital have severe sepsis, and half of these are treated in the intensive care unit (ICU), accounting for 10% of ICU admissions. Similar data on ICU patients are found in other high-income countries. Both community-acquired and health care-n-associated infections precede severe sepsis, with pneumonia that most common cause, followed by intra-abdominal and urinary tract infections. Only a third of patients have positive blood cultures, and up to a third have negative cultures from all sites. The most common gram-positive isolates are *Staphylococcus aureus* and *Streptococcus pneumoniae*; with *Escherichia coli*, klebsiella species, and *Pseudomonas aeruginosa* the most common gram-negative isolates. Sixty-two percent of patients with severe sepsis had positive cultures for gram-negative bacteria, 47% for gram-positive bacteria, and 19% for fungi.

Clinical Features.—Clinical manifestations are a function of the initial site of infection, causative organism, pattern of acute organ involvement, patient's underlying health status, and wait before treatment begins. Signs of infection and organ dysfunction can be subtle, so the list of warning signs is long. Classic manifestations include acute dysfunction of the respiratory and cardiovascular systems; central nervous system dysfunction occurring as obtundation or delirium; and kidney injury indicated by decreased urine output and increased serum creatinine levels.

Pathophysiology.—Evidence indicates that infection triggers a complex, variable, and prolonged host response involving pro-inflammatory and anti-inflammatory mechanisms. The specific response depends on the causative pathogen, the host, and the location. Pathogens activate immune cells, including inflammasomes and alarmins. Severe sepsis is usually associated with altered coagulation as well. The humoral, cellular, and neural mechanisms in the immune system can attenuate the potentially harmful effects of pro-inflammatory response mechanisms. Patients who survive early sepsis but remain in the ICU have immunosuppressed systems. As a result, they often have sustained infectious foci or latent viral infections that can be reactivated. Their blood leukocytes have reduced responsiveness to pathogens and demonstrate impaired spleen cells and immunosuppression of the lungs. Impaired tissue oxygenation plays a key role in organ dysfunction, accompanied by contributions from hypotension, reduced red blood cell deformability, and microvascular thrombus. Mitochondrial damage caused by oxidative stress and other mechanisms alters cellular oxygen use. Alarmins in the extracellular environment can activate neutrophils and cause more tissue injury.

Treatment and Outcomes.—The guidelines for treatment recommend two bundles of care that are associated with improved outcomes for sepsis patients. The initial management bundle is accomplished in the first 6 hours after presentation, whereas the management bundle is done in the ICU. Patients are provided with cardiorespiratory resuscitation and mitigate immediate threats of uncontrolled infection during the initial phase. A probable diagnosis is formed, cultures are obtained, and empirical antimicrobial therapy and source control are done. Once the patient moves to a site for ongoing care, he or she is closely monitored and receives organ function support. The goal is to avoid complications and step care down as appropriate. The initial broad-spectrum therapy is de-escalated to minimize the emergence of resistant organisms, the risk of drug toxicity, and the cost. A short course of hydrocortisone (200 to 300 mg/day for up to 7 days or until vasopressor support is discontinued) can be helpful for patients with refractory septic shock. With advanced training, surveillance and monitoring, and prompt initiation of therapy for the underlying infection, along with support for failing organs, mortality is about 20% to 30% for many patients. However, patients who survive to discharge are at increased risk for death for several months or years thereafter.

Conclusions.—Clinicians can reduce the risk of death associated with sepsis through advances in intensive care, awareness of the problem, and the widespread availability of evidence-based treatment. However, patients who survive sepsis appear to be an increased risk for death in the next few months or years. New therapeutic agents and better approaches to the design and execution of clinical trials are needed.

▶ The authors are experts in this field and do an excellent job of outlining the current thought in the area. Figs 1 and 2 in the original article are invaluable in cartooning the current concepts of pathophysiology as to why sepsis and septic shock occur in some, but not all, patients. Clearly, however, there is still great need for further knowledge in pathophysiology and therapy, as the mortality rate remains unacceptably high.

J. A. Barker, MD, FACP, FCCP

PART SIX

HEART AND CARDIOVASCULAR DISEASE

MICHAEL R. GOLD, MD, PHD

39 Chronic Coronary Artery Disease

National Trends in Heart Failure Hospitalization After Acute Myocardial Infarction for Medicare Beneficiaries 1998–2010

Chen J, Hsieh AF-C, Dharmarajan K, et al (Mid-Atlantic Permanente Res Inst, Rockville MD; Yale-New Haven Hosp, CT; et al)

Circulation 128:2577-2584, 2013

Background.—Previous studies have reported conflicting findings regarding how the incidence of heart failure (HF) after acute myocardial infarction (AMI) has changed over time, and data on contemporary national trends are sparse.

Methods and Results.—Using a complete national sample of 2 789 943 AMI hospitalizations of Medicare fee-for-service beneficiaries from 1998 through 2010, we evaluated annual changes in the incidence of subsequent HF hospitalization and mortality using Poisson and survival analysis models. The number of patients hospitalized for HF within 1 year after AMI declined modestly from 16.1 per 100 person-years in 1998 to 14.2 per 100 person years in 2010 ($P < 0.001$). After adjusting for demographic factors, a relative 14.6% decline for HF hospitalizations after AMI was observed over the study period (incidence risk ratio, 0.854; 95% confidence interval, 0.809–0.901). Unadjusted 1-year mortality following HF hospitalization after AMI was 44.4% in 1998, which decreased to 43.2% in 2004 to 2005, but then increased to 45.5% by 2010. After adjusting for demographic factors and clinical comorbidities, this represented a 2.4% relative annual decline (hazard ratio, 0.976; 95% confidence interval, 0.974–0.978) from 1998 to 2007, but a 5.1% relative annual increase from 2007 to 2010 (hazard ratio, 1.051; 95% confidence interval, 1.039–1.064).

Conclusions.—In a national sample of Medicare beneficiaries, HF hospitalization after AMI decreased from 1998 to 2010, which may indicate improvements in the management of AMI. In contrast, survival after HF following AMI remains poor, and has worsened from 2007 to 2010, demonstrating that challenges still remain for the treatment of this high-risk condition after AMI (Figs 1 and 2).

▶ Mortality from cardiovascular causes has decreased dramatically over the past 30 years. Much of this benefit has been attributed to aggressive treatment

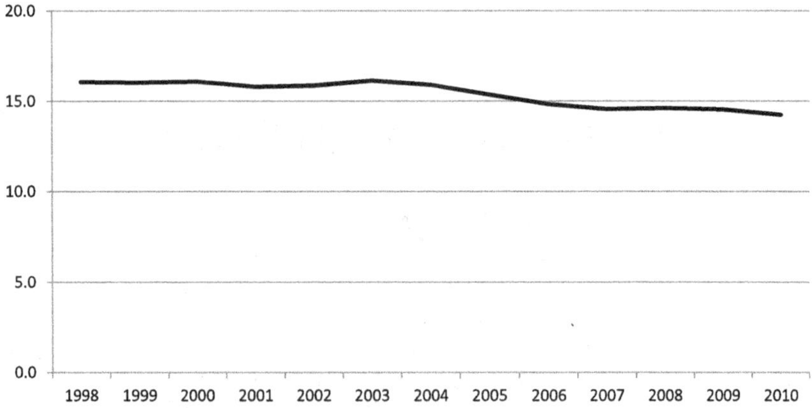

FIGURE 1.—Heart failure hospitalizations after acute myocardial infarction, per 100-patient years. (Reprinted from Chen J, Hsieh AF-C, Dharmarajan K, et al. National trends in heart failure hospitalization after acute myocardial infarction for Medicare beneficiaries 1998–2010. *Circulation.* 2013;128:2577-2584, Copyright 2013, with permission from American Heart Association, Inc.)

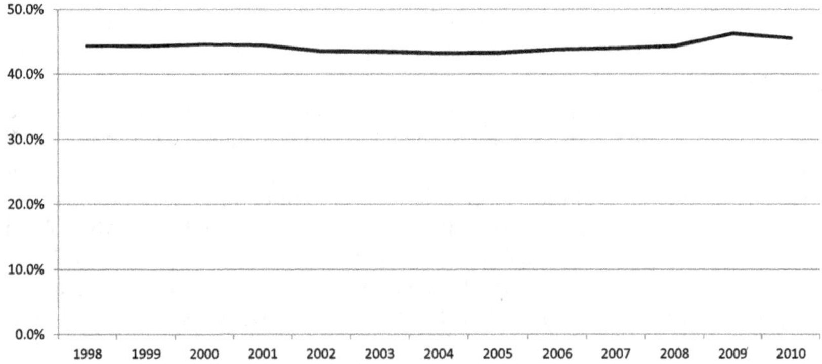

FIGURE 2.—One-year mortality for heart failure hospitalization after acute myocardial infarction. (Reprinted from Chen J, Hsieh AF-C, Dharmarajan K, et al. National trends in heart failure hospitalization after acute myocardial infarction for Medicare beneficiaries 1998–2010. *Circulation.* 2013;128:2577-2584, Copyright 2013, with permission from American Heart Association, Inc.)

of coronary artery disease (CAD) risk factors, including lipid-lowering therapy and smoking cessation. In addition, early revascularization at the time of acute myocardial infarction and improved medical therapy post-myocardial infarction (MI) also contribute to this benefit. With the improved survival after MI, the incidence of long-term complications has increased, such as heart failure (HF) with preserved or reduced ejection fraction and atrial fibrillation. It is less clear, however, whether early HF hospitalizations have decreased post-MI and whether the prognosis has changed for these episodes. To address this issue, a comprehensive analysis of the Medicare database was performed including more than 2.7 million hospitalizations. Over the period of 1998 to 2010, there was a modest decline in HF hospitalization in the first year post-MI

(Fig 1). However, the 1-year mortality after such hospitalization remains high at about 45% and may even be increasing (Fig 2). These observations indicate that HF in the first year post-MI remains a major clinical problem with a poor prognosis. Despite the advances made in prevention and treatment of coronary artery disease, more work is need to identify optimal strategies for MI associated with early HF.

M. Gold, MD

Cost-Effectiveness of Percutaneous Coronary Intervention in Patients With Stable Coronary Artery Disease and Abnormal Fractional Flow Reserve

Fearon WF, on behalf of the Fractional Flow Reserve Versus Angiography for Multivessel Evaluation 2 (FAME 2) Investigators (Stanford Univ School of Medicine, CA; et al)

Circulation 128:1335-1340, 2013

Background.—The Fractional Flow Reserve Versus Angiography for Multivessel Evaluation (FAME) 2 trial demonstrated a significant reduction in subsequent coronary revascularization among patients with stable angina and at least 1 coronary lesion with a fractional flow reserve ≤0.80 who were randomized to percutaneous coronary intervention (PCI) compared with best medical therapy. The economic and quality-of-life implications of PCI in the setting of an abnormal fractional flow reserve are unknown.

Methods and Results.—We calculated the cost of the index hospitalization based on initial resource use and follow-up costs based on Medicare reimbursements. We assessed patient utility using the EQ-5D health survey with US weights at baseline and 1 month and projected quality-adjusted life-years assuming a linear decline over 3 years in the 1-month utility improvements. We calculated the incremental cost-effectiveness ratio based on cumulative costs over 12 months. Initial costs were significantly higher for PCI in the setting of an abnormal fractional flow reserve than with medical therapy ($9927 versus $3900, $P < 0.001$), but the $6027 difference narrowed over 1-year follow-up to $2883 ($P < 0.001$), mostly because of the cost of subsequent revascularization procedures. Patient utility was improved more at 1 month with PCI than with medical therapy (0.054 versus 0.001 units, $P < 0.001$). The incremental cost-effectiveness ratio of PCI was $36 000 per quality-adjusted life-year, which was robust in bootstrap replications and in sensitivity analyses.

Conclusions.—PCI of coronary lesions with reduced fractional flow reserve improves outcomes and appears economically attractive compared with best medical therapy among patients with stable angina (Fig 1).

▶ The best initial treatment for patients with stable, but symptomatic, coronary artery disease remains a matter of debate.[1,2] Although the COURAGE trial

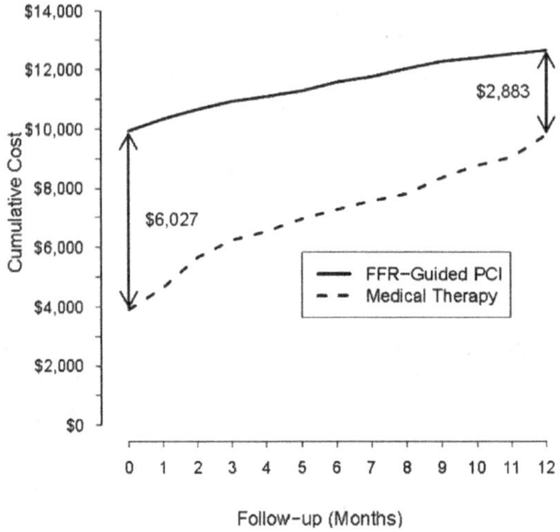

FIGURE 1.—Cumulative medical costs (vertical axis) of a strategy of percutaneous coronary intervention (PCI) in the setting of an abnormal fractional flow reserve (FFR; solid line) and a medical therapy strategy (dashed line) over 12 months of follow-up (horizontal axis). (Reprinted from Fearon WF, on behalf of the Fractional Flow Reserve Versus Angiography for Multivessel Evaluation 2 (FAME 2) Investigators. Cost-effectiveness of percutaneous coronary intervention in patients with stable coronary artery disease and abnormal fractional flow reserve. *Circulation.* 2013;128:1335-1340, Copyright 2013, with permission from American Heart Association, Inc.)

found that an initial strategy of medical therapy alone is equivalent to that of percutaneous coronary intervention (PCI) plus medical therapy, one of the limitations of this study was the angiographic assessment of disease (and therefore, the ischemic burden) in a stable and low-risk population. Fractional flow reserve (FFR) is an adjunct to angiography that allows an invasive and direct assessment of lesion severity and ischemia. The FAME trial evaluated patients with multivessel disease to angiographic driven PCI versus FFR-guided angioplasty and found improved outcomes in patients treated with FFR guided-PCI. FAME-2 evaluated patients with documented ischemia by FFR and randomly assigned them to PCI plus medical therapy or medical therapy alone. It was stopped early because of increased events in the medical therapy group compared with the PCI group. The current analysis reflects the cost effectiveness of the 2 strategies. Initial costs were significantly higher for patients treated with PCI than with medical therapy ($9927 vs $3900, $P < .001$), but the $6027 difference narrowed over 1-year follow-up to $2883 ($P < .001$) (Fig 1). The convergence of cost was largely because of increased revascularization in the medically treated patients. The overall cost per quality-adjusted life-year saved was favorable at 1 year. Overall, this study suggests that in patients with symptomatic coronary disease and a functionally significant lesion by FFR, an initial strategy of PCI is appropriate with acceptable cost effectiveness.

D. Steinberg, MD

References

1. Boden WE, O'Rourke RA, Teo KK, et al. Optimal medical therapy with or without PCI for stable coronary disease. *N Engl J Med.* 2007;356:1503-1516.
2. Tonino PA, De Bruyne B, Pijls NH, et al. Fractional flow reserve versus angiography for guiding percutaneous coronary intervention. *N Engl J Med.* 2009;360: 213-214.

C-Reactive Protein, but not Low-Density Lipoprotein Cholesterol Levels, Associate With Coronary Atheroma Regression and Cardiovascular Events After Maximally Intensive Statin Therapy

Puri R, Nissen SE, Libby P, et al (Cleveland Clinic, OH; Brigham and Women's Hosp, Boston, MA; et al)

Circulation 128:2395-2403, 2013

Background.—Baseline C-reactive protein (CRP) levels predict major adverse cardiovascular events (MACE: death, myocardial infarction, stroke, coronary revascularization, and hospitalization for unstable angina). The association between changes in CRP levels with plaque progression and MACE in the setting of maximally intensive statin therapy is unknown.

Methods and Results.—The Study of Coronary Atheroma by Intravascular Ultrasound: Effect of Rosuvastatin Versus Atorvastatin (SATURN) used serial intravascular ultrasound measures of coronary atheroma volume in patients treated with rosuvastatin 40 mg or atorvastatin 80 mg for 24 months. The treatment groups did not differ significantly in the change from baseline of percent atheroma volume on intravascular ultrasound, CRP-modulating effects, or MACE rates, thus allowing for a (prespecified) post hoc analysis to test associations between the changes in CRP levels with coronary disease progression and MACE. Patients with nonincreasing CRP levels (n = 621) had higher baseline (2.3 [1.1–4.7] versus 1.1 [0.5–1.8] mg/L; $P < 0.001$) and lower follow-up CRP levels (0.8 [0.5–1.7] versus 1.6 [0.7–4.1] mg/L; $P < 0.001$) versus those with increasing CRP levels (n = 364). Multivariable analysis revealed a nonincreasing CRP level to independently associate with greater percent atheroma volume regression ($P = 0.01$). Although the (log) change in CRP did not associate with MACE (hazard ratio, 1.18; 95% confidence interval, 0.93–1.50; $P = 0.17$), the (log) on-treatment CRP associated significantly with MACE (hazard ratio, 1.28; 95% confidence interval, 1.04–1.56; $P = 0.02$). On-treatment low-density lipoprotein cholesterol levels did not correlate with MACE (hazard ratio, 1.09; 95% confidence interval, 0.88–1.35; $P = 0.45$).

Conclusions.—Following 24 months of potent statin therapy, on-treatment CRP levels associated with MACE. Inflammation may be an

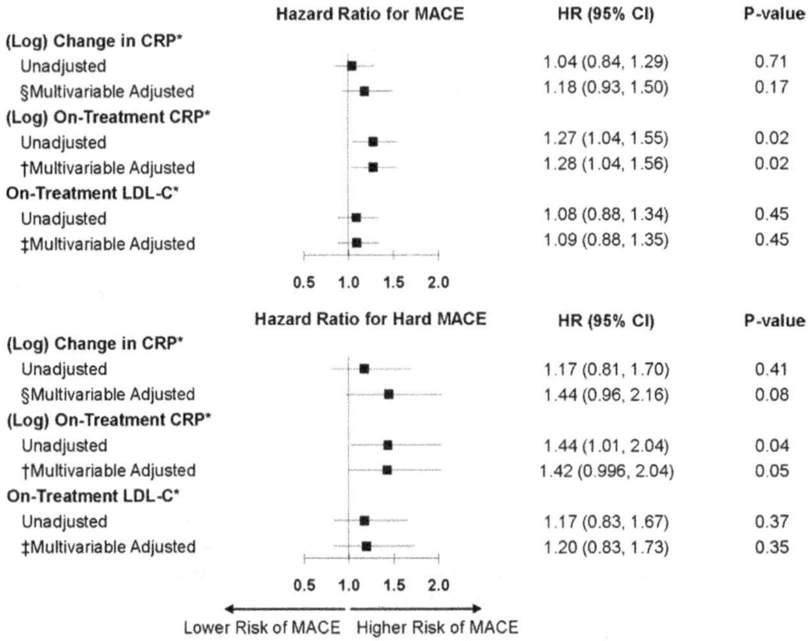

Hazard Ratio for MACE
HR (95% CI)
P-value
(Log) Change in CRP*
Unadjusted
1.04 (0.84, 1.29)
0.71
§Multivariable Adjusted
1.18 (0.93, 1.50)
0.17
(Log) On-Treatment CRP*
Unadjusted
1.27 (1.04, 1.55)
0.02
†Multivariable Adjusted
1.28 (1.04, 1.56)
0.02
On-Treatment LDL-C*
Unadjusted
1.08 (0.88, 1.34)
0.45
‡Multivariable Adjusted
1.09 (0.88, 1.35)
0.45
0.5 1.0 1.5 2.0
Hazard Ratio for Hard MACE
HR (95% CI)
P-value
(Log) Change in CRP*
Unadjusted
1.17 (0.81, 1.70)
0.41
§Multivariable Adjusted
1.44 (0.96, 2.16)
0.08
(Log) On-Treatment CRP*
Unadjusted
1.44 (1.01, 2.04)
0.04
†Multivariable Adjusted
1.42 (0.996, 2.04)
0.05
On-Treatment LDL-C*
Unadjusted
1.17 (0.83, 1.67)
0.37
‡Multivariable Adjusted
1.20 (0.83, 1.73)
0.35
0.5 1.0 1.5 2.0
Lower Risk of MACE
Higher Risk of MACE

FIGURE 1.—Cox proportional hazard ratios for time to first MACE or hard MACE, according to the change from baseline of CRP levels, on-treatment CRP levels, or on-treatment LDL-C levels. *Values of log-transformed change in CRP, on-treatment CRP, and on-treatment LDL-C were per standard deviation. §Adjusted for history of diabetes mellitus, concomitant ACE inhibitor use, and log-transformed baseline CRP. †Adjusted for history of diabetes mellitus, history of acute coronary syndrome, and concomitant use of ACE inhibitor. ‡Adjusted for history of diabetes mellitus, history of acute coronary syndrome, concomitant ACE inhibitor use, and log-transformed on-treatment CRP. ACE indicates angiotensin-converting enzyme; CI, confidence interval; CRP, C-reactive protein; HR, hazard ratio; LDL-C, low-density lipoprotein cholesterol; and MACE, major adverse cardiovascular events. (Reprinted from Puri R, Nissen SE, Libby P, et al. C-reactive protein, but not low-density lipoprotein cholesterol levels, associate with coronary atheroma regression and cardiovascular events after maximally intensive statin therapy. *Circulation.* 2013;128:2395-2403, Copyright 2013, with permission from American Heart Association, Inc.)

important driver of residual cardiovascular risk in patients with coronary artery disease despite aggressive statin therapy.

Clinical Trial Registration.—URL: http://clinicaltrials.gov. Unique identifier: NCT000620542 (Figs 1 and 2).

▶ Although statin therapy has been shown to improve clinical outcomes, many individuals demonstrate coronary atheroma progression despite guideline-directed medical therapy. The association between changes in C-reactive protein (CRP) with plaque progression and major adverse cardiovascular events (MACEs) in the setting of optimal statin therapy is unknown. Thus, the primary objective of this study was to assess the effect of CRP on both atheroma progression and MACEs in patients after 24 months of maximal stain therapy. This was a prespecified post hoc analysis of the SATURN Study and evaluated subgroups based on CRP change. Subjects with increasing levels of CRP from baseline demonstrated less plaque regression than those whose CRP levels

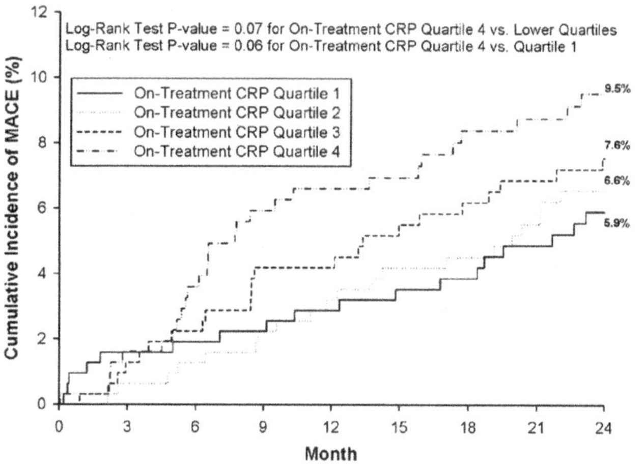

No. Patients At Risk									
On-Treatment CRP Quartile 1	315	308	306	303	299	294	290	284	272
On-Treatment CRP Quartile 2	316	312	309	304	299	293	290	278	270
On-Treatment CRP Quartile 3	316	309	305	295	295	282	277	272	265
On-Treatment CRP Quartile 4	316	303	290	282	277	269	253	245	235

FIGURE 2.—Kaplan—Meier survival curve analysis of quartiles of on-treatment CRP levels and MACE. The cumulative incidence of MACE in patients with the lowest quartile of on-treatment CRP was 5.9% in comparison with 9.5% in those with the highest quartile of baseline coronary PAV ($P = 0.06$). CRP indicates C-reactive protein; MACE, major adverse cardiovascular events; and PAV, percent atheroma volume. (Reprinted from Puri R, Nissen SE, Libby P, et al. C-reactive protein, but not low-density lipoprotein cholesterol levels, associate with coronary atheroma regression and cardiovascular events after maximally intensive statin therapy. *Circulation.* 2013;128:2395-2403, Copyright 2013, with permission from American Heart Association, Inc.)

did not increase (−0.910.15% vs −1.420.11%, $P = .007$). Changes in CRP did not associate significantly with MACE (multivariate adjusted hazard ratio [HR] 1.18; 0.93–1.50; $P = .17$); however, on-treatment CRP level was significantly and independently associated with MACE (multivariate adjusted HR 1.28; 1.04–1.56; $P = .02$). In contrast, on-treatment low-density lipoprotein levels were not significantly associated with MACE (Fig 1). Kaplan-Meier survival analysis according to quartiles of on-treatment CRP levels and MACE show a stepwise relationship between increasing CRP and MACE (Fig 2). These results highlight the potential importance of using on-treatment CRP levels to determine residual cardiovascular risk in patients already on maximally intensive statin therapy. Further studies are needed to determine whether potential interventions to alter on-treatment CRP can reduce MACE.

T. Todoran, MD, MSc

40 Risk Factors

A Randomized Trial of Colchicine for Acute Pericarditis

Imazio M, for the ICAP Investigators (Maria Vittoria Hosp, Turin, Italy)

N Engl J Med 369:1522-1528, 2013

Background.—Colchicine is effective for the treatment of recurrent pericarditis. However, conclusive data are lacking regarding the use of colchicine during a first attack of acute pericarditis and in the prevention of recurrent symptoms.

Methods.—In a multicenter, double-blind trial, eligible adults with acute pericarditis were randomly assigned to receive either colchicine (at a dose of 0.5 mg twice daily for 3 months for patients weighing >70 kg or 0.5 mg once daily for patients weighing ≤70 kg) or placebo in addition to conventional antiinflammatory therapy with aspirin or ibuprofen. The primary study outcome was incessant or recurrent pericarditis.

Results.—A total of 240 patients were enrolled, and 120 were randomly assigned to each of the two study groups. The primary outcome occurred in 20 patients (16.7%) in the colchicine group and 45 patients (37.5%) in the placebo group (relative risk reduction in the colchicine group, 0.56; 95% confidence interval, 0.30 to 0.72; number needed to treat, 4; $P < 0.001$). Colchicine reduced the rate of symptom persistence at 72 hours (19.2% vs. 40.0%, $P = 0.001$), the number of recurrences per patient (0.21 vs. 0.52, $P = 0.001$), and the hospitalization rate (5.0% vs. 14.2%, $P = 0.02$). Colchicine also improved the remission rate at 1 week (85.0% vs. 58.3%, $P < 0.001$). Overall adverse effects and rates of study-drug discontinuation were similar in the two study groups. No serious adverse events were observed.

Conclusions.—In patients with acute pericarditis, colchicine, when added to conventional anti-inflammatory therapy, significantly reduced the rate of incessant or recurrent pericarditis. (Funded by former Azienda Sanitaria Locale 3 of Turin [now Azienda Sanitaria Locale 2] and Acarpia; ICAP ClinicalTrials.gov number, NCT00128453.)

▶ For symptomatic management of patients with acute pericarditis, nonsteroidal anti-inflammatory drugs (NSAIDs) have long been a mainstay of therapy. Although colchicine is known to reduce recurrences, its role in acute management is not well established. This study sought to examine the efficacy of colchicine for the treatment of acute pericarditis by randomizing 240 patients to either colchicine 0.5 mg twice daily (or once daily for patients under 70 kg) vs placebo for 3 months; all patients were followed for at least 18 months. The primary endpoint was incessant or recurrent pericarditis. As shown in Fig 2 in the original article, colchicine therapy was associated with significant reductions in the primary outcome (16.7% colchicine vs 37.5% placebo, relative risk 0.56 (0.3–0.72), $P < .0001$), as well as symptom persistence at 72 hours (19.2% colchicine vs 40.0% placebo, $P = .001$), recurrences per patient (0.21 colchicine vs 0.52 placebo, $P = .001$) and hospitalization rates (5.0% vs 14.2%, $P = .02$). The drug was well tolerated with no serious adverse events observed. The authors concluded that, for patients with acute pericarditis, early treatment with colchicine in addition to NSAIDs may be effective in reducing incessant or recurrent pericarditis. This study should add to our armamentarium for treating pericarditis.

D. Steinberg, MD

Efficacy and Safety of Longer-Term Administration of Evolocumab (AMG 145) in Patients With Hypercholesterolemia: 52-Week Results From the Open-Label Study of Long-Term Evaluation Against LDL-C (OSLER) Randomized Trial

Koren MJ, for the OSLER Investigators (Jacksonville Ctr for Clinical Res, FL; et al)

Circulation 129:234-243, 2014

Background.—Evolocumab (AMG 145), a monoclonal antibody against proprotein convertase subtilisin/kexin type 9 (PCSK9), significantly reduced low-density lipoprotein cholesterol (LDL-C) in phase 2 studies of 12 weeks' duration. The longer-term efficacy and safety of PCSK9 inhibition remain undefined.

Methods and Results.—Of 1359 randomized and dosed patients in the 4 evolocumab phase 2 parent studies, 1104 (81%) elected to enroll into the Open-Label Study of Long-term Evaluation Against LDL-C (OSLER) study. Regardless of their treatment assignment in the parent study, patients were randomized 2:1 to receive either open-label subcutaneous evolocumab 420 mg every 4 weeks with standard of care (SOC) (evolocumab+ SOC, n = 736) or SOC alone (n = 368). Ninety-two percent of patients in the evolocumab+SOC group and 89% of patients in the SOC group completed 52 weeks of follow-up. Patients who first received evolocumab in OSLER experienced a mean 52.3% [SE, 1.8%] reduction in LDL-C at week 52 ($P < 0.0001$). Patients who received 1 of 6 dosing regimens of evolocumab in the parent studies and received evolocumab+SOC in OSLER had persistent LDL-C reductions (mean reduction, 50.4% [SE, 0.8%] at the end of the parent study versus 52.1% [SE, 1.0%] at 52 weeks; $P = 0.31$). In patients who discontinued evolocumab on entry into OSLER, LDL-C levels returned to near baseline levels. Adverse events and serious adverse events occurred in 81.4% and 7.1% of the evolocumab+SOC group patients and 73.1% and 6.3% of the SOC group patients, respectively.

Conclusion.—Evolocumab dosed every 4 weeks demonstrated continued efficacy and encouraging safety and tolerability over 1 year of

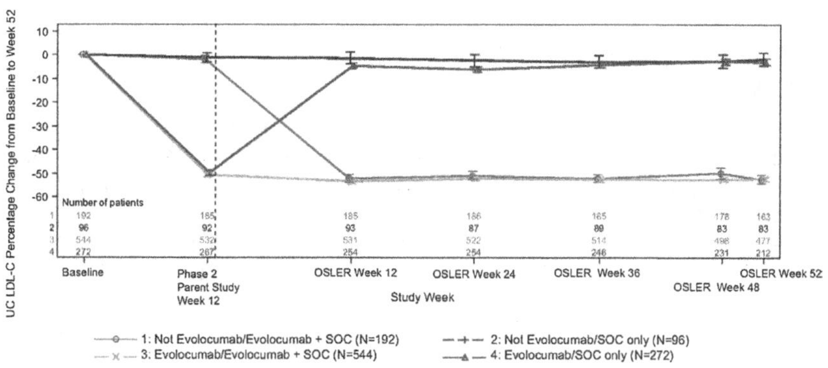

FIGURE 2.—Ultracentrifugation low-density lipoprotein cholesterol (UC LDL-C) percentage change from the phase 2 parent study baseline to week 52. Dashed vertical line indicates time between phase 2 parent and Open-Label Study of Long-term Evaluation Against LDL-C (OSLER) studies. Error bars represent standard error. Plot is based on observed data, and no imputation was used for missing values. SOC indicates standard of care. (Reprinted from Koren MJ, for the OSLER Investigators. Efficacy and safety of longer-term administration of evolocumab (AMG 145) in patients with hypercholesterolemia: 52-week results from the open-label study of long-term evaluation against LDL-C (OSLER) randomized trial. *Circulation.* 2014;129:234-243, Copyright 2014, with permission from American Heart Association, Inc.)

treatment in the largest and longest evaluation of a PCSK9 inhibitor in hypercholesterolemic patients to date.

Clinical Trial Registration.—URL: http://clinicaltrials.gov. Unique identifier: NCT01439880 (Fig 2).

▶ Despite the tremendous improvements in cardiovascular outcomes associated with HMG-CoA reductase inhibitors (statins), many patients still have suboptimal control of their low-density lipoprotein cholesterol (LDL-C). The reasons for this include more severe hyperlipidemia or statin intolerance. The proprotein convertase subtilisin/kexin type 9 (PCSK9) inhibitors represent an exciting novel target for LDL-C reduction, and the phase 2 trials of subcutaneous Evolocumab showed early benefit with good safety profiles. The OSLER trial evaluated 1104 of the 1359 patients enrolled into phase 2 trials and randomized them 2:1 to either continued subcutaneous Evolocumab 420 mg every 4 weeks + standard of care (SOC) or SOC alone. The medication was well tolerated, and 92% of Evolocumab patients completed 52-week follow-up compared with 89% of the SOC alone patients, with similarly low serious adverse event rates in both groups. Patients were divided into 4 groups for analysis based on whether they originally received Evolocumab in the phase 2 trials (vs placebo) and whether they continued on Evolocumab. The LDL-C reduction seen with Evolocumab was approximately 50%. As shown in Fig 2, patients who never received Evolocumab had LDL-C levels that stayed at baseline, and those that received Evolocumab in the parent trials but SOC alone in OSLER had their LDL-C levels return to baseline. Patients who received Evolocumab in the phase 2 trials and continued on it during OSLER had persistent benefit of decreased LDL-C, and those who first started Evolocumab as part of OSLER had reductions in LDL-C similar to those who continued. The findings demonstrate that Evolocumab may represent a well-tolerated, safe, and effective novel option for LDL-C reduction beyond what is achievable with statins as standard of care.

D. Steinberg, MD

Increased risk of coronary heart disease among individuals reporting adverse impact of stress on their health: the Whitehall II prospective cohort study

Nabi H, Kivimäki M, Batty GD, et al (Centre for Res in Epidemiology and Population Health, Villejuif, France; Univ College London, UK; et al)
Eur Heart J 34:2697-2705, 2013

Aim.—Response to stress can vary greatly between individuals. However, it remains unknown whether perceived impact of stress on health is associated with adverse health outcomes. We examined whether individuals who report that stress adversely affects their health are at increased risk of coronary heart disease (CHD) compared with those who report that stress has no adverse health impact.

Methods and Results.—Analyses are based on 7268 men and women (mean age: 49.5 years, interquartile range: 11 years) from the British Whitehall II cohort study. Over 18 years of follow-up, there were 352 coronary deaths or first non-fatal myocardial infarction (MI) events. After adjustment for sociodemographic characteristics, participants who reported at baseline that stress has affected their health 'a lot or extremely' had a 2.12 times higher (95% CI 1.52–2.98) risk of coronary death or incident non-fatal MI when compared with those who reported no effect of stress on their health. This association was attenuated but remained statistically significant after adjustment for biological, behavioural, and other psychological risk factors including perceived stress levels, and measures of social support; fully adjusted hazard ratio: 1.49 (95% CI 1.01–2.22).

Conclusions.—In this prospective cohort study, the perception that stress affects health, different from perceived stress levels, was associated with an increased risk of coronary heart disease. Randomized controlled trials are needed to determine whether disease risk can be reduced by increasing clinical attention to those who complain that stress greatly affects their health (Figs 1 and 2).

▶ Previous studies suggest that exposure to stress is associated with adverse clinical outcomes including cardiovascular disease. To date, most studies have focused on quantifying stress. The aim of this study was to examine whether individuals' perceptions of the impact of stress on their health is associated with risk of coronary heart disease (CHD). The study cohort was 7268 men and women from the British Whitehall II study. As part of this trial, patients were asked the question: "to what extent do you feel that your stress or pressure you have experienced in your life has affected your health?" Overall, 39% of participants reported that stress has affected their health not at all, 53% slightly or moderately, and 8% a lot or extremely. The survival curve for incident CHD among participants who

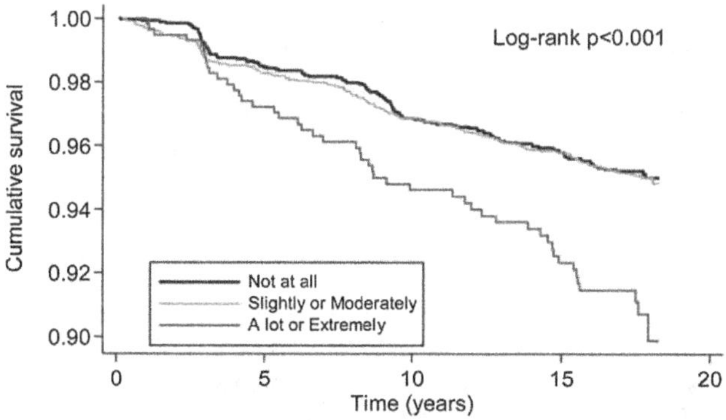

Number at risk

	0	5	10	15	20
Not at all	2835	2725	2497	2276	0
Slightly or Moderately	3849	3694	3402	3093	0
A lot or Extremely	584	549	490	431	0

FIGURE 1.—Unadjusted Kaplan–Meier survival curves showing the association between perceived impact of stress and incident CHD. (Reprinted from Nabi H, Kivimäki M, Batty GD, et al. Increased risk of coronary heart disease among individuals reporting adverse impact of stress on their health: the Whitehall II prospective cohort study. *Eur Heart J.* 2013;34:2697-2705, by permission of The European Society of Cardiology.)

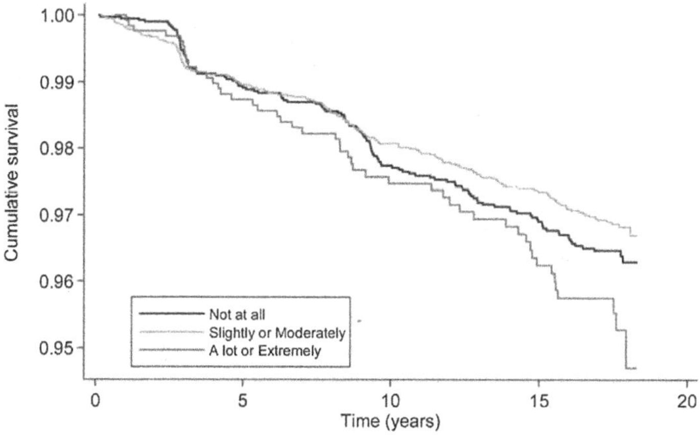

FIGURE 2.—Kaplan–Meier survival curves showing the association between perceived impact of stress and incident CHD adjusted for sociodemographics, health behaviours, biological cardiovascular disease risk factors, self-rated health, negative affect, psychological distress, social support, and perceived levels of stress. (Reprinted from Nabi H, Kivimäki M, Batty GD, et al. Increased risk of coronary heart disease among individuals reporting adverse impact of stress on their health: the Whitehall II prospective cohort study. *Eur Heart J.* 2013;34:2697-2705, by permission of The European Society of Cardiology.)

reported that stress affected their health a lot or extremely differed significantly ($P < .001$) from those in the other 2 groups (Fig 1). After adjusting for covariates, the survival disadvantage in participants who reported that stress affected their health a lot or extremely was maintained, although the difference between groups was smaller (Fig 2). These subjects had a 1.49 times higher (95% confidence interval, 101–2.22; $P = .04$) risk of cardiovascular death or nonfatal myocardial infarction compared with those who reported no effect of stress on their health. This study is unique in that it is an assessment of individuals' perceptions of stress impact on their health rather than their perceived stress levels. This represents the first trial to measure this in a large population cohort. Whether CHD risk can be reduced in individuals who believe that stress is greatly affecting their health is unknown, and randomized trials are needed.

T. Todoran, MD, MSc

Effects of Visit-to-Visit Variability in Systolic Blood Pressure on Macrovascular and Microvascular Complications in Patients With Type 2 Diabetes Mellitus: The ADVANCE Trial

Hata J, on behalf of the ADVANCE Collaborative Group (Univ of Sydney, Australia; et al)

Circulation 128:1325-1334, 2013

Background.—Recent evidence suggests that visit-to-visit variability in systolic blood pressure (SBP) and maximum SBP are predictors of cardiovascular disease. However, it remains uncertain whether these parameters predict the risks of macrovascular and microvascular complications in patients with type 2 diabetes mellitus.

Methods and Results.—The Action in Diabetes and Vascular Disease: Preterax and Diamicron Modified Release Controlled Evaluation (ADVANCE) was a factorial randomized controlled trial of blood pressure lowering and blood glucose control in patients with type 2 diabetes mellitus. The present analysis included 8811 patients without major macrovascular and microvascular events or death during the first 24 months after randomization. SBP variability (defined as standard deviation) and maximum SBP were determined during the first 24 months after randomization. During a median 2.4 years of follow-up from the 24-month visit, 407 major macrovascular (myocardial infarction, stroke, or cardiovascular death) and 476 microvascular (new or worsening nephropathy or retinopathy) events were observed. The association of major macrovascular and microvascular events with SBP variability was continuous even after adjustment for mean SBP and other confounding factors (both $P < 0.05$ for trend). Hazard ratios (95% confidence intervals) for the highest tenth of SBP variability were 1.54 (0.99–2.39) for macrovascular events and 1.84 (1.19–2.84) for microvascular events in comparison with the lowest tenth. For maximum SBP, hazard ratios (95% confidence intervals) for the highest tenth were 3.64 (1.73–7.66) and 2.18 (1.04–4.58), respectively.

Conclusion.—Visit-to-visit variability in SBP and maximum SBP were independent risk factors for macrovascular and microvascular complications in type 2 diabetes mellitus.

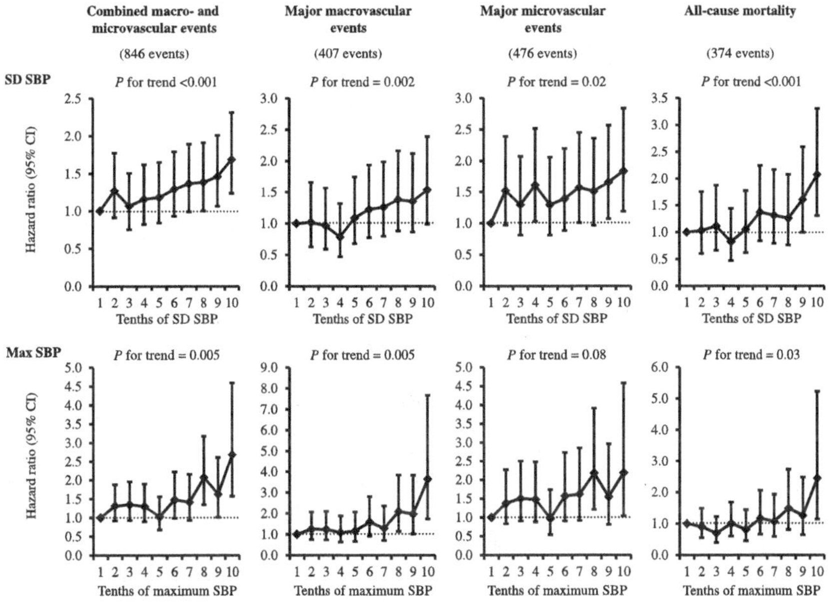

FIGURE 2.—Hazard ratios and 95% confidence intervals (CIs) for major macrovascular and microvascular events and death according to tenths of standard deviation (SD) or maximum (Max) of systolic blood pressure (SBP). SBP values measured at 6 occasions (from 3–24 months after randomization) were used to determine SD and maximum SBP. Each parameter was categorized into 10 groups according to the tenths within each BP-lowering treatment group. The ranges of SD SBP were 0.6 to 5.2, 5.3 to 6.8, 6.9 to 8.1, 8.2 to 9.3, 9.4 to 10.5, 10.6 to 11.7, 11.8 to 13.2, 13.3 to 15.2, 15.3 to 18.0, and 18.1 to 47.3 mm Hg in the placebo group; 0.4 to 5.0, 5.1 to 6.6, 6.7 to 7.7, 7.8 to 8.8, 8.9 to 9.9, 10.0 to 11.0, 11.1 to 12.5, 12.6 to 14.2, 14.3 to 16.7, and 16.8 to 33.5 mm Hg in the active group. The ranges of maximum SBP were 97.5 to 133.5, 134.0 to 140.0, 140.5 to 144.5, 145.0 to 149.5, 150.0 to 153.5, 154.0 to 158.5, 159.0 to 164.0, 164.5 to 171.0, 171.5 to 180.0, and 180.5 to 263.0 mm Hg in the placebo group; 91.0 to 127.0, 127.5 to 133.5, 134.0 to 138.0, 138.5 to 142.0, 142.5 to 146.5, 147.0 to 150.5, 151.0 to 156.0, 156.5 to 162.5, 163.0 to 172.5, and 173.0 to 247.0 mm Hg in the active group. Hazard ratios were adjusted for age, sex, randomized blood pressure–lowering intervention, randomized glucose control intervention, region of residence, duration of diabetes mellitus, current smoking, current alcohol drinking, heart rate, total cholesterol, log of triglycerides, body mass index, use of β-blockers, use of calcium-channel blockers, and mean SBP during the measurement period. (Reprinted from Hata J, on behalf of the ADVANCE Collaborative Group. Effects of visit-to-visit variability in systolic blood pressure on macrovascular and microvascular complications in patients with type 2 diabetes mellitus: the advance trial. *Circulation.* 2013;128:1325-1334, Copyright 2013, with permission from American Heart Association, Inc.)

Clinical Trial Registration.—URL: http://www.clinicaltrials.gov. Unique Identifier: NCT00145925 (Fig 2).

► Recent studies have demonstrated that visit-to-visit variability in systolic blood pressure (SBP) and maximal SBP are associated with future risks of stroke and other cardiovascular events, independent of mean SBP and comorbidities. However, there is little evidence that these effects influence macrovascular (stroke, myocardial infarction, and cardiovascular death) and microvascular (new or worsening retinopathy or nephropathy) complications in patients with type 2 diabetes mellitus (DM). In this study, 8011 patients (mean age 66 years, 42% female, 37% Asian) with type 2 DM and no major macrovascular or microvascular events or death during the first 24 months after randomization in the ADVANCE study were analyzed. After adjustment for mean SBP and other cardiovascular risk factors, visit-to-visit variability SBP was positively associated with risks of combined, major macrovascular and microvascular events and all-cause mortality ($P < .05$ for trend). Higher maximum SPB was positively associated with risks of combined events, major macrovascular events, and all-cause mortality ($P < .05$ for trend) but not major microvascular events ($P = .08$; Fig 2). After adjustment, the highest visit-to-visit variability SBP group was associated with increased combined events (hazard ratio [HR] 1.69), major macrovascular events (HR 1.54), major macrovascular events (HR 1.84), and all-cause mortality (HR 2.08) compared with the lowest group. Highest maximum SBP group was associated with increased combined events (HR 2.68), macrovascular events (HR 3.64), microvascular events (HR 2.18), and all-cause mortality (HR 2.44). This study represents one of the largest observational studies demonstrating the predictive value of visit-to-visit variability and maximal SBP on risks of macro- and microvascular complications and mortality in a cohort of patients with type 2 DM. Translating this information into clinical practice of management of blood pressure remains to be determined and will require further clinical trials but suggests that labile BP may be a risk factor for complications from hypertension.

T. Todoran, MD, MSc

41 Arrhythmias

Effect of Yoga on Arrhythmia Burden, Anxiety, Depression, and Quality of Life in Paroxysmal Atrial Fibrillation: The YOGA My Heart Study

Lakkireddy D, Atkins D, Pillarisetti J, et al (Univ of Kansas Hosp & Med Ctr; et al)

J Am Coll Cardiol 61:1177-1182, 2013

Objectives.—The purpose of this study was to examine the impact of yoga on atrial fibrillation (AF) burden, quality of life (QoL), depression, and anxiety scores.

Background.—Yoga is known to have significant benefit on cardiovascular health. The effect of yoga in reducing AF burden is unknown.

Methods.—This single-center, pre-post study enrolled patients with symptomatic paroxysmal AF with an initial 3-month noninterventional observation period followed by twice-weekly 60-min yoga training for next 3 months. AF episodes during the control and study periods as well as SF-36, Zung self-rated anxiety, and Zung self-rated depression scores at baseline, before, and after the study phase were assessed.

Results.—Yoga training reduced symptomatic AF episodes (3.8 ± 3 vs. 2.1 ± 2.6, $p < 0.001$), symptomatic non-AF episodes (2.9 ± 3.4 vs. 1.4 ± 2.0; $p < 0.001$), asymptomatic AF episodes (0.12 ± 0.44 vs. 0.04 ± 0.20; $p < 0.001$), and depression and anxiety ($p < 0.001$), and improved the QoL parameters of physical functioning, general health, vitality, social functioning, and mental health domains on SF-36 ($p = 0.017$, $p < 0.001$, $p < 0.001$, $p = 0.019$, and $p < 0.001$, respectively). There was significant decrease in heart rate, and systolic and diastolic blood pressure before and after yoga ($p < 0.001$).

Conclusions.—In patients with paroxysmal AF, yoga improves symptoms, arrhythmia burden, heart rate, blood pressure, anxiety and depression scores, and several domains of QoL (Fig 1).

► Most therapies in cardiovascular care involve pharmacologic, surgical, or device interventions. However, it has become clear more recently that support groups, alternative medicine, and holistic approaches can be effective treatment modalities. Atrial fibrillation (AF) is the most common arrhythmia, with many challenging aspects of care, including only modest benefit of antiarrhythmic drugs and significant morbidity and recurrences with ablation techniques. Accordingly, complementary treatment options are needed. In the present study, yoga is evaluated in a cohort of patients with symptomatic AF. There were 49 patients who completed the study, serving as their own controls. The

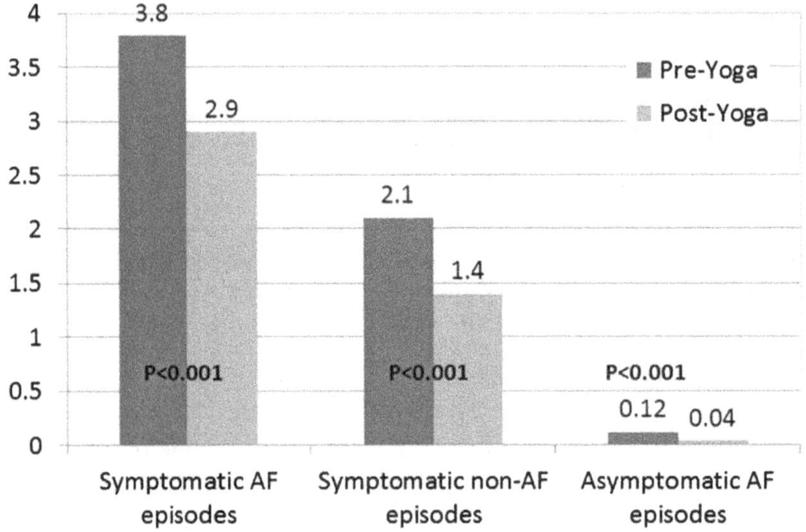

FIGURE 1.—Differences in primary efficacy outcomes measures between the control and intervention phase. Values are mean ± SD. (Reprinted from the Journal of the American College of Cardiology. Lakkireddy D, Atkins D, Pillarisetti J, et al. Effect of yoga on arrhythmia burden, anxiety, depression, and quality of life in paroxysmal atrial fibrillation: the YOGA my heart study. *J Am Coll Cardiol.* 2013;61:1177-1182, Copyright 2013, with permission from the American College of Cardiology.)

use of yoga reduced both symptomatic and asymptomatic episodes (Fig 1). It also reduced anxiety and depression, while improving quality of life and decreasing heart rate. These provocative results suggest that yoga and other meditation disciplines may have an important role in the management of symptomatic arrhythmias. However, this was an nonrandomized and unblended study, so further confirmation is needed.

M. Gold, MD

Syncope in High-Risk Cardiomyopathy Patients With Implantable Defibrillators: Frequency, Risk Factors, Mechanisms, and Association With Mortality: Results From the Multicenter Automatic Defibrillator Implantation Trial–Reduce Inappropriate Therapy (MADIT-RIT) Study

Ruwald MH, Okumura K, Kimura T, et al (Univ of Rochester Med Ctr, NY; Hirosaki Univ Hosp, Japan; Kyoto Univ Hosp, Japan; et al)

Circulation 129:545-552, 2014

Background.—There is a relative paucity of studies investigating the mechanisms of syncope among heart failure patients with implantable cardioverter-defibrillators, and it is controversial whether nonarrhythmogenic syncope is associated with increased mortality.

Methods and Results.—The Multicenter Automatic Defibrillator Implantation Trial-Reduce Inappropriate Therapy (MADIT-RIT) randomized

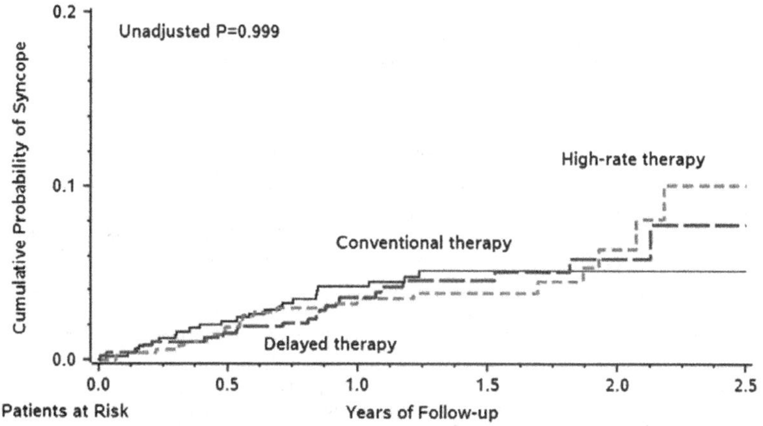

Patients at Risk						
Conv therapy	514	475 (0.02)	358 (0.04)	184 (0.05)	74 (0.05)	12 (0.05)
High-rate therapy	500	456 (0.02)	336 (0.04)	188 (0.04)	70 (0.06)	15 (0.10)
Delayed therapy	486	454 (0.01)	346 (0.04)	182 (0.05)	81 (0.06)	10 (0.08)

FIGURE 1.—Cumulative probability of first occurrence of all-cause syncope according to treatment arm. Kaplan–Meier estimates of the cumulative probability of a first occurrence of all-cause syncope are shown for patients randomly assigned to implantable cardioverter-defibrillator (ICD) programming of either conventional ICD therapy at a heart rate of ≥170 bpm, high-rate cutoff ICD therapy at a heart rate of ≥200 bpm and a monitoring zone between 170 and 199 bpm, or delayed ICD therapy with prolonged monitored zones at a heart rate >170 bpm. Conv indicates conventional. (Reprinted from Ruwald MH, Okumura K, Kimura T, et al. Syncope in high-risk cardiomyopathy patients with implantable defibrillators: frequency, risk factors, mechanisms, and association with mortality: results from the Multicenter Automatic Defibrillator Implantation Trial–Reduce Inappropriate Therapy (MADIT-RIT) Study. *Circulation.* 2014;129:545-552, Copyright 2014, with permission from American Heart Association, Inc.)

1500 patients to 3 different implantable cardioverter-defibrillator programming arms: (1) Conventional programming with therapy for ventricular tachycardia ≥170 bpm; (2) high-rate cutoff with therapy for ventricular tachycardia ≥200 bpm and a monitoring zone at 170 to 199 bpm, and (3) prolonged 60-second delay with a monitoring zone before therapy. Syncope was a prespecified safety end point that was adjudicated independently. Multivariable Cox models were used to identify risk factors associated with syncope and to analyze subsequent risk of mortality. During follow-up, 64 of 1500 patients (4.3%) had syncope. The incidence of syncope was similar across the 3 treatment arms. Prognostic factors for all-cause syncope included the presence of ischemic cardiomyopathy (hazard ratio [HR], 2.48; 95% confidence interval [CI], 1.42-4.34; $P = 0.002$), previous ventricular arrhythmias (HR, 2.99; 95% CI, 1.18-7.59; $P = 0.021$), left ventricular ejection fraction ≤25% (HR, 1.65; 95% CI, 0.98-2.77; $P = 0.059$), and younger age (by 10 years; HR, 1.25; 95% CI, 1.00-1.52; $P = 0.046$). Syncope was associated with increased risk of death regardless of its cause (arrhythmogenic syncope: HR, 4.51; 95% CI, 1.39-14.64, $P = 0.012$; non-arrhythmogenic syncope: HR, 2.97; 95% CI, 1.07-8.28, $P = 0.038$).

Conclusions.—Innovative programming of implantable cardioverter-defibrillators with therapy for ventricular tachycardia ≥200 bpm or a

TABLE 6.—Risk Factors Associated With All-Cause Death by Arrhythmogenic, Nonarrhythmogenic, and All-Cause Syncope in Univariable and Multivariable Cox Regression Models

Variable	Univariable HR (95% CI)	*P* Value	Multivariable* HR (95% CI)	*P* Value	Events: Death/Syncope, n (%)
Arrhythmogenic syncope	3.94 (1.23–12.61)	0.021	4.51 (1.39–14.64)	0.012	3/25 (12)
Nonarrhythmogenic syncope	3.26 (1.18–9.04)	0.023	2.97 (1.07–8.28)	0.038	4/39 (10)
All-cause syncope	3.70 (1.67–8.18)	0.001	3.65 (1.64–8.12)	0.002	7/64 (11)

Total deaths, n = 71.
CI indicates confidence interval; and HR, hazard ratio.
*Adjusted for treatment arm B, age, diastolic blood pressure, diabetes mellitus, treatment with implantable cardioverter-defibrillator or cardiac resynchronization therapy defibrillator, New York Heart Association class II or III, and ejection fraction ≤25%.
Reprinted from Ruwald MH, Okumura K, Kimura T, et al. Syncope in high-risk cardiomyopathy patients with implantable defibrillators: frequency, risk factors, mechanisms, and association with mortality: results from the Multicenter Automatic Defibrillator Implantation TrialeReduce Inappropriate Therapy (MADIT-RIT) Study. Circulation. 2014;129:545-552, Copyright 2014, with permission from American Heart Association, Inc.

long delay is not associated with increased risk of arrhythmogenic or all-cause syncope, and syncope caused by slow ventricular tachycardias (<200 bpm) is a rare event. The clinical risk factors associated with syncope are related to increased cardiovascular risk profile, and syncope is associated with increased mortality irrespective of the cause.

Clinical Trial Registration.—URL: http://www.clinicaltrials.gov. Unique identifier: NCT00947310 (Fig 1, Table 6).

▶ Syncope is a common clinical problem. Cardiac syncope has been shown to have a worse prognosis than most other etiologies. Therefore, syncope in the presence of structural heart disease is particularly worrisome. Often unexplained syncope in cardiac patients is considered an indication for pacemaker in the presence of conduction disease or implantable cardioverter-defibrillator in the presence of structural heart disease (systolic heart failure, hypertrophic cardiomyopathy, long QT syndrome, etc). However, it is clear that there are nonarrhythmic causes of syncope, which complicates medical decision making. Our understanding of management of these patiens is further challenged by the paucity of prospective, randomized clinical studies of this cohort. With regard to ICDs, syncope did not qualify for secondary prevention in the absence of documented ventricular arrhythmias, and these subjects were considered too high risk for primary prevention studies. To help understand this problem better, a retrospective analysis of the MADIT-RIT trial was performed. Over the course of this study, 4.3% of the 1500 randomized patients had syncope. The incidence was independent of the randomized programming of ICDs in this trial, which is reassuring given the aggressive strategies used, including treating no arrhythmias < 200 beats per minute or delaying 60 seconds to treat slow arrhythmias. Thus, programming to markedly reduce inappropriate shocks is not associated with increased syncope (Fig 1). In addition, the etiology of syncope (arrhythmogenic vs non-arrhythmogenic) had a similar adverse impact on prognosis (Table 6). Thus, syncope is a marker of decreased survival among subjects with a reduced left ventricular ejection fraction. Further studies are needed to explore treatment options to improve outcomes in these subjects.

M. Gold, MD

Safety and Efficacy of a Totally Subcutaneous Implantable-Cardioverter Defibrillator

Weiss R, Knight BP, Gold MR, et al (The Ohio State Univ, Columbus; Northwestern Univ, Chicago, IL; Med Univ of South Carolina, Charleston; et al)

Circulation 128:944-953, 2013

Background.—The most frequent complications associated with implantable cardioverter-defibrillators (ICDs) involve the transvenous leads. A subcutaneous implantable cardioverter-defibrillator (S-ICD) has been developed as an alternative system. This study evaluated the safety and effectiveness of the S-ICD System (Cameron Health/Boston Scientific) for the treatment of life-threatening ventricular arrhythmias (ventricular tachycardia/ventricular fibrillation).

Methods and Results.—This prospective, nonrandomized, multicenter trial included adult patients with a standard indication for an ICD, who neither required pacing nor had documented pace-terminable ventricular tachycardia. The primary safety end point was the 180-day S-ICD System complication-free rate compared with a prespecified performance goal of 79%. The primary effectiveness end point was the induced ventricular fibrillation conversion rate compared with a prespecified performance goal of 88%, with success defined as 2 consecutive ventricular fibrillation conversions of 4 attempts. Detection and conversion of spontaneous episodes were also evaluated. Device implantation was attempted in 321 of 330 enrolled patients, and 314 patients underwent successful implantation. The cohort was followed for a mean duration of 11 months. The study population was 74% male with a mean age of 52 ± 16 years and mean left ventricular ejection fraction of 36 ± 16%. A previous transvenous ICD had been implanted in 13%. Both primary end points were met: The 180-day system complication-free rate was 99%, and sensitivity analysis of the acute ventricular fibrillation conversion rate was >90% in the entire cohort. There were 38 discrete spontaneous episodes of ventricular tachycardia/ventricular fibrillation recorded in 21 patients (6.7%), all of which successfully converted. Forty-one patients (13.1%) received an inappropriate shock.

Conclusions.—The findings support the efficacy and safety of the S-ICD System for the treatment of life-threatening ventricular arrhythmias (Fig 3, Table 3).

▶ The implantable cardioverter-defibrillator (ICD) is an effective therapy for the primary or secondary prevention of sudden death. However, short- and long-term complications from these devices increase costs and limit their adoption.

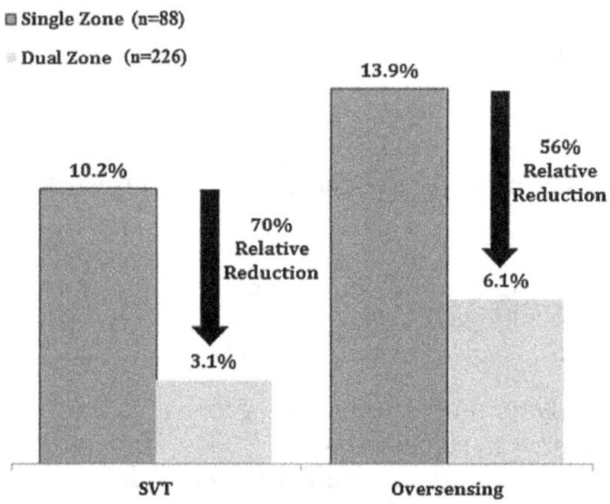

FIGURE 3.—Relative reduction of inappropriate shocks (for supraventricular tachyarrhythmias [SVT] or oversensing) associated with programming an arrhythmia discrimination zone at discharge. (Reprinted from Weiss R, Knight BP, Gold MR, et al. Safety and efficacy of a totally subcutaneous implantable-cardioverter defibrillator. *Circulation.* 2013;128:944-953, Copyright 2013, with permission from American Heart Association, Inc.)

TABLE 3.—Induced Ventricular Tachycardia/Ventricular Fibrillation Detection Sensitivity

Testing Time Point	Treated/Shock Delivered (%)
Acute VF conversion testing	808/809 (99.9)
Chronic conversion testing	89/90 (98.9)
Total	897/899 (99.8)

VF indicates ventricular fibrillation.

Reprinted from Weiss R, Knight BP, Gold MR, et al. Safety and efficacy of a totally subcutaneous implantablecardioverter defibrillator. Circulation. 2013;128:944-953, Copyright 2013, with permission from American Heart Association, Inc.

In response to this problem, a totally subcutaneous system (S-ICD) has been developed, which avoids the need for intravascular leads. The present prospective study is the largest trial to date of this technology. The results show a high efficacy for the detection of ventricular fibrillation (Table 3) despite much smaller subcutaneous signals compared with intracardiac signals. The device is also effective at terminating both induced and spontaneous arrhythmias, although the output of 80 J is higher than for transvenous ICDs. Finally, the discrimination algorithm markedly reduces inappropriate shocks (Fig 3). These results establish the S-ICD as an important alternative to traditional defibrillators for patients who do not require pacing for bradycardia, tachycardia, or resynchronization. Further clinical experience will help identify the patients best suited for this device.

M. R. Gold, MD, PhD

Edoxaban versus Warfarin in Patients with Atrial Fibrillation

Giugliano RP, for the ENGAGE AF-TIMI 48 Investigators (Brigham and Women's Hosp and Harvard Med School, Boston, MA; et al)

N Engl J Med 369:2093-2104, 2013

Background.—Edoxaban is a direct oral factor Xa inhibitor with proven antithrombotic effects. The long-term efficacy and safety of edoxaban as compared with warfarin in patients with atrial fibrillation is not known.

Methods.—We conducted a randomized, double-blind, double-dummy trial comparing two once-daily regimens of edoxaban with warfarin in 21,105 patients with moderate-to-high-risk atrial fibrillation (median follow-up, 2.8 years). The primary efficacy end point was stroke or systemic embolism. Each edoxaban regimen was tested for noninferiority to warfarin during the treatment period. The principal safety end point was major bleeding.

Results.—The annualized rate of the primary end point during treatment was 1.50% with warfarin (median time in the therapeutic range, 68.4%), as compared with 1.18% with high-dose edoxaban (hazard ratio, 0.79; 97.5% confidence interval [CI], 0.63 to 0.99; $P < 0.001$ for noninferiority) and 1.61% with low-dose edoxaban (hazard ratio, 1.07; 97.5% CI, 0.87 to 1.31; $P = 0.005$ for noninferiority). In the intention-to-treat analysis, there was a trend favoring high-dose edoxaban versus warfarin (hazard ratio, 0.87; 97.5% CI, 0.73 to 1.04; $P = 0.08$) and an unfavorable trend with low-dose edoxaban versus warfarin (hazard ratio, 1.13; 97.5% CI, 0.96 to 1.34; $P = 0.10$). The annualized rate of major bleeding was 3.43% with warfarin versus 2.75% with high-dose edoxaban (hazard ratio, 0.80; 95% CI, 0.71 to 0.91; $P < 0.001$) and 1.61% with low-dose edoxaban (hazard ratio, 0.47; 95% CI, 0.41 to 0.55; $P < 0.001$). The corresponding annualized rates of death from cardiovascular causes were 3.17% versus 2.74% (hazard ratio, 0.86; 95% CI, 0.77 to 0.97; $P = 0.01$), and 2.71% (hazard ratio, 0.85; 95% CI, 0.76 to 0.96; $P = 0.008$), and the corresponding rates of the key secondary end point (a composite of stroke, systemic embolism, or death from cardiovascular causes) were 4.43% versus 3.85% (hazard ratio, 0.87; 95% CI, 0.78 to 0.96; $P = 0.005$), and 4.23% (hazard ratio, 0.95; 95% CI, 0.86 to 1.05; $P = 0.32$).

Conclusions.—Both once-daily regimens of edoxaban were noninferior to warfarin with respect to the prevention of stroke or systemic embolism and were associated with significantly lower rates of bleeding and death from cardiovascular causes. (Funded by Daiichi Sankyo Pharma Development; ENGAGE AF-TIMI 48 ClinicalTrials.gov number, NCT00781391.) (Fig 1)

► Stroke remains one of the most serious consequences of atrial fibrillation. Anticoagulation is the most effective strategy to prevent stroke in high-risk subjects, as determined by the CHADS or CHADSVASc scoring systems. Although left atrial appendage closure devices may provide a nonpharmacologic treatment for stroke prevention, anticoagulation is clearly the primary treatment modality.

A Stroke or Systemic Embolic Event

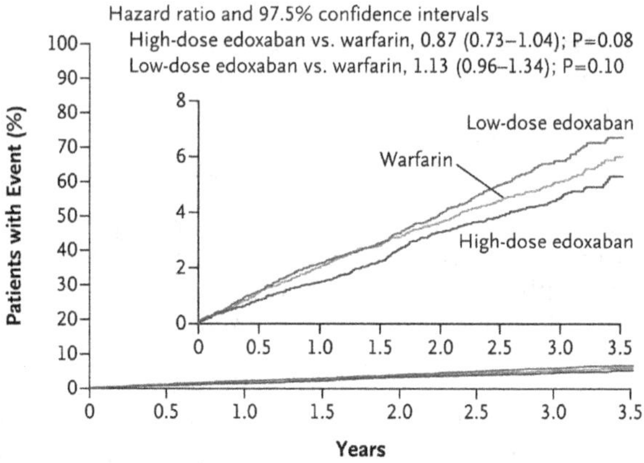

No. at Risk

Warfarin	7036	6798	6615	6406	6225	4593	2333	536
High-dose edoxaban	7035	6816	6650	6480	6283	4659	2401	551
Low-dose edoxaban	7034	6815	6631	6461	6277	4608	2358	534

B Major Bleeding

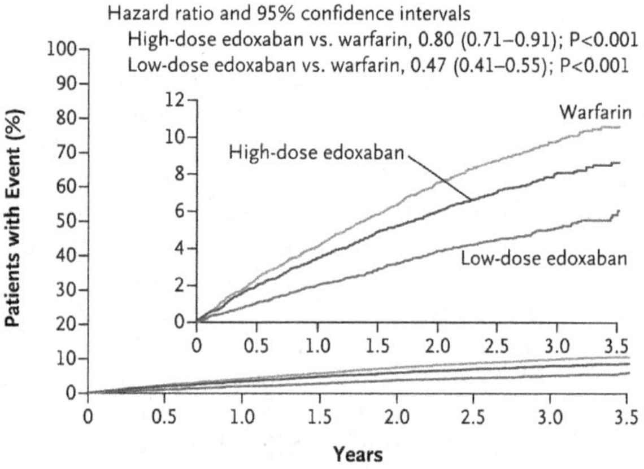

No. at Risk

Warfarin	7012	6116	5630	5278	4941	3446	1687	370
High-dose edoxaban	7012	6039	5594	5232	4910	3471	1706	345
Low-dose edoxaban	7002	6218	5791	5437	5110	3635	1793	386

FIGURE 1.—Kaplan–Meier curves for the primary efficacy and principal safety end points. Panel A shows the cumulative event rates for stroke or systemic embolism in the intention-to-treat population (all patients who underwent randomization) during the overall study period (i.e., beginning from the time of randomization to the end of the double-blind treatment period); data from the overall study period, rather than the treatment period only, were used in the superiority analyses of efficacy. Panel B shows the principal safety outcome of major bleeding, defined according to the criteria of the International Society on Thrombosis and Haemostasis,[10] in the safety population during the treatment period. The Kaplan–Meier curve was drawn without interval censoring for treatment interruptions. The inset in each panel shows the same data on an enlarged segment of the y axis. *Editor's Note*: Please refer to original journal article for full references. (Reprinted from Giugliano RP, for the ENGAGE AF-TIMI 48 Investigators, Edoxaban versus warfarin in patients with atrial fibrillation. *N Engl J Med*. 2013;369:2093-2104, Copyright 2013, with permission from Massachusetts Medical Society.)

Despite the effectiveness of warfarin for stroke protection in atrial fibrillation, it is a difficult drug to manage clinically, with dietary restrictions, many drug interactions and the need for chronic testing of anticoagulation status among patients. This has led to the development of a series of novel oral anticoagulants (NOACs) that act as either direct thrombin inhibitors or factor Xa inhibitors. Edoxaban is now the fourth such agent to complete large-scale clinical trials. The ENGAGE AF-TIMI 48 trial was a prospective, multinational, randomized trial of 21 105 subjects that included 2 once-daily doses of edoxaban. Both doses were noninferior to warfarin for preventing stroke or systemic embolus while significantly reducing major bleeding (Fig 1). High-dose edoxaban was more effective than low-dose edoxaban, but it was associated with more major bleeding events. Finally, the net clinical benefit, which is an important measure of overall risks and benefit of new therapies, was significantly increased with both dosages compared with warfarin. This study clearly supports the use of edoxaban as another once-daily anticoagulant in atrial fibrillation.

M. Gold, MD

Catheter ablation vs. antiarrhythmic drug treatment of persistent atrial fibrillation: a multicentre, randomized, controlled trial (SARA study)

Mont L, on behalf of SARA investigators (Hosp Clínic, Barcelona, Catalonia, Spain; et al)

Eur Heart J 35:501-507, 2014

Background.—Catheter ablation (CA) is a highly effective therapy for the treatment of paroxysmal atrial fibrillation (AF) when compared with antiarrhythmic drug therapy (ADT). No randomized studies have compared the two strategies in persistent AF. The present randomized trial aimed to compare the effectiveness of CA vs. ADT in treating persistent AF.

Methods and Results.—Patients with persistent AF were randomly assigned to CA or ADT (excluding patients with long-standing persistent AF). Primary endpoint at 12-month follow-up was defined as any episode of AF or atrial flutter lasting >24 h that occurred after a 3-month blanking period. Secondary endpoints were any atrial tachyarrhythmia lasting >30 s, hospitalization, and electrical cardioversion. In total, 146 patients were included (aged 55 ± 9 years, 77% male). The ADT group received class Ic (43.8%) or class III drugs (56.3%). In an intention-to-treat analysis, 69 of 98 patients (70.4%) in the CA group and 21 of 48 patients (43.7%) in the ADT group were free of the primary endpoint ($P = 0.002$), implying an absolute risk difference of 26.6% (95% CI 10.0–43.3) in favour of CA. The proportion of patients free of any recurrence (>30 s) was higher in the CA group than in the ADT group (60.2 vs. 29.2%; $P < 0.001$) and cardioversion was less frequent (34.7 vs. 50%, respectively; $P = 0.018$).

Conclusion.—Catheter ablation is superior to medical therapy for the maintenance of sinus rhythm in patients with persistent AF at 12-month follow-up.

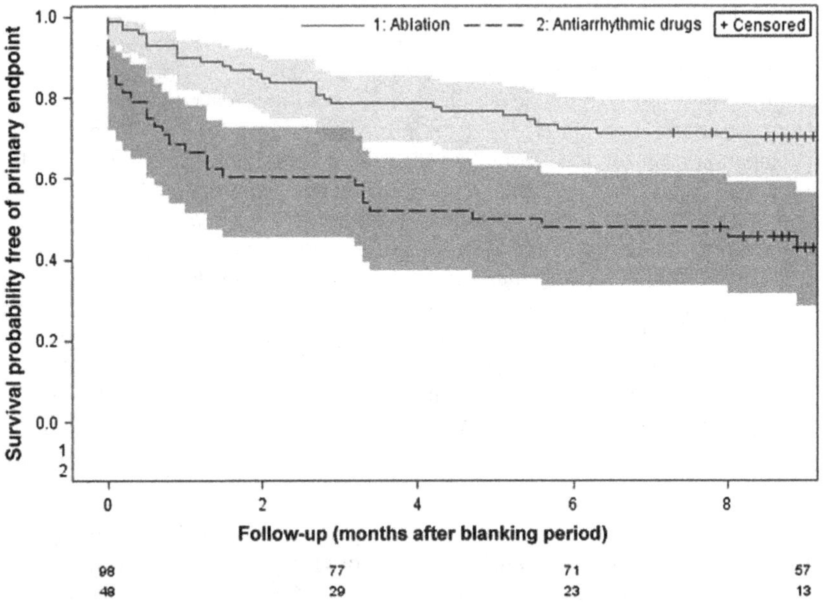

FIGURE 2.—Survival curves for the primary endpoint. (Reprinted from Mont L, on behalf of SARA investigators. Catheter ablation vs. antiarrhythmic drug treatment of persistent atrial fibrillation: a multicentre, randomized, controlled trial (SARA study). *Eur Heart J*. 2014;35:501-507, by permission of The European Society of Cardiology.)

Clinical Trial Registration Information.—NCT00863213 (http://clinicaltrials.gov/ct2/show/NCT00863213) (Fig 2).

▶ Atrial fibrillation (AF) is the most common pathologic arrhythmia. The prevalence of AF is increasing rapidly as the population ages and comorbidities such as hypertension and diabetes increase. The role of anticoagulation to reduce the risk of stroke among high-risk patients with AF is clear. However, controversy still exists with regard to antiarrhythmic therapy versus rate control. The advent of AF catheter ablation has added to the therapeutic dilemma for treatment. Ablation is found to be superior to drug antiarrhythmic therapy for patients with symptomatic, paroxysmal AF. However, both ablation and drugs are less efficacious for persistent AF. Accordingly, the SARA study was the first multicenter, randomized study to compare ablation and drugs. There were 146 patients randomly selected in this trial, which showed that the ablation was more effective for preventing less than 24-hour recurrences of atrial tachyarrhythmias between 3 and 12 months, the primary endpoint (Fig 2). Cardioversions and shorter episodes of AF were also less common in the ablation group. Although these results are encouraging in support of ablation, there were some unusual aspects of the trial, such as the high use of class Ic agents (44%) and the young age of the cohort (mean, 55 years). Whether ablation is superior to drugs when class III agents are used, which are preferred for persistent AF, and for an older population, remains to be determined. Nevertheless, SARA is another important advance helping define optimal strategies for the rapidly growing AF population.

M. Gold, MD

Incident Atrial Fibrillation Among Asians, Hispanics, Blacks, and Whites

Dewland TA, Olgin JE, Vittinghoff E, et al (Univ of California, San Francisco)

Circulation 128:2470-2477, 2013

Background.—Because the association between atrial fibrillation (AF) and race has only been rigorously compared in population-based studies that dichotomized participants as white or black, it is unclear whether white race confers elevated AF risk or black race affords AF protection.

Methods and Results.—The Healthcare Cost and Utilization Project was used to identify patients receiving hospital-based care in California between January 1, 2005 and December 31, 2009. The association between race and incident AF was examined using Cox proportional hazards models. Interaction analyses were performed to elucidate the mechanism underlying the race-AF association. Among 13 967 949 patients, 375 318 incident AF episodes were observed over a median 3.2 (interquartile range 1.8-4.3) years. In multivariable Cox models adjusting for patient demographics and established AF risk factors, blacks (hazard ratio, 0.84; 95% confidence interval, 0.82—0.85; $P < 0.001$), Hispanics (hazard ratio, 0.78; 95% confidence interval, 0.77—0.79; $P < 0.001$), and Asians (hazard ratio, 0.78; 95% confidence interval, 0.77—0.79; $P < 0.001$) each exhibited a lower AF risk compared with whites. AF risk among whites was disproportionately higher in the absence of acquired cardiovascular risk factors and diminished or reversed in the presence of comorbid diseases. Although Hispanics and Asians also had a lower adjusted risk of incident atrial flutter compared with whites, the risk of flutter was significantly higher among blacks.

Conclusions.—In a large hospital-based cohort, whites have an increased risk of AF whether compared with blacks, Asians, or Hispanics. The heightened AF risk among whites is most pronounced in the absence of cardiovascular comorbidities (Fig 3).

▶ Atrial fibrillation (AF) is a common arrhythmia and is associated with significant morbidity and long-term mortality. Comorbidities associated with AF, such as hypertension, heart failure, and diabetes, are well established. Aggressive treatment and prevention of these conditions are a mainstay of AF prevention. However, recent studies have shown that AF is not uniformly distributed in the population. Specifically, blacks have less AF than whites, despite more frequent comorbidities. This suggests a potential genetic predisposition to this arrhythmia. Less is known with regard to other ethnic and racial associations with the incidence of AF. Accordingly, the present study evaluated a large database of patients hospitalized in California over a 5-year period. Almost 14 million patients were evaluated with more than 375 000 AF episodes documented. AF

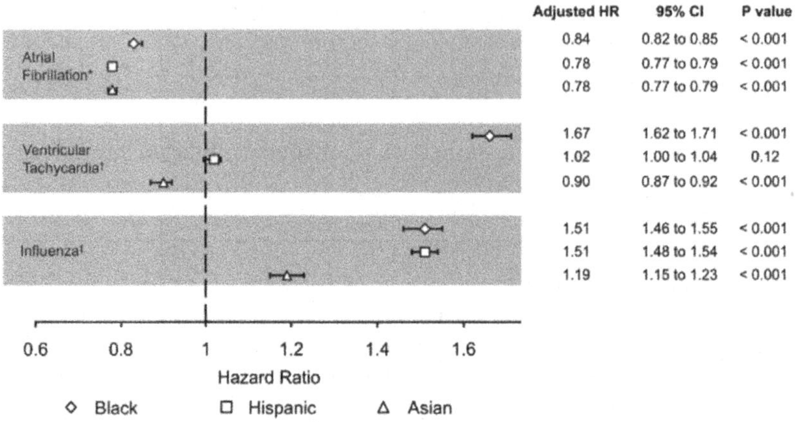

FIGURE 3.—Adjusted association between race and medical diagnoses. Adjusted hazard ratios (HR) for atrial fibrillation, ventricular tachycardia, and influenza among blacks, Hispanics, and Asians using white race as reference group for all analyses. *Adjusted for age, sex, insurance payer, income, history of cardiothoracic surgery, and presence of hypertension, heart failure, coronary artery disease, valvular heart disease, pulmonary disease, chronic kidney disease, and diabetes mellitus. †Adjusted for age, sex, insurance payer, income, and history of coronary artery disease and heart failure. ‡Adjusted for age, sex, insurance payer, income, and history of pulmonary disease. Error bars denote 95% confidence intervals (CI). (Reprinted from Dewland TA, Olgin JE, Vittinghoff E, et al. Incident atrial fibrillation among Asians, hispanics, blacks, and whites. *Circulation.* 2013;128:2470-2477, with permission from American Heart Association, Inc.)

was more common among white patients, compared with blacks, Asians, or Hispanics, even with adjustment for comorbidities (Fig 3). In fact, in the presence of comorbidities, the difference in the incidence of AF between groups was reduced. These observational data suggest that rather than a protective effect in blacks from developing AF, there may be a facilitatory process in whites independent of traditional risk factors for this arrhythmia.

M. Gold, MD

Effect of Weight Reduction and Cardiometabolic Risk Factor Management on Symptom Burden and Severity in Patients With Atrial Fibrillation: A Randomized Clinical Trial

Abed HS, Wittert GA, Leong DP, et al (Univ of Adelaide, Australia; et al)
JAMA 310:2050-2060, 2013

Importance.—Obesity is a risk factor for atrial fibrillation. Whether weight reduction and cardiometabolic risk factor management can reduce the burden of atrial fibrillation is not known.

Objective.—To determine the effect of weight reduction and management of cardiometabolic risk factors on atrial fibrillation burden and cardiac structure.

Design, Setting, and Patients.—Single-center, partially blinded, randomized controlled study conducted between June 2010 and December 2011 in Adelaide, Australia, among overweight and obese ambulatory patients (N = 150) with symptomatic atrial fibrillation. Patients underwent a median of 15 months of follow-up.

Interventions.—Patients were randomized to weight management (intervention) or general lifestyle advice (control). Both groups underwent intensive management of cardiometabolic risk factors.

Main Outcomes and Measures.—The primary outcomes were Atrial Fibrillation Severity Scale scores: symptom burden and symptom severity. Scores were measured every 3 months from baseline to 15 months. Secondary outcomes performed at baseline and 12 months were total atrial fibrillation episodes and cumulative duration measured by 7-day Holter, echocardiographic left atrial area, and interventricular septal thickness.

Results.—Of 248 patients screened, 150 were randomized (75 per group) and underwent follow-up. The intervention group showed a significantly greater reduction, compared with the control group, in weight (14.3 and 3.6 kg, respectively; $P < .001$) and in atrial fibrillation symptom burden scores (11.8 and 2.6 points, $P < .001$), symptom severity scores (8.4 and 1.7 points, $P < .001$), number of episodes (2.5 and no change, $P = .01$), and cumulative duration (692-minute decline and 419-minute increase, $P = .002$). Additionally, there was a reduction in interventricular septal thickness in the intervention and control groups (1.1 and 0.6 mm, $P = .02$) and left atrial area (3.5 and 1.9 cm^2, $P = .02$).

Conclusions and Relevance.—In this study, weight reduction with intensive risk factor management resulted in a reduction in atrial fibrillation symptom burden and severity and in beneficial cardiac remodeling. These findings support therapy directed at weight and risk factors in the management of atrial fibrillation.

Trial Registration.—anzctr.org.au Identifier: ACTRN12610000497000.

▶ The incidence of atrial fibrillation (AF) continues to increase as the population ages and risk factors become more prevalent. Most treatment strategies are directed to preventing embolic events and controlling symptoms. Control of hypertension and ischemia and treatment of sleep apnea are all advocated as preventative measures. However, lifestyle changes have received relatively little attention in the routine treatment of AF, other than to avoid excess alcohol consumption and cigarettes. The present study was a randomized trial of weight reduction and metabolic risk factor management in a cohort with symptomatic AF. The results were dramatic: the active treatment group lost 14.3 kg on average and had marked reductions in symptoms (Fig 3 in the original article) and AF burden. The study demonstrates, with a rigorous design, that lifestyle and risk-factor modification can have a significant impact on AF severity. This indicates that interventions such as these should become routine in arrhythmia management. However, it is important to note that this was likely a very motivated cohort, because weight reduction was greater than that observed in many other studies.

M. Gold, MD

42 Acute Coronary Syndromes

Racial/Ethnic and Gender Gaps in the Use of and Adherence to Evidence-Based Preventive Therapies Among Elderly Medicare Part D Beneficiaries After Acute Myocardial Infarction

Lauffenburger JC, Robinson JG, Oramasionwu C, et al (Univ of North Carolina at Chapel Hill; Univ of Iowa)

Circulation 129:754-763, 2014

Background.—It is unclear whether gender and racial/ethnic gaps in the use of and patient adherence to β-blockers, angiotensin-converting enzyme inhibitors/angiotensin receptor blockers, and statins after acute myocardial infarction have persisted after establishment of the Medicare Part D prescription program.

Methods and Results.—This retrospective cohort study used 2007 to 2009 Medicare service claims among Medicare beneficiaries ≥65 years of age who were alive 30 days after an index acute myocardial infarction hospitalization in 2008. Multivariable logistic regression models examined racial/ethnic (white, black, Hispanic, Asian, and other) and gender differences in the use of these therapies in the 30 days after discharge and patient adherence at 12 months after discharge, adjusting for patient baseline sociodemographic and clinical characteristics. Of 85 017 individuals, 55%, 76%, and 61% used angiotensin-converting enzyme inhibitors/angiotensin receptor blockers, β-blockers, and statins, respectively, within 30 days after discharge. No marked differences in use were found by race/ethnicity, but women were less likely to use angiotensin-converting enzyme inhibitors/angiotensin receptor blockers and β-blockers compared with men. However, at 12 months after discharge, compared with white men, black and Hispanic women had the lowest likelihood (≈30%–36% lower; $P < 0.05$) of being adherent, followed by white, Asian, and other women and black and Hispanic men (≈9%–27% lower; $P < 0.05$). No significant difference was shown between Asian/other men and white men.

Conclusions.—Although minorities were initially no less likely to use the therapies after acute myocardial infarction discharge compared with white patients, black and Hispanic patients had significantly lower

TABLE 3.—Association Between Use of ACEIs/ARBs, β-Blockers, and Statins Within 30 Days After Discharge From AMI Hospitalization and Race/Ethnicity and Gender Categories

	ACEIs/ARBs* (n = 47 124)		β-Blockers* (n = 64 939)		Statins* (n = 52 185)	
Race/Ethnicity and Gender	Adjusted OR†	95% CI (*P* Value)	Adjusted OR†	95% CI (*P* Value)	Adjusted OR†	95% CI (*P* Value)
White men	Referent	...	Referent	...	Referent	...
White women	0.91	0.88–0.94 (<0.001)	0.93	0.90–0.97 (<0.001)	0.98	0.95–1.02 (0.26)
Black men	1.06	0.99–1.13 (0.08)	0.96	0.90–1.03 (0.28)	1.04	0.97–1.11 (0.26)
Black women	0.98	0.89–1.07 (0.64)	0.85	0.77–0.94 (0.001)	1.08	0.98–1.18 (0.12)
Hispanic men	1.04	0.92–1.17 (0.52)	1.03	0.90–1.17 (0.70)	1.02	0.90–1.15 (0.81)
Hispanic women	1.20	1.05–1.37 (0.009)	1.09	0.94–1.27 (0.25)	1.04	0.90–1.20 (0.60)
Asian men	0.98	0.84–1.14 (0.76)	0.97	0.82–1.14 (0.70)	0.95	0.81–1.11 (0.53)
Asian women	1.01	0.87–1.17 (0.89)	0.94	0.80–1.11 (0.46)	1.20	1.02–1.41 (0.03)
Other men	0.98	0.82–1.17 (0.81)	0.84	0.70–1.02 (0.08)	1.04	0.86–1.25 (0.71)
Other women	1.00	0.81–1.24 (0.99)	0.91	0.70–1.13 (0.36)	1.02	0.82–1.27 (0.87)

ACEI indicates angiotensin-converting enzyme inhibitor; AMI, acute myocardial infarction; ARB, angiotensin receptor blocker; CI, confidence interval; and OR, odds ratio.

*Of all 85 017 beneficiaries.

†Adjusted for all the measured demographic, clinical, and baseline characteristics listed in Table 1.

TABLE 5.—Medication Adherence to ACEIs/ARBs, β-Blockers, and Statins After Discharge From AMI Hospitalization by Race/Ethnicity and Gender

Race/Ethnicity and Gender	ACEIs/ARBs (n = 47 124) Adjusted OR*	ACEIs/ARBs 95% CI (*P* Value)	β-Blockers (n = 64 939) Adjusted OR*	β-Blockers 95% CI (*P* Value)	Statins (n = 52 185) Adjusted OR*	Statins 95% CI (*P* Value)
White men	Referent	...	Referent	...	Referent	...
White women	0.91	0.87–0.95 (<0.001)	0.90	0.86–0.93 (<0.001)	1.05	1.01–1.09 (0.03)
Black men	0.88	0.81–0.96 (0.004)	0.74	0.69–0.79 (<0.001)	0.73	0.67–0.79 (<0.001)
Black women	0.70	0.62–0.78 (<0.001)	0.64	0.58–0.71 (<0.001)	0.72	0.66–0.89 (<0.001)
Hispanic men	0.95	0.82–1.11 (0.53)	0.81	0.71–0.92 (0.002)	0.77	0.66–0.89 (<0.001)
Hispanic women	0.85	0.72–1.00 (0.05)	0.70	0.60–0.80 (<0.001)	0.71	0.61–0.83 (<0.001)
Asian men	1.06	0.88–1.28 (0.53)	1.06	0.89–1.26 (0.50)	1.15	0.95–1.40 (0.14)
Asian women	0.92	0.77–1.11 (0.39)	0.83	0.70–0.97 (0.02)	0.95	0.80–1.13 (0.58)
Other men	1.10	0.87–1.40 (0.42)	0.86	0.70–1.06 (0.16)	1.08	0.86–1.36 (0.53)
Other women	0.85	0.65–1.11 (0.24)	0.76	0.60–0.95 (0.02)	0.74	0.58–0.95 (0.02)

ACEI indicates angiotensin-converting enzyme inhibitor; AMI, acute myocardial infarction; ARB, angiotensin receptor blocker; CI, confidence interval; and OR, odds ratio.

*Adjusted for all the measured demographic, clinical, and baseline characteristics listed in Table 1.

adherence over 12 months. Strategies to address gender and racial/ethnic gaps in the elderly are needed (Tables 3 and 5).

► As a result of improvement in medical therapies such as lipid-lowering agents, angiotensin-converting enzyme inhibitor (ACEI), angiotensin receptor blocker (ARB) and β-blockers, mortality from acute myocardial infarction (AMI) has declined in the general population. Despite these advances, both initial use and long-term adherence of medical therapy after AMI is disappointingly low. Moreover, there are gender and racial/ethnic disparities in outcomes. The purpose of this study was to assess whether there were gender and racial/ethnic gaps in the use of and patient adherence to evidence-based medical therapy after a hospitalization for AMI in a cohort of elderly patients. There were 85 017 individuals included in this large Medicare cohort. Within 30 days after a hospitalization for AMI, 47 124 (55%) used ACEI/ARB, 64 939 (76%) used beta-blockers, and 52 185 (61%) used statins. Compared with white men, there were no marked differences in medical therapy across racial/ethnic and gender groups. A few exceptions were that white women were less likely to use ACEI/ARB and β-blockers, and black women were less likely to use β-blockers compared with white men. Conversely, Hispanic women and Asian women were more likely to use ACEI/ARB and statins, respectively (Table 3). For ACEI/ARB, compared with white men, black women had the lowest likelihood (30% lower) of adherence 12 months after discharge followed by white women and black men (approximately 10% lower). In β-blocker use, black and Hispanic women had the lowest likelihood (36% and 30% lower respectively) of adherence compared with white men followed by black men (26% lower), Hispanic men (19% lower), and white women (10% lower). For statin therapy, black men and women along with Hispanic men and women had approximately 30% lower likelihood of adherence compared with white men (Table 5). This study shows no difference in initiation of ACEI/ARB, β-blocker, or statin therapy after discharge within 30 days after an AMI. At 12 months, however, adherence to these medications is significantly less in minority patients compared with white patients. Minority women, particularly black and Hispanic women, had the lowest adherence to all 3 therapies. Furthermore, these findings highlight the need for interventions to improve adherence of medical therapy after discharge, particularly for minority women.

T. Todoran, MD, MSc

Bivalirudin Started during Emergency Transport for Primary PCI

Steg PG, for the EUROMAX Investigators (Université Paris-Diderot, France; et al)

N Engl J Med 369:2207-2217, 2013

Background.—Bivalirudin, as compared with heparin and glycoprotein IIb/IIIa inhibitors, has been shown to reduce rates of bleeding and death in patients undergoing primary percutaneous coronary intervention (PCI). Whether these benefits persist in contemporary practice characterized by prehospital initiation of treatment, optional use of glycoprotein IIb/IIIa inhibitors and novel $P2Y_{12}$ inhibitors, and radial-artery PCI access use is unknown.

Methods.—We randomly assigned 2218 patients with ST-segment elevation myocardial infarction (STEMI) who were being transported for primary PCI to receive either bivalirudin or unfractionated or low-molecular-weight heparin with optional glycoprotein IIb/IIIa inhibitors (control group). The primary outcome at 30 days was a composite of death or major bleeding not associated with coronary-artery bypass grafting (CABG), and the principal secondary outcome was a composite of death, reinfarction, or non-CABG major bleeding.

Results.—Bivalirudin, as compared with the control intervention, reduced the risk of the primary outcome (5.1% vs. 8.5%; relative risk, 0.60; 95% confidence interval [CI], 0.43 to 0.82; $P = 0.001$) and the principal secondary outcome (6.6% vs. 9.2%; relative risk, 0.72; 95% CI, 0.54 to 0.96; $P = 0.02$). Bivalirudin also reduced the risk of major bleeding (2.6% vs. 6.0%; relative risk, 0.43; 95% CI, 0.28 to 0.66; $P < 0.001$). The risk of acute stent thrombosis was higher with bivalirudin (1.1% vs. 0.2%; relative risk, 6.11; 95% CI, 1.37 to 27.24; $P = 0.007$). There was no significant difference in rates of death (2.9% vs. 3.1%) or reinfarction (1.7% vs. 0.9%). Results were consistent across subgroups of patients.

Conclusions.—Bivalirudin, started during transport for primary PCI, improved 30-day clinical outcomes with a reduction in major bleeding but with an increase in acute stent thrombosis. (Funded by the Medicines Company; EUROMAX ClinicalTrials.gov number, NCT01087723.)

▶ In patients with ST-segment elevation myocardial infarction (STEMI), antithrombotic therapy with bivalirudin has been found to significantly reduce bleeding and improve mortality compared with therapy heparin and glycoprotein IIb/IIa inhibitors (GPI) at the cost of a slightly higher risk of stent thrombosis. The question remains whether this benefit translates to more modern practice, which includes bleeding reduction strategies, such as decreased routine GPI use, increased utilization of transradial access, and improved antiplatelet therapies, such as prasugrel and ticagrelor. This trial randomly selected 2218 patients with STEMI to prehospital treatment with either bivalirudin or heparin and optional GPI before primary percutaneous coronary intervention (PCI) with the primary endpoint of death or major bleeding. Almost half of the patients in each group were treated via transradial access, most patients in each group were treated with either prasugrel or ticagrelor, and GPI use was 11.5% in the bivalirudin group versus 69.1% in the heparin/GPI group. Patients treated with bivalirudin had improved death or major bleeding (5.1% bivalirudin vs 8.5% heparin; relative risk [RR], 0.60; 95% confidence interval [CI], 0.43–0.82; $P = .001$) compared with the heparin group, and this difference was almost entirely due to a reduction in major bleeding (Fig 1 in the original article). Death rate was similar between the 2 groups, and there was an increased risk of stent thrombosis in the patients treated with bivalirudin (1.1% vs 0.2%; RR, 6.1; 95% CI, 1.4–27.2; $P = .007$). These findings extend the evidence that treatment with bivalirudin is associated with decreased bleeding in patients undergoing primary PCI for STEMI; however, there does not appear to be significant mortality benefit, and bivalirudin treatment is associated with increased rates of stent thrombosis.

D. Steinberg, MD

Randomized Trial of Preventive Angioplasty in Myocardial Infarction

Wald DS, for the PRAMI Investigators (Queen Mary Univ of London, UK; et al)
N Engl J Med 369:1115-1123, 2013

Background.—In acute ST-segment elevation myocardial infarction (STEMI), the use of percutaneous coronary intervention (PCI) to treat the artery responsible for the infarct (infarct, or culprit, artery) improves prognosis. The value of PCI in noninfarct coronary arteries with major stenoses (preventive PCI) is unknown.

Methods.—From 2008 through 2013, at five centers in the United Kingdom, we enrolled 465 patients with acute STEMI (including 3 patients with left bundle-branch block) who were undergoing infarct-artery PCI and randomly assigned them to either preventive PCI (234 patients) or no preventive PCI (231 patients). Subsequent PCI for angina was recommended only for refractory angina with objective evidence of ischemia. The primary outcome was a composite of death from cardiac causes, nonfatal myocardial infarction, or refractory angina. An intention-to-treat analysis was used.

Results.—By January 2013, the results were considered conclusive by the data and safety monitoring committee, which recommended that the trial be stopped early. During a mean follow-up of 23 months, the primary outcome occurred in 21 patients assigned to preventive PCI and in 53 patients assigned to no preventive PCI (infarct-artery- only PCI), which translated into rates of 9 events per 100 patients and 23 per 100, respectively (hazard ratio in the preventive-PCI group, 0.35; 95% confidence interval [CI], 0.21 to 0.58; $P < 0.001$). Hazard ratios for the three components of the primary outcome were 0.34 (95% CI, 0.11 to 1.08) for death from cardiac causes, 0.32 (95% CI, 0.13 to 0.75) for nonfatal myocardial infarction, and 0.35 (95% CI, 0.18 to 0.69) for refractory angina.

Conclusions.—In patients with STEMI and multivessel coronary artery disease undergoing infarctartery PCI, preventive PCI in noninfarct coronary arteries with major stenoses significantly reduced the risk of adverse cardiovascular events, as compared with PCI limited to the infarct artery. (Funded by Barts and the London Charity; PRAMI Current Controlled Trials number, ISRCTN73028481.)

► Primary percutaneous coronary intervention (PCI) is well established as the standard therapy for patients with acute ST-segment elevation myocardial infarction (STEMI). For patients with multivessel disease at the time of STEMI, PCI of noninfarct arteries during the index procedure is largely contraindicated with a class III guideline indication (no benefit or harm) unless the patient is hemodynamically compromised. There is some debate as to whether patients benefit from staged revascularization of noninfarct arteries after STEMI. The PRAMI trial aimed to answer this question by randomly selecting patients undergoing primary PCI for STEMI to receive either immediate preventative PCI for noninfarct arteries or medical therapy with further revascularization only in cases of objective ischemia. The primary outcome of this trial was a composite of death, myocardial infarction, and refractory angina, and there was a planned enrollment of 600 patients. The study was stopped by the Data and Safety Monitoring Board after 465 patients were enrolled because of a highly significant difference in outcomes between the 2 groups favoring preventive PCI. Event rates were lower in the preventive PCI group (hazard ratio [HR], 0.35 [95% confidence interval (CI), 0.21–0.58]; $P < .01$) with significant differences in combined death or myocardial infarction (HR, 0.36 [95% CI, 0.18–0.73]; $P = .004$) and nonsignificant trend toward reduced cardiovascular mortality (Fig 2 in the original article). This study suggests that preventive PCI of noninfarct arteries may have benefit in patients undergoing primary PCI for STEMI, which will have a large effect on clinical practice.

D. Steinberg, MD

Derivation and Validation of a Risk Standardization Model for Benchmarking Hospital Performance for Health-Related Quality of Life Outcomes After Acute Myocardial Infarction

Arnold SV, Masoudi FA, Rumsfeld JS, et al (Saint Luke's Mid America Heart Inst, Kansas City, MO; Univ of Colorado, Denver)
Circulation 129:313-320, 2014

Background.—Before outcomes-based measures of quality can be used to compare and improve care, they must be risk-standardized to account for variations in patient characteristics. Despite the importance of health-related quality of life (HRQL) outcomes among patients with acute myocardial infarction (AMI), no risk-standardized models have been developed.

Methods and Results.—We assessed disease-specific HRQL using the Seattle Angina Questionnaire at baseline and 1 year later in 2693 unselected AMI patients from 24 hospitals enrolled in the Translational Research Investigating Underlying disparities in acute Myocardial infarction Patients' Health status (TRIUMPH) registry. Using 57 candidate sociodemographic, economic, and clinical variables present on admission, we developed a parsimonious, hierarchical linear regression model to predict HRQL. Eleven variables were independently associated with poor HRQL after AMI, including younger age, previous coronary artery bypass graft surgery, depressive symptoms, and financial difficulties ($R^2 = 20\%$). The model demonstrated excellent internal calibration and reasonable calibration in an independent sample of 1890 AMI patients in a separate registry, although the model slightly overpredicted HRQL scores in the higher deciles. Among the 24 TRIUMPH hospitals, 1-year unadjusted HRQL scores ranged from 67–89. After risk-standardization, HRQL score variability

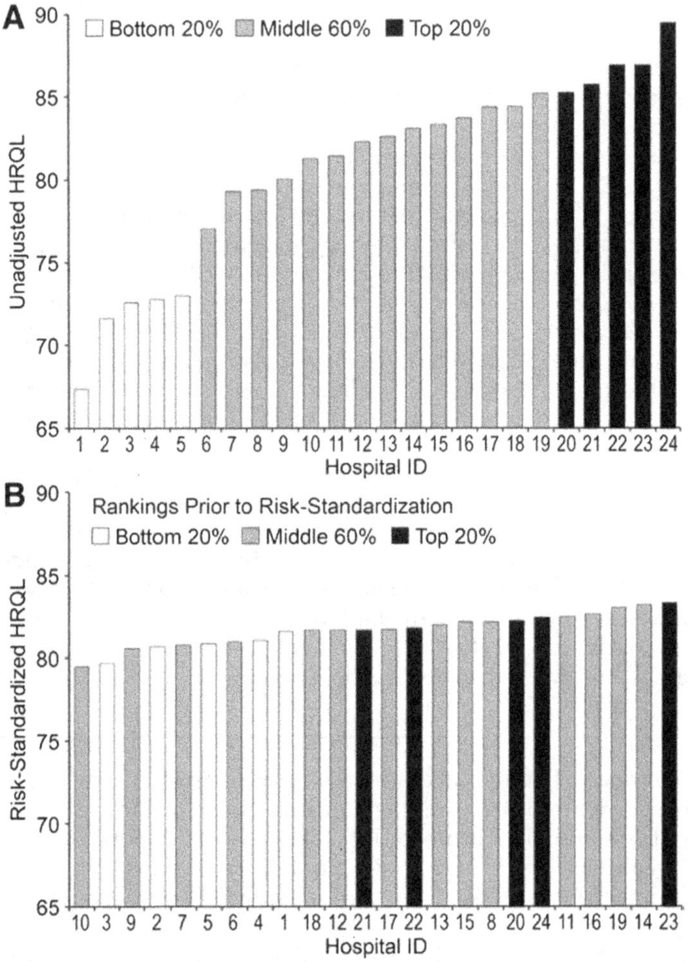

FIGURE 3.—Unadjusted (A) and risk-standardized (B) 1-year health-related quality of life (HRQL) outcomes by site. (Reprinted from Arnold SV, Masoudi FA, Rumsfeld JS, et al. Derivation and validation of a risk standardization model for benchmarking hospital performance for health-related quality of life outcomes after acute Myocardial infarction. *Circulation.* 2014;129:313-320, Copyright 2014, with permission from American Heart Association, Inc.)

narrowed substantially (range = 79−83), and the group of hospital performance (bottom 20%/middle 60%/top 20%) changed in 14 of the 24 hospitals (58% reclassification with risk-standardization).

Conclusions.—In this predictive model for HRQL after AMI, we identified risk factors, including economic and psychological characteristics, associated with HRQL outcomes. Adjusting for these factors substantially altered the rankings of hospitals as compared with unadjusted comparisons. Using this model to compare risk-standardized HRQL outcomes across hospitals may identify processes of care that maximize this important patient-centered outcome (Fig 3).

▶ When using patient outcomes to assess, compare, and improve quality, it is important to adjust for patient characteristics that are present before the delivery of care. Risk adjustment allows hospitals to be graded on the quality of care they provide rather than the type of patients they treat. The aim of this study was to develop a predictive model for health-related quality of life (HRQL) after acute myocardial infarction (AMI) and apply this model to AMI patients from 24 hospitals enrolled in the TRIUMPH registry. The 1-year unadjusted HRQL across hospitals was 67.4 to 89.5. After risk standardization, the median risk-standardized HRQL was 81.7 and the range was narrower (79.5–83.3). Comparing unadjusted to risk-standardized rankings, the median absolute change was 4 places (range 1–9) and 14 of the 24 hospitals (58.3%) had a change in their ranking category of top 20%, middle 60%, or bottom 20% (Fig 3). Adjusting for factors such as demographics, psychosocial status, economic status, comorbidities, and baseline health status altered the rankings of the hospitals compared with unadjusted comparisons. Many of these factors are not modifiable and thus allowed for a fair comparison of outcomes among hospitals. This study represents the first development and validation of a model to risk-standardize 1-year HRQL after AMI. It is important because it permits comparison hospital performance independent of type of patients treated; such outcome measures are becoming more important for assessment of quality and comparisons between institutions and are linked to reimbursement.

T. Todoran, MD, MSc

43 Coronary Intervention Procedures

A Prospective Randomized Trial of Everolimus-Eluting Stents Versus Bare-Metal Stents in Octogenarians: The XIMA Trial (Xience or Vision Stents for the Management of Angina in the Elderly)

de Belder A, on behalf of the XIMA Investigators (Brighton and Sussex Univ Hosps Natl Health Service Trust, England; et al)

J Am Coll Cardiol 63:1371-1375, 2014

Objectives.—The aim of this study was to determine whether drug-eluting stents (DES) are superior to bare-metal stents (BMS) in octogenarian patients with angina.

Background.—Patients >80 years of age frequently have complex coronary disease warranting DES but have a higher risk of bleeding from prolonged dual antiplatelet therapy.

Methods.—gr1This multicenter randomized trial was conducted in 22 centers in the United Kingdom and Spain. Patients ≥80 years of age underwent stent placement for angina. The primary endpoint was a 1-year composite of death, myocardial infarction, cerebrovascular accident, target vessel revascularization, or major hemorrhage.

Results.—In total, 800 patients (83.5 ± 3.2 years of age) were randomized to BMS (n = 401) or DES (n = 399) for treatment of stable angina (32%) or acute coronary syndrome (68%). Procedural success did not differ between groups (97.7% for BMS vs. 95.4% for DES; $p = 0.07$). Thirty-eight percent of patients had ≥2-vessel percutaneous coronary intervention, and 66% underwent complete revascularization. Patients who received BMS had shorter stent implants (24.0 ± 13.4 mm vs. 26.6 ± 14.3 mm; $p = 0.01$). Rates of dual antiplatelet therapy at 1 year were 32.2% for patients in the BMS group and 94.0% for patients in the DES group. The primary endpoint occurred in 18.7% of patients in the BMS group versus 14.3% of patients in the DES group ($p = 0.09$). There was no difference in death (7.2% vs. 8.5%; $p = 0.50$), major hemorrhage (1.7% vs. 2.3%; $p = 0.61$), or cerebrovascular accident (1.2% vs. 1.5%; $p = 0.77$). Myocardial infarction (8.7% vs. 4.3%; $p = 0.01$) and target

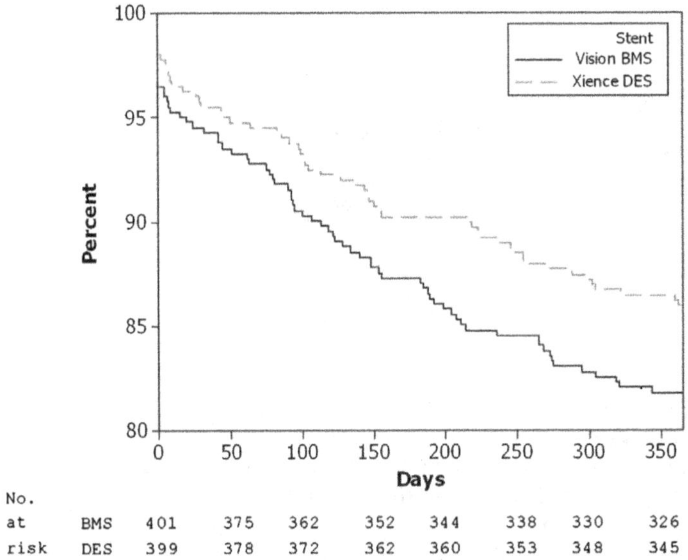

FIGURE 1.—Kaplan-Meier survival plot. Kaplan-Meier survival plot for time to first primary endpoint event for the DES and BMS groups. BMS = bare-metal stent(s); DES = drug-eluting stent(s). (Reprinted from the Journal of the American College of Radiology. de Belder A, on behalf of the XIMA Investigators. A prospective randomized trial of everolimus-eluting stents versus bare-metal stents in octogenarians: the XIMA trial (xience or vision stents for the management of angina in the elderly). *J Am Coll Cardiol.* 2014;63:1371-1375, Copyright 2014, with permission from the American College of Radiology.)

vessel revascularization (7.0% vs. 2.0%; $p = 0.001$) occurred more often in patients in the BMS group.

Conclusions.—BMS and DES offer good clinical outcomes in this age group. DES were associated with a lower incidence of myocardial infarction and target vessel revascularization without increased incidence of major hemorrhage. (Xience or Vision Stent-Management of Angina in the Elderly [XIMA]; ISRCTN92243650) (Fig 1).

▶ Patients aged older than 80 years are presenting more commonly with stable coronary artery disease (CAD) and acute coronary syndromes (ACS). Although coronary artery stenting is feasible, it is associated with higher complication rates in the elderly, particularly bleeding in the setting of long-term dual antiplatelet therapy. Furthermore, little is known regarding the incremental benefit of drug-eluting stents (DES) compared with bare-metal stents (BMS) because many clinical trials excluded these patients. In this prospective study, 800 octogenarian patients (83.5 ± 3.2 years of age) with stable CAD and ACS that warranted treatment with DES (lesion length greater than or equal to 15 mm or vessel diameter less than 3 mm) were randomized to BMS (n = 401) or DES (n = 399). The composite primary end point of all-cause death, myocardial infarction, target vessel revascularization, stroke, and major bleeding was higher in the BMS group compared with the DES group (18.7% vs 14.3%, $P = .09$). Time to first event is shown in the Kaplan-Meier analysis (Fig 1). The difference in primary end point between groups was driven primarily by a difference in myocardial infarction (8.7% vs 4.3%, *P* = .01) and target vessel revascularization (7.0% vs 2.0%, *P* = .001) for BMS and DES, respectively. This study supports the use of DES in octogenarians undergoing coronary stent placement for symptomatic CAD. When compared with BMS, DES resulted in a reduction of myocardial infarction and target vessel revascularization without increase in stroke or major bleeding. Potential confounders of mortality and bleeding in this study are the higher number of noncardiac deaths in the DES group compared with the BMS group and the relatively large percentage of patients in the BMS group on dual antiplatelet therapy at 1 year (32%).

T. Todoran, MD, MSc

Intra-aortic balloon counterpulsation in acute myocardial infarction complicated by cardiogenic shock (IABP-SHOCK II): final 12 month results of a randomised, open-label trial

Thiele H, on behalf of the Intraaortic Balloon Pump in cardiogenic shock II (IABP-SHOCK II) trial investigators (Univ of Leipzig—Heart Centre, Germany; et al)

Lancet 382:1638-1645, 2013

Background.—In current international guidelines the recommendation for intra-aortic balloon pump (IABP) use has been downgraded in cardiogenic shock complicating acute myocardial infarction on the basis of registry data. In the largest randomised trial (IABP-SHOCK II), IABP support did not reduce 30 day mortality compared with control. However, previous trials in cardiogenic shock showed a mortality benefit only at extended follow-up. The present analysis therefore reports 6 and 12 month results.

Methods.—The IABP-SHOCK II trial was a randomised, open-label, multicentre trial. Patients with cardiogenic shock complicating acute myocardial infarction who were undergoing early revascularisation and optimum medical therapy were randomly assigned (1:1) to IABP versus control via a central web-based system. The primary efficacy endpoint was 30 day all-cause mortality, but 6 and 12 month follow-up was done in addition to quality-of-life assessment for all survivors with the Euroqol-5D questionnaire. A masked central committee adjudicated clinical outcomes. Patients and investigators were not masked to treatment allocation. Analysis was by intention to treat. This trial is registered at ClinicalTrials.gov, NCT00491036.

Findings.—Between June 16, 2009, and March 3, 2012, 600 patients were assigned to IABP (n = 301) or control (n = 299). Of 595 patients completing 12 month follow-up, 155 (52%) of 299 patients in the IABP group and 152 (51%) of 296 patients in the control group had died (relative risk [RR] 1·01, 95% CI 0·86–1·18, $p = 0·91$). There were no significant differences in reinfarction (RR 2·60, 95% CI 0·95–7·10, $p = 0·05$),

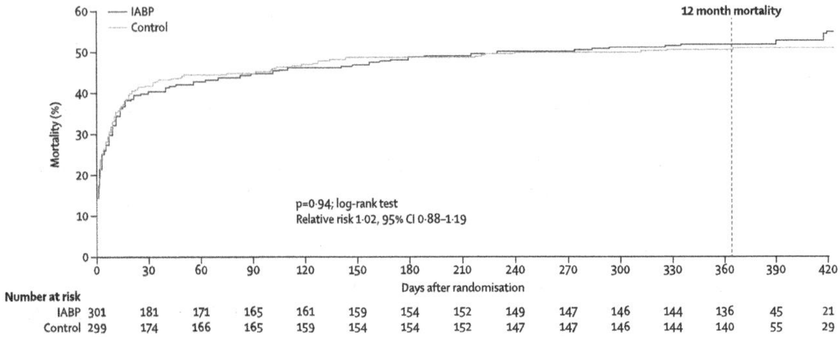

FIGURE 2.—Time-to-event curves for all-cause mortality up to 12 months. Event rates represent Kaplan-Meier estimates. Two patients in the IABP group died at days 388 and 419 postrandomisation, which is represented in the Kaplan-Meier curves. IABP = intra-aortic balloon pump. (Reprinted from Thiele H, on behalf of the Intraaortic Balloon Pump in cardiogenic shock II (IABP-SHOCK II) trial investigators, Intra-aortic balloon counterpulsation in acute myocardial infarction complicated by cardiogenic shock (IABP-SHOCK II): final 12 month results of a randomised, open-label trial. *Lancet.* 2013;382:1638-1645, Copyright 2013, with permission from Elsevier.)

recurrent revascularisation (0·91, 0·58–1·41, $p = 0{\cdot}77$), or stroke (1·50, 0·25–8·84, $p = 1{\cdot}00$). For survivors, quality-of-life measures including mobility, self-care, usual activities, pain or discomfort, and anxiety or depression did not differ significantly between study groups.

Interpretation.—In patients undergoing early revascularisation for myocardial infarction complicated by cardiogenic shock, IABP did not reduce 12 month all-cause mortality (Fig 2).

▶ Despite advances in treatment of myocardial infarction, such as early revascularization, mortality in acute myocardial infarction complicated by cardiogenic shock remains high. Intra-aortic balloon pump (IABP) counterpulsation has been the most widely used mechanical hemodynamic support device for decades for shock, but only one large, randomized trial has been performed on this technology. The short-term follow-up data at 30 days from the IABP-SHOCK II trial was previously reported showing no survival benefit with IABP support compared with control. However, other trials have shown a benefit of therapy in cardiogenic shock only with long-term follow-up. The IABP SHOCK II trial was a randomized, open-labeled, multicenter trial. Six hundred patients with acute myocardial infarction complicated by cardiogenic shock and undergoing early revascularization were randomly assigned 1:1 to IABP (n = 301) versus control (n = 299). There were 595 (99%) patients completing 12-month follow-up. Mortality did not differ significantly between the IABP and control groups at 6 months (48.7% vs 49.2%; relative risk [RR], 0.99; 95% confidence interval [CI], 0.85–1.16; $P = .91$) and 12 months (51.8% vs 51.4%; RR, 1.01; 95% CI, 0.86–1.18; $P = .91$) after randomization (Fig 2). Additionally, there were no significant differences in reinfarction (RR, 2.60; 95% CI, 0.95–7.10; $P = .05$), repeat revascularization (RR, 0.91; 95% CI, 0.58–1.41; $P = .77$), or stroke (RR, 1.50; 95% CI, 0.25–8.84; $P = 1.00$). Among survivors, quality-of-life assessment did not differ between treatment groups. Despite early revascularization, the mortality rate is nearly 50% at 12 months. Although this study contrasts survival benefit at long-term follow-up of earlier trials, it represents the largest randomized trial in the primary percutaneous coronary intervention era and thus provides important information in defining that there is a limited role of IABP in the treatment of myocardial infarction complicated by cardiogenic shock.

T. Todoran, MD, MSc

Cessation of dual antiplatelet treatment and cardiac events after percutaneous coronary intervention (PARIS): 2 year results from a prospective observational study

Mehran R, Baber U, Steg PG, et al (Icahn School of Medicine at Mount Sinai, NY; Hôpital Bichat-Claude Bernard, Paris, France; et al)

Lancet 382:1714-1722, 2013

Background.—Dual antiplatelet therapy (DAPT) cessation increases the risk of adverse events after percutaneous coronary intervention (PCI). Whether risk changes over time, depends on the underlying reason for DAPT cessation, or both is unknown. We assessed associations between different modes of DAPT cessation and cardiovascular risk after PCI.

Methods.—The PARIS (patterns of non-adherence to anti-platelet regimens in stented patients) registry is a prospective observational study of patients undergoing PCI with stent implantation in 15 clinical sites in the USA and Europe between July 1, 2009, and Dec 2, 2010. Adult patients (aged 18 years or older) undergoing successful stent implantation in one or more native coronary artery and discharged on DAPT were eligible for enrolment. Patients were followed up at months 1, 6, 12, and 24 after implantation. Prespecified categories for DAPT cessation included physicianrecommended discontinuation, brief interruption (for surgery), or disruption (non-compliance or because of bleeding). All adverse events and episodes of DAPT cessation were independently adjudicated. Using Cox models with time-varying covariates, we examined the effect of DAPT cessation on major adverse events (MACE [composite of cardiac death, definite or probable stent thrombosis, myocardial infarction, or target-lesion revascularisation]). Incidence rates for DAPT cessation and adverse events were calculated as Kaplan-Meier estimates of time to the first event. This study is registered with ClinicalTrials.gov, number NCT00998127.

Findings.—We enrolled 5031 patients undergoing PCI, including 5018 in the final study population. Over 2 years, the overall incidence of any DAPT cessation was 57·3%. Rate of any discontinuation was 40·8%, of interruption was 10·5%, and of disruption was 14·4%. The corresponding overall 2 year MACE rate was 11·5%, most of which (74%) occurred while patients were taking DAPT. Compared with those on DAPT, the adjusted hazard ratio (HR) for MACE due to interruption was 1·41 (95% CI 0·94–2·12; $p = 0{\cdot}10$) and to disruption was 1·50

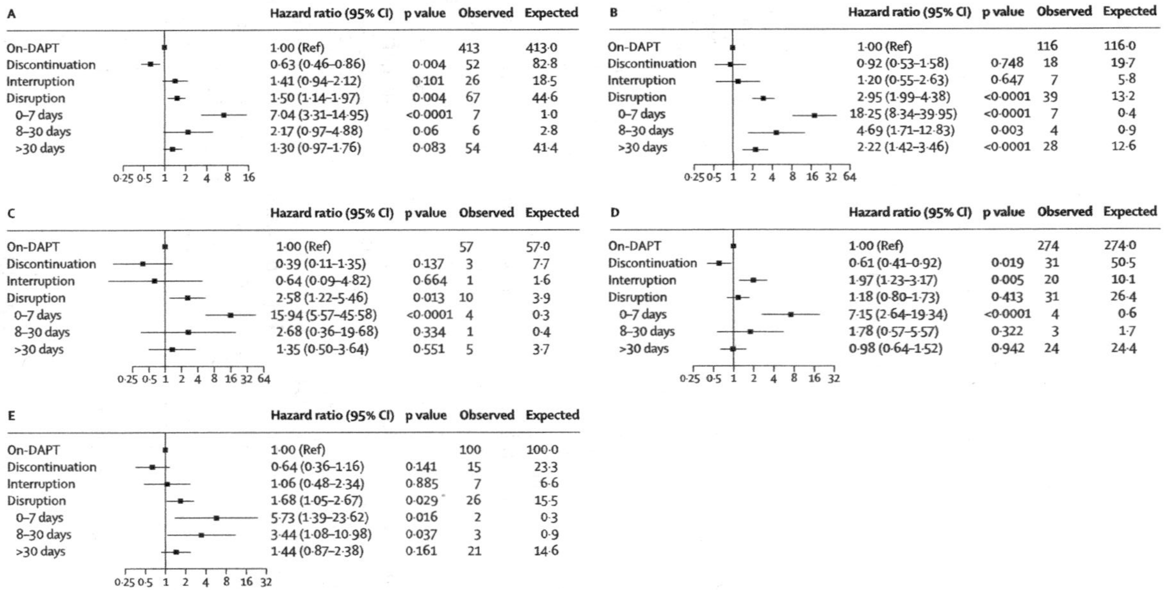

FIGURE 3.—Risk of ischaemic endpoints. Results of Cox model analyses for risk of major adverse cardiovascular event (MACE; A), spontaneous myocardial infarction (B), definite or probable stent thrombosis (C), target lesion revascularisation (D), and cardiac death (E). Boxes are hazard ratio point estimates and error bars are 95% CIs. DAPT = dual antiplatelet therapy. (Reprinted from The Lancet. Mehran R, Baber U, Steg PG, et al. Cessation of dual antiplatelet treatment and cardiac events after percutaneous coronary intervention (PARIS): 2 year results from a prospective observational study. *Lancet.* 2013;382:1714-1722, Copyright 2013, with permission from Elsevier.)

(1·14–1.97; $p = 0·004$). Within 7 days, 8–30 days, and more than 30 days after disruption, adjusted HRs were 7·04 (3·31–14·95), 2·17 (0·97–4·88), and 1·3 (0·97–1·76), respectively. By contrast with patients who remained on DAPT, those who discontinued had lower MACE risk (0·63 [0·46–0·86]). Results were similar after excluding patients receiving bare metal stents and using an alternative MACE definition that did not include target lesion revascularisation.

Interpretation.—In a real-world setting, for patients undergoing PCI and discharged on DAPT, cardiac events after DAPT cessation depend on the clinical circumstance and reason for cessation and attenuates over time. While most events after PCI occur in patients on DAPT, early risk for events due to disruption is substantial irrespective of stent type (Fig 3).

▶ After percutaneous coronary intervention (PCI), the lack of dual antiplatelet therapy (DAPT) is perhaps the most significant predictor of stent thrombosis, especially in the first few months after implantation of a drug-eluting stent. There are multiple reasons why patients stop dual antiplatelet therapy, and the impact of these reasons and the timing of events are not well defined. This prospective, multicenter, observational study evaluated 5018 PCI patients over 2 years. The overall rate of DAPT cessation was 57.3%, and DAPT therapy was discontinued (based on physician recommendation) in 40.8%, interrupted (due to medical necessity but restarted within 14 days) in 10.5%, and disrupted (due to bleeding or noncompliance) in 14.4%. The combined 2-year event rate (death, stent thrombosis, myocardial infarction, revascularization) was 11.5%, and 74% of these events occurred in patients on DAPT. DAPT discontinuation was actually associated with a lower event rate (hazard ratio [HR], 0.63; 95% confidence interval [CI], 0.48–0.86), whereas there was no significant difference for DAPT interruption. DAPT disruption was associated with a higher event rate (HR, 1.51; 95% CI, 1.14–1.97), especially within 7 days of disruption (Fig 3). These findings suggest that DAPT can be safely discontinued as appropriate after stent implantation, and short interruptions are also safe when necessary. Early disruption of therapy remains predictive of adverse events.

D. Steinberg, MD

Optimal Duration of Dual Antiplatelet Therapy After Drug-Eluting Stent Implantation: A Randomized, Controlled Trial

Lee CW, Ahn J-M, Park D-W, et al (Univ of Ulsan College of Medicine, Seoul, South Korea; et al)

Circulation 129:304-312, 2014

Background.—The risks and benefits of long-term dual antiplatelet therapy remain unclear.

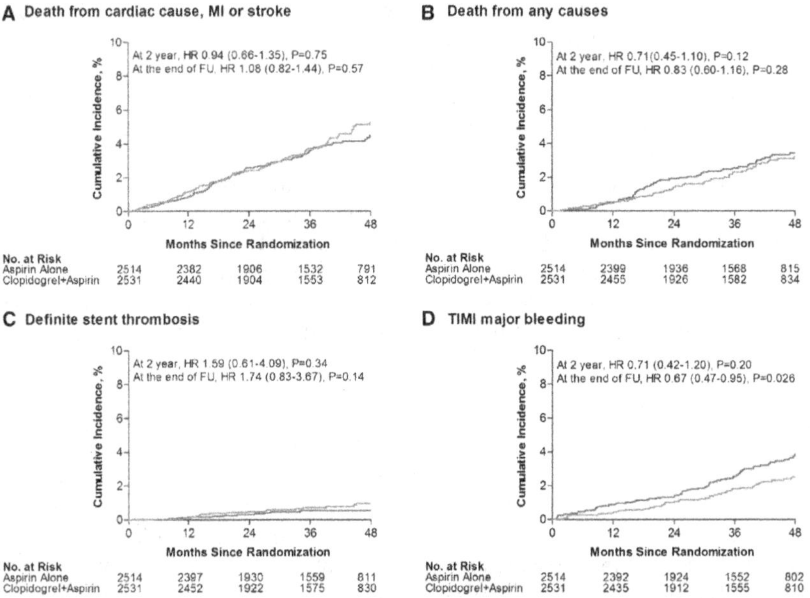

FIGURE 2.—Kaplan–Meier estimates of primary and secondary end points at the end of follow-up (FU). Shown are the cumulative incidences of the primary end point of death resulting from cardiac causes, myocardial infarction (MI), or stroke (**A**); death resulting from any cause (**B**); definite stent thrombosis (C); and Thrombolysis in Myocardial Infarction (TIMI) major bleeding (**D**). The dual-therapy group is shown in blue and aspirin-alone group in red. HR indicates hazard ratio. For interpretation of the references to color in this figure legend, the reader is referred to web version of this article. (Reprinted from Lee CW, Ahn J-M, Park D-W, et al. Optimal duration of dual antiplatelet therapy after drug-eluting stent implantation: a randomized, controlled trial. *Circulation.* 2014;129:304-312, with permission from American Heart Association, Inc.)

Methods and Results.—This prospective, multicenter, open-label, randomized comparison trial was conducted in 24 clinical centers in Korea. In total, 5045 patients who received drug-eluting stents and were free of major adverse cardiovascular events and major bleeding for at least 12 months after stent placement were enrolled between July 2007 and July 2011. Patients were randomized to receive aspirin alone (n = 2514) or clopidogrel plus aspirin (n = 2531). The primary end point was a composite of death resulting from cardiac causes, myocardial infarction, or stroke 24 months after randomization. At 24 months, the primary end point occurred in 57 aspirin-alone group patients (2.4%) and 61 dual-therapy group patients (2.6%; hazard ratio, 0.94; 95% confidence interval, 0.66–1.35; $P = 0.75$). The 2 groups did not differ significantly in terms of the individual risks of death resulting from any cause, myocardial infarction, stent thrombosis, or stroke. Major bleeding occurred in 24 (1.1%) and 34 (1.4%) of the aspirin-alone group and dual-therapy group patients, respectively (hazard ratio, 0.71; 95% confidence interval, 0.42–1.20; $P = 0.20$).

Conclusions.—Among patients who were on 12-month dual antiplatelet therapy without complications, an additional 24 months of dual antiplatelet therapy versus aspirin alone did not reduce the risk of the composite end point of death from cardiac causes, myocardial infarction, or stroke.

Clinical Trial Registration.—URL: http://www.clinicaltrials.gov. Unique identifier: NCT01186146. (Fig 2).

▶ Compared with bare metal stents, drug-eluting stents (DES) have dramatically reduced neointimal proliferation and clinical in-stent restenosis. However, because of delayed and often incomplete stent endothelialization, a small but real increase in late (up to 1 year) or very late (after 1 year) stent thrombosis exists. As a result, extended dual antiplatelet therapy (DAPT) with aspirin and an adenosine diphosphate receptor inhibitor is standard, but the optimal duration of such therapy remains in question. Current US guidelines recommend 1 year of DAPT, and whereas European guidelines suggest shorter durations are reasonable, many studies of extended DAPT are still ongoing. The current study evaluated 5045 patients who underwent percutaneous coronary intervention with a DES and were free from events over the ensuing 12 months while on DAPT. Patients were randomized to either aspirin alone ($n = 2514$) or continued DAPT ($n = 2531$) with aspirin plus clopidogrel for an additional 24 months with a primary end point of cardiac death, myocardial infarction, or stroke. Major bleeding was also evaluated. As shown in Fig 2, at 24 months, there were no significant differences between the 2 groups with regard to the primary end point (2.4% aspirin vs 2.6% DAPT, hazard ratio [HR] 0.94 (0.66–1.35), $P = .75$). Major bleeding was also similar between groups (1.1% aspirin, 1.4% DAPT, HR 0.71 (0.42–1.20), $P = .20$). The authors concluded that extended DAPT does not reduce the risk of death, myocardial infarction, or stroke in patients treated with DES. These findings are in line with a growing body of evidence supporting no more than 1 year of DAPT after DES implantation.

D. Steinberg, MD

44 Cardiomyopathy

Heart Failure–Associated Hospitalizations in the United States

Blecker S, Paul M, Taksler G, et al (New York Univ School of Medicine)

J Am Coll Cardiol 61:1259-1267, 2013

Objectives.—This study sought to characterize temporal trends in hospitalizations with heart failure as a primary or secondary diagnosis.

Background.—Heart failure patients are frequently admitted for both heart failure and other causes.

Methods.—Using the Nationwide Inpatient Sample (NIS), we evaluated trends in heart failure hospitalizations between 2001 and 2009. Hospitalizations were categorized as either primary or secondary heart failure hospitalizations based on the location of heart failure in the discharge diagnosis. National estimates were calculated using the sampling weights of the NIS. Age- and sex-standardized hospitalization rates were determined by dividing the number of hospitalizations by the U.S. population in a given year and using direct standardization.

Results.—The number of primary heart failure hospitalizations in the United States decreased from 1,137,944 in 2001 to 1,086,685 in 2009, whereas secondary heart failure hospitalizations increased from 2,753,793 to 3,158,179 over the same period. Age- and sex-adjusted rates of primary heart failure hospitalizations decreased steadily from 2001 to 2009, from 566 to 468 per 100,000 people. Rates of secondary heart failure hospitalizations initially increased from 1,370 to 1,476 per 100,000 people from 2001 to 2006, then decreased to 1,359 per 100,000 people in 2009. Common primary diagnoses for secondary heart failure hospitalizations included pulmonary disease, renal failure, and infections.

Conclusions.—Although primary heart failure hospitalizations declined, rates of hospitalizations with a secondary diagnosis of heart failure were stable in the past decade. Strategies to reduce the high burden of hospitalizations of heart failure patients should include consideration of both cardiac disease and noncardiac conditions (Fig 1).

▶ Heart failure (HF) remains one of the leading causes for hospitalization in the United States and many other countries. There was a rapid increase in the number of HF admissions for several decades. However, several studies have shown that this trend has slowed or reversed. This has been attributed to many factors, including better adherence to guideline-based therapies and close follow-up of patients. However, these studies have focused on hospitalization for HF as the primary diagnosis. The present study used the Nationwide Inpatient Sample to

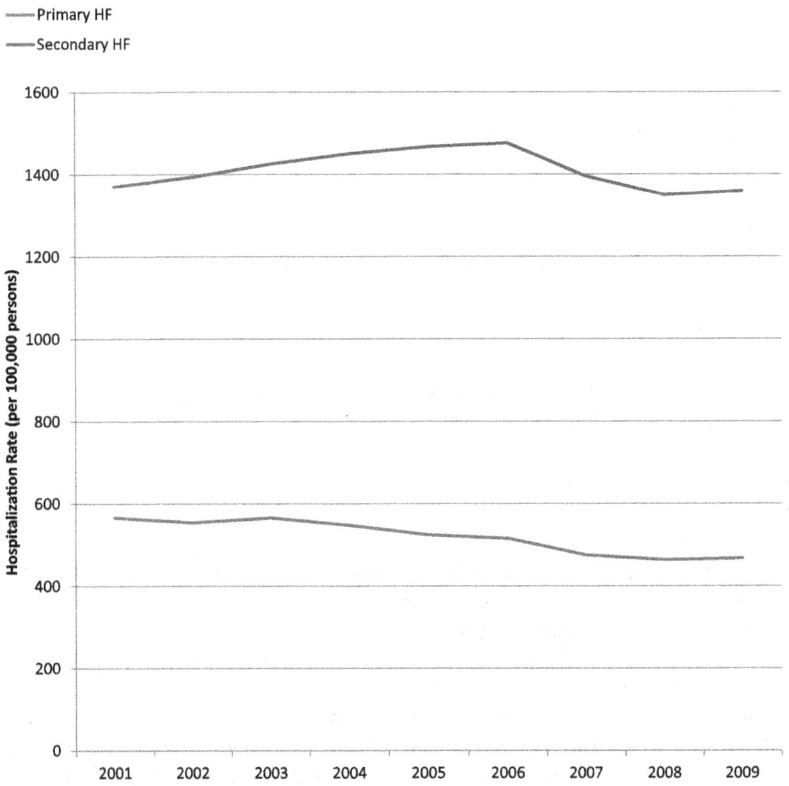

FIGURE 1.—Rates of heart failure–related hospitalization. Annual age- and sex-adjusted rates of hospitalizations in the United States with a diagnosis of heart failure (HF) in the primary versus secondary position are shown. (Reprinted from the Journal of the American College of Cardiology. Blecker S, Paul M, Taksler G, et al. Heart failure–associated hospitalizations in the United States. *J Am Coll Cardiol.* 2013;61:1259-1267, Copyright 2013, with permission from the American College of Cardiology.)

evaluate the frequency of HF admissions as both a primary and secondary diagnosis over an 8-year period. The decline in HF admissions as a primary diagnosis was confirmed; however, there is nearly a 3-fold increase in HF admissions as a secondary diagnosis (Fig 1). Moreover, the rate HF admissions as a secondary diagnosis did not decline over this period. There were multiple comorbidities associated with HF, most prominently respiratory disease, renal disease, and infection. These interesting data indicate that strategies to treat such comorbidities are important to decrease the total number of HF hospital admissions.

M. Gold, MD

Spironolactone for Heart Failure with Preserved Ejection Fraction

Pitt B, for the TOPCAT Investigators (Univ of Michigan School of Medicine, Ann Arbor; et al)

N Engl J Med 370:1383-1392, 2014

Background.—Mineralocorticoid-receptor antagonists improve the prognosis for patients with heart failure and a reduced left ventricular ejection fraction. We evaluated the effects of spironolactone in patients with heart failure and a preserved left ventricular ejection fraction.

Methods.—In this randomized, double-blind trial, we assigned 3445 patients with symptomatic heart failure and a left ventricular ejection fraction of 45% or more to receive either spironolactone (15 to 45 mg daily) or placebo. The primary outcome was a composite of death from cardiovascular causes, aborted cardiac arrest, or hospitalization for the management of heart failure.

Results.—With a mean follow-up of 3.3 years, the primary outcome occurred in 320 of 1722 patients in the spironolactone group (18.6%) and 351 of 1723 patients in the placebo group (20.4%) (hazard ratio, 0.89; 95% confidence interval [CI], 0.77 to 1.04; $P = 0.14$). Of the components of the primary outcome, only hospitalization for heart failure had a significantly lower incidence in the spironolactone group than in the placebo group (206 patients [12.0%] vs. 245 patients [14.2%]; hazard ratio, 0.83; 95% CI, 0.69 to 0.99, $P = 0.04$). Neither total deaths nor hospitalizations for any reason were significantly reduced by spironolactone. Treatment with spironolactone was associated with increased serum creatinine levels and a doubling of the rate of hyperkalemia (18.7%, vs. 9.1% in the placebo group) but reduced hypokalemia. With frequent monitoring, there were no significant differences in the incidence of serious adverse events, a serum creatinine level of 3.0 mg per deciliter (265 μmol per liter) or higher, or dialysis.

Conclusions.—In patients with heart failure and a preserved ejection fraction, treatment with spironolactone did not significantly reduce the incidence of the primary composite outcome of death from cardiovascular causes, aborted cardiac arrest, or hospitalization for the management of heart failure. (Funded by the National Heart, Lung, and Blood Institute; TOPCAT ClinicalTrials.gov number, NCT00094302.) (Fig 1).

▶ Heart failure (HF) is the leading cause of hospitalization in the United States. The most rapidly growing segment of HF patients and hospitalizations is the group with preserved ejection fraction (HFpEF). In heart failure with reduced ejection fraction, many drugs have been found to reduce mortality or hospitalization, including β blockers, angiotensin-converting-enzyme inhibitors, angiotensin II receptor blockers, and spironolactone. In contrast, no drug therapy has been found to be effective for HFpEF. The TOPCAT trial was a prospective, double-blind, randomized trial evaluating the role of spironolactone in this population. There were 3445 patients randomly selected in this study, which failed to show a reduction in the composite primary endpoint (cardiovascular death,

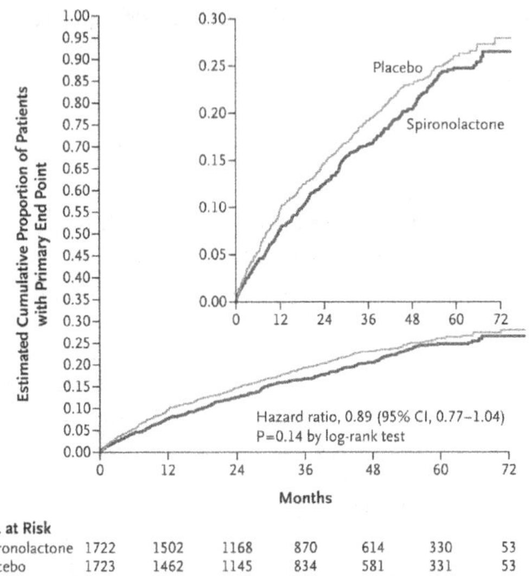

FIGURE 1.—Kaplan–Meier Plot of Time to the First Confirmed Primary-Outcome Event. The primary outcome was a composite of death from cardiovascular causes, aborted cardiac arrest, or hospitalization for the management of heart failure. The inset shows the same data on an expanded y axis. (Reprinted from Pitt B, for the TOPCAT Investigators. Spironolactone for heart failure with preserved ejection fraction. *N Engl J Med.* 2014;370:1383-1392, Copyright 2014, with permission from Massachusetts Medical Society.)

aborted cardiac arrest, or HF hospitalization; Fig 1). There was a significant but modest reduction in HF hospitalization with spironolactone, but this therapy was associated with worsening renal function and doubling of the rate of hyperkalemia. TOPCAT represents another disappointing result for drug therapy to treat HFpEF. Currently, the best therapy for this problem remains aggressive treatment of comorbidities, including hypertension, diabetes, and coronary artery disease.

M. Gold, MD

An individual patient meta-analysis of five randomized trials assessing the effects of cardiac resynchronization therapy on morbidity and mortality in patients with symptomatic heart failure

Cleland JG, Abraham WT, Linde C, et al (Univ of Hull, Kingstonupon-Hull, UK; The Ohio State Univ, Columbus, OH; Karolinska Univ Hosp, Stockholm, Sweden; et al)
Eur Heart J 34:3547-3556, 2013

Aims.—Cardiac resynchronization therapy (CRT) with or without a defibrillator reduces morbidity and mortality in selected patients with heart failure (HF) but response can be variable. We sought to identify pre-implantation variables that predict the response to CRT in a meta-analysis using individual patient-data.

Methods and Results.—An individual patient meta-analysis of five randomized trials, funded by Medtronic, comparing CRT either with no active device or with a defibrillator was conducted, including the following baseline variables: age, sex, New York Heart Association class, aetiology, QRS morphology, QRS duration, left ventricular ejection fraction (LVEF), and systolic blood pressure. Outcomes were all-cause mortality and first hospitalization for HF or death. Of 3782 patients in sinus rhythm, median (inter-quartile range) age was 66 (58–73) years, QRS duration was 160 (146–176) ms, LVEF was 24 (20–28)%, and 78% had left bundle branch block. A multivariable model suggested that only QRS duration predicted the magnitude of the effect of CRT on outcomes. Further analysis produced estimated hazard ratios for the effect of CRT on all-cause mortality and on the composite of first hospitalization for HF or death that suggested increasing benefit with increasing QRS duration, the 95% confidence bounds excluding 1.0 at ~140 ms for each endpoint, suggesting a high probability of substantial benefit from CRT when QRS duration exceeds this value.

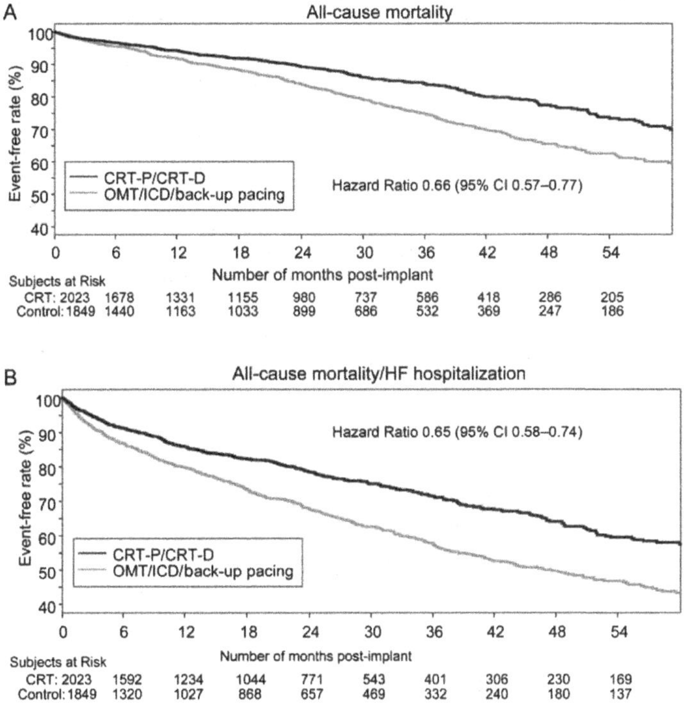

FIGURE 2.—Overall effect of cardiac resynchronization therapy vs. control on all-cause mortality (*A*) and on death or heart failure hospitalization (*B*). (Reprinted from Cleland JG, Abraham WT, Linde C, et al. An individual patient meta-analysis of five randomized trials assessing the effects of cardiac resynchronization therapy on morbidity and mortality in patients with symptomatic heart failure. *Eur Heart J.* 2013;34:3547-3556, by permission of The European Society of Cardiology.)

Conclusion.—QRS duration is a powerful predictor of the effects of CRT on morbidity and mortality in patients with symptomatic HF and left ventricular systolic dysfunction who are in sinus rhythm. QRS morphology did not provide additional information about clinical response.

ClinicalTrials.gov Numbers.—NCT00170300, NCT00271154, NCT00251251 (Fig 2).

▶ Cardiac resynchronization therapy (CRT) is well-accepted therapy for the treatment of systolic heart failure. Initially, this treatment was restricted to patients with advanced heart failure (New York Heart Association III/IV), but more recent studies have found similar benefit among patients with mild heart failure. Despite this expansion of CRT indications, the nonresponder rate has remained stable at about 30%. Despite controversy with regard to the classification of nonresponders and the implications of such designation, it is clear that optimizing CRT response is important for this invasive, expensive therapy. Individual prospective, randomized studies have found that female gender, nonischemic cardiomyopathy, left bundle branch block, and QRS duration, in particular >150 msec, predict good outcomes. This study was an individual meta-analysis in which individual patient data, rather than summary data, are used to analyze clinical predictors of response. QRS duration was the most powerful predictor of response. Moreover, this was a continuous relationship with no threshold effect noted at the traditional cutoff of 150 msec (Fig 2). This study emphasizes the value of individual meta-analyses to provide increased power to identify predictors of response caused by the large number of patients included (n = 3782). It also reinforces the value of QRS to predict response but challenges the appropriateness of 150 msec as the optimal cutoff.

M. Gold, MD

Low-Dose Dopamine or Low-Dose Nesiritide in Acute Heart Failure With Renal Dysfunction: The ROSE Acute Heart Failure Randomized Trial

Chen HH, for the NHLBI Heart Failure Clinical Research Network (Mayo Clinic, Rochester, MN; et al)

JAMA 310:2533-2543, 2013

Importance.—Small studies suggest that low-dose dopamine or low-dose nesiritide may enhance decongestion and preserve renal function in patients with acute heart failure and renal dysfunction; however, neither strategy has been rigorously tested.

Objective.—To test the 2 independent hypotheses that, compared with placebo, addition of low-dose dopamine (2 μg/kg/min) or low-dose nesiritide (0.005 μg/kg/min without bolus) to diuretic therapy will enhance decongestion and preserve renal function in patients with acute heart failure and renal dysfunction.

Design, Setting, and Participants.—Multicenter, double-blind, placebo-controlled clinical trial (Renal Optimization Strategies Evaluation [ROSE]) of 360 hospitalized patients with acute heart failure and renal dysfunction (estimated glomerular filtration rate of 15-60 mL/min/1.73 m^2), randomized within 24 hours of admission. Enrollment occurred from September 2010 to March 2013 across 26 sites in North America.

Interventions.—Participants were randomized in an open, 1:1 allocation ratio to the dopamine or nesiritide strategy. Within each strategy, participants were randomized in a double-blind, 2:1 ratio to active treatment or placebo. The dopamine (n = 122) and nesiritide (n = 119) groups were independently compared with the pooled placebo group (n = 119).

Main Outcomes and Measures.—Coprimary end points included 72-hour cumulative urine volume (decongestion end point) and the change in serum cystatin C from enrollment to 72 hours (renal function end point).

Results.—Compared with placebo, low-dose dopamine had no significant effect on 72-hour cumulative urine volume (dopamine, 8524 mL; 95% CI, 7917-9131 vs placebo, 8296 mL; 95% CI, 7762-8830; difference, 229 mL; 95% CI, −714 to 1171 mL; P =.59) or on the change in cystatin C level (dopamine, 0.12 mg/L; 95% CI, 0.06-0.18 vs placebo, 0.11 mg/L; 95% CI, 0.06-0.16; difference, 0.01; 95% CI, −0.08 to 0.10; P =.72). Similarly, low-dose nesiritide had no significant effect on 72-hour cumulative urine volume (nesiritide, 8574 mL; 95% CI, 8014-9134 vs placebo, 8296 mL; 95% CI, 7762-8830; difference, 279 mL; 95% CI, −618 to 1176 mL; P =.49) or on the change in cystatin C level (nesiritide, 0.07 mg/L; 95% CI, 0.01-0.13 vs placebo, 0.11 mg/L; 95% CI, 0.06-0.16; difference, −0.04; 95% CI, −0.13 to 0.05; P =.36). Compared with placebo, there was no effect of low-dose dopamine or nesiritide on secondary end points reflective of decongestion, renal function, or clinical outcomes.

Conclusion and Relevance.—In participants with acute heart failure and renal dysfunction, neither low-dose dopamine nor low-dose nesiritide enhanced decongestion or improved renal function when added to diuretic therapy.

Trial Registration.—clinicaltrials.gov Identifier: NCT01132846 (Table 2).

▶ The incidence of heart failure (HF) continues to increase despite advances in medical therapy. HF is now the leading cause of hospitalization in the United States. In response to the increasing number of HF admissions, 30-day readmission has now been established as a performance metric. One of the best predictors of successful treatment of HF to prevent readmissions is achieving decongestion as measured by reduced left ventricular filling pressure. Thus, diuresis remains one of the mainstay treatments for acute HF exacerbations. Patients with underlying renal dysfunction are challenging to treat with diuresis, as further exacerbation of renal function is common. For this reason, adjunctive therapies, including low-dose dopamine and nesiritide, are commonly used in this setting. The ROSE study was double-blind, randomized trial to evaluate the role of these agents among patients admitted with acute HF. Importantly, both subjects with preserved and reduced ejection fraction were included in this trial. Neither agent improved renal function or diuresis in this study (Table 2). Subgroup analyses indicated that dopamine was less effective than

TABLE 2.—Coprimary End Points: Effect of Low-Dose Dopamine vs Placebo or Low-Dose Nesiritide vs Placebo on Cumulative Urine Volume During 72 Hours and Change in Cystatin C Level From Baseline to 72 Hours

	Mean (95% CI)			
	Placebo	Drug	Treatment Difference	*P* Value
Dopamine strategy	Placebo (n = 119)	Dopamine (n = 122)		
Cumulative urine volume from randomization to 72 h, mL	8296 (7762 to 8830)	8524 (7917 to 9131)	229 (−714 to 1171)	.59
Change in cystatin C level from randomization to 72 h, mg/L	0.11 (0.06 to 0.16)	0.12 (0.06 to 0.18)	0.01 (−0.08 to 0.10)	.72
Nesiritide strategy	Placebo (n = 119)	Nesiritide (n = 119)		
Cumulative urine volume from randomization to 72 h, mL	8296 (7762 to 8830)	8574 (8014 to 9134)	279 (−618 to 1176)	.49
Change in cystatin C level from randomization to 72 h, mg/L	0.11 (0.06 to 0.16)	0.07 (0.01 to 0.13)	−0.04 (−0.13 to 0.05)	.36

placebo for promoting diuresis among patients with preserved ejection fraction, whereas nesiritide was more effective than placebo for preserving renal function in the low ejection fraction cohort. However, overall this well-designed study reinforces the need for additional therapies for the treatment of acute HF.

M. Gold, MD

45 Valvular Heart Disease

Impact of Preoperative Moderate/Severe Mitral Regurgitation on 2-Year Outcome After Transcatheter and Surgical Aortic Valve Replacement: Insight From the Placement of Aortic Transcatheter Valve (PARTNER) Trial Cohort A

Barbanti M, on behalf of the Placement of Aortic Transcatheter Valve (PARTNER) Trial Investigators (St. Paul's Hosp, Vancouver, British Columbia, Canada; et al)

Circulation 128:2776-2784, 2013

Background.—The effect of preoperative mitral regurgitation (MR) on clinical outcomes of patients undergoing transcatheter aortic valve replacement (TAVR) is controversial. This study sought to examine the impact of moderate and severe MR on outcomes after TAVR and surgical aortic valve replacement (SAVR).

Methods and Results.—Data were drawn from the randomized Placement of Aortic Transcatheter Valve (PARTNER) Trial cohort A patients with severe, symptomatic aortic stenosis undergoing either TAVR (n = 331) or SAVR (n = 299). Both TAVR and SAVR patients were dichotomized according to the degree of preoperative MR (moderate/severe versus none/mild). At baseline, moderate or severe MR was reported in 65 TAVR patients (19.6%) and 63 SAVR patients (21.2%). At 30 days, among survivors who had isolated SAVR/TAVR, moderate/severe MR had improved in 25 SAVR patients (69.4%) and 30 TAVR patients (57.7%), was unchanged in 10 SAVR patients (27.8%) and 19 TAVR patients (36.5%), and worsened in 1 SAVR patient (2.8%) and 4 TAVR patients (5.8%; all $P = NS$). Mortality at 2 years was higher in SAVR patients with moderate or severe MR than in those with mild or less MR (49.8% versus 28.1%; adjusted hazard ratio, 1.73; 95% confidence interval, 1.01–2.96; $P = 0.04$). In contrast, MR severity at baseline did not affect mortality in TAVR patients (37.0% versus 32.7%, moderate/severe versus none/mild; hazard ratio, 1.14; 95% confidence interval, 0.72-1.78; $P = 0.58$; P for interaction = 0.05).

Conclusions.—Both TAVR and SAVR were associated with a significant early improvement in MR in survivors. However, moderate or severe MR at baseline was associated with increased 2-year mortality after SAVR but

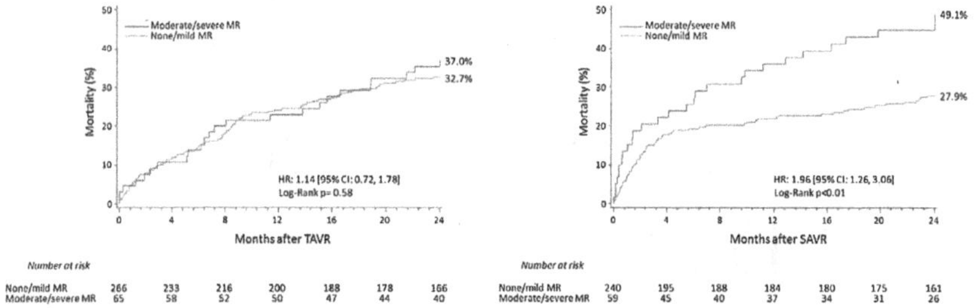

FIGURE 2.—Kaplan-Meier curves showing cumulative death rate through 2 years for transcatheter aortic valve replacement (TAVR) and surgical aortic valve replacement (SAVR). Comparison of the cumulative death rate through 1 year in patients with no/mild periprocedural mitral regurgitation (MR) compared with patients with moderate/severe periprocedural MR. TAVR cohort A only (**A**); SAVR cohort A only (**B**). CI indicates confidence interval; and HR, hazard ratio. (Reprinted from Barbanti M, on behalf of the Placement of Aortic Transcatheter Valve (PARTNER) Trial Investigators. Impact of preoperative moderate/severe mitral regurgitation on 2-year outcome after transcatheter and surgical aortic valve replacement insight from the placement of aortic transcatheter valve (PARTNER) trial cohort a. *Circulation.* 2013;128:2776-2784, Copyright 2013, with permission from American Heart Association, Inc.)

not after TAVR. TAVR may be a reasonable option in selected patients with combined aortic and mitral valve disease.

Clinical Trial Registration.—URL: http://www.clinicaltrials.gov. Unique identifier: NCT00530894 (Fig 2).

▶ Patients with severe aortic stenosis and elevated surgical risk referred for transcatheter aortic valve replacement (TAVR) often have some degree of mitral regurgitation. When mitral regurgitation is secondary to increased afterload, it often improves after aortic valve replacement, but if it is the primary pathology, then the mitral regurgitation may not improve; in the latter situation, double valve replacement is often needed. The effect of preoperative mitral regurgitation on patients undergoing TAVR was examined in an analysis of the PARTNER Cohort A trial evaluating TAVR versus surgical aortic valve replacement (SAVR) in 730 high-risk patients. Patients were divided into no/mild and moderate/severe mitral regurgitation for purposes of comparison. Moderate/severe mitral regurgitation was present in 65 TAVR patients and 63 SAVR patients. At 30 days, the degree of mitral regurgitation improved in 57.7% of TAVR patients and 69.4% of SAVR patients. As shown in Fig 2, compared with no/mild mitral regurgitation, moderate/severe mitral regurgitation at baseline was not associated with increased 2-year mortality in TAVR patients (37.0% vs 32.7%; relative risk [RR], 95% confidence interval [CI], 1.14 [0.72–1.78]; $P = .58$), but in SAVR patients, there was an increase in mortality (49.8% vs 28.1%; RR, 1.73 [95% CI, 1.01–2.96]; $P = .04$) for patients with moderate/severe mitral regurgitation at baseline. Functional class improvement was seen in all patients, regardless of severity of baseline mitral regurgitation or the type of therapy received. These findings suggest that, regardless of baseline mitral regurgitation severity, TAVR may be reasonable for patients with severe aortic stenosis and elevated surgical risk.

D. Steinberg, MD

Mitral-Valve Repair versus Replacement for Severe Ischemic Mitral Regurgitation

Acker MA, for the CTSN (Univ of Pennsylvania School of Medicine, Philadelphia; et al)

N Engl J Med 370:23-32, 2014

Background.—Ischemic mitral regurgitation is associated with a substantial risk of death. Practice guidelines recommend surgery for patients with a severe form of this condition but acknowledge that the supporting evidence for repair or replacement is limited.

Methods.—We randomly assigned 251 patients with severe ischemic mitral regurgitation to undergo either mitral-valve repair or chordal-sparing replacement in order to evaluate efficacy and safety. The primary end point was the left ventricular end-systolic volume index (LVESVI) at 12 months, as assessed with the use of a Wilcoxon rank-sum test in which deaths were categorized below the lowest LVESVI rank.

Results.—At 12 months, the mean LVESVI among surviving patients was 54.6 ± 25.0 ml per square meter of body-surface area in the repair group and 60.7 ± 31.5 ml per square meter in the replacement group (mean change from baseline, −6.6 and −6.8 ml per square meter, respectively). The rate of death was 14.3% in the repair group and 17.6% in the replacement group (hazard ratio with repair, 0.79; 95% confidence interval, 0.42 to 1.47; $P = 0.45$ by the log-rank test). There was no significant between-group difference in LVESVI after adjustment for death (z score, 1.33; $P = 0.18$). The rate of moderate or severe recurrence of mitral regurgitation at 12 months was higher in the repair group than in the replacement group (32.6% vs. 2.3%, $P < 0.001$). There were no significant between-group differences in the rate of a composite of major adverse cardiac or cerebrovascular events, in functional status, or in quality of life at 12 months.

Conclusions.—We observed no significant difference in left ventricular reverse remodeling or survival at 12 months between patients who underwent mitral-valve repair and those who underwent mitral-valve replacement. Replacement provided a more durable correction of mitral regurgitation, but there was no significant between-group difference in clinical outcomes. (Funded by the National Institutes of Health and the Canadian Institutes of Health; ClinicalTrials.gov number, NCT00807040.)

► Among patients with degenerative mitral regurgitation, mitral valve repair is favored over mitral valve replacement when feasible. When performed by experienced surgeons, repair is associated with excellent long-term outcomes and freedom from reoperation approaching 90% at 10 years. However, outcomes following mitral valve repair for ischemic mitral regurgitation are not as durable, largely because ischemic mitral regurgitation is secondary to left ventricular dysfunction as opposed to primary valvular pathology. In view of this, there is debate as to whether chordal sparing replacement (preserving of the mitral valve apparatus) is equivalent or favorable to repair in this population. This study randomized 251 patients to either repair or replacement with a primary outcome of reverse remodeling measured by left ventricular end systolic volume index (LVESVI). At 12 months, the mean change in LVESVI was −6.6 mL in the repair group and −6.8 in the replacement group; this difference was not significant between groups. Mortality was similar between groups (14.3% repair vs 17.6% replacement, hazard ratio 0.79 [0.42–1.47], $P = .45$). Importantly, 12-month recurrent moderate or severe mitral regurgitation was more common in the repair group (32.6% vs 2.3%, $P < .001$), and 3 patients in the repair group underwent mitral valve replacement for severe recurrent mitral regurgitation. Other clinical end points such as functional class or recurrent hospitalization were not different between groups during follow-up. The results of this study suggest that chordal sparing mitral valve replacement is equivalent and may be favorable to mitral valve repair in patients with severe ischemic mitral regurgitation owing to a lower recurrence of moderate or severe mitral regurgitation.

D. Steinberg, MD

Comparison of Balloon-Expandable vs Self-expandable Valves in Patients Undergoing Transcatheter Aortic Valve Replacement: The CHOICE Randomized Clinical Trial

Abdel-Wahab M, for the CHOICE investigators (Heart Ctr, Bad Segeberg, Germany; et al)

JAMA 311:1503-1514, 2014

Importance.—Transcatheter aortic valve replacement (TAVR) is an effective treatment option for high-risk patients with severe aortic stenosis. Different from surgery, transcatheter deployment of valves requires either a balloon-expandable or self-expandable system. A randomized comparison of these 2 systems has not been performed.

Objective.—To determine whether the balloon-expandable device is associated with a better success rate than the self-expandable device.

Design, Setting, and Patients.—The CHOICE study was an investigator-initiated trial in high-risk patients with severe aortic stenosis and an anatomy suitable for the transfemoral TAVR procedure. One hundred twenty-one patients were randomly assigned to receive a balloon-expandable valve (Edwards Sapien XT) and 120 were assigned to receive a self-expandable valve (Medtronic CoreValve). Patients were enrolled between March 2012 and December 2013 at 5 centers in Germany.

Interventions.—Transfemoral TAVR with a balloon-expandable or self-expandable device.

Main Outcomes and Measures.—The primary end point was device success, which is a composite end point including successful vascular access and deployment of the device and retrieval of the delivery system, correct position of the device, intended performance of the heart valve without moderate or severe regurgitation, and only 1 valve implanted in the proper anatomical location. Secondary end points included cardiovascular mortality, bleeding and vascular complications, postprocedural pacemaker placement, and a combined safety end point at 30 days, including all-cause mortality, major stroke, and other serious complications.

Results.—Device success occurred in 116 of 121 patients (95.9%) in the balloon-expandable valve group and 93 of 120 patients (77.5%) in the self-expandable valve group (relative risk [RR], 1.24, 95% CI, 1.12-1.37, $P < .001$). This was attributed to a significantly lower frequency of residual more-than-mild aortic regurgitation (4.1% vs 18.3%; RR, 0.23; 95% CI, 0.09-0.58; $P < .001$) and the less frequent need for implanting more than 1 valve (0.8% vs 5.8%, $P = .03$) in the balloon-expandable valve group. Cardiovascular mortality at 30 days was 4.1% in the balloon-expandable valve group and 4.3% in the self-expandable valve group (RR, 0.97; 95% CI, 0.29-3.25; $P = .99$). Bleeding and vascular complications were not significantly different, and the combined safety end point occurred in 18.2% of those in the balloon-expandable valve group and 23.1% of the self-expandable valve group (RR, 0.79; 95% CI, 0.48-1.30; $P = .42$). Placement of a new permanent pacemaker was less frequent in the balloon-expandable valve group (17.3%vs 37.6%, $P = .001$).

Conclusions and Relevance.—Among patients with high-risk aortic stenosis undergoing TAVR, the use of a balloon-expandable valve resulted in a greater rate of device success than use of a self-expandable valve.

Trial Registration.—clinicaltrials.gov Identifier: NCT01645202.

▶ Transcatheter aortic valve replacement (TAVR) has had a dramatic impact on treatment options for patients with aortic stenosis who have elevated or prohibitive surgical risk. The balloon expandable valve (Edwards-Sapien) and self-expanding valve (Medtronic CoreValve) are the 2 most widely used devices in Europe, with the latter device recently approved in the United States. Whereas outcomes with the 2 TAVR devices seems comparable in registries, randomized head-to-head data have been lacking before this study. In the CHOICE trial, investigators at 5 German centers randomized 241 patients with severe aortic stenosis and elevated surgical risk to either the balloon expandable or the self-expanding valve. The primary endpoint was a successful procedure (defined as proper device deployment and positioning, retrieval of the delivery system, and freedom from moderate-severe aortic insufficiency, greater than 1 valve implant, and vascular access complications). Secondary endpoints included cardiovascular mortality and the need for pacemaker implantation. The primary endpoint of a successful procedure was more common in the balloon expandable patients (95.9% vs 77.5%, relative risk 1.24 [1.12–1.37], $P < .001$), and this was primarily related to increased rates of moderate-severe aortic insufficiency and multiple valve implants in the patients treated with a self-expanding valve (Table 4 in the original article). Cardiovascular mortality was similar between the 2 groups, but, consistent with other trials, more patients in the self-expanding group (37.6%) required permanent pacemaker implantation compared with the balloon-expandable group (17.3%)

with a *P* value of .001. These findings suggest that the balloon-expandable valve is associated with increased procedural success compared with the self-expanding valve with no significant difference mortality.

D. Steinberg, MD

PART SEVEN

THE DIGESTIVE SYSTEM

KENNETH R. DEVAULT, MD

46 Esophagus

Central Obesity in Asymptomatic Volunteers Is Associated With Increased Intrasphincteric Acid Reflux and Lengthening of the Cardiac Mucosa

Robertson EV, Derakhshan MH, Wirz AA, et al (Univ of Glasgow, UK; et al)

Gastroenterology 145:730-739, 2013

Background & Aims.—In the West, a substantial proportion of subjects with adenocarcinoma of the gastric cardia and gastroesophageal junction have no history of reflux. We studied the gastroesophageal junction in asymptomatic volunteers with normal and large waist circumferences (WCs) to determine if central obesity is associated with abnormalities that might predispose individuals to adenocarcinoma.

Methods.—We performed a study of 24 healthy, *Helicobacter pylori*–negative volunteers with a small WC and 27 with a large WC. Abdominal fat was quantified by magnetic resonance imaging. Jumbo biopsy specimens were taken across the squamocolumnar junction (SCJ). High-resolution pH-metry (12 sensors) and manometry (36 sensors) were performed in upright and supine subjects before and after a meal; the SCJ was visualized fluoroscopically.

Results.—The cardiac mucosa was significantly longer in the large WC group (2.5 vs 1.75 mm; $P = .008$); its length correlated with intra-abdominal ($R = 0.35$; $P = .045$) and total abdominal ($R = 0.37$; $P = .034$) fat. The SCJ was closer to the upper border of the lower esophageal sphincter (LES) in subjects with a large WC (2.77 vs 3.54 cm; $P = .02$). There was no evidence of excessive reflux 5 cm above the LES in either group. Gastric acidity extended more proximally within the LES in the large WC group, compared with the upper border (2.65 vs 4.1 cm; $P = .027$) and peak LES pressure (0.1 cm proximal vs 2.1 cm distal; $P = .007$). The large WC group had shortening of the LES, attributable to loss of the distal component (total LES length, 3 vs 4.5 cm; $P = .043$).

Conclusions.—Central obesity is associated with intrasphincteric extension of gastric acid and cardiac mucosal lengthening. The latter might arise through metaplasia of the most distal esophageal squamous epithelium and this process might predispose individuals to adenocarcinoma.

▶ Central obesity has been associated with benign conditions such as gastroesophageal reflux disease (GERD), but has also been associated with multiple intra-abdominal malignancies and premalignant conditions including Barrett's esophagus and esophageal adenocarcinoma (EAC). This study provides some explanation of why this association might exist.

The findings that normal volunteers had increased acid in the lower esophageal sphincter (LES) region and had an increase in the length of their cardia could result in an unstable area that predisposes to the development of carcinoma. In addition, there are many patients who develop cancer at the esophagogastric junction who may or may not have underlying Barrett's type metaplasia and even more frequently do not have symptoms consistent with reflux. If acid refluxing into, but not substantially above, the LES truly results in metaplasia of the distal esophageal mucosa, then perhaps asymptomatic reflux might also lead to adenocarcinoma. One cannot discount other mechanisms including humoral and inflammatory mechanisms associated with the metabolism within intra-abdominal fat tissue. There was also an increase in the length of this segment with age, which is another important risk factor for these malignancies. In addition to the interaction between obesity and cancer, obesity increases the risk for symptomatic GERD and makes reflux surgery difficult to the point that many centers do not offer fundoplication to patients with body mass index > 30. All of this together gives us even more information to present to patients in an attempt to have them better control their weight.

K. R. DeVault, MD

Comparing omeprazole with fluoxetine for treatment of patients with heartburn and normal endoscopy who failed once daily proton pump inhibitors: Double-blind placebo-controlled trial

Ostovaneh MR, Saeidi B, Hajifathalian K, et al (Johns Hopkins Med Institutions, Baltimore, MD; Tehran Univ of Med Sciences, Iran; Harvard Univ, Boston, MA)

Neurogastroenterol Motil 26:670-678, 2014

Background.—Patients with heartburn but without esophageal erosion respond less well to proton pump inhibitors (PPIs). There is a growing body of evidence implicating the role of psychological comorbidities in producing reflux symptoms. Pain modulators improve symptoms in patients with other functional gastrointestinal disorders. We aimed to compare the efficacy of fluoxetine with omeprazole and placebo to achieve symptomatic relief in patients with heartburn and normal endoscopy who failed once daily PPIs.

Methods.—Endoscopy-negative patients with heartburn who failed once daily PPIs were randomly allocated to receive 6 weeks treatment of fluoxetine, omeprazole, or placebo. Random allocation was stratified according to ambulatory pH monitoring study. Percentage of heartburn-free days and symptom severity was assessed.

Key Results.—Sixty patients with abnormal and 84 patients with normal pH test were randomized. Subjects receiving fluoxetine experienced more improvement in percentage of heartburn-free days (median 35.7, IQR 21.4–57.1) than those on omeprazole (median 7.14, IQR 0–50, $p < 0.001$) or placebo (median 7.14, IQR 0–33.6, $p < 0.001$). In normal pH subgroup, fluoxetine was superior to both omeprazole and placebo regarding percentage of heartburn-free days (median improvement, 57.1, IQR 35.7–57.1 vs 13.9, IQR, 0–45.6 and 7.14, 0–23.8, respectively, $p < 0.001$), but no significant difference was observed between medications in abnormal pH subgroup.

Conclusions & Inferences.—Fluoxetine was superior to omeprazole for improving the symptoms of patients with heartburn and normal endoscopy who failed once daily PPIs. The superiority of fluoxetine was mostly attributed to those with normal esophageal pH rather than those with abnormal pH (ClinicalTrials.gov, number NCT01269788).

▶ Proton pump inhibitor (PPI) therapy provides outstanding relief of heartburn, but ongoing or refractory symptoms can be expected in 10% to 40% of patients. Many of these patients do not have esophagitis and often require extensive testing to confirm their disease and are often subjected to prolonged high-dose PPI trials and even reflux surgery in attempts to control those refractory symptoms. Some of these patients have excess acid and normal endoscopies (nonerosive reflux disease), whereas others have both normal acid exposure and normal endoscopy (functional heartburn). The optimal approach to both groups have not been defined, but there does appear to be increased esophageal sensitivity in at least a subset and treating with agents that lower sensitivity has been proposed. This article is a unique, blinded trial comparing continued PPI and placebo to an antidepressant in a group of heartburn patients who have failed a PPI trial. About half of the patients in this study had abnormal acid exposure, and the other half was normal. Fluoxetine produced more heartburn-free days compared with both placebo and omeprazole. This difference was predominantly in the group who were pH-negative; the 3 arms were not statistically different in the pH-positive patients.

When should the use of fluoxetine or other agents that lower visceral sensitivity be considered in heartburn patients? Although symptomatic treatment without endoscopy is a reasonable, initial approach to heartburn, significant esophagitis and Barrett esophagus should be excluded before considering this therapy. A more difficult question is whether pH testing should be used to guide therapy, and this will vary between centers and patient populations. Another question is whether the endoscopy and pH-negative patients should be required to fail a PPI trial before fluoxetine, but this is probably a moot point because most patients would have had a therapeutic trial before endoscopy or pH testing. Finally, particularly in the pH-positive patients, is there a role for adding fluoxetine to the PPI rather than switching? There are obviously as many questions as answers here, but this study does provide support for attempting to alter visceral sensitivity in at least a subset of heartburn patients.

K. R. DeVault, MD

Long-term Efficacy and Safety of Endoscopic Resection for Patients With Mucosal Adenocarcinoma of the Esophagus

Pech O, May A, Manner H, et al (Univ of Regensburg, Germany; Univ of Mainz, Wiesbaden, Germany; et al)

Gastroenterology 146:652-660e1, 2014

Background & Aims.—Barrett's esophagus-associated high-grade dysplasia is commonly treated by endoscopy. However, most guidelines offer no recommendations for endoscopic treatment of mucosal adenocarcinoma of the esophagus (mAC). We investigated the efficacy and safety of endoscopic resection in a large series of patients with mAC.

Methods.—We collected data from 1000 consecutive patients (mean age, 69.1 ± 10.7 years; 861 men) with mAC (481 with short-segment and 519 with long-segment Barrett's esophagus) who presented at a tertiary care center from October 1996 to September 2010. Patients with low-grade and high-grade dysplasia and submucosal or more advanced cancer were excluded. All patients underwent endoscopic resection of mACs. Patients found to have submucosal cancer at their first endoscopy examination were excluded from the analysis.

Results.—After a mean follow-up period of 56.6 ± 33.4 months, 963 patients (96.3%) had achieved a complete response; surgery was necessary in 12 patients (3.7%) after endoscopic therapy failed. Metachronous lesions or recurrence of cancer developed during the follow-up period in 140 patients (14.5%) but endoscopic re-treatment was successful in 115, resulting in a long-term complete remission rate of 93.8%; 111 died of concomitant disease and 2 of Barrett's esophagus-associated cancer. The calculated 10-year survival rate of patients who underwent endoscopic resection of mACs was 75%. Major complications developed in 15 patients (1.5%) but could be managed conservatively.

Conclusions.—Endoscopic therapy is highly effective and safe for patients with mAC, with excellent long-term results. In an almost 5-year follow-up of 1000 patients treated with endoscopic resection, there was no mortality and less than 2% had major complications. Endoscopic therapy should become the standard of care for patients with mAC.

▶ The treatment of esophageal adenocarcinoma (EAC) has traditionally been based on the stage of disease and might include initial surgery in patients with early cancer, radiation, and chemotherapy followed by surgery in intermediate-stage cancer and palliation in those with advanced disease. Endoscopic mucosal resection (EMR) of neoplastic lesions is being performed in many areas of the gastrointestinal tract and have demonstrated good long-term efficacy.

This study provides strong support for this therapy for early-stage adenocarcinoma of the esophagus with good efficacy and a low rate of serious side effects. Patients with these lesions should be referred to centers with expertise in EMR, and if the lesion appears amenable to EMR, then the resection can both provide the most accurate staging, but also potential cure. After the lesion is resected, then additional therapy may be needed to control the cancer if the sample indicates any invasion. Even the if the cancer is "cured," there is often residual Barrett's esophagus, which should either be resected using EMR or ablated in some other manner. The major challenge in the widespread adoption of this approach is the limited number of endoscopists well trained in the technique, but more are becoming adept at the procedure in both large and small centers.

K. R. DeVault, MD

Radiofrequency Ablation vs Endoscopic Surveillance for Patients With Barrett Esophagus and Low-Grade Dysplasia: A Randomized Clinical Trial

Phoa KN, van Vilsteren FGI, Weusten BLAM, et al (Univ of Amsterdam, the Netherlands; St Antonius Hosp, Nieuwegein, the Netherlands; et al)

JAMA 311:1209-1217, 2014

Importance.—Barrett esophagus containing low-grade dysplasia is associated with an increased risk of developing esophageal adenocarcinoma, a cancer with a rapidly increasing incidence in the western world.

Objective.—To investigate whether endoscopic radiofrequency ablation could decrease the rate of neoplastic progression.

Design, Setting, and Participants.—Multicenter randomized clinical trial that enrolled 136 patients with a confirmed diagnosis of Barrett esophagus containing low-grade dysplasia at 9 European sites between June 2007 and June 2011. Patient follow-up ended May 2013.

Interventions.—Eligible patients were randomly assigned in a 1:1 ratio to either endoscopic treatment with radiofrequency ablation (ablation) or endoscopic surveillance (control). Ablation was performed with the balloon device for circumferential ablation of the esophagus or the focal device for targeted ablation, with a maximum of 5 sessions allowed.

Main Outcomes and Measures.—The primary outcomewas neoplastic progression to high-grade dysplasia or adenocarcinoma during a 3-year follow-up since randomization. Secondary outcomes were complete eradication of dysplasia and intestinal metaplasia and adverse events.

Results.—Sixty-eight patients were randomized to receive ablation and 68 to receive control. Ablation reduced the risk of progression to high-grade dysplasia or adenocarcinoma by 25.0% (1.5% for ablation vs 26.5% for control; 95% CI, 14.1%-35.9%; $P < .001$) and the risk of progression to adenocarcinoma by 7.4% (1.5% for ablation vs 8.8% for control; 95% CI, 0%-14.7%; $P = .03$). Among patients in the ablation group, complete eradication occurred in 92.6% for dysplasia and 88.2% for intestinal metaplasia compared with 27.9% for dysplasia and 0.0% for intestinal metaplasia among patients in the control group ($P < .001$). Treatment-related adverse events occurred in 19.1% of patients receiving ablation ($P < .001$). The most common adverse event was stricture, occurring in 8 patients receiving ablation (11.8%), all resolved by endoscopic dilation (median, 1 session). The data and safety monitoring board recommended early termination of the trial due to superiority of ablation for the primary outcome and the potential for patient safety issues if the trial continued.

Conclusions and Relevance.—In this randomized trial of patients with Barrett esophagus and a confirmed diagnosis of low-grade dysplasia, radiofrequency ablation resulted in a reduced risk of neoplastic progression over 3 years of follow-up.

Trial Registration.—trialregister.nl Identifier: NTR1198.

▶ Barrett's esophagus (BE) is the primary precursor of esophageal adenocarcinoma, which has markedly increased in prevalence in the past decades. BE progresses to cancer through various degrees of metaplasia and dysplasia (metaplasia to low-grade dysplasia [LGD] to high-grade dysplasia to cancer). Patients with BE are often enrolled in surveillance programs in an effort to identify histologic changes at a point in that progression where an intervention can prevent cancer. Before the development of ablative techniques, once high-grade dysplasia or early cancer was identified, the patient was offered an esophagectomy, which is a procedure with considerable morbidity and mortality. Several methods of ablation, including radiofrequency ablation (RFA), have been shown to prevent advanced cancer in patients with high-grade dysplasia. Whether this approach can be extended to those with low-grade dysplasia is addressed in this trial.

This study demonstrated that RFA could reduce both the progression from low- to high-grade dysplasia as well as the development of carcinoma. The impressive results led to the study being stopped early. The major side effect of RFA is stricture, but this can be dealt with effectively in most patients. Should this change our practice? The answer is a cautious "yes." It is now reasonable to offer RFA to patients with LGD. It is of great importance that the LGD is confirmed, ideally by an expert pathologist and perhaps during more than 1 endoscopy (histologic downgrading from LGD to nondysplastic BE has been reported in biopsies initially read in a community session and subsequently referred to an expert pathologist). It is also important to remember that the LGD resolved in 28% of the control patients and that the surveillance program did prevent progression to advanced disease even in the control group. Thus, surveillance remains an appropriate, alternative strategy. There are no similar data for nondysplastic BE, although there are ongoing studies looking at that much larger population.

K. R. DeVault, MD

47 Stomach

A Comparative Study of Sequential Therapy and Standard Triple Therapy for *Helicobacter pylori* Infection: A Randomized Multicenter Trial

Zhou L, Zhang J, Chen M, et al (Peking Univ Third Hosp, Beijing, China; Chinese Ctr for Disease Control and Prevention, Beijing, China; First Affiliated Hosp of Sun Yat-sen Univ, Guangzhou, China; et al)

Am J Gastroenterol 109:535-541, 2014

Objectives.—Studies conducted in large populations of patients and providing full information on *Helicobacter pylori* (*H. pylori*) antibiotic resistance are needed to determine the efficacy of sequential therapy (SQT) against this pathogen. This study compared eradication rates with SQT and standard triple therapy (STT), and evaluated the impact of antibiotic resistance on outcomes.

Methods.—The study population included adults with positive *H. pylori* culture presenting at four centers in China between March 2008 and December 2010. Patients were randomly assigned to 10 days of treatment with esomeprazole, amoxicillin, and clarithromycin (STT; $n = 140$) or to 5 days of treatment with esomeprazole and amoxicillin, followed by 5 days of esomeprazole, clarithromycin, and tinidazole (SQT; $n = 140$). Eradication was assessed 8–12 weeks after treatment.

Results.—There was no significant difference between the eradication rates achieved with STT (66.4% (95% confidence interval (CI) 59.3–74.3)) and SQT (72.1% (65.0–79.3); $P = 0.300$) in either the intention-to-treat analysis or the per-protocol analysis (72.7% (65.6–79.7) and 76.5% (69.7–83.3), respectively; $P = 0.475$). Clarithromycin resistance (CLA-R, odds ratio (OR) = 8.34 (3.13–22.26), $P < 0.001$) and metronidazole resistance (MET-R, OR = 7.14 (1.52–33.53), $P = 0.013$) both independently predicted treatment failure in the SQT group. Patients in the SQT group with dual CLA-R and MET-R had a lower eradication rate (43.9%) than those with isolated CLA-R (88.9%, $P = 0.024$) or isolated MET-R (87.8%, $P < 0.001$).

Conclusions.—*H. pylori* eradication rates with STT and SQT were compromised by antibiotic resistance. SQT may be suitable in regions with high prevalence of isolated CLA-R, but it is unsatisfactory when both CLA-R and MET-R are present.

▶ *Helicobacter pylori* remain a common cause of gastric mucosal disease including gastritis, peptic ulcer, and gastric carcinoma. Eradication of the infection has become more challenging because of antibiotic resistance. This resistance is present in both developed and less developed countries. Standard therapy has used multiple medications given together for 7 to 14 days. Sequential therapy involves a change in medications at some point in the course of treatment. Although previous studies have suggested superiority for sequential therapy, there was no difference in eradication in this study between standard therapy (66.4%) and sequential therapy (76.5%).

There is much to learn from this study, despite its negative outcome. The significant compromise in *H. pylori* eradication brought about by antibiotic resistance is a fact throughout the world. Resistance rates included clarithromycin, 39% to 41%; metronidazole, 65% to 69%, and amoxicillin (4% to 5%), which appear to be high in China, but not out of the range seen in other countries. A 25% to 50% failure rate (highest with multiresistent strains) is difficult for patients and providers to accept in a world where we believe infections can be eliminated with modern antibiotics. Basing therapy on culture and sensitivity testing is difficult and not widely available, but if these resistance trends continue, it may be reasonable to put efforts into extending that availability. In conclusion, health care providers should understand the resistance rate in their area and council patients that there is no perfect treatment for *H pylori*. Lack of eradication should be considered in any patient with persistent symptoms after treatment of this infection.

K. R. DeVault, MD

Acute Gastroenteritis and the Risk of Functional Dyspepsia: a Systematic Review and Meta-Analysis

Pike BL, Porter CK, Sorrell TJ, et al (Naval Med Res Ctr, Silver Spring, MD)
Am J Gastroenterol 108:1558-1563, 2013

Objectives.—The objective of this systematic review and meta-analysis was to estimate the risk of developing functional dyspepsia (FD) following acute infectious gastroenteritis (IGE).

Methods.—Eligible studies were identified through PubMed and EMBASE searches. Data and quality indicators were extracted by two authors from nine studies examining the risk of FD following IGE in 5,755 exposed individuals.

Results.—Estimates of FD risk following IGE based on a random effects model yielded a pooled odds ratio (OR) of 2.18 (95% confidence interval (CI): 1.70–2.81). Subanalyses revealed differences in the odds of FD following self-reported IGE (OR: 2.83, 95% CI: 2.10–3.81) compared with documented IGE medical encounters (OR: 1.81, 95% CI: 1.26–2.58), and a decreasing FD risk with time from IGE (≤12 months: OR: 4.76, 95% CI: 2.47–9.20 and >12 months: OR: 1.97, 95% CI: 1.51–2.56).

Conclusions.—Taken together, these data suggest that the risk of developing FD is significantly increased following IGE.

▶ Many patients present with upper gastrointestinal symptoms and are eventually diagnosed with functional dyspepsia (FD). This disorder is defined as 1 or more of the following chronic symptoms in a patient with no evidence of structural disease: bothersome postprandial fullness, early satiety, or epigastric pain or burning. The cause of FD is not clear at all; however, many, but not all, patients seem to have developed their symptoms after an acute gastrointestinal illness. Because FD is often diagnosed months or even years after that illness, it is often difficult to identify and characterize the initiating illness. This systematic review and meta-analysis found that there was roughly double the chance of developing FD after an episode of acute gastroenteritis.

This study confirms our assumption that acute gastroenteritis predisposes to FD, but there are some confounding issues in the 9 studies included in this analysis. Several of the studies had a predominately young, male (military) population, but FD seems to be more common in women and perhaps in older individuals. Many of these studies used questionnaires to diagnose FD and the findings in those presenting to a health care provider might well be different. Despite those concerns, it seems reasonable that 10% or more of patients with an acute gastrointestinal illness might go on to develop FD. In addition to FD, there are similar data on irritable bowel syndrome. These associations are difficult for patients and often drive the search for a "chronic infection," which is rarely identified. Further studies are needed to better characterize this risk and perhaps begin to develop strategies to decrease that risk.

K. R. DeVault, MD

48 Small Bowel

Systematic review: sprue-like enteropathy associated with olmesartan

Ianiro G, Bibbò S, Montalto M, et al (Catholic Univ, Rome, Italy)
Aliment Pharmacol Ther 40:16-23, 2014

Background.—The onset of a sprue-like enteropathy in association with olmesartan therapy has been recently reported.

Aims.—To perform a systematic review of the literature and describe three additional cases of olmesartan-associated enteropathy.

Methods.—Electronic and manual bibliographic searches were performed to identify original reports in which subjects who were undertaking olmesartan developed a sprue-like enteropathy. Because of the scarcity of studies with adequate sample size, case series with less than 10 patients and case reports were also considered. Data extraction was performed independently by two reviewers.

Results.—A total of 11 publications met our pre-defined inclusion criteria, for an overall number of 54 patients (including our series). Almost all patients presented with diarrhoea and weight loss. Normocytic normochromic anaemia and hypoalbuminaemia were the commonest laboratory defects at presentation. Antibody testing for coeliac disease was always negative. Variable degrees of duodenal villous atrophy were present in 98% of patients, while increased intra-epithelial lymphocytes were documented in only 65% of cases. After discontinuation of olmesartan, all reported patients achieved resolution of signs and symptoms.

Conclusions.—Although the available evidence is limited, the olmesartan-associated sprue-like enteropathy may be considered as a distinct clinical entity, and should be included in the differential diagnosis when serological testing for coeliac disease is negative.

▶ Gluten sensitivity and celiac disease are important and increasing health care problems. The most common diagnostic dilemma is when the patient is gluten sensitive but has no mucosal or serological evidence of celiac disease, which has been labeled gluten sensitivity. This study looks at a different situation in which a patient has symptoms and endoscopic evidence of celiac disease but negative serology. An association between a commonly prescribed antihypertensive (olmesartan) and a sprue (celiac)-like enteropathy has been reported and is reviewed systematically.

When a patient taking olmesartan presents with significant gastrointestinal symptoms, this association should be considered. The syndrome is best diagnosed via endoscopy with appropriately obtained biopsies and, at times, serology to exclude celiac disease. It was interesting that more than 70% of patients who had human leukocyte antigen (HLA) testing for DQ2 or 8 had a positive test. These haplotypes are presents in 30% to 40% of the normal population, so there may be some connection with this sensitivity. Tissue transglutaminase was always negative in the reported cases, but positive HLA testing (especially if the patient was already on a gluten-free diet) might suggest that some of these patients could have easily been misclassified as having classic celiac disease. In fact, the majority had attempted a gluten-free diet, and many had been treated with topical or systemic steroids. Thankfully, all of the patients recovered their intestinal absorptive capacity after stopping olmesartan.

K. R. DeVault, MD

A Diet Low in FODMAPs Reduces Symptoms of Irritable Bowel Syndrome

Halmos EP, Power VA, Shepherd SJ, et al (Monash Univ, Box Hill, Victoria, Australia)
Gastroenterology 146:67-75, 2014

Background & Aims.—A diet low in fermentable oligosaccharides, disaccharides, monosaccharides, and polyols (FODMAPs) often is used to manage functional gastrointestinal symptoms in patients with irritable bowel syndrome (IBS), yet there is limited evidence of its efficacy, compared with a normal Western diet. We investigated the effects of a diet low in FODMAPs compared with an Australian diet, in a randomized, controlled, single-blind, cross-over trial of patients with IBS.

Methods.—In a study of 30 patients with IBS and 8 healthy individuals (controls, matched for demographics and diet), we collected dietary data from subjects for 1 habitual week. Participants then randomly were assigned to groups that received 21 days of either a diet low in FODMAPs or a typical Australian diet, followed by a washout period of at least 21 days, before crossing over to the alternate diet. Daily symptoms were rated using a 0- to 100-mm visual analogue scale. Almost all food was provided during the interventional diet periods, with a goal of less than 0.5 g intake of FODMAPs per meal for the low-FODMAP diet. All stools were collected from days 17–21 and assessed for frequency, weight, water content, and King's Stool Chart rating.

Results.—Subjects with IBS had lower overall gastrointestinal symptom scores (22.8; 95% confidence interval, 16.7–28.8 mm) while on a diet low in FODMAPs, compared with the Australian diet (44.9; 95% confidence interval, 36.6–53.1 mm; $P < .001$) and the subjects' habitual diet. Bloating, pain, and passage of wind also were reduced while IBS patients were on the low-FODMAP diet. Symptoms were minimal and unaltered by either diet among controls. Patients of all IBS subtypes had greater satisfaction with stool consistency while on the low-FODMAP diet, but diarrhea-predominant IBS was the only subtype with altered fecal frequency and King's Stool Chart scores.

Conclusions.—In a controlled, cross-over study of patients with IBS, a diet low in FODMAPs effectively reduced functional gastrointestinal symptoms. This high-quality evidence supports its use as a first-line therapy. Clinical Trial number: ACTRN12612001185853 (Fig 1A).

▶ Irritable bowel syndrome (IBS) is 1 of the more frequently diagnosed gastrointestinal conditions. It results in substantial health care costs and lowers quality of life. Dietary manipulation is often recommended, but data are weak, and recommendations vary greatly from practitioner to practitioner. Recently, the concept of a group of sugars as an initiating factor for IBS has been introduced. These agents are described as FODMAPs (fermentable oligosaccharides, disaccharides, monosaccharides, and polyols), which are poorly absorbed short-chain carbohydrates including fructose (in excess of glucose), lactose, polyols, fructans, and galacto-oligosaccharides. This trial randomized IBS patients to either a routine diet or a diet low in FODMAPs and showed lower IBS symptoms in a low FODMAP diet (Fig 1). The results are more impressive than many studies because the control population were not on a FODMAP-enhanced diet, just taking in what would be considered a normal amount of these sugars.

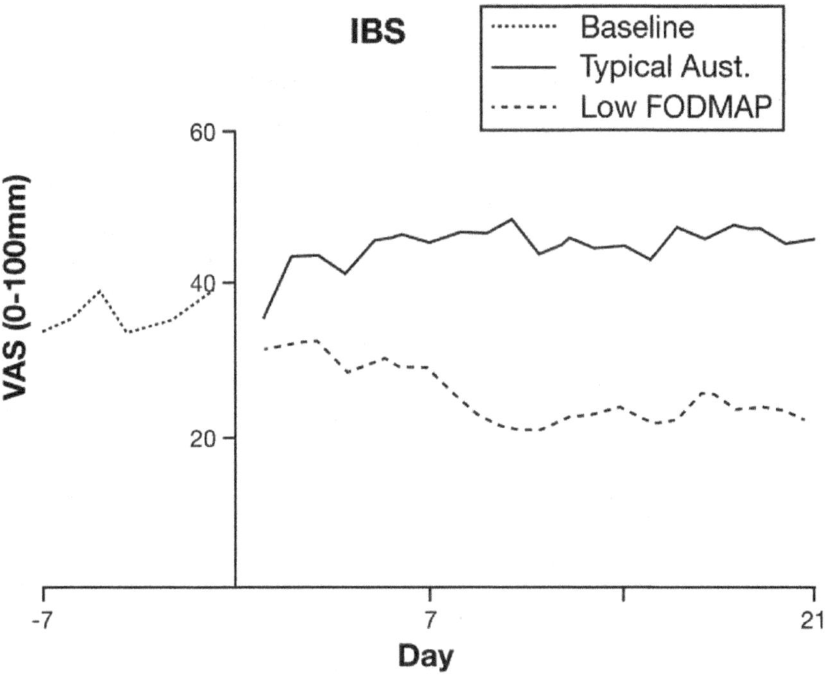

FIGURE 1.—Mean overall gastrointestinal symptoms from the (*A*) IBS cohort, low FODMAP and typical Australian diets. Symptoms improved significantly on low FODMAP compared with baseline and the typical Australian diet for the IBS cohort. No differences were observed between any of the diets in the healthy cohort. (Reprinted from Gastroenterology. Halmos EP, Power VA, Shepherd SJ, et al. A diet low in FODMAPs reduces symptoms of irritable bowel syndrome. *Gastroenterology.* 2014;146:67-75, Copyright 2014, with permission from the AGA Institute.)

The authors suggested this as a frontline therapy for IBS; is that reasonable? I would offer a qualified "yes." There are multiple printable guidelines for lowering FODMAPs, but it is not clear that patient-driven changes will work as well as the more intense intervention in a clinical trial. Perhaps, dieticians trained in this dietary maneuver will become an important part of the IBS treatment team. Interestingly, the diet improvement was noted almost immediately and persisted through the trial. This makes this even more attractive because such a short trial can be both diagnostic and therapeutic. Patients and providers should also understand that low-gluten diets may also be low-FODMAP diets, so, in some patients, gluten sensitivity might actually be FODMAP-induced IBS.

K. R. DeVault, MD

Celiac Disease or Non-Celiac Gluten Sensitivity? An Approach to Clinical Differential Diagnosis

Kabbani TA, Vanga RR, Leffler DA, et al (Beth Israel Deaconess Med Ctr, Boston, MA)

Am J Gastroenterol 109:741-746, 2014

Objectives.—Differentiating between celiac disease (CD) and non-celiac gluten sensitivity (NCGS) is important for appropriate management but is often challenging.

Methods.—We retrospectively reviewed records from 238 patients who presented for the evaluation of symptoms responsive to gluten restriction without prior diagnosis or exclusion of CD. Demographics, presenting symptoms, serologic, genetic, and histologic data, nutrient deficiencies, personal history of autoimmune diseases, and family history of CD were recorded. NCGS was defined as symptoms responsive to a gluten-free diet (GFD) in the setting of negative celiac serology and duodenal biopsies while on a gluten-containing diet or negative human leukocyte antigen (HLA) DQ2/DQ8 testing.

Results.—Of the 238 study subjects, 101 had CD, 125 had NCGS, 9 had non-celiac enteropathy, and 3 had indeterminate diagnosis. CD subjects presented with symptoms of malabsorption 67.3% of the time compared with 24.8% of the NCGS subjects ($P < 0.0001$). In addition, CD subjects were significantly more likely to have a family history of CD ($P = 0.004$), personal history of autoimmune diseases ($P = 0.002$), or nutrient deficiencies ($P < 0.0001$). The positive likelihood ratio for diagnosis of CD of a >2× upper limit of normal IgA *trans*-glutaminase antibody (tTG) or IgA/IgG deaminated gliadan peptide antibody (DGP) with clinical response to GFD was 130 (confidence interval (CI): 18.5–918.3). The positive likelihood ratio of the combination of gluten-responsive symptoms and negative IgA tTG or IgA/IgG DGP on a regular diet for NCGS was 9.6 (CI: 5.5–16.9). When individuals with negative IgA tTG or IgA/IgG DGP also lacked symptoms of malabsorption (weight loss, diarrhea, and nutrient deficiencies) and CD risk factors (personal history of autoimmune diseases and family history of CD), the positive likelihood ratio for NCGS increased to 80.9.

Conclusions.—On the basis of our findings, we have developed a diagnostic algorithm to differentiate CD from NCGS. Subjects with negative celiac serologies (IgA tTG or IgA/IgG DGP) on a regular diet are unlikely to have CD. Those with negative serology who also lack clinical evidence of malabsorption and CD risk factors are highly likely to have NCGS and may not require further testing. Those with equivocal serology should undergo HLA typing to determine the need for biopsy (Fig 2).

▶ Celiac disease (CD) is a well-characterized autoimmune process that is associated with the intake of gluten-containing foods. Interestingly, some patients who do not seem to have true Celiac disease may respond to low or gluten-free diets creating diagnostic uncertainty. It is important to sort this out because patients with CD should strictly avoid even the smallest amount of gluten whereas those with nonceliac gluten sensitivity can follow a more symptom-driven approach. In addition, nonceliac patients do not seem at risk of nutritional or malignant complications that have been associated with CD. Testing for these disorders can be both expensive (serology and human leukocyte antigen testing) and invasive (endoscopy). This article suggests an approach to this conundrum, which is demonstrated in the Fig 2.

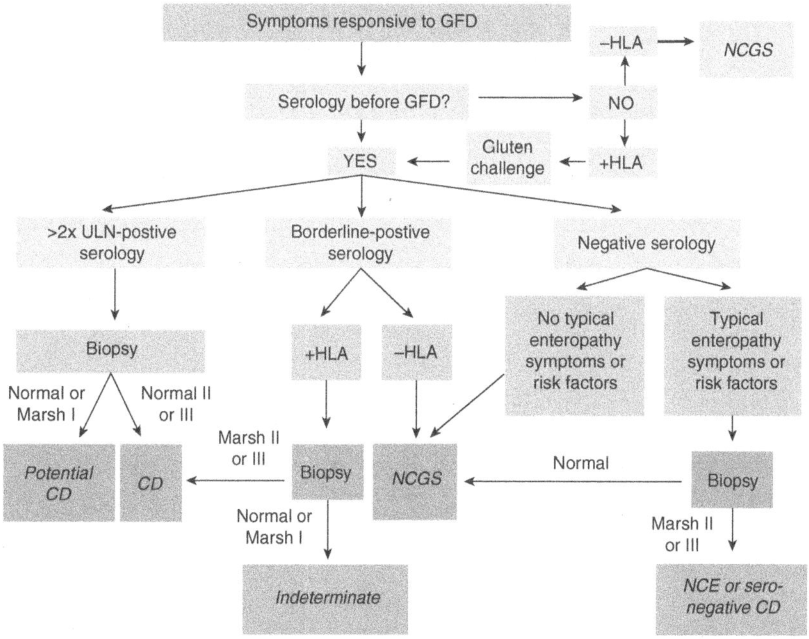

FIGURE 2.—Diagnostic model for symptoms responsive to gluten exclusion. CD, celiac disease; NCE, non-celiac enteropathy; NCGS, non-celiac gluten sensitivity; ULN, upper limit of normal. (Reprinted by permission from Macmillan Publishers Ltd: American Journal of Gastroenterology. Kabbani TA, Vanga RR, Leffler DA, et al. Celiac disease or non-celiac gluten sensitivity? An approach to clinical differential diagnosis. *Am J Gastroenterol.* 2014;109:741-746, Copyright 2014.)

The study clearly suggests that the initial presentation can help begin to classify patients. CD patients are more likely to have a personal history of autoimmune disorders, diarrhea, weight loss, and nutrition deficiencies. This model still relies on a gluten challenge in many patients. I have frequently experienced resistance to that challenge. I try to reassure patients that it is safe, although I have seen a single case of kidney failure due to severe diarrhea that developed during a gluten challenge. It also clearly shows that serology before a gluten-free diet is most helpful, but, of course, is less common these days given the lay public's interest in gluten and frequent self-directed trials. A patient with negative serology (on gluten) and lack of significant malabsorptive signs or symptoms will benefit little from endoscopy, so following this guideline would result in lower cost of care. It provides some data-driven clarification to a common and difficult diagnostic dilemma.

K. R. DeVault, MD

49 Colon

ACG Clinical Guideline: Management of Benign Anorectal Disorders

Wald A, Bharucha AE, Cosman BC, et al (Univ of Wisconsin School of Medicine and Public Health, Madison; Mayo Clinic, Rochester, MN; Univ of California San Diego School of Medicine; et al)

Am J Gastroenterol 109:1141-1157, 2014

These guidelines summarize the definitions, diagnostic criteria, differential diagnoses, and treatments of a group of benign disorders of anorectal function and/or structure. Disorders of function include defecation disorders, fecal incontinence, and proctalgia syndromes, whereas disorders of structure include anal fissure and hemorrhoids. Each section reviews the definitions, epidemiology and/or pathophysiology, diagnostic assessment, and treatment recommendations of each entity. These recommendations reflect a comprehensive search of all relevant topics of pertinent English language articles in PubMed, Ovid Medline, and the National Library of Medicine from 1966 to 2013 using appropriate terms for each subject. Recommendations for anal fissure and hemorrhoids lean heavily on adaptation from the American Society of Colon and Rectal Surgeons Practice Parameters from the most recent published guidelines in 2010 and 2011 and supplemented with subsequent publications through 2013. We used systematic reviews and meta-analyses when available, and this was supplemented by review of published clinical trials.

▶ Complaints related to the rectum are common in both gastroenterology and general practice. Guidelines for these disorders are published in this article. Key, clinically relevant concepts include the following:

1 Disordered defecation (DD) is a common cause of constipation. Diagnosis of this disorder requires a combination of clinical history, careful rectal examination, and selected confirmatory testing. Biofeedback (the approach is outlined in article) is the preferred treatment for patients with DD.

2 Chronic proctalgia presents with recurring rectal pain and tenderness on rectal exam. Some patients require exclusion of structure disorders using selected tests. It also can respond to biofeedback therapy.

3 Fecal incontinence (FI) is a common, life-altering symptom. Obtaining a history of FI is sometimes difficult because of the stigma of that condition and should be specifically questioned, particularly in patients presenting with "diarrhea." Common causes are outlined in the table. When conservative treatment (directed at firming stool) fails, anorectal manometry and anal

ultrasound may aid in the diagnosis. Pelvic floor rehabilitation is helpful in many patients. Injectable agents may have a role in patients with symptoms refractory to the foregoing options. Surgical treatments are available and outlined in the article.

4 Anal fissures should initially be treated with sitz baths, fiber, and bulking agents. Topical nitrates and calcium blockers are second-line therapies. Intrasphincteric botulinum toxin injection and surgery are reserved for refractory cases.

5 Hemorrhoids are diagnosed by history and examination. If thrombosed, early surgical referral is appropriate. Routine hemorrhoids can be managed with increased fiber and fluid intake. Persistent lesions should be managed endoscopically or surgically.

K. R. DeVault, MD

Efficacy of Pharmacological Therapies for the Treatment of Opioid-Induced Constipation: Systematic Review and Meta-Analysis

Ford AC, Brenner DM, Schoenfeld PS (St James's Univ Hosp, Leeds, UK; Northwestern Memorial Hosp, Chicago, IL; Univ of Michigan School of Medicine, Ann Arbor)

Am J Gastroenterol 108:1566-1574, 2013

Objectives.—There has been no definitive synthesis of the evidence for any benefit of available pharmacological therapies in opioid-induced constipation (OIC). We conducted a systematic review and meta-analysis to address this deficit.

Methods.—We searched MEDLINE, EMBASE, EMBASE Classic, and the Cochrane central register of controlled trials through to December 2012 to identify placebo-controlled trials of μ-opioid receptor antagonists, prucalopride, lubiprostone, and linaclotide in the treatment of adults with OIC. No minimum duration of therapy was required. Trials had to report a dichotomous assessment of overall response to therapy, and data were pooled using a random effects model. Effect of pharmacological therapies was reported as relative risk (RR) of failure to respond to therapy, with 95% confidence intervals (CIs).

Results.—Fourteen eligible randomized controlled trials (RCTs) of μ-opioid receptor antagonists, containing 4,101 patients, were identified. These were superior to placebo for the treatment of OIC (RR of failure to respond to therapy = 0.69; 95 % CI 0.63–0.75). Methylnaltrexone (six RCTs, 1,610 patients, RR = 0.66; 95 % CI 0.54–0.84), naloxone (four trials, 798 patients, RR = 0.64; 95 % CI 0.56–0.72), and alvimopan (four RCTs, 1,693 patients, RR = 0.71; 95 % CI 0.65–0.78) were all superior to placebo. Total numbers of adverse events, diarrhea, and abdominal pain were significantly commoner when data from all RCTs were pooled. Reversal of analgesia did not occur more frequently with active therapy. Only one trial of prucalopride was identified, with a nonsignificant trend toward higher responder rates with active therapy. Two RCTs of lubiprostone were found, with significantly higher responder rates with lubiprostone in both, but reporting of data precluded meta-analysis.

Conclusions.—μ-Opioid receptor antagonists are safe and effective for the treatment of OIC. More data are required before the role of prucalopride or lubiprostone in the treatment of OIC are clear.

▶ Constipation is a common symptom that may be caused or worsened by the use of opioids when they are taken on either a short- or long-term basis. Treatment is often difficult, but several agents have been developed over the past few years that may be helpful in this situation.

Over-the-counter laxative use is common in opioid-induced constipation (OIC) but have poor efficacy. Three prescription agents have been studied in OIC, are the subject of this analysis, and are available in some, but not all, countries. They are u-opioid antagonists (naloxone, alvimopan, and methylnaltrexone), lubiprostone, and prucalopride. All 3 of the opioid antagonists were found to be superior to placebo, and there were efficacy trends for the other 2 agents.

A possible approach to patients with OIC would be as follows:

1 Routine laxatives and attempting to minimize narcotic dose is an appropriate first step, despite their poor efficacy in clinical trials.
2 If that fails, adding an oral agent is reasonable. Although not yet well studied, linaclotide might also have some efficacy.
3 Subcutaneous injections using methylnaltrexone should be reserved for those failing conservative and oral medications but can produce substantial improvement in a subset of patients. The current indications for this agent in the United States are somewhat limited but hopefully will be expanded in the future.

K. R. DeVault, MD

50 Liver

Simple Noninvasive Systems Predict Long-term Outcomes of Patients With Nonalcoholic Fatty Liver Disease

Angulo P, Bugianesi E, Bjornsson ES, et al (Univ of Kentucky Med Ctr, Lexington; Univ of Torino, Italy; Natl Univ Hosp, Reykjavik, Iceland; et al)
Gastroenterology 145:782-789, 2013

Background & Aims.—Some patients with nonalcoholic fatty liver disease (NAFLD) develop liver-related complications and have higher mortality than other patients with NAFLD. We determined the accuracy of simple, noninvasive scoring systems in identification of patients at increased risk for liver-related complications or death.

Methods.—We performed a retrospective, international, multicenter cohort study of 320 patients diagnosed with NAFLD, based on liver biopsy analysis through 2002 and followed through 2011. Patients were assigned to mild-, intermediate-, or high-risk groups based on cutoff values for 2 of the following: NAFLD fibrosis score, aspartate aminotransferase/platelet ratio index, FIB-4 score, and BARD score. Outcomes included liver-related complications and death or liver transplantation. We used multivariate Cox proportional hazard regression analysis to adjust for relevant variables and calculate adjusted hazard ratios (aHRs).

Results.—During a median follow-up period of 104.8 months (range, 3–317 months), 14% of patients developed liver-related events and 13% died or underwent liver transplantation. The aHRs for liver-related events in the intermediate-risk and high-risk groups, compared with the low-risk group, were 7.7 (95% confidence interval [CI]: 1.4–42.7) and 34.2 (95% CI: 6.5–180.1), respectively, based on NAFLD fibrosis score; 8.8 (95% CI: 1.1–67.3) and 20.9 (95% CI: 2.6–165.3) based on the aspartate aminotransferase/platelet ratio index; and 6.2 (95% CI: 1.4–27.2) and 6.6 (95% CI: 1.4–31.1) based on the BARD score. The aHRs for death or liver transplantation in the intermediate-risk and high-risk groups compared with the low-risk group were 4.2 (95% CI: 1.3–13.8) and 9.8 (95% CI: 2.7–35.3), respectively, based on the NAFLD fibrosis scores. Based on aspartate aminotransferase/platelet ratio index and FIB-4 score, only the high-risk group had a greater risk of death or liver transplantation (aHR = 3.1; 95% CI: 1.1–8.4 and aHR = 6.6; 95% CI: 2.3–20.4, respectively).

Conclusions.—Simple noninvasive scoring systems help identify patients with NAFLD who are at increased risk for liver-related complications or death. NAFLD fibrosis score appears to be the best indicator of patients at risk, based on HRs. The results of this study require external validation.

▶ Nonalcoholic fatty liver disease (NAFLD) is a common consideration in the evaluation of patients (especially overweight patients) with elevated liver function testing. The range of severity in this condition can vary from an inconsequential elevation of blood tests to cirrhosis and end-stage liver disease, which is now one of the top indications for liver transplantation in the United States. Judging the severity of damage in patients with NAFLD has been difficult, requiring expensive imaging, liver biopsy, or both. This makes noninvasive scoring systems, as presented in this article, highly desirable.

All of the scoring systems were able to predict patients with NAFLD who went on to develop liver-related complications, liver transplantation, or death, although 1 (the NAFLD fibrosis score) was perhaps mildly superior. All overweight patients with abnormal liver tests should be encouraged to loose weight and ideally be placed in a formal weight loss program. Unfortunately, the success of those programs are low but should still be pursued. Application of these scoring systems will help identify patients who should undergo additional testing to both evaluate their current condition and to provide prognostic information.

K. R. DeVault, MD

Ledipasvir and Sofosbuvir for 8 or 12 Weeks for Chronic HCV without Cirrhosis

Kowdley KV, for the ION-3 Investigators (Virginia Mason Med Ctr, Seattle, WA; et al)

N Engl J Med 370:1879-1888, 2014

Background.—High rates of sustained virologic response were observed among patients with hepatitis C virus (HCV) infection who received 12 weeks of treatment with the nucleotide polymerase inhibitor sofosbuvir combined with the NS5A inhibitor ledipasvir. This study examined 8 weeks of treatment with this regimen.

Methods.—In this phase 3, open-label study, we randomly assigned 647 previously untreated patients with HCV genotype 1 infection without cirrhosis to receive ledipasvir and sofosbuvir (ledipasvir–sofosbuvir) for 8 weeks, ledipasvir–sofosbuvir plus ribavirin for 8 weeks, or ledipasvir–sofosbuvir for 12 weeks. The primary end point was sustained virologic response at 12 weeks after the end of therapy.

Results.—The rate of sustained virologic response was 94% (95% confidence interval [CI], 90 to 97) with 8 weeks of ledipasvir–sofosbuvir, 93% (95% CI, 89 to 96) with 8 weeks of ledipasvir–sofosbuvir plus ribavirin, and 95% (95% CI, 92 to 98) with 12 weeks of ledipasvir–sofosbuvir. As compared with the rate of sustained virologic response in the group that received 8 weeks of ledipasvir–sofosbuvir, the rate in the 12-week group was 1 percentage point higher (97.5% CI, −4 to 6) and the rate in the group that received 8 weeks of ledipasvir–sofosbuvir with ribavirin was

1 percentage point lower (95% CI, −6 to 4); these results indicated noninferiority of the 8-week ledipasvir—sofosbuvir regimen, on the basis of a noninferiority margin of 12 percentage points. Adverse events were more common in the group that received ribavirin than in the other two groups. No patient who received 8 weeks of only ledipasvir—sofosbuvir discontinued treatment owing to adverse events.

Conclusions.—Ledipasvir—sofosbuvir for 8 weeks was associated with a high rate of sustained virologic response among previously untreated patients with HCV genotype 1 infection without cirrhosis. No additional benefit was associated with the inclusion of ribavirin in the regimen or with extension of the duration of treatment to 12 weeks. (Funded by Gilead Sciences; ION-3 ClinicalTrials.gov number, NCT01851330.)

▶ The treatment of hepatitis C virus (HCV) infection has improved markedly over the past 20 years. Shortly after the virus was discovered, the infection was treated using daily dosing of interferon, which had an adverse side-effect profile and poor efficacy. Combining longer-acting forms of interferon with ribavirin produced greater efficacy but still with a fairly difficult set of side effects. New oral agents have recently been released that have a favorable profile and may not require interferon coadministration. This particular study used 2 oral antiviral agents with or without ribavirin and no interferon in any arm. They found 8 weeks of the combination therapy to be effective and did not see any benefit to adding ribavirin or of extending the therapy for an additional 4 weeks. Side effects were less common in the groups that did not receive ribavirin.

This is one of several studies showing that a fairly short course of new oral agents to be highly effective in the treatment of HCV. This study was in previously untreated, noncirrhotic patients with HCV genotype 1. It is becoming increasing clear that many HCV patients will have good results with antivirals such as this combination. In fact, many hepatologists have been delaying treating HCV patients in anticipation of these agents. The biggest down side may be the high drug cost: sofosbuvir alone may cost up to $80 000 for 12 weeks of therapy in the United States! Limiting treatment to 8 rather than 12 weeks certainly lowers that still-substantial cost. Other studies cited in the discussion of this article have suggested that 8 weeks may be the minimum duration of therapy. These noninterferon/nonribavirin-based treatments are truly revolutionary and will continue to change the way we view and treat HCV infection.

K. R. DeVault, MD

ACG Clinical Guideline: The Diagnosis and Management of Idiosyncratic Drug-Induced Liver Injury

Chalasani NP, on behalf of the Practice Parameters Committee of the American College of Gastroenterology (Indiana Univ School of Medicine, Indianapolis; et al)
Am J Gastroenterol 109:950-966, 2014

Idiosyncratic drug-induced liver injury (DILI) is a rare adverse drug reaction and it can lead to jaundice, liver failure, or even death.

Antimicrobials and herbal and dietary supplements are among the most common therapeutic classes to cause DILI in the Western world. DILI is a diagnosis of exclusion and thus careful history taking and thorough work-up for competing etiologies are essential for its timely diagnosis. In this ACG Clinical Guideline, the authors present an evidence-based approach to diagnosis and management of DILI with special emphasis on DILI due to herbal and dietary supplements and DILI occurring in individuals with underlying liver disease.

▶ Elevated liver tests are some of the most common side effects of drug therapy. This is now characterized as drug-induced liver injury (DILI). The outcomes of patients with DILI can range from asymptomatic recovery to end-stage liver disease and death. This review and guideline statement provides guidance for anyone treating patients with medications when there is possibility of DILI. Some of the more important summary statements from this guideline include (some are summarized):

1 Certain variables such as age, gender, and alcohol consumption may increase risk for DILI in a drug-specific fashion.
2 DILI is a diagnosis of exclusion, and thus appropriate competing etiologies should be excluded in a systematic fashion.
3 In general, outcomes of idiosyncratic DILI are good, with only approximately 10% reaching the threshold of acute liver failure (ALF; coagulopathy and encephalopathy).
4 DILI that does evolve to ALF carries a poor prognosis, with 40% requiring liver transplantation and 42% dying of the episode. Advanced coma grade and high Model for End-Stage Liver Disease scores are associated with bad outcomes.
5 Re-exposure to a drug thought likely to have caused hepatotoxicity is strongly discouraged, especially if the initial liver injury was associated with significant aminotransferase elevation. An exception to this recommendation is in cases of life-threatening situations in which there is no suitable alternative.
6 In individuals with suspected DILI, especially when liver biochemistries are rising rapidly or there is evidence of liver dysfunction, suspected agent(s) should be promptly stopped.
7 No definitive therapies are available either for idiosyncratic DILI with or without ALF: however, n-acetylcysteine may be considered in adults with early-stage ALF, given its good safety profile and some evidence for efficacy in early coma stage patients.
8 Chronic DILI occurs in about 15% to 20% of cases of acute DILI.
9 Patients experiencing DILI due to prescription medications, dietary supplements, or herbal products should be followed clinically and biochemically to complete resolution.
10 DILI patients with severe acute cholestatic liver injury appear to be at increased risk of developing chronic liver injury and require careful long-term follow-up.

11 Herbal and dietary supplements account for an increasing proportion of DILI events in the United States, with body-building and weight-loss supplements being the most commonly implicated.

K. R. DeVault, MD

Systematic review with meta-analysis: the effects of rifaximin in hepatic encephalopathy

Kimer N, Krag A, Møller S, et al (Copenhagen Univ Hosp Hvidovre, Denmark; Univ of Southern Denmark, Odense, Denmark)

Aliment Pharmacol Ther 40:123-132, 2014

Background.—Rifaximin is recommended for prevention of hepatic encephalopathy (HE). The effects of rifaximin on overt and minimal HE are debated.

Aim.—To perform a systematic review and meta-analysis of randomised controlled trials (RCTs) on rifaximin for HE.

Methods.—We performed electronic and manual searches, gathered information from the U.S. Food and Drug Administration Home Page, and obtained unpublished information on trial design and outcome measures from authors and pharmaceutical companies. Meta-analyses were performed and results presented as risk ratios (RR) with 95% confidence intervals (CI) and the number needed to treat. Subgroup, sensitivity, regression and sequential analyses were performed to evaluate the risk of bias and sources of heterogeneity.

Results.—We included 19 RCTs with 1370 patients. Outcomes were recalculated based on unpublished information of 11 trials. Overall, rifaximin had a beneficial effect on secondary prevention of HE (RR: 1.32; 95% CI 1.06–1.65), but not in a sensitivity analysis on rifaximin after TIPSS (RR: 1.27; 95% CI 1.00–1.53). Rifaximin increased the proportion of patients who recovered from HE (RR: 0.59; 95% CI: 0.46–0.76) and reduced mortality (RR: 0.68, 95% CI 0.48–0.97). The results were robust to adjustments for bias control. No small study effects were identified. The sequential analyses only confirmed the results of the analysis on HE recovery.

Conclusions.—Rifaximin has a beneficial effect on hepatic encephalopathy and may reduce mortality. The combined evidence suggests that rifaximin may be considered in the evidence-based management of hepatic encephalopathy.

▶ Hepatic encephalopathy (HE) is a common complication of end-stage liver disease that results in considerable loss of quality of life, morbidity, and mortality. Treatment is directed at lowering ammonia concentrations. Laxative therapy using lactulose is effective but poorly tolerated. Some studies have suggested protein limitation as an approach, but it can result in worsening outcome due to malnutrition. Ammonia is produced by intestinal bacteria, so antibiotic therapy has been studied. Systemically absorbed agents can be effective but have side effects and can promote bacterial resistance. Rifaximin is a nonabsorbable antibiotic that lowers gut bacteria but has little systemic uptake or effect.

This analysis suggested that rifaximin is effective in the prevention and treatment of HE as well as mortality from HE. It has good efficacy and few side effects. This medication also has a beneficial effect on spontaneous bacterial peritonitis and perhaps other complications of liver disease. The duration of therapy varied in the studies with acute HE often treated with short courses and longer courses in the treatment of chronic HE. Rifaximin is an expensive medication, and it may be more cost-effective to try other medications such as lactulose and reserve rifaximin for failures. On the other hand, the medication has such a high benefit-to-risk ratio that cost might well be offset by other savings when the global cost of patient care is considered.

K. R. DeVault, MD

ABT-450/r–Ombitasvir and Dasabuvir with Ribavirin for Hepatitis C with Cirrhosis

Poordad F, Hezode C, Trinh R, et al (Texas Liver Inst–Univ of Texas Health Science Ctr, San Antonio; Univ Paris-Est, Créteil, France; AbbVie, North Chicago, IL; et al)
N Engl J Med 370:1973-1982, 2014

Background.—Interferon-containing regimens for the treatment of hepatitis C virus (HCV) infection are associated with increased toxic effects in patients who also have cirrhosis. We evaluated the interferon-free combination of the protease inhibitor ABT-450 with ritonavir (ABT-450/r), the NS5A inhibitor ombitasvir (ABT-267), the nonnucleoside polymerase inhibitor dasabuvir (ABT-333), and ribavirin in an open-label phase 3 trial involving previously untreated and previously treated adults with HCV genotype 1 infection and compensated cirrhosis.

Methods.—We randomly assigned 380 patients with Child–Pugh class A cirrhosis to receive either 12 or 24 weeks of treatment with ABT-450/r–ombitasvir (at a once-daily dose of 150 mg of ABT-450, 100 mg of ritonavir, and 25 mg of ombitasvir), dasabuvir (250 mg twice daily), and ribavirin administered according to body weight. The primary efficacy end point was a sustained virologic response 12 weeks after the end of treatment. The rate of sustained virologic response in each group was compared with the estimated rate with a telaprevir-based regimen (47%; 95% confidence interval [CI], 41 to 54). A noninferiority margin of 10.5 percentage points established 43% as the noninferiority threshold; the superiority threshold was 54%.

Results.—A total of 191 of 208 patients who received 12 weeks of treatment had a sustained virologic response at post-treatment week 12, for a rate of 91.8% (97.5% CI, 87.6 to 96.1). A total of 165 of 172 patients who received 24 weeks of treatment had a sustained virologic response at post-treatment week 12, for a rate of 95.9% (97.5% CI, 92.6 to 99.3). These rates were superior to the historical control rate. The three most common adverse events were fatigue (in 32.7% of patients in the 12-week group and 46.5% of patients in the 24-week group), headache (in 27.9% and 30.8%, respectively), and nausea (in 17.8% and 20.3%, respectively). The hemoglobin level was less than 10 g per deciliter in 7.2% and 11.0% of patients in the respective groups. Overall, 2.1% of patients discontinued treatment owing to adverse events.

Conclusions.—In this phase 3 trial of an oral, interferon-free regimen evaluated exclusively in patients with HCV genotype 1 infection and cirrhosis, multitargeted therapy with the use of three new antiviral agents and ribavirin resulted in high rates of sustained virologic response. Drug discontinuations due to adverse events were infrequent. (Funded by AbbVie; TURQUOISE-II ClinicalTrials.gov number, NCT01704755.)

▶ This study looked at a new oral combination therapy combined with ribavirin, but avoiding any type of interferon, and found outstanding efficacy and a low rate of adverse effects in hepatitis C (HCV) genotype 1 patients with documented cirrhosis. Cirrhosis is present in up to 25% of adults infected with HCV in the United States. Early in the history of HCV, cirrhosis was a relative and, in some centers, absolute contraindication for attempted HCV eradication. Over the years, several studies supported a benefit for eradicating the virus in patients with established cirrhosis, but the adverse-effect profile is problematic in this group.

New, oral anti-HCV agents represent a major advance for most patients with HCV infection. It is important to note that this study contained both treatment-naïve patients and patients previously treated with interferon-based therapy and found similar outstanding results in both groups. Twelve weeks of therapy had similar efficacy to 24 weeks, which was another important finding that may result in lower cost and fewer adverse effects when therapy is limited to 12 weeks. There were some genotype-specific trends, perhaps suggesting longer therapy for previously treated patients with genotype 1a. The rate of study discontinuation due to side effects was only 2.1%, which is remarkably low when compared with previous, interferon-based treatment. This and other oral treatment regimens are a tremendous advancement in this field, and all hepatitis C patients should have this treatment option considered either on an open-label basis or as part of a clinical trial as these agents become available.

K. R. DeVault, MD

PART EIGHT

ENDOCRINOLOGY, DIABETES, AND METABOLISM

DEREK LeROITH, MD, PHD

Introduction

During 2014 there have been phenomenal advances in endocrinology, both at the basic science levels and in the clinical therapeutic arena.

Looking at the number of outstanding studies that have been published, it is clear that endocrinology is still a leader in new discoveries and our ability to bring to clinical practice newer agents for our patients and their varied conditions.

Obviously, there are too many studies to address in this edition, and therefore I have chosen a few select ones that hopefully will give the reader some insights into both basic and clinically applicable topics.

Derek LeRoith, MD, PhD

51 Calcium and Bone Metabolism

In Vivo Assessment of Bone Quality in Postmenopausal Women with Type 2 Diabetes

Farr JN, Drake MT, Amin S, et al (Mayo Clinic, Rochester, MN)
J Bone Miner Res 29:787-795, 2014

While patients with type 2 diabetes (T2D) are at significant risk for well recognized diabetic complications, including macrovascular disease, retinopathy, nephropathy, and neuropathy, it is also clear that T2D patients are at increased risk for fragility fractures. Furthermore, fragility fractures in patients with T2D occur at higher bone mineral density (BMD) values compared to non-diabetic controls, suggesting abnormalities in bone material strength (BMS) and/or bone microarchitecture (bone "quality"). Thus, we performed *in vivo* microindentation testing of the tibia to directly measure BMS in 60 postmenopausal women (age range, 50–80 yrs) including 30 patients diagnosed with T2D for >10 yrs and 30 age-matched, non-diabetic controls. Regional BMD was measured by DXA; cortical and trabecular bone microarchitecture was assessed from HRpQCT images of the distal radius and tibia. Compared to controls, T2D patients had significantly lower BMS: unadjusted (−11.7%; $p < 0.001$); following adjustment for BMI (−10.5%; $p < 0.001$); and following additional adjustment for age, hypertension, nephropathy, neuropathy, retinopathy, and vascular disease (−9.2%; $p = 0.022$). By contrast, after adjustment for confounding by BMI, T2D patients had bone microarchitecture and BMD that were not significantly different than controls; however, radial cortical porosity tended to be higher in the T2D patients. In addition, patients with T2D had significantly reduced serum markers of bone turnover (all $p < 0.001$) compared to controls. Of note, in patients with T2D, the average glycated hemoglobin level over the previous 10 yrs was negatively correlated with BMS ($r = -0.41$; $p = 0.026$). In conclusion, these findings represent the first demonstration of compromised bone material strength in patients with T2D. Furthermore, our results confirm previous studies demonstrating low bone turnover in patients with T2D and highlight the potential detrimental effects of prolonged hyperglycemia on bone quality. Thus, the skeleton needs to be recognized as another important target tissue subject to diabetic complications.

▶ Patients with type 2 diabetes mellitus have an increased risk of fragility fractures at the hip, spine, and wrist,[1-5] despite having normal or increased bone mineral density (BMD) normalized for body mass index (BMI).[6,7] Data from 3 large prospective observational studies in the United States have recently shown that BMD and the Fracture Risk Assessment Tool (FRAX) underestimate fracture risk for a given femoral neck T-score and age in patients with type 2 diabetes mellitus.[8,9] These observations suggest that an underlying skeletal microstructural or bone material strength abnormalities may be present to explain the increased fracture risk in type 2 diabetes mellitus, but no abnormalities have been identified to date.

This study used *in vivo* microindentation testing of the tibia to assess bone material strength (BMS), dual-energy x-ray absorptiometry (DXA) BMD, and high-resolution peripheral quantitative computed tomography (HRpQCT) scanning to assess microstructural abnormalities in 60 postmenopausal women, 30 of whom had type 2 diabetes mellitus, and 30 of whom were healthy age-matched nondiabetic controls. Patients with type 2 diabetes mellitus had 11.7% lower BMS, 10.5% lower BMS after adjustment for BMI, and 9.2% lower BMS after further adjustment for age, hypertension, nephropathy, neuropathy, retinopathy, and vascular disease compared with the healthy controls. In contrast, DXA BMD and bone microstructure were not different in the diabetics compared with the controls, with radial cortical porosity nonsignificantly mildly increased in the diabetics. Serum markers of bone turnover were all decreased in the diabetics. Average glycated hemoglobin over the preceding 10 years was inversely correlated with BMS.

These findings represent the first demonstration of reduced BMS in postmenopausal women with type 2 diabetes mellitus. The study confirms previous findings of low serum markers of bone turnover in adults with type 2 diabetes mellitus, and the findings suggest that prolonged hyperglycemia may have detrimental effects on the skeleton. Further studies will be required to assess whether abnormalities in bone material strength alone completely explain the increased fracture risk seen in patients with type 2 diabetes mellitus.

B. L. Clarke, MD

References

1. Schwartz AV, Sellmeyer DE, Ensrud KE, et al. Older women with diabetes have an increased risk of fracture: a prospective study. *J Clin Endocrinol Metab*. 2001;86: 32-38.
2. Strotmeyer ES, Cauley JA, Schwartz AV, et al. Nontraumatic fracture risk with diabetes mellitus and impaired fasting glucose in older white and black adults: the health, aging, and body composition study. *Arch Intern Med*. 2005;165:1612-1617.
3. Bonds DE, Larson JC, Schwartz AV, et al. Risk of fracture in women with type 2 diabetes: the Women's Health Initiative Observational Study. *J Clin Endocrinol Metab*. 2006;91:3404-3410.
4. Melton LJ, Leibson CL, Achenbach SJ, Therneau TM, Khosla S. Fracture risk in type 2 diabetes: update of a population-based study. *J Bone Miner Res*. 2008; 23:1334-1342.

5. Janghorbani M, Van Dam RM, Willett WC, Hu FB. Systematic review of type 1 and type 2 diabetes mellitus and risk of fracture. *Am J Epidemiol.* 2007;166: 495-505.
6. Vestergaard P. Discrepancies in bone mineral density and fracture risk in patients with type 1 and type 2 diabetes—a meta-analysis. *Osteoporos Int.* 2007;18: 427-444.
7. Strotmeyer ES, Cauley JA, Schwartz AV, et al. Diabetes is associated independently of body composition with BMD and bone volume in older white and black men and women: The Health, Aging, and Body Composition Study. *J Bone Miner Res.* 2004;19:1084-1091.
8. Schwartz AV, Vittinghoff E, Bauer DC, et al. Association of BMD and FRAX score with risk of fracture in older adults with type 2 diabetes. *JAMA.* 2011;305: 2184-2192.
9. Dawson-Hughes B, Tosteson AN, Melton LJ 3rd, et al. Implications of absolute fracture risk assessment for osteoporosis practice guidelines in the USA. *Osteoporos Int.* 2008;19:449-458.

Fracture risk following bariatric surgery: a population-based study

Nakamura KM, Haglind EGC, Clowes JA, et al (Mayo Clinic, Rochester, MN)
Osteoporos Int 25:151-158, 2014

The effects of bariatric surgery on skeletal health are poorly understood. We found that bariatric surgery patients are more prone to fracture when compared to the general population. While further studies of fracture risk in this population are needed, bone health should be discussed in bariatric surgery clinics.

Introduction.—Bariatric surgery is an increasingly common treatment for medically complicated obesity. Adverse skeletal changes after bariatric surgery have been reported, but their clinical importance remains unknown. We hypothesized that bariatric surgery patients are at increased risk of fracture.

Methods.—We conducted a historical cohort study of fracture incidence among 258 Olmsted County, Minnesota, residents who underwent a first bariatric surgery in 1985–2004. Relative fracture risk was expressed as standardized incidence ratios (SIRs), while potential risk factors were evaluated by hazard ratios (HR) obtained from a time-to-fracture regression model.

Results.—The mean (±SD) body mass index at bariatric surgery was 49.0 ± 8.4 kg/m^2, with an average age of 44 ± 10 years and 82 % (212) females. Gastric bypass surgery was performed in 94 % of cases. Median follow-up was 7.7 years (range, 6 days to 25 years), during which 79 subjects experienced 132 fractures. Relative risk for any fracture was increased 2.3-fold (95 % confidence interval (CI), 1.8–2.8) and was elevated for a first fracture at the hip, spine, wrist, or humerus (SIR, 1.9; 95 % CI, 1.1–2.9), as well as for a first fracture at any other site (SIR, 2.5; 95 % CI, 2.0–3.2). Better preoperative activity status was associated with a lower age-adjusted risk (HR, 0.4; 95 % CI, 0.2–0.8) while prior fracture history was not associated with postoperative fracture risk.

Conclusions.—Bariatric surgery, which is accompanied by substantial biochemical, hormonal, and mechanical changes, is associated with an increased risk of fracture.

▶ Bariatric surgery is increasingly frequently recommended as treatment for obesity in patients with body mass index ≥ 40 kg/m^2, or ≥35 kg/m^2 when complicated by type 2 diabetes mellitus or other disorders.[1-3] In the United States in 2009, 220 000 bariatric surgeries were performed, representing a greater than 10-fold increase over those performed in the previous decade.[4] Long-term skeletal outcomes of bariatric surgery are not well defined. Two previous studies reported increased fracture risk after bariatric surgery,[5,6] whereas evaluation of a large population-based cohort in the United Kingdom showed no evidence of increased fractures after this type of surgery.[7] Malabsorption of calcium, vitamin D, and other nutrients after bariatric surgery could potentially lead to bone loss and increased fractures.

This study was done to assess fracture risk after bariatric surgery in a population-based study of 258 patients in Olmsted County, Minnesota. Most subjects had gastric bypass procedures. Over a median follow-up of 7.7 years, with a range of 6 days to 25 years, 79 patients in the study had 132 fractures. These observations led to an estimate of a 2.3-fold increased first fracture risk after surgery, with increased fractures of the hip, spine, wrist, and humerus observed. First fractures at other sites were also increased by 2.5-fold. More than half of the fractures identified occurred more than 5 years after the surgical procedure. Lesser preoperative physical activity and vitamin D deficiency were associated with increased age-adjusted risk of fracture, whereas presurgical fracture history did not increase postsurgical fracture risk. The study concluded that bariatric surgery led to an increase in fracture risk.

These findings provide further evidence that bariatric surgery may cause adverse skeletal outcomes years after the procedure. The pathophysiologic mechanisms causing the increased fracture risk appeared to be activated early after surgery, and appeared to be sustained over many years, given the relatively uniform divergence in cumulative fracture incidence after surgery compared with expected fracture incidence in the general population. This is the only population-based study to estimate fracture incidence during a long period of follow-up in women and men who have undergone bariatric surgery.

B. L. Clarke, MD

References

1. Centers for Disease Control and Prevention. *Overweight and Obesity,* http://www.cdc.gov/obesity; 2011. Accessed February 21, 2014.
2. Sjöström L, Lindroos AK, Peltonen M, et al. Lifestyle, diabetes, and cardiovascular risk factors 10 years after bariatric surgery. *N Engl J Med.* 2004;351:2683-2693.
3. Adams TD, Gress RE, Smith SC, et al. Long-term mortality after gastric bypass surgery. *N Engl J Med.* 2007;357:753-761.
4. American Society for Metabolic and Bariatric Surgery. *Fact Sheet: Metabolic and Bariatric Surgery,* http://asmbs.org/; 2010. Accessed February 21, 2014.
5. Berarducci A, Haines K, Murr MM. Incidence of bone loss, falls, and fractures after Roux-en-Y gastric bypass for morbid obesity. *Appl Nurs Res.* 2009;22:35-41.

6. Abu-Lebdeh HS, Paat JJ. Are post bariatric surgery fractures different from fractures in severely obese subjects? In: IOF World Congress on Osteoporosis. Florence, Italy. 2010.
7. Lalmohamed A, de Vries F, Bazelier MT, et al. Risk of fracture after bariatric surgery in the United Kingdom: population based, retrospective cohort study. *BMJ*. 2011;345:e5085.

Gonadal Steroids and Body Composition, Strength, and Sexual Function in Men

Finkelstein JS, Lee H, Burnett-Bowie S-AM, et al (Massachusetts General Hosp, Boston)
N Engl J Med 369:1011-1022, 2013

Background.—Current approaches to diagnosing testosterone deficiency do not consider the physiological consequences of various testosterone levels or whether deficiencies of testosterone, estradiol, or both account for clinical manifestations.

Methods.—We provided 198 healthy men 20 to 50 years of age with goserelin acetate (to suppress endogenous testosterone and estradiol) and randomly assigned them to receive a placebo gel or 1.25 g, 2.5 g, 5 g, or 10 g of testosterone gel daily for 16 weeks. Another 202 healthy men received goserelin acetate, placebo gel or testosterone gel, and anastrozole (to suppress the conversion of testosterone to estradiol). Changes in the percentage of body fat and in lean mass were the primary outcomes. Subcutaneous- and intraabdominal-fat areas, thigh-muscle area and strength, and sexual function were also assessed.

Results.—The percentage of body fat increased in groups receiving placebo or 1.25 g or 2.5 g of testosterone daily without anastrozole (mean testosterone level, 44 ± 13 ng per deciliter, 191 ± 78 ng per deciliter, and 337 ± 173 ng per deciliter, respectively). Lean mass and thigh-muscle area decreased in men receiving placebo and in those receiving 1.25 g of testosterone daily without anastrozole. Leg-press strength fell only with placebo administration. In general, sexual desire declined as the testosterone dose was reduced.

Conclusions.—The amount of testosterone required to maintain lean mass, fat mass, strength, and sexual function varied widely in men. Androgen deficiency accounted for decreases in lean mass, muscle size, and strength; estrogen deficiency primarily accounted for increases in body fat; and both contributed to the decline in sexual function. Our findings support changes in the approach to evaluation and management of hypogonadism in men. (Funded by the National Institutes of Health and others; ClinicalTrials.gov number, NCT00114114.)

▶ Hypogonadism in men remains difficult to define. In most cases, a low serum testosterone level and clinical symptoms of hypogonadism are required to make the diagnosis, and much emphasis is placed on the serum testosterone level, especially in older men.[1,2] Usually serum total testosterone more than 2 standard deviations below the mean value in normal young men is considered deficient. Because more than 80% of circulating estradiol in men is derived from aromatization of testosterone,[3] estradiol levels decrease as testosterone levels decline.[4,5] Testosterone treatment is usually given to treat nonspecific symptoms, such as fatigue, lack of energy, or sexual dysfunction, when the serum testosterone level is less than the laboratory reference range.

This study evaluated the relative degree of testosterone deficiency, estradiol deficiency, or both at which undesirable changes in body composition, strength, and sexual function occurred and whether these changes were caused by androgen or estrogen deficiency or both. About 400 men were given the GnRH agonist goserelin acetate to suppress endogenous testosterone and estradiol production. They were then randomly selected to receive different doses of testosterone gel or placebo, with or without anastrozole to inhibit aromatization of testosterone into estradiol, for 16 weeks. Changes in the percentage of body fat, lean mass, subcutaneous and intra-abdominal fat, thigh muscle area and strength, and sexual function were assessed at baseline and at the end of treatment. The study found that lean mass, muscle size, and muscle strength were regulated by androgens, fat accumulation was stimulated by estrogen deficiency, and sexual function was regulated by both androgens and estrogens. However, the amount of testosterone required for an effect varied widely among men.

The findings of this significant study suggest that testosterone replacement alone may not adequately treat the full syndrome of testosterone deficiency. Goal levels of serum testosterone during therapy should likely be individualized based on symptoms in response to treatment. Definition of the degrees of hypogonadism at which each adverse consequence develops and of the relative roles of androgens and estrogens in each outcome will help develop more logical approaches to the diagnosis and treatment of hypogonadism in men.

B. L. Clarke, MD

References

1. Liverman CT, Blazer DG. *Testosterone and Aging: Clinical Research Directions.* Washington, DC: National Academy of Sciences; 2004.
2. Harman SM, Metter EJ, Tobin JD, Pearson J, Blackman MR. Longitudinal effects of aging on serum total and free testosterone levels in healthy men. *J Clin Endocrinol Metab.* 2001;86:724-731.
3. Longcope C, Kato T, Horton R. Conversion of blood androgens to estrogens in normal adult men and women. *J Clin Invest.* 1969;48:2191-2201.
4. Khosla S, Melton LJ III, Atkinson EJ, O'Fallon WM, Klee GG, Riggs BL. Relationship of serum sex steroid levels and bone turnover markers with bone mineral density in men and women: a key role for bioavailable estrogen. *J Clin Endocrinol Metab.* 1998;83:2266-2274.
5. van den Beld AW, de Jong FH, Grobbee DE, Pols HA, Lamberts SW. Measures of bioavailable serum testosterone and estradiol and their relationships with muscle strength, bone density, and body composition in elderly men. *J Clin Endocrinol Metab.* 2000;85:3276-3282.

Persistent Hyperparathyroidism Is a Major Risk Factor for Fractures in the Five Years After Kidney Transplantation

Perrin P, Caillard S, Javier RM, et al (Univ Hosp, Strasbourg, France)

Am J Transplant 13:2653-2663, 2013

The risk of fractures after kidney transplantation is high. Hyperparathyroidism frequently persists after successful kidney transplantation and contributes to bone loss, but its impact on fracture has not been demonstrated. This longitudinal study was designed to evaluate hyperparathyroidism and its associations with mineral disorders and fractures in the 5 posttransplant years. We retrospectively analyzed 143 consecutive patients who underwent kidney transplantation between August 2004 and April 2006. The biochemical parameters were determined at transplantation and at 3, 12 and 60 months posttransplantation, and fractures were recorded. The median intact parathyroid hormone (PTH) level was 334 ng/L (interquartile 151–642) at the time of transplantation and 123 ng/L (interquartile 75–224) at 3 months. Thirty fractures occurred in 22 patients. The receiver operating characteristic (ROC) curve analysis for PTH at 3 months (area under the ROC curve = 0.711, p = 0.002) showed that a good threshold for predicting fractures was 130 ng/L (sensitivity = 81%, specificity = 57%). In a multivariable analysis, independent risk factors for fracture were PTH > 130 ng/L at 3 months (adjusted hazard ratio [AHR] = 7.5, 95% CI 2.18–25.50), and pretransplant osteopenia (AHR = 2.7, 95% CI 1.07–7.26). In summary, this study demonstrates for the first time that persistent hyperparathyroidism is an independent risk factor for fractures after kidney transplantation.

▶ Kidney transplant recipients have higher fracture risk than dialysis patients or the general population.[1-3] Fractures in this population are associated with increased morbidity and mortality,[1] as in other populations. The increased risk of fractures after transplantation results from glucocorticoid therapy,[4] other immunosuppressive medications, diabetes,[5] female sex, and older age.[2] Pre-existing renal osteodystrophy may also play a role, as fracture incidence is associated with duration of dialysis before renal transplantation.[6] After renal transplantation, hyperparathyroidism persists in many patients and contributes to bone loss.[7] The effect of persistent hyperparathyroidism on fractures in renal transplant patients has not yet been found.

This report shows for the first time that persistent hyperparathyroidism is an independent risk factor for fractures after kidney transplantation. The study evaluated fractures in 143 consecutive kidney transplant recipients at an academic medical center over 5 years after transplantation. Measured parathyroid hormone levels were increased at the time of transplantation and gradually decreased over time. Thirty fractures occurred in 22 patients, with fracture risk increased with parathyroid hormone levels greater than 130 pg/mL at 3 months after transplant and with pretransplant osteopenia.

These findings indicate that persistent hyperparathyroidism during the first 5 years after renal transplantation may be associated with increased fracture risk. The study suggests that better control of pre- and posttransplant hyperparathyroidism may help reduce fractures. Randomized studies will be required to show whether cinacalcet reduces fracture risk in renal transplant patients with persistent hyperparathyroidism.

B. L. Clarke, MD

References

1. Abbott KC, Oglesby RJ, Hypolite IO, et al. Hospitalizations for fractures after renal transplantation in the United States. *Ann Epidemiol.* 2001;11:450-457.
2. Ball AM, Gillen DL, Sherrard D, et al. Risk of hip fracture among dialysis and renal transplant recipients. *JAMA.* 2002;288:3014-3018.
3. Grotz WH, Mundinger FA, Gugel B, Exner V, Kirste G, Schollmeyer PJ. Bone fracture and osteodensitometry with dual energy X-ray absorptiometry in kidney transplant recipients. *Transplantation.* 1994;58:912-915.
4. Nikkel LE, Hollenbeak CS, Fox EJ, Uemura T, Ghahramani N. Risk of fractures after renal transplantation in the United States. *Transplantation.* 2009;87:1846-1851.
5. Nisbeth U, Lindh E, Ljunghall S, Backman U, Fellström B. Increased fracture rate in diabetes mellitus and females after renal transplantation. *Transplantation.* 1999;67:1218-1222.
6. O'Shaughnessy EA, Dahl DC, Smith CL, Kasiske BL. Risk factors for fractures in kidney transplantation. *Transplantation.* 2002;74:362-366.
7. Akaberi S, Lindergård B, Simonsen O, Nyberg G. Impact of parathyroid hormone on bone density in long-term renal transplant patients with good graft function. *Transplantation.* 2006;82:749-752.

52 Adrenal Cortex

Reduced Cortisol Metabolism during Critical Illness

Boonen E, Vervenne H, Meersseman P, et al (KU Leuven, Belgium; et al)

N Engl J Med 368:1477-1488, 2013

Background.—Critical illness is often accompanied by hypercortisolemia, which has been attributed to stress-induced activation of the hypothalamic–pituitary–adrenal axis. However, low corticotropin levels have also been reported in critically ill patients, which may be due to reduced cortisol metabolism.

Methods.—In a total of 158 patients in the intensive care unit and 64 matched controls, we tested five aspects of cortisol metabolism: daily levels of corticotropin and cortisol; plasma cortisol clearance, metabolism, and production during infusion of deuterium-labeled steroid hormones as tracers; plasma clearance of 100 mg of hydrocortisone; levels of urinary cortisol metabolites; and levels of messenger RNA and protein in liver and adipose tissue, to assess major cortisol-metabolizing enzymes.

Results.—Total and free circulating cortisol levels were consistently higher in the patients than in controls, whereas corticotropin levels were lower ($P < 0.001$ for both comparisons). Cortisol production was 83% higher in the patients ($P = 0.02$). There was a reduction of more than 50% in cortisol clearance during tracer infusion and after the administration of 100 mg of hydrocortisone in the patients ($P \leq 0.03$ for both comparisons). All these factors accounted for an increase by a factor of 3.5 in plasma cortisol levels in the patients, as compared with controls ($P < 0.001$). Impaired cortisol clearance also correlated with a lower cortisol response to corticotropin stimulation. Reduced cortisol metabolism was associated with reduced inactivation of cortisol in the liver and kidney, as suggested by urinary steroid ratios, tracer kinetics, and assessment of liver-biopsy samples ($P \leq 0.004$ for all comparisons).

Conclusions.—During critical illness, reduced cortisol breakdown, related to suppressed expression and activity of cortisol-metabolizing enzymes, contributed to hypercortisolemia and hence corticotropin suppression. The diagnostic and therapeutic implications for critically ill patients are unknown. (Funded by the Belgian Fund for Scientific Research and others; ClinicalTrials.gov numbers, NCT00512122 and NCT00115479;

and Current Controlled Trials numbers, ISRCTN49433936, ISRCTN 49306926, and ISRCTN08083905.)

▶ This study is noteworthy because it adds significant information to our knowledge of generation and metabolization of cortisol in critically ill patients. With its part on cortisol metabolism, it extends other investigations into the diagnosis of adrenal reserve or glucocorticoid application in intensive care unit (ICU) patients.

The starting point was that patients had very low adrenocorticotropic hormone (ACTH) plasma levels. This is also true for other studies.[1] On the other hand, normal subjects had rather high basal ACTH levels that made the difference between patients and controls unbelievable. Nonetheless, the elevated cortisol levels in ICU patients did not seem to be explained by plasma ACTH values, although ACTH concentrations were inadequately high for plasma cortisol concentrations. This observation stimulated metabolic studies using labeled D4-cortisol (deuterated) showing that the clearance of cortisol is reduced. Although this has been known since the 1950s, the authors elegantly determined the amount or activities of cortisol metabolizing enzymes, including 11β-hydroxysteroid dehydrogenases and 5α and 5β-reductases, which was not possible at that time, and they showed that the activities of these enzymes were reduced indeed. Thus, urinary excretion of glucocorticoids was rather high, but diuresis of inactivated glucocorticoids remained rather low. This result is in support of the initial finding of relatively low ACTH levels as a relative minor causative agent for increased cortisol concentrations in ICU patients. This view is supported by findings of others showing low androgen precursor levels in patients with sepsis.[2] As an alternative explanation, the authors offer that cytokines, including interleukin-6, have a direct influence on adrenal steroidogenesis in critically ill patients. Thus, the results are in concordance with those of an earlier study on the influence of interleukin-6 on corticotropin and its dissociation from cortisol secretion in ill subjects.

H. S. Willenberg, MD

References

1. Marx C, Petros S, Bornstein SR, et al. Adrenocortical hormones in survivors and nonsurvivors of severe sepsis: diverse time course of dehydroepiandrosterone, dehydroepiandrosterone-sulfate, and cortisol. *Crit Care Med.* 2003;31:1382-1388.
2. Mastorakos G, Chrousos GP, Weber JS. Recombinant interleukin-6 activates the hypothalamic-pituitary-adrenal axis in humans. *J Clin Endocrinol Metab.* 1993; 77:1690-1694.

Detection of Circulating Tumor Cells in Patients With Adrenocortical Carcinoma: A Monocentric Preliminary Study

Pinzani P, Scatena C, Salvianti F, et al (Univ of Florence, Italy)
J Clin Endocrinol Metab 98:3731-3738, 2013

Context.—Adrenocortical carcinoma (ACC) is a rare malignancy, the prognosis of which is mainly dependent on stage at diagnosis. The identification of disease-associated markers for early diagnosis and drug monitoring is mandatory. Circulating tumor cells (CTCs) are released into the bloodstream from primary tumor/metastasis. CTC detection in blood samples may have enormous potential for assisting in the diagnosis of malignancy, estimating prognosis, and monitoring the disease.

Objective.—The aim of the study was to investigate the presence of CTCs in blood samples of patients with ACC or benign adrenocortical adenoma (ACA).

Setting.—We conducted the study at a university hospital.

Intervention.—CTC analysis was performed in blood samples from 14 ACC patients and 10 ACA patients. CTCs were isolated on the basis of cell size by filtration through ScreenCell devices, followed by identification according to validated morphometric criteria and immunocytochemistry.

Main Outcome Measure.—We measured the difference in CTC detection between ACC and ACA.

Results.—CTCs were detected in all ACC samples, but not in ACA samples. Immunocytochemistry confirmed the adrenocortical origin. When ACC patients were stratified according to the median value of tumor diameter and metastatic condition, a statistically significant difference was found in the number of CTCs detected after surgery. A significant correlation between the number of CTCs in postsurgical samples and clinical parameters was found for tumor diameter alone.

Conclusions.—Our findings provide the first evidence for adrenocortical tumors that CTCs may represent a useful marker to support differential diagnosis between ACC and ACA. The correlation with some clinical parameters suggests a possible relevance of CTC analysis for prognosis and noninvasive monitoring of disease progression and drug response.

▶ Sometimes it is difficult to safely distinguish between benign or malignant adrenocortical carcinoma (ACC) lesions preoperatively. Usually, computed tomography and magnetic resonance imaging studies are used for characterization of such adrenal lesions. More recently, these techniques have been combined with the information from positron emission tomography studies or with the results of steroid profiling in 24-hour urine samples. Here, the authors tried a different technique, which seemed to be suitable to distinguish malignant from benign disease. They screened blood samples of patients with ACC or benign adrenocortical tumors for the appearance of supposedly circulating tumor cells (CTC) of adrenocortical origin and malignant behavior. This supports the concept of others who used this technique for other tumor types.

However, before such an approach is put into place or facilities offering such a service are established to aid clinicians in their decision process, it is necessary to show that a blinded analysis of blood samples for the presence of CTCs renders similar results. In addition, it is also important to demonstrate that the cells identified as CTCs behave malignantly. Above all, however, it needs to be shown in prospective trials that patients with ACC do not have CTCs when they remain free of disease over the long term when other patients who have CTCs will relapse.

If this technique works reliably, it may become useful in the care of patients with adrenocortical tumors.

H. S. Willenberg, MD

Hypothalamo-pituitary and immune-dependent adrenal regulation during systemic inflammation

Kanczkowski W, Alexaki V-I, Tran N, et al (Technical Univ Dresden, Germany; Univ Dresden, Germany; Univ Hosp Frankfurt, Germany; et al)

Proc Natl Acad Sci U S A 110:14801-14806, 2013

Inflammation-related dysregulation of the hypothalamic–pituitary–adrenal (HPA) axis is central to the course of systemic inflammatory response syndrome or sepsis. The underlying mechanisms, however, are not well understood. Initial activation of adrenocortical hormone production during early sepsis depends on the stimulation of hypothalamus and pituitary mediated by cytokines; in late sepsis, there is a shift from neuroendocrine to local immune–adrenal regulation of glucocorticoid production. Therefore, the modulation of the local immune–adrenal cross talk, and not of the neuroendocrine circuits involved in adrenocorticotropic hormone production, may be more promising in the prevention of the adrenal insufficiency associated with prolonged sepsis. In the present work, we investigated the function of the crucial Toll-like receptor (TLR) adaptor protein myeloid differentiation factor 88 (MyD88) in systemic and local activation of adrenal gland inflammation and glucocorticoid production mediated by lipopolysachharides (LPSs). To this end, we used mice with a conditional MyD88 allele. These mice either were interbred with Mx1 Cre mice, resulting in systemic MyD88 deletion, predominantly in the liver and hematopoietic system, or were crossed with Akr1b7 Cre transgenic mice, resulting thereby in deletion of MyD88, which was adrenocortical-specific. Although reduced adrenal inflammation and HPA-axis activation mediated by LPS were found in $Mx1^{Cre+}$-$MyD88^{fl/fl}$ mice, adrenocortical-specific MyD88 deletion did not alter the adrenal inflammation or HPA-axis activity under systemic inflammatory response syndrome conditions. Thus, our data suggest an important role of immune cell rather than adrenocortical MyD88 for adrenal inflammation and HPA-axis activation mediated by LPS.

▶ In sepsis, the activation of the hypothalamo-pituitary-adrenal (HPA) axis serves the organism for the concentration of its energy metabolism on absolutely essential functions and to prevent a potentially harmful overactivation of the immune system. The stimulation of HPA axis is believed to be mediated by cytokines to a large extent and seems to happen on several levels, including directly in the adrenal gland. This also seems to be the case in experimental animal models using lipopolysaccharides (LPS) as pathogenic agents. LPS particles are ligands of pattern recognition receptors such as toll-like receptors (TLRs), which are expressed on adrenocortical cells as well as immune and other cells. Absence of TLRs has been found to correlate with increased basal levels of corticotropin (TLR2 knock-down) or corticosterone and an enlargement of the adrenal cortex (TLR4 knock-down). In addition, it is associated with a reduced adrenal response in steroidogenesis to LPS. Myeloid differentiation factor 88 (MyD88) is important for TLR signaling and consequent activation of nuclear factor κB. Based on these thoughts, the contribution of adrenal TLR activation to the overall response of the HPA axis to LPS exposure was studied in genetically modified mice models.

The authors found that inactivation of MyD88 in hematopoietic cells, but not in adrenocortical cells, resulted in a decreased secretion of both corticotropin and corticosterone in response to LPS. In addition, mice without MyD88 in their hematopoietic cells displayed reduced LPS-mediated, inflammation-triggered neutrophil recruitment to the adrenal gland and had decreased concentrations of proinflammatory cytokines and chemokines in the adrenal gland as well as in the circulation. However, such observations were not made when MyD88 was absent in adrenocortical cells. Thus, surprisingly, this study suggests that immune cells likely recruited to the adrenal gland rather than steroid-producing cells are the major regulators of the immune-adrenal cross talk as seen in experimental sepsis.

H. S. Willenberg, MD

Mitotane Therapy in Adrenocortical Cancer Induces CYP3A4 and Inhibits 5α-Reductase, Explaining the Need for Personalized Glucocorticoid and Androgen Replacement

Chortis V, Taylor AE, Schneider P, et al (Univ of Birmingham, UK; et al)
J Clin Endocrinol Metab 98:161-171, 2013

Context.—Mitotane [1-(2-chlorophenyl)-1-(4-chlorophenyl)-2,2-dichloro ethane] is the first-line treatment for metastatic adrenocortical carcinoma (ACC) and is also regularly used in the adjuvant setting after presumed complete removal of the primary tumor. Mitotane is considered an adrenolytic substance, but there is limited information on distinct effects on steroidogenesis. However, adrenal insufficiency and male hypogonadism are widely recognized side effects of mitotane treatment.

Objective.—Our objective was to define the impact of mitotane treatment on *in vivo* steroidogenesis in patients with ACC.

Setting and Design.—At seven European specialist referral centers for adrenal tumors, we analyzed 24-h urine samples ($n = 127$) collected from patients with ACC before and during mitotane therapy in the adjuvant setting ($n = 23$) or for metastatic ACC ($n = 104$). Urinary steroid metabolite excretion was profiled by gas chromatography/mass spectrometry in comparison with healthy controls ($n = 88$).

Results.—We found a sharp increase in the excretion of 6β-hydroxycortisol over cortisol ($P < 0.001$), indicative of a strong induction of the major drug-metabolizing enzyme cytochrome P450 3A4. The contribution of 6β-hydroxycortisol to total glucocorticoid metabolites increased from 2% (median, interquartile range 1–4%) to 56% (39–71%) during mitotane treatment. Furthermore, we documented strong inhibition of systemic 5α-reductase activity, indicated by a significant decrease in 5α-reduced steroids, including 5α-tetrahydrocortisol, 5α-tetrahydrocorticosterone, and androsterone (all $P < 0.001$). The degree of inhibition was similar to that in patients with inactivating 5α-reductase type 2 mutations (n = 23) and patients receiving finasteride (n = 5), but cluster analysis of steroid data revealed a pattern of inhibition distinct from these two groups. Longitudinal data showed rapid onset and long-lasting duration of the observed effects.

Conclusions.—Cytochrome P4503A4 induction by mitotane results in rapid inactivation of more than 50% of administered hydrocortisone, explaining the need for doubling hydrocortisone replacement in mitotane-treated patients. Strong inhibition of 5α-reductase activity is in line with the clinical observation of relative inefficiency of testosterone replacement in mitotane-treated men, calling for replacement by 5α-reduced androgens.

▶ Adrenocortical cancer (ACC) is a tumor with high mortality. It harms patients through its malignant behavior and tumor complications but also through other mechanisms, one of which is excess hormone secretion in a substantial number of cases. Treatment of ACC may help patients to prevent tumor-related problems but may also put the patient at risk for medication side effects. The latter includes reversal of hormone excess, increased binding of glucocorticoids, a higher inactivation rate of glucocorticoids, and the formation of intermediate steroids that may interfere with cortisol immunoassays. All these properties of mitotane may facilitate manifestation of adrenal insufficiency. Therefore, every study that better characterizes the action of this compound and the mechanism through which side effects develop is most welcome. The study by Chortis et al yields an explanation for why male patients on mitotane come down with hypogonadism and why testosterone treatment is less effective in such patients than others. This is because 5α-reductase activity declines in the presence of mitotane. Of note, overall steroidogenesis seems to be inhibited by mitotane without affecting 11β-hydroxylase activity, as seen by the decrease in the sum of total androgen and mineralocorticoid metabolites excreted into the urine.

In addition, this study elegantly confirms the incremental inactivation of glucocorticoids and androstenedione through CYP3A4 when mitotane is administered.

H. S. Willenberg, MD

53 Reproductive Endocrinology

In Older Men an Optimal Plasma Testosterone Is Associated With Reduced All-Cause Mortality and Higher Dihydrotestosterone With Reduced Ischemic Heart Disease Mortality, While Estradiol Levels Do Not Predict Mortality

Yeap BB, Alfonso H, Chubb SAP, et al (Univ of Western Australia, Perth, Australia; et al)

J Clin Endocrinol Metab 99:E9-E18, 2014

Context.—Testosterone (T) levels decline with age and lower T has been associated with increased mortality in aging men. However, the associations of its metabolites, dihydrotestosterone (DHT) and estradiol (E_2), with mortality are poorly defined.

Objective.—We assessed associations of T, DHT, and E_2 with all-cause and ischemic heart disease (IHD) mortality in older men.

Participants.—Participants were community-dwelling men aged 70 to 89 years who were residing in Perth, Western Australia.

Main Outcome Measures.—Plasma total T, DHT, and E_2 were assayed using liquid chromatographytandem mass spectrometry in early morning samples collected in 2001 to 2004 from 3690 men. Deaths to December 2010 were ascertained by data linkage.

Results.—There were 974 deaths (26.4%), including 325 of IHD. Men who died had lower baseline T (12.8 ± 5.1 vs 13.2 ± 4.8 nmol/L [mean ± SD], $P = .013$), DHT (1.4 ± 0.7 vs 1.5 ± 0.7 nmol/L, $P = .002$), and E_2 (71.6 ± 29.3 vs 74.0 ± 29.0 pmol/L, $P = .022$). After allowance for other risk factors, T and DHT were associated with all-cause mortality (T: quartile [Q] Q2:Q1, adjusted hazard ratio [HR] = 0.82, $P = .033$; Q3:Q1, HR = 0.78, $P = .010$; Q4:Q1, HR = 0.86, $P > .05$; DHT: Q3:Q1, HR = 0.76, $P = .003$; Q4:Q1, HR = 0.84, $P > .05$). Higher DHT was associated with lower IHD mortality (Q3:Q1, HR = 0.58, $P = .002$; Q4:Q1, HR = 0.69, $P = .026$). E_2 was not associated with either all-cause or IHD mortality.

Conclusions.—Optimal androgen levels are a biomarker for survival because older men with midrange levels of T and DHT had the lowest death rates from any cause, whereas those with higher DHT had lower

IHD mortality. Further investigations of the biological basis for these associations including randomized trials of T supplementation are needed.

▶ Serum testosterone is the main circulating androgen in adult men, but most is bound to sex hormone binding globulin (SHBG), whereas some is bound to albumin, with a lesser amount being free. There is a decline in serum testosterone concentrations as men age but SHBG concentrations increase, which modulates the total concentration and lowers the free testosterone. Whether serum testosterone concentrations are a risk factor for coronary artery disease and death is unresolved. Studies have associated lower testosterone values with poorer health outcomes, including cardiovascular disease (CVD) and mortality. However, men with normal values for testosterone also suffer from CVD and mortality. Correcting low testosterone in men has been associated with lower mortality during follow-up. It is not disputed that testosterone replacement increases lean body mass, lowers body fat, and improves bone health in men. Yeap and associates observed that older men with optimal plasma testosterone concentrations had reduced all-cause mortality and higher dihydrotestosterone (DHT). Ischemic heart disease mortality was also reduced. Estradiol was not a predictor of mortality. Older men with midrange values of testosterone and DHT had the lowest death rates from any cause.[1-7]

A. W. Meikle, MD

References

1. Magnani JW, Moser CB, Murabito JM, et al. Association of sex hormones, aging, and atrial fibrillation in men: the framingham heart study. *Circ Arrhythm Electrophysiol.* 2014;7:307-312.
2. Yeap BB, Flicker L. Hormones and cardiovascular disease in older men. *J Am Med Dir Assoc.* 2014 Feb 11 [Epub ahead of print].
3. Kaplan AL, Trinh QD, Sun M, et al. Testosterone replacement therapy following the diagnosis of prostate cancer: outcomes and utilization trends. *J Sex Med.* 2014; 11:1063-1070.
4. Hilbert-Walter A, Buttner R, Sieber C, Bollheimer C. Testosterone in old age: an up-date. *Dtsch Med Wochenschr.* 2012;137:2117-2122.
5. Yeap BB. Hormones and health outcomes in aging men. *Exp Gerontol.* 2013;48: 677-681.
6. Morris PD, Channer KS. Testosterone and cardiovascular disease in men. *Asian J Androl.* 2012;14:428-435.
7. Lerchbaum E, Pilz S, Boehm BO, Grammer TB, Obermayer-Pietsch B, März W. Combination of low free testosterone and low vitamin D predicts mortality in older men referred for coronary angiography. *Clin Endocrinol (Oxf).* 2012;77:475-483.

Longitudinal Changes in Testosterone Over Five Years in Community-Dwelling Men

Shi Z, Araujo AB, Martin S, et al (Univ of Adelaide, South Australia, Australia; New England Res Insts, Inc, Watertown, MA; et al)
J Clin Endocrinol Metab 98:3289-3297, 2013

Context.—There are few population-based studies reporting longitudinal changes in total T, LH, FSH, and SHBG levels, and there is limited information on risk factors for their change.

Objective.—The objective of the study was to examine 5-year changes in serum T, LH, FSH, and SHBG levels among Australian men.

Design.—The study initially included a randomly selected, community-based cohort of 1588 men age 35 years or older at recruitment (mean age, 54 ± 11 y) with available data at 2 visits. Men on medications known to affect, or with established pathology of, the hypothalamo-pituitary-gonadal axis were excluded, leaving 1382 for analysis.

Results.—Mean baseline and follow-up T levels were 16.2 ± 1.4 and 15.6 ± 1.4 nmol/L, a change of −0.13 nmol/L/y. Annualized T changes were associated with obesity, being unmarried, and smoking at baseline, but not with diabetes, hypertension, or cardiovascular disease. T declined in men who had persistent depression or developed chronic disease, and it increased in men who were married, as compared to unmarried, at both time points. In the multivariate analysis, smoking cessation, development of central obesity (waist ≥100 cm), or generalized obesity (body mass index ≥30 kg/m^2) resulted in T decreases of 0.36, 0.25, and 0.20 nmol/L/y, respectively. Quitting smoking, developing obesity, and having persisting depression were inversely related to SHBG change.

Conclusions.—An age-related decline in T levels is not inevitable but is largely explained by smoking behavior and intercurrent changes in health status, particularly obesity and depression.

▶ Serum testosterone concentrations are determined by many factors, including hypothalamic-pituitary-testicular function, but are also affected by age, obesity, cardiovascular disease, type 2 diabetes, hypertension, depression, smoking, and insulin resistance. Treatment of men with low testosterone has been associated with a reduced risk of mortality over about 2 years. Shi et al did a longitudinal study in men over 5 years and quantitated serum testosterone concentration by mass spectrometry. They evaluated the influence of multiple factors to determine if the decline in testosterone was independent of aging and related to identifiably factors. Lifestyle factors and chronic conditions were found to contribute to the testosterone decline. The strength of the study was that it was a large randomly selected population with accurate measurement of serum testosterone. On the other hand, the study was limited to mainly urban-dwelling white men. Further investigation is required to determine whether reversal of the adverse factors would result in elevation of testosterone.[1-5]

A. W. Meikle, MD

References

1. Meldrum DR. Aging gonads, glands, and gametes: immutable or partially reversible changes? *Fertil Steril.* 2013;99:1-4.
2. Kim YS, Hong D, Lee DJ, Joo NS, Kim KM. Total testosterone may not decline with ageing in Korean men aged 40 years or older. *Clin Endocrinol (Oxf).* 2012; 77:296-301.
3. O'Connor DB, Lee DM, Corona G, et al. The relationships between sex hormones and sexual function in middle-aged and older European men. *J Clin Endocrinol Metab.* 2011;96:E1577-E1587.
4. Grossmann M. Low testosterone in men with type 2 diabetes: significance and treatment. *J Clin Endocrinol Metab.* 2011;96:2341-2353.

5. Bhasin S, Pencina M, Jasuja GK, et al. Reference ranges for testosterone in men generated using liquid chromatography tandem mass spectrometry in a community-based sample of healthy nonobese young men in the Framingham Heart Study and applied to three geographically distinct cohorts. *J Clin Endocrinol Metab*. 2011;96:2430-2439.

Bone Marrow Fat Composition as a Novel Imaging Biomarker in Postmenopausal Women With Prevalent Fragility Fractures

Patsch JM, Li X, Baum T, et al (Univ of California San Francisco)

J Bone Miner Res 28:1721-1728, 2013

The goal of this magnetic resonance (MR) imaging study was to quantify vertebral bone marrow fat content and composition in diabetic and nondiabetic postmenopausal women with fragility fractures and to compare them with nonfracture controls with and without type 2 diabetes mellitus. Sixty-nine postmenopausal women (mean age 63 ± 5 years) were recruited. Thirty-six patients (47.8%) had spinal and/or peripheral fragility fractures. Seventeen fracture patients were diabetic. Thirty-three women (52.2%) were nonfracture controls. Sixteen women were diabetic nonfracture controls. To quantify vertebral bone marrow fat content and composition, patients underwent MR spectroscopy (MRS) of the lumbar spine at 3 Tesla. Bone mineral density (BMD) was determined by dual-energy X-ray absorptiometry (DXA) of the hip and lumbar spine (LS) and quantitative computed tomography (QCT) of the LS. To evaluate associations of vertebral marrow fat content and composition with spinal and/or peripheral fragility fractures and diabetes, we used linear regression models adjusted for age, race, and spine volumetric bone mineral density (vBMD) by QCT. At the LS, nondiabetic and diabetic fracture patients had lower vBMD than controls and diabetics without fractures ($p = 0.018$; $p = 0.005$). However, areal bone mineral density (aBMD) by DXA did not differ between fracture and nonfracture patients. After adjustment for age, race, and spinal vBMD, the prevalence of fragility fractures was associated with −1.7% lower unsaturation levels (confidence interval [CI] −2.8% to −0.5%, $p = 0.005$) and +2.9% higher saturation levels (CI 0.5% to 5.3%, $p = 0.017$). Diabetes was associated with −1.3% (CI −2.3% to −0.2%, $p = 0.018$) lower unsaturation and +3.3% (CI 1.1% to 5.4%, $p = 0.004$) higher saturation levels. Diabetics with fractures had the lowest marrow unsaturation and highest saturation. There were no associations of marrow fat content with diabetes or fracture. Our results suggest that altered bone marrow fat composition is linked with fragility fractures and diabetes. MRS of spinal bone marrow fat may therefore serve as a novel tool for BMD-independent fracture risk assessment (Fig 2).

▶ Links between bone and adipose tissue have been investigated. One link is that mesenchymal stem cells and osteoblasts and adipocytes have a common origin. Another link is that aging and estrogen deficiency, which are associated

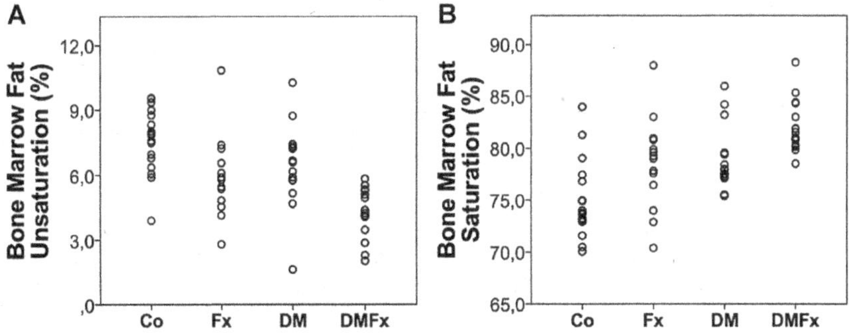

FIGURE 2.—Bone marrow fat composition in controls (Co), postmenopausal women with fragility fractures (Fx), diabetic postmenopausal women without fractures (DM), and diabetic postmenopausal women with fragility fractures (DMFx). (*A*) Unsaturation levels. (*B*) Saturation levels. (Reproduced from Journal of Bone and Mineral Research. Patsch JM, Li X, Baum T, et al. Bone marrow fat composition as a novel imaging biomarker in postmenopausal women with prevalent fragility fractures. *J Bone Miner Res.* 2013;28:1721-1728, with permission from the American Society for Bone and Mineral Research.)

with osteoporosis, are associated with lower osteogenic and more fat cell linage derived from mesenchymal stem cells. Disorders associated with alteration in fat or fat distribution are observed to have lower bone density. With an interest in bone marrow fat and osteoporosis, noninvasive imaging techniques, such as magnetic resonance spectroscopy, are being used to assess bone quality. Patsch et al investigated the bone marrow fat composition with new imaging techniques with the goal of evaluating fragility fractures. They found that altered bone marrow fat was associated with fragility fractures and diabetes. How lower unsaturated fat and higher saturation concentrations of bone marrow predispose to fragility fractures requires additional investigation. Total marrow fat content did not differ between those with fractures and those without, irrespective of diabetes. Another surprising finding was that lower unsaturated fat and higher saturated fat components predisposed to a higher fracture risk.

A. W. Meikle, MD

Abrupt decrease in serum testosterone levels after an oral glucose load in men: implications for screening for hypogonadism

Caronia LM, Dwyer AA, Hayden D, et al (Massachusetts General Hosp, Boston; Centre Hospitalier Universitaire Vaudois, Lausanne, Switzerland; et al)
Clin Endocrinol 78:291-296, 2013

Objective.—This study examines the physiological impact of a glucose load on serum testosterone (T) levels in men with varying glucose tolerance (GT).

Design.—Cross-sectional study.

Patients and Methods.—74 men (19–74 years, mean 51·4 ± 1·4 years) underwent a standard 75-g oral glucose tolerance test with blood sampling at 0, 30, 60, 90 and 120 min. Fasting serum glucose, insulin, total T (and calculated free T), LH, SHBG, leptin and cortisol were measured.

Results.—57% of the men had normal GT, 30% had impaired GT and 13% had newly diagnosed type 2 diabetes. Glucose ingestion was associated with a 25% decrease in mean T levels (delta = −4·2 ± 0·3 nm, $P < 0{\cdot}0001$). T levels remained suppressed at 120 min compared with baseline (13·7 ± 0·6 vs 16·5 ± 0·7 nm, $P < 0{\cdot}0001$) and did not differ across GT or BMI. Of the 66 men with normal T levels at baseline, 10 (15%) had levels that decreased to the hypogonadal range (<9·7 nm) at one or more time points. SHBG, LH and cortisol levels were unchanged. Leptin levels decreased from baseline at all time points ($P < 0{\cdot}0001$).

Conclusions.—Glucose ingestion induces a significant reduction in total and free T levels in men, which is similar across the spectrum of glucose tolerance. This decrease in T appears to be because of a direct testicular defect, but the absence of compensatory changes in LH suggests an additional central component. Men found to have low nonfasting T levels should be re-evaluated in the fasting state (Fig 1).

▶ Several factors affect serum testosterone concentrations in men. Dysfunction of the hypothalamus, pituitary, and Leydig cells are well-characterized abnormalities. Others are less likely to be fully characterized for a mechanism. The associations with testosterone deficiency include obesity, the metabolic syndrome, type 2 diabetes associated with insulin resistance, aging, circadian variation, and nutrient ingestion, which was associated with a 15% to 40% postprandial decline in testosterone or no change.[1-4] The study by Caronia et al observed a decrease in serum testosterone concentration after oral ingestion of glucose. They invoked a direct glucose effect on the testes, but also a possible central effect because there was no apparent change in serum luteinizing hormone. The authors suggest that dietary intake should be taken into

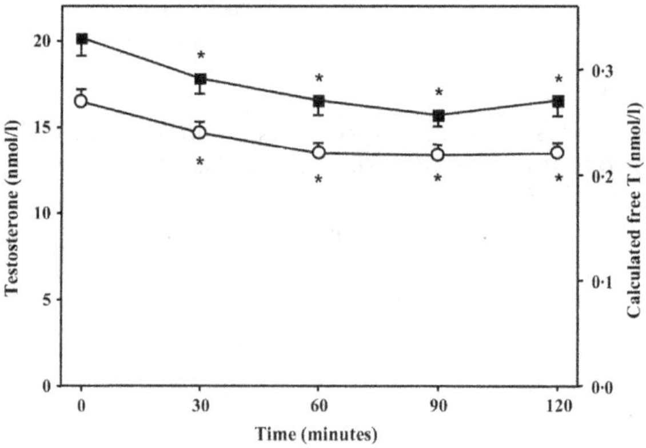

FIGURE 1.—Changes in total testosterone (○) and calculated free testosterone (■) in response to a 75-g oral glucose load ($n = 74$). Each time point represents mean ± SEM, asterisks (*) denote change from baseline ($P < 0{\cdot}0001$). (Reprinted from Caronia LM, Dwyer AA, Hayden D, et al. Abrupt decrease in serum testosterone levels after an oral glucose load in men: implications for screening for hypogonadism. *Clin Endocrinol.* 2013;78:291-296, with acknowledgement of Wiley-Blackwell.)

consideration when measuring serum testosterone concentrations in men being evaluated for deficiency. A morning blood collection should be taken before breakfast in men suspected of testosterone deficiency. This would control for dietary as well as circadian variation in testosterone secretion.

A. W. Meikle, MD

References

1. Bhasin S, Cunningham GR, Hayes FJ, et al. Testosterone therapy in men with androgen deficiency syndromes: an Endocrine Society clinical practice guideline. *J Clin Endocrinol Metab.* 2010;95:2536-2559.
2. Meikle AW, Stringham JD, Woodward MG, et al. Effects of a fat-containing meal on sex hormones in men. *Metabolism.* 1990;39:943-946.
3. Habito RC, Ball MJ. Postprandial changes in sex hormones after meals of different composition. *Metabolism.* 2001;50:505-511.
4. Volek JS, Gómez AL, Love DM, Avery NG, Sharman MJ, Kraemer WJ. Effects of a high-fat diet on postabsorptive and postprandial testosterone responses to a fat-rich meal. *Metabolism.* 2001;50:1351-1355.

Determinants of testosterone recovery after bariatric surgery: is it only a matter of reduction of body mass index?

Luconi M, Samavat J, Seghieri G, et al (Univ of Florence, Italy; General Hosp, Pistoia, Italy; et al)

Fertil Steril 99:1872-1879.e1, 2013

Objective.—To explore the correlation models between body mass index (BMI) and sex hormones constructed from a male cross-sectional survey and evaluate the effects of surgery-induced weight loss on sex hormones in morbidly obese subjects that are not predicted by the constructed BMI correlation models.

Design.—Cross-sectional population and longitudinal studies.

Setting.—Bariatric surgery center in a university hospital.

Patient(s).—A cross-sectional survey of a male general population of 161 patients (BMI median [interquartile range] = 29.2 [24.8–41.9] kg/m^2) in addition to 24 morbidly obese subjects (BMI = 43.9 [40.8–53.8] kg/m^2) who were undergoing bariatric surgery were prospectively studied for 6 and 12 months.

Intervention(s).—Bariatric surgery on 24 morbidly obese men.

Main Outcome Measure(s).—Cross-sectional population: construction of the best-fitting models describing the relationship between baseline BMI with total (TT) and calculated free (cFT) testosterone, E_2, sex hormone–binding globulin (SHBG), FSH, and LH levels. Longitudinal study deviation between the observed sex hormone levels at 6- and 12-month follow-up and those expected on BMI bases.

Result(s).—The correlation of BMI with sex hormones was not univocally linear (E_2), but the best-fitting model was exponential for TT, cFT, FSH, LH, and TT/E_2 and power for SHBG. In addition to the significant improvement of all parameters observed after surgery in the longitudinal cohort, the increase in TT and SHBG, but not in cFT, was significantly higher than expected from the corresponding weight loss at 6 months from surgery (14.80 [12.30–19.00] nM vs. 12.77 [10.92–13.64] nM and 40.0 [28.9–54.5] nM vs. 24.7 [22.5–25.8] nM for TT and SHBG, respectively), remaining rather stable at 12 months.

Conclusion(s).—The increase in TT and SHBG, but not the increase in cFT, after bariatric surgery is greater than expected based on weight loss (Fig 1).

▶ Obesity in men is associated with several alterations in endocrine and reproductive abnormalities. Total testosterone and sex hormone binding globulin (SHBG) are reduced and estrogen is increased. There is failure of a compensatory increase in gonadotropins. Other factors affecting the gonads in obese men are leptin, kisspeptin, and adipokines. The mechanism for this alteration requires additional study. Few studies have investigated men with morbid obesity before and after weight loss from bariatric surgery.[1-5] Luconi et al extended prior studies by using mathematical models correlating body mass index with different sex hormones or assessing determinates of changes in sex hormone with losing weight. Surgery did not produce a significantly higher recovery of

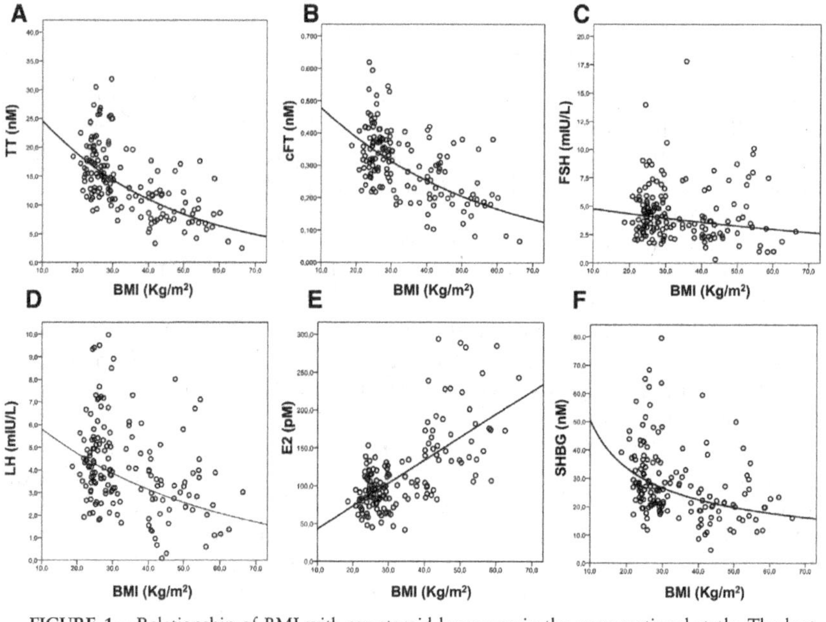

FIGURE 1.—Relationship of BMI with sex steroid hormones in the cross-sectional study. The best-fitting regression curves are shown for the relationship between BMI and TT (A, exponential model), cFT (B, exponential model), FSH (C, exponential model), LH (D, exponential model), E_2 (E, linear model), and SHBG (F, power model) in the cross-sectional cohort of subjects composed of population- and clinic-based samples. Relative equations and parameters are reported in Table 2. (Reprinted from Fertility and Sterility. Luconi M, Samavat J, Seghieri G, et al. Determinants of testosterone recovery after bariatric surgery: is it only a matter of reduction of body mass index? *Fertil Steril.* 2013;99:1872-1879.e1, Copyright 2013, with permission from American Society for Reproductive Medicine.)

gonadotropins as observed for SHGB and total testosterone. They postulated that the recovery of the hypothalamic-pituitary-gonadal axis after weight loss has a longer latency requiring a longer follow-up. The study has several limitations, including surgery-induced weight loss, total testosterone, and SHBG in morbid obesity. Confirmation of the results requires a larger study and a longer follow-up.

A. W. Meikle, MD

References

1. Corona G, Rastrelli G, Monami M, et al. Body weight loss reverts obesity-associated hypogonadotropic hypogonadism: a systematic review and meta-analysis. *Eur J Endocrinol.* 2013;168:829-843.
2. Hammoud AO, Meikle AW, Reis LO, Gibson M, Peterson CM, Carrell DT. Obesity and male infertility: a practical approach. *Semin Reprod Med.* 2012;30: 486-495.
3. Hammoud A, Gibson M, Hunt SC, et al. Effect of Roux-en-Y gastric bypass surgery on the sex steroids and quality of life in obese men. *J Clin Endocrinol Metab.* 2009;94:1329-1332.
4. Hammoud AO, Gibson M, Peterson CM, Meikle AW, Carrell DT. Impact of male obesity on infertility: a critical review of the current literature. *Fertil Steril.* 2008; 90:897-904.
5. Hammoud AO, Wilde N, Gibson M, Parks A, Carrell DT, Meikle AW. Male obesity and alteration in sperm parameters. *Fertil Steril.* 2008;90:2222-2225.

Symptomatic Reduction in Free Testosterone Levels Secondary to Crizotinib Use in Male Cancer Patients

Weickhardt AJ, Doebele RC, Purcell WT, et al (Univ of Colorado Anschutz Med Campus, Aurora; et al)

Cancer 119:2383-2390, 2013

Background.—Crizotinib is a tyrosine kinase inhibitor active against *ALK*, *MET*, and *ROS1*. We previously reported that crizotinib decreases testosterone in male patients. The detailed etiology of the effect, its symptomatic significance, and the effectiveness of subsequent testosterone replacement have not been previously reported.

Methods.—Male cancer patients treated with crizotinib had total testosterone levels measured and results compared with non-crizotinib-treated patients. Albumin, sex hormone-binding globulin (SHBG), follicle-stimulating hormone (FSH), and/or luteinizing hormone (LH) were tracked longitudinally. A subset of patients had free testosterone levels measured and a hypogonadal screening questionnaire administered. Patients receiving subsequent testosterone supplementation were assessed for symptomatic improvement.

Results.—Mean total testosterone levels were −25% below the lower limit of normal (LLN) in 32 crizotinib-treated patients (27 of 32 patients below LLN, 84%) compared with +29% above LLN in 19 non-crizotinib-treated patients (6 of 19 below LLN, 32%), $P = .0012$. Levels of albumin and SHBG (which both bind testosterone) declined rapidly with crizotinib,

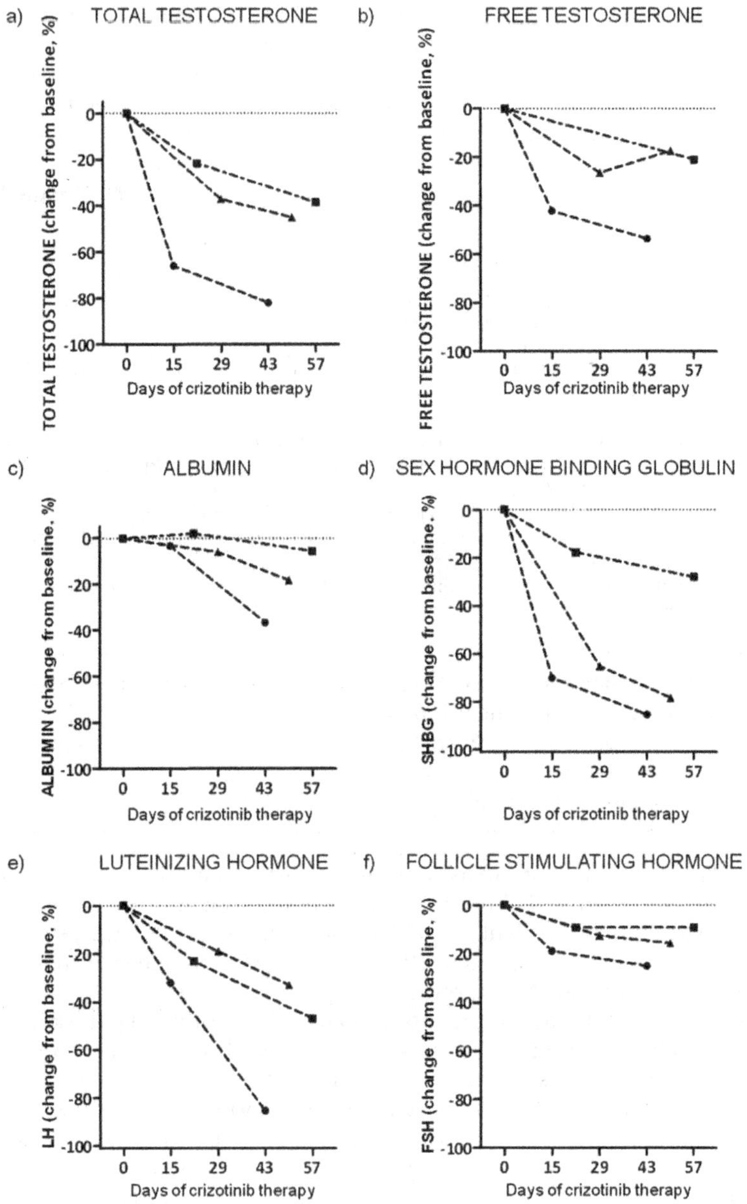

FIGURE 4.—Dynamic assessment of sex hormones and testosterone-binding proteins in 3 patients commenced on crizotinib, showing decrease in total and free testosterone relative to baseline measurement, as well as rapid decreases in LH and FSH, albumin, and sex hormone-binding globulin. (Reprinted from Cancer. Weickhardt AJ, Doebele RC, Purcell WT, et al. Symptomatic reduction in free testosterone levels secondary to crizotinib use in male cancer patients. *Cancer.* 2013;119:2383-2390, Copyright 2013, American Cancer Society. This material is reproduced with permission of Wiley-Liss, Inc., a subsidiary of John Wiley & Sons, Inc., www.interscience.wiley.com.)

but so did FSH, LH, and free testosterone, suggesting a centrally mediated, true hypogonadal effect. Mean free testosterone levels were, −17% below LLN (19 of 25 patients below LLN, 76%). Eighty-four percent (16 of 19) with low free levels, and 79% (19/24) with low total levels had symptoms of androgen deficiency. Five of 9 patients (55%) with low testosterone given testosterone supplementation had improvement in symptoms, coincident with increases in testosterone above LLN.

Conclusions.—Symptoms of androgen deficiency and free or total/free testosterone levels should be tracked in male patients on crizotinib with consideration of testosterone replacement as appropriate (Fig 4).

▶ Crizotinib is an inhibitor of tyrosine kinases and is used to treat various tumors, including anaplastic lymphoma and non-small cell lung cancer.[1] The drug was also observed to decrease serum testosterone concentrations to less than normal in men. The effect on testosterone was reversible and appeared to be suppressed by a central mechanism. It is uncertain whether some of the side effects of crizotinib are drug related or from testosterone deficiency. The study by Weickhardt et al investigated the mechanism for the reduction in testosterone after treatment with crizotinib.[2] They observed that the main binding proteins for testosterone (sex hormone-binding globulin and albumin) declined rapidly, but so did follicle-stimulating hormone, luteinizing hormone, and free testosterone, suggesting that the effect of crizotinib was central. It is unresolved if the effect of crizotinib is at the pituitary or hypothalamic level.[3] Additional studies are needed to determine the mechanism of crizotinib on inhibiting testosterone secretion, and it will likely involve the hypothalamus.

A. W. Meikle, MD

References

1. Timm A, Kolesar JM. Crizotinib for the treatment of non-small-cell lung cancer. *Am J Health Syst Pharm.* 2013;70:943-947.
2. Weickhardt AJ, Rothman MS, Salian-Mehta S, et al. Rapid-onset hypogonadism secondary to crizotinib use in men with metastatic nonsmall cell lung cancer. *Cancer.* 2012;118:5302-5309.
3. Ramalingam SS, Shaw AT. Hypogonadism related to crizotinib therapy: implications for patient care. *Cancer.* 2012;118:E1-E2.

54 Pediatric Endocrinology

Parathyroid Hormone as a Functional Indicator of Vitamin D Sufficiency in Children

Maguire JL, Birken C, Thorpe KE, et al (Univ of Toronto, Ontario, Canada; et al)

JAMA Pediatr 2014 [Epub ahead of print]

There has been debate on what constitutes physiologically normal 25-hydroxyvitamin D serum levels in children. The Institute of Medicine and the American Academy of Pediatrics have recommended that 25-hydroxyvitamin D levels in children be more than 50 nmol/L. The Canadian Paediatric Society has suggested that 25-hydroxyvitamin D levels be more than 75 nmol/L. Given the long time course for the development of chronic health outcomes that may be related to low vitamin D levels in children, physiological indicators of vitamin D sufficiency would be helpful.

One physiological indicator of bone health is parathyroid hormone (PTH). Studies of adults have identified that PTH levels cease to decline at 25-hydroxyvitamin D levels typically more than 75 nmol/L, suggesting physiological vitamin D sufficiency. In children, identifying such a plateau has been elusive. To address this, we conducted a study of healthy young children to determine whether a 25-hydroxyvitamin D plateau exists above which serum PTH is minimized (Fig).

▶ A potential deleterious effect of vitamin D insufficiency on human health has been a hot topic for quite a long time. This is hardly surprising when one considers the multitude of conditions for which insufficient vitamin D has been implicated as a risk factor. These have included everything from type 1 diabetes to schizophrenia to numerous cancers to multiple sclerosis to an earlier age of menarche in girls! Although these observations do not establish causality, the sheer magnitude of the evidence linking low serum vitamin D concentrations to adverse outcomes highlights that ensuring vitamin D sufficiency in children is paramount. Despite general unanimity on this issue, defining the precise level that signifies that 25-hydroxy vitamin D stores are replete has been enigmatic. Thus, this report represents an important contribution to this area. Particular strengths include the large sample size, the inclusion of subjects on vitamin D supplementation, and the young age of the participants. As seen in the figure, the inflection point for parathyroid hormone occurred at an approximate vitamin

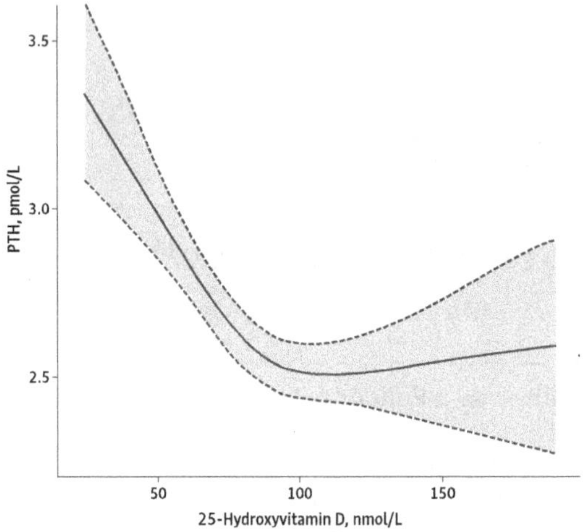

FIGURE.—Plot of the Regression Model for 25-Hydroxyvitamin D and Parathyroid Hormone (PTH). Shaded areas inside the dashed lines represent 95% confidence intervals. (Reprinted from Maguire JL, Birken C, Thorpe KE, et al. Parathyroid hormone as a functional indicator of vitamin D sufficiency in children. *JAMA Pediatr.* 2014;[Epub ahead of print], with permission from American Medical Association.)

D concentration of 100 nmol/L (40 ng/dL). Not surprisingly, this is considerably higher than has been observed in adults. Additional studies such as this in older children and adolescents would be wonderful. In the meantime, this study finally provides concrete guidance to pediatricians regarding target serum vitamin D concentrations in our young patients.

E. Eugster, MD

Onset of Breast Development in a Longitudinal Cohort

Biro FM, Greenspan LC, Galvez MP, et al (Cincinnati Children's Hosp Med Ctr, OH; Kaiser Permanente, San Francisco, CA; Mount Sinai School of Medicine, NY; et al)

Pediatrics 132:1019-1027, 2013

Background and Objectives.—There is growing evidence of pubertal maturation occurring at earlier ages, with many studies based on cross-sectional observations. This study examined age at onset of breast development (thelarche), and the impact of BMI and race/ethnicity, in the 3 puberty study sites of the Breast Cancer and the Environment Research Program, a prospective cohort of >1200 girls.

Methods.—Girls, 6 to 8 years at enrollment, were followed longitudinally at regular intervals from 2004 to 2011 in 3 geographic areas: the San Francisco Bay Area, Greater Cincinnati, and New York City. Sexual maturity assessment using Tanner staging was conducted by using standardized observation and palpation methods by trained and certified staff. Kaplan-Meier analyses were used to describe age at onset of breast maturation by covariates.

Results.—The age at onset of breast stage 2 varied by race/ethnicity, BMI at baseline, and site. Median age at onset of breast stage 2 was 8.8, 9.3, 9.7, and 9.7 years for African American, Hispanic, white non-Hispanic, and Asian participants, respectively. Girls with greater BMI reached breast stage 2 at younger ages. Age-specific and standardized prevalence of breast maturation was contrasted to observations in 2 large cross-sectional studies conducted 10 to 20 years earlier (Pediatric Research in Office Settings and National Health and Nutrition Examination Survey III) and found to have occurred earlier among white, non-Hispanic, but not African American girls.

Conclusions.—We observed the onset of thelarche at younger ages than previously documented, with important differences associated with race/ethnicity and BMI, confirming and extending patterns seen previously. These findings are consistent with temporal changes in BMI (Fig 1).

► This is yet another study from the Breast Cancer and the Environment Research Program that joins a squad of similar reports implicating an earlier onset of puberty in girls. Particular strengths of this project include its substantive sample size, prospective nature, and inclusion of subjects with a range of ethnicities, body mass indexes (BMIs), and geographical settings. One of the main aspects of this particular study, which investigated average age at thelarche in girls, was a comparison of the current findings with those reported from 2 previous cross-sectional studies of pubertal timing in girls, one of which was published more than 16 years ago. Although the authors tout their

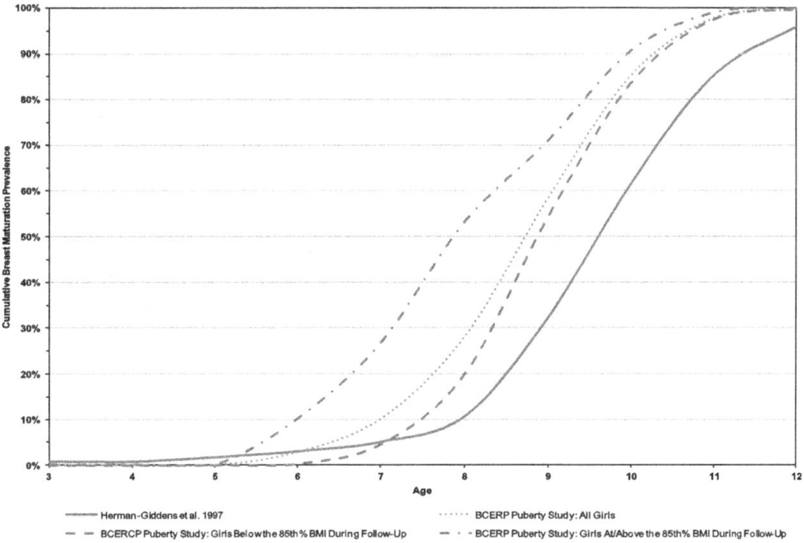

FIGURE 1.—Comparing the cumulative prevalence of Breast Stage 2+ for non-Hispanic white participants between the BCERP Puberty Study and PROS.[9] *Editor's Note*: Please refer to original journal article for full references. (Reproduced with permission from Pediatrics. Biro FM, Greenspan LC, Galvez MP, et al. Onset of breast development in a longitudinal cohort. *Pediatrics*. 2013;132:1019-1027, Copyright 2013, with permission from American Academy of Pediatrics.)

finding of overall earlier breast development in white girls as evidence for a continued secular trend, in fact, no difference was seen in this metric in girls with BMIs less than 85th percentile between the 2 studies, as seen in Fig 1. This observation, along with the finding of similar ages of Tanner II breast development in African-American girls in the current as well as the previous study, argues against any such trend. As has been noted in a plethora of similar reports, a higher BMI was statistically associated with earlier breast development, suggesting a direct relationship between the obesity epidemic and pubertal onset in girls. Whether this is caused by actual HPG axis activation or is occurring as a result of endocrine disrupting chemicals remains to be elucidated. An even more fundamental question, however, is whether the observed breast enlargement truly represents glandular breast tissue rather than adipose, particularly in the overweight cohort. Until studies such as this one incorporate objective biochemical markers such as kisspeptin, peak stimulated or random ultrasensitive luteinizing hormone, or pelvic ultrasound scans, it is likely premature to conclude that the controversy[1] regarding whether pubertal timing is continuing to decline is behind us!

E. Eugster, MD

Reference

1. Herman-Giddens ME. The enigmatic pursuit of puberty in girls. *Pediatrics*. 2013; 132:1125-1126.

55 Neuroendocrinology

Progression of Vertebral Fractures Despite Long-Term Biochemical Control of Acromegaly: A Prospective Follow-up Study

Claessen KMJA, Kroon HM, Pereira AM, et al (Leiden Univ Med Ctr, The Netherlands)

J Clin Endocrinol Metab 98:4808-4815, 2013

Background.—In active acromegaly, pathologically elevated GH and IGF-1 levels are associated with increased bone turnover and a high bone mass, the latter being sustained after normalization of GH values. In a cross-sectional study design, we have previously reported a high prevalence of vertebral fractures (VFs) of about 60% in patients with controlled acromegaly, despite normal mean bone mineral density (BMD) values. Whether these fractures occur during the active acromegaly phase or after remission is achieved is not known.

Objective.—Our objective was to study the natural progression of VFs and contributing risk factors in patients with controlled acromegaly over a 2.5-year follow-up period.

Methods.—Forty-nine patients (mean age 61.3 ± 11.1 years, 37% female) with controlled acromegaly for ≥2 years after surgery, irradiation, and/or medical therapy and not using bisphosphonates were included in the study. Conventional spine radiographs including vertebrae Th4–L4 were assessed for VFs according to the Genant method. VF progression was defined as development of new/incident fractures and/or a minimum 1-point increase in the Genant scoring of preexisting VFs. BMD was assessed by dual-energy x-ray absorptiometry (Hologic 4500).

Results.—Prevalence of baseline VFs was 63%, being highest in men, and fractures were unrelated to baseline BMD. VF progression was documented in 20% of patients, especially in men and in case of ≥2 VFs at baseline. VF progression was not related to BMD values or BMD changes over time.

Conclusion.—Findings from this longitudinal study show that VFs progress in the long term in 20% of patients with biochemically controlled acromegaly in the absence of osteoporosis or osteopenia. These data suggest that an abnormal bone quality persists in these patients after remission, possibly related to pretreatment long-term exposure to high circulating levels of GH.

▶ Acromegaly is a devastating disease affecting many organs. Clinically relevant consequences include acral changes, metabolic disturbances, heart disease, sleep apnea syndrome, and tumor development. With respect to bone, it is still unclear whether development of osteoporosis in some patients is due to growth hormone excess or the presence of hypogonadism. Importantly, there appears to be a dissociation between bone mineral density usually used to screen for osteoporosis and real incidence of vertebral fractures. This study demonstrates vertebral fractures in nearly two-thirds of patients with controlled acromegaly (without any relation to bone mineral density), with additional fractures developing in 20% over a follow-up period of 2.5 years. Therefore, risk factors for vertebral fractures appear to persist even with long-term control of acromegaly, making bone changes one of the most debilitating long-term consequences of acromegaly.

Because assessment of bone mineral density was not able to predict the risk for bone fractures in those patients and other clear predictive parameters are not apparent, screening for vertebral fractures in patients with acromegaly by conventional spine radiographs should be included in the routine follow-up programs.

S. Petersenn, MD

A Cross-Sectional Study of the Prevalence of Cardiac Valvular Abnormalities in Hyperprolactinemic Patients Treated With Ergot-Derived Dopamine Agonists

Drake WM, on behalf of the UK Dopamine Agonist Valvulopathy Group (St Bartholomew's Hosp, London, UK; et al)
J Clin Endocrinol Metab 99:90-96, 2014

Context.—Concern exists in the literature that the long-term use of ergot-derived dopamine agonist drugs for the treatment of hyperprolactinemia may be associated with clinically significant valvular heart disease.

Objective.—The aim of the study was to determine the prevalence of valvular heart abnormalities in patients taking dopamine agonists as treatment for lactotrope pituitary tumors and to explore any associations with the cumulative dose of drug used.

Design.—A cross-sectional echocardiographic study was performed in a large group of patients who were receiving dopamine agonist therapy for hyperprolactinemia. Studies were performed in accordance with the British Society of Echocardiography minimum dataset for a standard adult transthoracic echocardiogram. Poisson regression was used to calculate relative risks according to quartiles of dopamine agonist cumulative dose using the lowest cumulative dose quartile as the reference group.

Setting.—Twenty-eight centers of secondary/tertiary endocrine care across the United Kingdom participated in the study.

Results.—Data from 747 patients (251 males; median age, 42 y; interquartile range [IQR], 34–52 y) were collected. A total of 601 patients had taken cabergoline alone; 36 had been treated with bromocriptine alone; and 110 had received both drugs at some stage. The median cumulative dose for cabergoline was 152 mg (IQR, 50–348 mg), and for bromocriptine it was 7815 mg (IQR, 1764–20 477 mg). A total of 28 cases of moderate valvular stenosis or regurgitation were observed in 24 (3.2%) patients. No associations were observed between cumulative doses of dopamine agonist used and the age-corrected prevalence of any valvular abnormality.

Conclusion.—This large UK cross-sectional study does not support a clinically concerning association between the use of dopamine agonists for the treatment of hyperprolactinemia and cardiac valvulopathy.

▶ Surgery is considered the primary treatment option for many pituitary adenomas, offering the chance of cure. However, potential side effects include pituitary insufficiency and local complications. Furthermore, tumors extending into the lateral cavernous sinus may not be completely resectable even in the hands of the most experienced neurosurgeon. Interestingly, for prolactinoma, one of the most frequent entities of pituitary adenomas, medical treatment with a dopamine agonist has been well established. It offers both control of prolactin hypersecretion and tumor proliferation and is well tolerated by most patients. However, because treatment is lifelong in the majority of patients, some side effects may be recognized only after many years, as recently demonstrated for clinically significant valvular heart disease in patients treated with high doses of dopamine agonists for Parkinson disease.[1,2]

Those publications posed new questions with respect to the medical treatment of prolactinoma and whether surgery should be reconsidered in patients with resectable tumors. Although most studies did not find an increased risk for the lower doses of dopamine agonists used for prolactinoma, the underlying analyses may have had insufficient power to detect theses changes because of the relatively small number of patients and years of follow-up.

A recent large cohort study[3] from Denmark did not find any increased incidence of valve heart disease but relied on diagnosis encoded in the Danish National Registry of Patients, without any sufficient information on both the frequency of echocardiography in these patients and clinically undetected valve disease.

The current study of 28 centers of endocrine care across the United Kingdom required a transthoracic echocardiogram in all patients. Again, no clear association was found between cumulative doses of bromocriptine and cabergoline and the prevalence of valvular abnormalities. These data may assure patients that treatment doses used for prolactinoma do not pose a significant risk for valvular heart disease. However, we probably have to wait for reports of longer treatment times because the follow-up times are still relatively short compared with the life expectancy of patients after diagnosis of prolactinoma. Furthermore, we need more information on other dopamine agonists; for example, quinagolide is thought not to cause valvular changes because of its receptor selectivity.

S. Petersenn, MD

References

1. Zanettini R, Antonini A, Gatto G, Gentile R, Tesei S, Pezzoli G. Valvular heart disease and the use of dopamine agonists for Parkinson's disease. *N Engl J Med.* 2007;356:39-46.
2. Schade R, Andersohn F, Suissa S, Haverkamp W, Garbe E. Dopamine agonists and the risk of cardiac-valve regurgitation. *N Engl J Med.* 2007;356:29-38.
3. Steffensen C, Maegbaek ML, Laurberg P, et al. Heart valve disease among patients with hyperprolactinemia: a nationwide population-based cohort study. *J Clin Endocrinol Metab.* 2012;97:1629-1634.

56 Lipoproteins and Atherosclerosis

Relation of Hepatic Steatosis to Atherogenic Dyslipidemia

Makadia SS, Blaha M, Keenan T, et al (Johns Hopkins Med Insts, Baltimore, MD; Johns Hopkins Ciccarone Preventative Cardiology Ctr, Baltimore, MD; et al)

Am J Cardiol 112:1599-1604, 2013

Hepatic steatosis is closely associated with the metabolic syndrome. We assessed for an independent association between hepatic steatosis and atherogenic dyslipidemia after adjustment for obesity, physical activity, hyperglycemia, and systemic inflammation. We studied 6,333 asymptomatic subjects without clinical cardiovascular disease undergoing a health screen in Brazil from November 2008 to July 2010. Hepatic steatosis was diagnosed by ultrasound. Atherogenic dyslipidemia was defined using 2 definitions: criteria for (1) metabolic syndrome or (2) insulin resistance (triglyceride/high-density–lipoprotein cholesterol ratio of ≥2.5 in women and ≥3.5 in men). In hierarchical multivariate regression models, we evaluated for an independent association of hepatic steatosis with atherogenic dyslipidemia. Hepatic steatosis was detected in 36% of participants (average age 43.5 years, 79% men, average body mass index 26.3 kg/m^2). Subjects with hepatic steatosis had similar levels of low-density–lipoprotein cholesterol, with significantly lower level of high-density-lipoprotein cholesterol and higher level of triglyceride compared with those without steatosis. Hepatic steatosis remained significantly independently associated with atherogenic dyslipidemia of both definitions (metabolic syndrome [odds ratio 2.47, 95% confidence interval 2.03 to 3.02] and insulin resistance [odds ratio 2.50, 95% confidence interval 2.13 to 2.91]) after multivariate adjustment. Stratified analyses showed a persistent independent association in nonobese subjects, those without metabolic syndrome, those with normal high-sensitivity C-reactive protein, nonalcohol abusers, and those with normal liver enzymes. Hepatic steatosis was significantly associated with atherogenic dyslipidemia independent of obesity, physical activity, hyperglycemia, and systemic inflammation after multivariate adjustment. In conclusion, this adds to the growing body of evidence that hepatic steatosis may play a direct

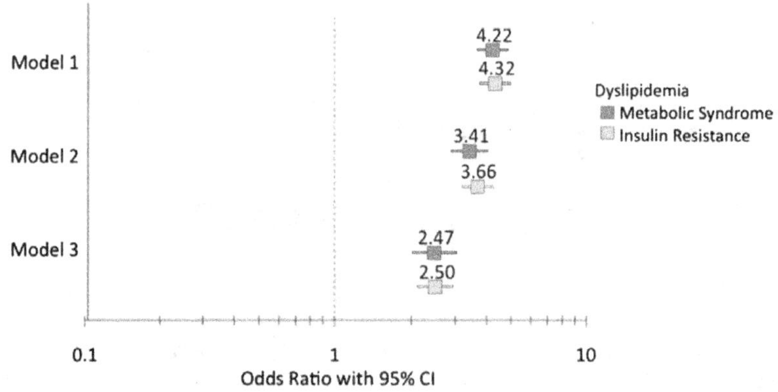

FIGURE 2.—ORs for atherogenic dyslipidemia in subjects with hepatic steatosis by sequential hierarchal regression. Model 1: unadjusted. Model 2: adjusted for age, gender, alcohol use, and physical activity. Model 3: adjusted for model 2 plus BMI, waist circumference, hypertension or antihypertensive medications, diabetes or use of diabetes medications, hyperglycemia, log hs-CRP, smoking, and use of lipid-lowering medications. Dyslipidemia (metabolic syndrome): levels of TG ≥150 mg/dl and HDL-C <40 mg/dl in men or <50 mg/dl in women or the use of lipidlowering medications. Dyslipidemia (insulin resistance): TG/HDL-C ratio of ≥2.5 in women and ≥3.5 in men. (Reprinted from the American Journal of Cardiology. Makadia SS, Blaha M, Keenan T, et al. Relation of hepatic steatosis to atherogenic dyslipidemia. *Am J Cardiol.* 2013;112:1599-1604, Copyright 2013, with permission from Elsevier.)

TABLE 2.—Difference Between Lipid Values in Patients with Hepatic Steatosis and those Without it in Multivariate Linear Regression

	Model 1	Model 2	Model 3
Lipid Parameter	β Coefficient (95% CI)	β Coefficient (95% CI)	β Coefficient (95% CI)
TC (mg/dl)	9.43 (7.50 to 11.37)	6.33 (4.15 to 8.51)	4.49 (1.87 to 7.12)
LDL-C (mg/dl)	7.39 (5.67 to 9.10)	3.28 (1.35 to 5.22)	0.73 (−1.58 to 3.03)
HDL-C (mg/dl)	−8.74 (−9.33 to −8.16)	−5.55 (−6.16 to −4.95)	−2.96 (−3.69 to −2.23)
TGs (mg/dl)*	0.40 (0.37 to 0.42)	0.31 (0.28 to 0.33)	0.23 (0.20 to 0.26)
Non-HDL-C (mg/dl)	18.2 (16.2 to 20.1)	11.9 (9.70 to 14.08)	7.47 (4.83 to 10.11)
TG/HDL ratio*	0.57 (0.54 to 0.61)	0.43 (0.39 to 0.46)	0.29 (0.25 to 0.34)
TC/HDL ratio*	0.22 (0.21 to 0.24)	0.15 (0.13 to 0.16)	0.09 (0.07 to 0.10)

Model 1: unadjusted; n = 6,333.
Model 2: adjusted for age, gender, alcohol use, and physical activity; n = 5,697.
Model 3: adjusted for model 2 plus BMI, waist circumference, hypertension or antihypertensive medications, diabetes or diabetes medications, hyperglycemia, log hs-CRP, smoking, and use of lipid-lowering medications; n = 4,825.
*Log transformed.
Reprinted from the American Journal of Cardiology. Makadia SS, Blaha M, Keenan T, et al. Relation of hepatic steatosis to atherogenic dyslipidemia. Am J Cardiol. 2013;112:1599-1604, Copyright 2013, with permission from Elsevier.

metabolic role in conferring increased cardiovascular risk (Fig 2, Tables 2 and 3).

▶ Hepatic steatosis is widely regarded as a reliable marker of insulin resistance (IR) and is frequently observed in the setting of metabolic syndrome (MS). Hepatic steatosis also correlates with increased risk of ectopic fat deposition in other tissues, such as the pancreas, epicardium, skeletal muscle, and myocardium.[1] Hepatic steatosis results from the excess influx of free fatty acid and inadequate

TABLE 3.—Stratified ORs of Hepatic Steatosis with Dyslipidemia in Multivariate Logistic Regression

	Dyslipidemia	
	Metabolic Syndrome	Insulin Resistance
Stratifications	OR (95% CI)	OR (95% CI)
Obesity*		
Yes, n = 1,122	2.51 (1.73 to 3.64)	2.20 (1.64 to 2.95)
No, n = 3,703	2.97 (2.39 to 3.68)	3.25 (2.73 to 3.87)
Systemic Inflammation*		
Yes, n = 930	2.74 (1.74 to 4.31)	3.20 (2.25 to 4.56)
No, n = 3,895	2.42 (1.94 to 3.01)	2.39 (2.01 to 2.85)
Metabolic Syndrome†		
Yes, n = 1,108	1.51 (1.12 to 2.03)	1.64 (1.18 to 2.28)
No, n = 4,310	2.26 (1.71 to 2.99)	2.25 (1.87 to 2.70)

Dyslipidemia (metabolic syndrome) is defined as HDL levels of <40 mg/dl in men and <50 mg/dl in women and TG level of ≥150 mg/dl.

Dyslipidemia (insulin resistance) is defined as a TG/HDL ratio of ≥2.5 in women and ≥3.5 in men.

Obesity is defined as a BMI of ≥30 kg/m^2 or waist circumference of >88 cm in women or >102 cm in men if BMI is ≥25 kg/m^2.

Systemic inflammation is defined as an hs-CRP level of ≥3.

*Adjusted for BMI (not in no obesity or obesity), waist circumference (not in no obesity or obesity), hypertension, hypertension medications, diabetes, diabetes medications, log hs-CRP (not in hs-CRP level < or ≥3), smoking, and lipid-lowering medications.

†Regression analysis for no metabolic syndrome or metabolic syndrome subgroups excluded those who met the Harmonizing Definition for metabolic syndrome.

capacity to dispose of this excess lipid via mitochondrial oxidation, increased gluconeogenesis, or augmented secretion within very-low-density lipoprotein particles. MS and IR are well known to be associated with several disturbances in lipid and lipoprotein metabolism.[2] In an elegant study by Makadia et al, the quantitative relationship between atherogenic dyslipidemia and hepatic steatosis was investigated using a cohort of 6333 patients in Sao Paolo, Brazil. Atherogenic dyslipidemia was defined according to (1) the National Cholesterol Education Program's criteria for MS (triglyceride ≥150 mg/dL, high-density lipoprotein cholesterol [HDL-C] less than 40 mg/dL in men and less than 50 mg/dL in women) and (2) established lipid-dependent definition for IR (triglyceride/HDL-C ratio ≥2.5 in women and ≥3.5 in men). Liver ultrasonography was used to establish or negate the presence of steatosis. For multivariable regression analyses, a hierarchical model was applied: model 1 is unadjusted; adjustments were first made for age, gender, alcohol use, and physical activity (model 2); in model 3, additional adjustments for obesity, components of the metabolic syndrome, systemic inflammation, body mass index, waist circumference, hypertension, antihypertensive medications, diabetes, diabetes medications, hyperglycemia, log hs–C-reactive protein (hs-CRP), smoking status, and lipid-lowering medications. The associations between hepatic steatosis and dyslipidemia were stratified by alcohol consumption, obesity, log hs-CRP, metabolic syndrome, and liver function studies. Hepatic steatosis correlated significantly with triglycerides, HDL-C, non–HDL-C, triglyceride/HDL-C, and total cholesterol/HDL-C across hierarchical adjustment (Table 2). Even after comprehensive adjustment for covariates (model 3), dyslipidemia correlated highly with hepatic steatosis (metabolic syndrome definition: odds ratio [OR], 2.47; 95% confidence interval [CI], 2.03 to 3.02 and insulin resistance definition: OR, 2.50; 95% CI, 2.13 to 2.91; Fig 2). In addition, in a subgroup analysis using model 3, there were statistically significant associations between hepatic steatosis and dyslipidemia for both MS and IR in subjects with and without obesity, with and without elevated hs-CRP levels, and with and without metabolic syndrome (Table 2). The results were significant even after adjusting for liver function studies.

This study establishes that dyslipidemia is independently associated with hepatic steatosis. Atherogenic dyslipidemia correlated highly with steatosis even after comprehensive multivariable adjustment. It also shows that hepatic steatosis can occur in the absence of obesity, evidence of systemic inflammation, and meeting criteria for MS. Increased serum levels of hepatic enzymes correlated poorly with steatosis.

P. P. Toth, MD, PhD

References

1. Toth PP. Epicardial steatosis, insulin resistance, and coronary artery disease. *Heart Fail Clin.* 2012;8:671-678.
2. Toth PP. Insulin resistance, small LDL particles, and risk for atherosclerotic disease. *Curr Vasc Pharmacol.* 2013 Apr 25 [Epub ahead of print].

Statin **Therapy in Patients With Chronic Kidney Disease Undergoing Percutaneous Coronary Intervention (from the Evaluation of Drug Eluting Stents and Ischemic Events Registry)**

Dasari TW, Cohen DJ, Kleiman NS, et al (Univ of Oklahoma Health Sciences Ctr; St Luke's Mid America Heart Inst, KS; Methodist DeBakey Heart & Vascular Ctr, Houston, TX; et al)
Am J Cardiol 113:621-625, 2014

Secondary prevention trials have demonstrated the efficacy of statins in reducing cardiovascular morbidity and mortality in patients with coronary artery disease and events after percutaneous coronary intervention (PCI). However, there are few data describing the clinical value of statins in patients with coronary artery disease and chronic kidney disease (CKD) undergoing PCI. Of 10,148 patients who entered into Evaluation of Drug Eluting Stents and Ischemic Events, a multicenter registry of unselected patients undergoing PCI from July 2004 to December 2007, we studied 2,306 patients with CKD (estimated glomerular filtration rate ≤60 ml/min based on the Modified Diet in Renal Disease calculation). Patients were stratified into those receiving statins at discharge (n = 1,833, 79%) or not (n = 473, 21%). Patients in the statin group had a greater prevalence of hypertension, recent myocardial infarction (MI), and use of β blockers and angiotensin-converting enzyme inhibitors. Outcomes were assessed from discharge through 1-year follow-up. One-year all-cause mortality was 5.7% in statin group versus 8.7% in the no statin group (adjusted hazard ratio 0.55, 95% confidence interval 0.34 to 0.88). The composite of death, MI, and repeat revascularization was lower in statin group (adjusted hazard ratio 0.71, 95% confidence interval 0.51 to 0.99). In conclusion, among patients with CKD undergoing PCI, the prescription of statins at hospital discharge was associated with a significant improvement in subsequent outcomes including mortality and composite end point of death, MI, and repeat revascularization (Figs 1 and 2, Table 1).

▶ Chronic kidney disease (CKD) is recognized by some specialty organizations as a coronary artery disease (CAD) risk equivalent. CKD is associated with multiple disturbances in lipid lipoprotein metabolism, including elevated triglycerides, low high-density lipoprotein cholesterol (HDL-C), and increased numbers of small, dense low-density lipoprotein (LDL) particles independent of insulin resistance. The Study of Heart and Renal Protection trial found that treatment with a combination of simvastatin and ezetimibe in patients with a mean glomerular filtration rate (GFR) of 27 mL/min reduced risk for cardiovascular events compared with placebo, although mortality was not decreased.[1] In contrast, statin therapy has not been found to be efficacious in patients with end-stage renal disease (ESRD) and receiving dialysis.[2,3] CKD is widely prevalent, and a significant percentage of patients undergoing percutaneous coronary intervention (PCI) have CKD. To date, there has been no investigation to ascertain if statin therapy in patients with CKD undergoing PCI reduces risk for mortality or cardiovascular events.

Dasari and coworkers evaluated this issue with the Evaluation of Drug Eluting Stents and Ischemic Events (EVENT) registry. Data were from 2306 patients with CKD. A total of 1833 patients were given a statin at the time of discharge, whereas 473 were not. The groups were not evenly matched for use of β

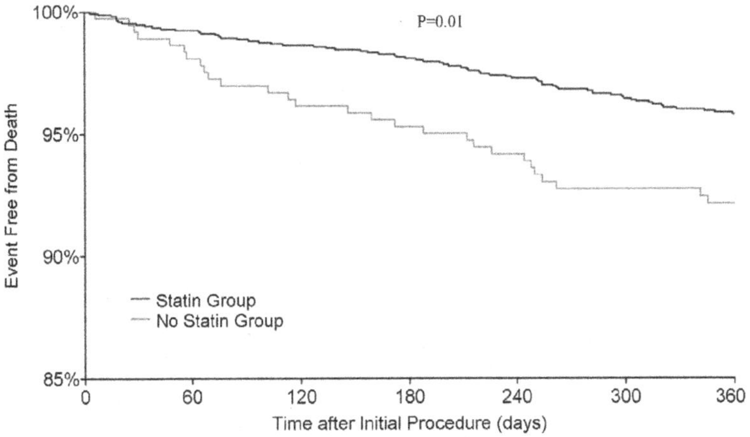

FIGURE 1.—All-cause mortality during follow-up. (Reprinted from the American Journal of Cardiology. Dasari TW, Cohen DJ, Kleiman NS, et al. *Statin* therapy in patients with chronic kidney disease undergoing percutaneous coronary intervention (from the Evaluation of Drug Eluting Stents and Ischemic Events Registry). *Am J Cardiol.* 2014;113:621-625, Copyright 2014, with permission from Elsevier.)

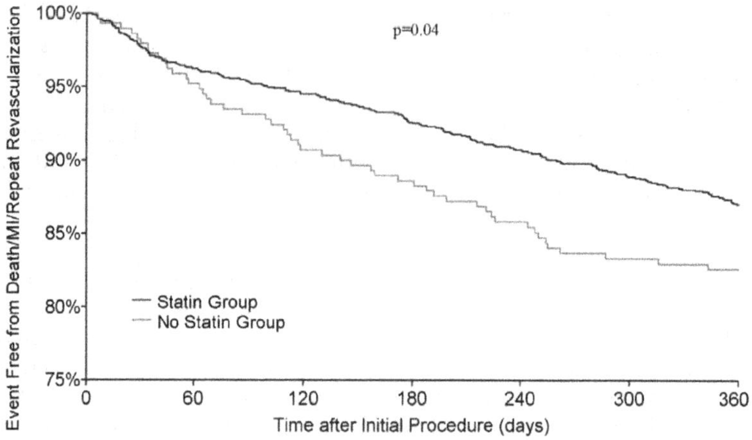

FIGURE 2.—Composite of death, MI, and repeat revascularization during follow-up. (Reprinted from Dasari TW, Cohen DJ, Kleiman NS, et al. *Statin* therapy in patients with chronic kidney disease undergoing percutaneous coronary intervention (from the Evaluation of Drug Eluting Stents and Ischemic Events Registry). *Am J Cardiol.* 2014;113:621-625, with permission from Elsevier.)

TABLE 1.—Baseline Demographic and Clinical Characteristics of the Study Population

Characteristic	Statin Therapy Yes (n = 1,833), %	No (n = 473), %	*p* Value
Age (yrs), mean ± SD	74 ± 10	75 ± 10	0.16
Men	54	48	0.01
Body mass index (mean ± SD)	27 ± 5	26 ± 5	0.12
Diabetes mellitus	36	37	0.66
Hypertension	87	82	0.004
Current smoker	14	13	0.59
Renal dialysis	7	7	0.58
Previous stroke	14	18	0.07
Heart failure	18	20	0.36
Peripheral arterial disease	17	19	0.45
Previous MI	41	36	0.06
Previous PCI	39	36	0.36
Previous coronary bypass	30	25	0.06
MI within 7 days	16	11	0.002
Number of narrowed coronary arteries			0.26
1	43	46	
2	30	29	
3	27	25	

blockade, angiotensin-converting enzyme inhibition, or nonstatin lipid lowering, but data were adjusted for these differences as well as for age, sex, hypertension, heart failure class, and recent myocardial infarction (MI) using multivariable Cox proportional hazard models (Table 1). Follow-up was for 1 year. At the end of 1 year, all-cause mortality was reduced significantly by 45% and the composite of death, MI, and need for revascularization was reduced significantly by 29% (Figs 1 and 2). Separation of the Kaplan-Meier survival curves for these outcomes was apparent within 30 days. Consistent with previous studies, patients receiving dialysis did not derive benefit from statin therapy.

Although these patients were not randomly selected, the magnitude of between-group differences is striking. This study provides the first evidence supporting the use of statin therapy in patients with CAD and CKD undergoing PCI. It will be of interest to better ascertain long-term outcomes in these patients. It remains poorly understood why statin therapy consistently offers no benefit in patients with ESRD. Until a randomized study is completed (unlikely to be performed), patients with CKD and not on dialysis undergoing PCI for CAD should receive a statin.

P. P. Toth, MD, PhD

References

1. Baigent C, Landray MJ, Reith C, et al. The effects of lowering LDL cholesterol with simvastatin plus ezetimibe in patients with chronic kidney disease (Study of Heart and Renal Protection): a randomised placebo-controlled trial. *Lancet.* 2011;377:2181-2192.
2. Fellström BC, Jardine AG, Schmieder RE, et al. Rosuvastatin and cardiovascular events in patients undergoing hemodialysis. *N Engl J Med.* 2009;360:1395-1407.
3. Wanner C, Krane V, März W, et al. Atorvastatin in patients with type 2 diabetes mellitus undergoing hemodialysis. *N Engl J Med.* 2005;353:238-248.

C-reactive Protein, but not Low-Density Lipoprotein Cholesterol Levels, Associate With Coronary Atheroma Regression and Cardiovascular Events After Maximally Intensive Statin Therapy

Puri R, Nissen SE, Libby P, et al (Cleveland Clinic, OH; Brigham and Women's Hosp, Boston, MA; et al)

Circulation 128:2395-2403, 2013

Background.—Baseline C-reactive protein (CRP) levels predict major adverse cardiovascular events (MACE: death, myocardial infarction, stroke, coronary revascularization, and hospitalization for unstable angina). The association between changes in CRP levels with plaque progression and MACE in the setting of maximally intensive statin therapy is unknown.

Methods and Results.—The Study of Coronary Atheroma by Intravascular Ultrasound: Effect of Rosuvastatin Versus Atorvastatin (SATURN) used serial intravascular ultrasound measures of coronary atheroma volume in patients treated with rosuvastatin 40 mg or atorvastatin 80 mg for 24 months. The treatment groups did not differ significantly in the change from baseline of percent atheroma volume on intravascular ultrasound, CRP-modulating effects, or MACE rates, thus allowing for a (prespecified) post hoc analysis to test associations between the changes in CRP levels with coronary disease progression and MACE. Patients with nonincreasing CRP levels (n = 621) had higher baseline (2.3 [1.1–4.7] versus 1.1 [0.5–1.8] mg/L; $P < 0.001$) and lower follow-up CRP levels (0.8 [0.5–1.7] versus 1.6 [0.7–4.1] mg/L; $P < 0.001$) versus those with increasing CRP levels (n = 364). Multivariable analysis revealed a nonincreasing CRP level to independently associate with greater percent atheroma volume regression ($P = 0.01$). Although the (log) change in CRP did not associate with MACE (hazard ratio, 1.18; 95% confidence interval, 0.93–1.50; $P = 0.17$), the (log) on-treatment CRP associated significantly with MACE (hazard ratio, 1.28; 95% confidence interval, 1.04–1.56; $P = 0.02$). On-treatment low-density lipoprotein cholesterol levels did not correlate with MACE (hazard ratio, 1.09; 95% confidence interval, 0.88–1.35; $P = 0.45$).

Conclusions.—Following 24 months of potent statin therapy, on-treatment CRP levels associated with MACE. Inflammation may be an important driver of residual cardiovascular risk in patients with coronary artery disease despite aggressive statin therapy.

Clinical Trial Registration.—URL: http://clinicaltrials.gov. Unique identifier: NCT000620542 (Figs 1 and 2, Table 3).

▶ Atherosclerosis is now widely acknowledged as an inflammatory disease. As arterial walls are exposed to cardiovascular disease risk factors, progressive

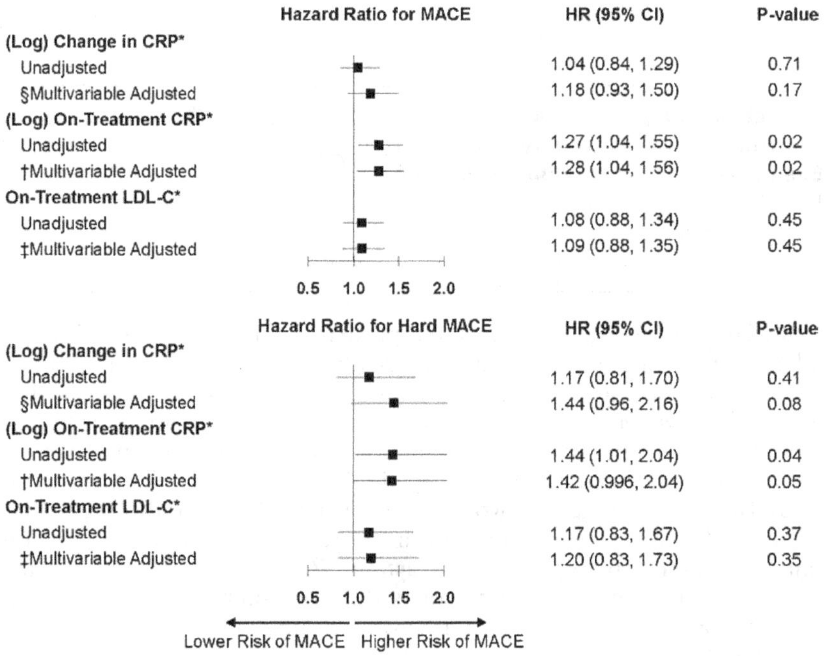

FIGURE 1.—Cox proportional hazard ratios for time to first MACE or hard MACE, according to the change from baseline of CRP levels, on-treatment CRP levels, or on-treatment LDL-C levels. *Values of log-transformed change in CRP, on-treatment CRP, and on-treatment LDL-C were per standard deviation. §Adjusted for history of diabetes mellitus, concomitant ACE inhibitor use, and log-transformed baseline CRP. †Adjusted for history of diabetes mellitus, history of acute coronary syndrome, and concomitant use of ACE inhibitor. ‡Adjusted for history of diabetes mellitus, history of acute coronary syndrome, concomitant ACE inhibitor use, and log-transformed on-treatment CRP. ACE indicates angiotensin-converting enzyme; CI, confidence interval; CRP, C-reactive protein; HR, hazard ratio; LDL-C, low-density lipoprotein cholesterol; and MACE, major adverse cardiovascular events. (Reprinted from Puri R, Nissen SE, Libby P, et al. C-reactive protein, but not low-density lipoprotein cholesterol levels, associate with coronary atheroma regression and cardiovascular events after maximally intensive statin therapy. *Circulation.* 2013;128:2395-2403, Copyright 2013, with permission from American Heart Association, Inc.)

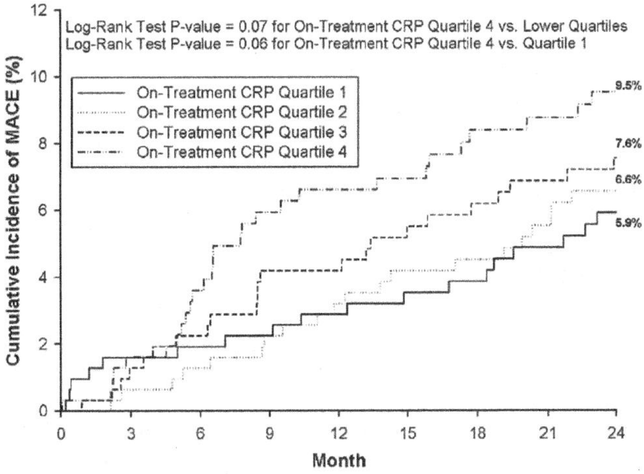

No. Patients At Risk									
On-Treatment CRP Quartile 1	315	308	306	303	299	294	290	284	272
On-Treatment CRP Quartile 2	316	312	309	304	299	293	290	278	270
On-Treatment CRP Quartile 3	316	309	305	295	295	282	277	272	265
On-Treatment CRP Quartile 4	316	303	290	282	277	269	253	245	235

FIGURE 2.—Kaplan–Meier survival curve analysis of quartiles of on-treatment CRP levels and MACE. The cumulative incidence of MACE in patients with the lowest quartile of on-treatment CRP was 5.9% in comparison with 9.5% in those with the highest quartile of baseline coronary PAV ($P = 0.06$). CRP indicates C-reactive protein; MACE, major adverse cardiovascular events; and PAV, percent atheroma volume. (Reprinted from Puri R, Nissen SE, Libby P, et al. C-reactive protein, but not low-density lipoprotein cholesterol levels, associate with coronary atheroma regression and cardiovascular events after maximally intensive statin therapy. *Circulation.* 2013;128:2395-2403, Copyright 2013, with permission from American Heart Association, Inc.)

TABLE 3.—Ultrasonic Measures of Atheroma Volume and Vascular Dimensions

IVUS Parameter	Total (n = 985)	Change From Baseline CRP: No Increase (n = 621)	Change From Baseline CRP: Increase (n = 364)	*P* Value*
Percent atheroma volume, %				
Baseline	36.4 ± 8.2	36.6 ± 8.0	36.0 ± 8.4	0.29
Change from baseline	−1.23 ± 0.09	−1.42 ± 0.11	−0.91 ± 0.15	0.007
P value for change from baseline	<0.001	<0.001	<0.001	
Lumen volume, mm^3				
Baseline	248.0 ± 87.8	248.8 ± 86.8	246.6 ± 89.7	0.54
Change from baseline	1.08 ± 0.93	2.30 ± 1.17	−1.00 ± 1.53	0.09
P value for change from baseline	0.25	0.05	0.52	
EEM volume, mm^3				
Baseline	392.2 ± 134.9	394.8 ± 134.6	387.7 ± 135.3	0.40
Change from baseline	−6.11 ± 1.17	−5.40 ± 1.47	−7.33 ± 1.92	0.43
P value for change from baseline	<0.001	<0.001	<0.001	

Baseline and follow-up values are reported as mean ± SD, and change values are reported as least squares mean ± SE. CRP indicates C-reactive protein; EEM, external elastic membrane; IVUS, intravascular ultrasound; SD, standard deviation; and SE, standard error.

**P* value reflects comparisons between groups dichotomized according to change in CRP level.

Reprinted from Puri R, Nissen SE, Libby P, et al. C-reactive protein, but not lowdensity lipoprotein cholesterol levels, associate with coronary atheroma regression and cardiovascular events after maximally intensive statin therapy. Circulation. 2013;128:2395-2403, Copyright 2013, with permission from American Heart Association, Inc.

endothelial dysfunction and lipid uptake into the subendothelial space are followed by a plethora of inflammatory responses driven by T lymphocytes and monocytes. The inflammatory response potentiates low-density lipoprotein (LDL) oxidation and macrophage scavenging, giving rise to foam cells and the progenitors to fatty streaks and atherosclerotic lesions.[1,2] Serum C-reactive protein (CRP) levels are highly correlated with risk for cardiovascular events. Post hoc analyses from the JUPITER, PROVE-IT, and A to Z trials all suggest that the patients who experienced the greatest reductions in risk for cardiovascular events were able to achieve both an LDL cholesterol <70 mg/dL and a CRP <1.0 mg/L.[3-5]

The Study of Coronary Atheroma by Intravascular Ultrasound: Effect of Rosuvastatin Versus Atorvastatin (SATURN) compared 2 high-dose regimens of statin therapy (rosuvastatin 40 mg daily and atorvastatin 80 mg daily) in patients with established coronary artery disease and evaluated their impact on rates of target atherosclerotic plaque progression.[6] There was a difference between groups in the primary outcome of change in percent atheroma volume. In this post hoc analysis, the authors evaluate the impact of on-treatment changes in CRP on disease progression. Compared with patients who experienced an increase of CRP during the course of the trial, those with no increase had significantly greater regression of target lesions (Table 1 in the original article). In both unadjusted and multivariable adjusted models, on-treatment CRP correlated with risk for major coronary events whereas LDL cholesterol did not (Fig 1). There was a rising gradient of risk for major coronary events as CRP levels rose (Fig 2).

These results are remarkable and suggest that CRP contributes significantly to likelihood of disease progression or regression. To date CRP is regarded as a risk biomarker. However, it is possible it may evolve into a target of therapy. Multiple trials are underway to test this hypothesis. In the meantime, it is reasonable to intensify lifestyle modification in patients whose CRP is elevated despite intensive background therapy for risk factor burden.

P. P. Toth, MD, PhD

References

1. Ross R. Atherosclerosis—an inflammatory disease. *N Engl J Med.* 1999;340:115-126.
2. Libby P. Inflammation in atherosclerosis. *Nature.* 2002;420:868-874.
3. Ridker PM, MacFadyen J, Libby P, Glynn RJ. Relation of baseline high-sensitivity C-reactive protein level to cardiovascular outcomes with rosuvastatin in the Justification for Use of statins in Prevention: an Intervention Trial Evaluating Rosuvastatin (JUPITER). *Am J Cardiol.* 2010;106:204-209.
4. Ridker PM, Cannon CP, Morrow D, et al. C-reactive protein levels and outcomes after statin therapy. *N Engl J Med.* 2005;352:20-28.
5. Morrow DA, de Lemos JA, Sabatine MS, et al. Clinical relevance of C-reactive protein during follow-up of patients with acute coronary syndromes in the Aggrastat-to-Zocor Trial. *Circulation.* 2006;114:281-288.
6. Nicholls SJ, Ballantyne CM, Barter PJ, et al. Effect of two intensive statin regimens on progression of coronary disease. *N Engl J Med.* 2011;365:2078-2087.

AMG145, a Monoclonal Antibody Against Proprotein Convertase Subtilisin Kexin Type 9, Significantly Reduces Lipoprotein(a) in Hypercholesterolemic Patients Receiving Statin Therapy: An Analysis From the LDL-C Assessment With Proprotein Convertase Subtilisin Kexin Type 9 Monoclonal Antibody Inhibition Combined With Statin Therapy (LAPLACE)–Thrombolysis in Myocardial Infarction (TIMI) 57 Trial

Desai NR, Kohli P, Giugliano RP, et al (Brigham and Women's Hosp, Boston, MA; et al)

Circulation 128:962-969, 2013

Background.—Lipoprotein(a) [Lp(a)] is an emerging risk factor for cardiovascular disease. Currently, there are few available therapies to lower Lp(a). We sought to evaluate the impact of AMG145, a monoclonal antibody against proprotein convertase subtilisin kexin type 9 (PCSK9), on Lp(a).

Methods and Results.—As part of the LDL-C Assessment With PCSK9 Monoclonal Antibody Inhibition Combined With Statin Therapy (LAPLACE)–Thrombolysis in Myocardial Infarction (TIMI) 57 trial, 631 patients with hypercholesterolemia receiving statin therapy were randomized to receive AMG145 at 1 of 3 different doses every 2 weeks or 1 of 3 different doses every 4 weeks versus placebo. Lp(a) and other lipid parameters were measured at baseline and at week 12. Compared with placebo,

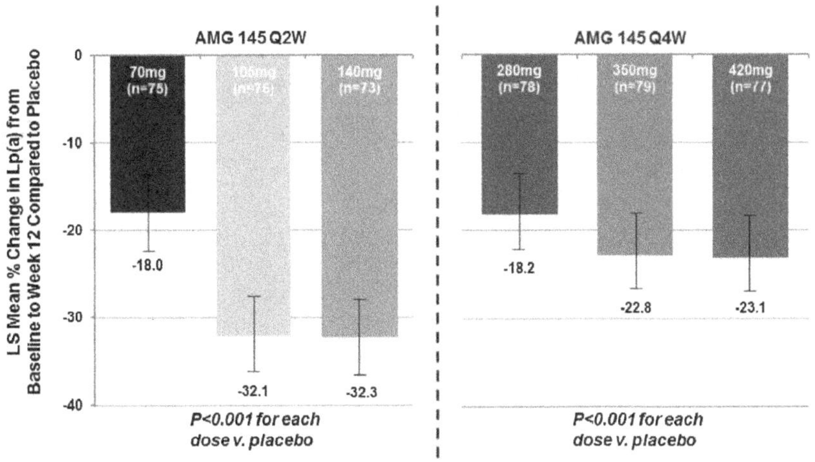

FIGURE 1.—Least squares (LS) mean percent change in lipoprotein(a) [Lp(a)] from baseline to week 12 among subjects with Lp(a) assessed at both of those time points (n = 612). The mean percent change was +3.4% for placebo every 2 weeks (Q2W) and −0.08% for placebo every 4 weeks (Q4W). The bars show the mean percent change by AMG145 treatment arm compared with the corresponding placebo. Error bars depict the standard error. (Reprinted from Desai NR, Kohli P, Giugliano RP, et al. AMG145, a monoclonal antibody against proprotein convertase subtilisin kexin type 9, significantly reduces lipoprotein(a) in hypercholesterolemic patients receiving statin therapy: an analysis from the LDL-C Assessment With Proprotein Convertase Subtilisin Kexin Type 9 Monoclonal Antibody Inhibition Combined With Statin Therapy (LAPLACE)–Thrombolysis in Myocardial Infarction (TIMI) 57 trial. *Circulation*. 2013;128:962-969, with permission from American Heart Association, Inc.)

AMG145 70 mg, 105 mg, and 140 mg every 2 weeks reduced Lp(a) at 12 weeks by 18%, 32%, and 32%, respectively ($P < 0.001$ for each dose versus placebo). Likewise, AMG145 280 mg, 350 mg, and 420 mg every 4 weeks reduced Lp(a) by 18%, 23%, and 23%, respectively ($P < 0.001$ for each dose versus placebo). The reduction in Lp(a) correlated with the reduction in low-density lipoprotein cholesterol ($\rho = 0.33$, $P < 0.001$). The effect of AMG145 on Lp(a) was consistent regardless of age, sex, race, history of diabetes mellitus, and background statin regimen. Patients with higher levels of Lp(a) at baseline had larger absolute reductions but comparatively smaller percent reductions in Lp(a) with AMG145 compared with those with lower baseline Lp(a) values.

Conclusions.—AMG145 significantly reduces Lp(a), by up to 32%, among subjects with hypercholesterolemia receiving statin therapy, offering an additional, complementary benefit beyond robust low-density

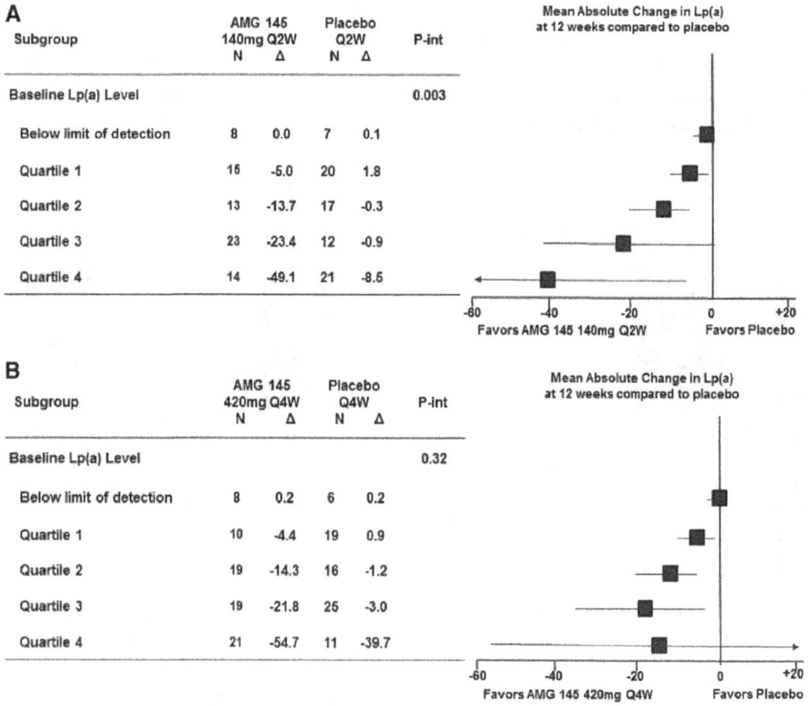

FIGURE 5.—Forest plot of the mean absolute change in lipoprotein(a) [Lp(a)] from baseline to week 12 for AMG145 140 mg every 2 weeks (Q2W; **A**) and AMG145 420 mg every 4 weeks (Q4W; **B**) across quartiles of baseline Lp(a). (Reprinted from Desai NR, Kohli P, Giugliano RP, et al. AMG145, a monoclonal antibody against proprotein convertase subtilisin kexin type 9, significantly reduces lipoprotein(a) in hypercholesterolemic patients receiving statin therapy: an analysis from the LDL-C Assessment With Proprotein Convertase Subtilisin Kexin Type 9 Monoclonal Antibody Inhibition Combined With Statin Therapy (LAPLACE)–Thrombolysis in Myocardial Infarction (TIMI) 57 trial. *Circulation.* 2013;128:962-969, Copyright 2013, with permission from American Heart Association, Inc.)

lipoprotein cholesterol reduction with regard to a patient's atherogenic lipid profile (Figs 1 and 5).

▶ Lipoprotein(a) is widely recognized as a risk factor for atherosclerotic disease.[1,2] Niacin is currently the only approved lipid-modifying agent that can reduce serum levels of Lp(a). However, there is no evidence that lowering Lp(a) with niacin impacts risk for atherosclerotic cardiovascular disease (ASCVD) events. Given the strength of association between Lp(a) levels and risk for ASCVD, new pharmacologic interventions that impact serum levels of this lipoprotein are urgently needed so we can better ascertain through prospective, randomized clinical trials whether reducing this moiety results in reduced risk for acute cardiovascular events.

The monoclonal antibodies against PCSK9 show significant capacity to reduce serum levels of Lp(a). Desai et al show in the LDL-C Assessment With PCSK9 Monoclonal Antibody Inhibition Combined With Statin Therapy (LAPLACE)—Thrombolysis in Myocardial Infarction (TIMI) 57 trial, that AMG 145 given every 2 weeks can reduce Lp(a) by about one-third (Fig 1). The magnitude of Lp(a) reduction is directly related to baseline level of this lipoprotein: higher levels correlate with larger absolute reductions from baseline (Fig 5).

With major outcomes trials underway with PCSK9 monoclonal antibodies, it is possible that benefit from Lp(a) reduction will be discerned. This would be an exciting development and a major advance toward reducing residual risk. It remains to be seen if different isoforms of Lp(a) are reduced to differing degrees by these agents.

P. P. Toth, MD, PhD

References

1. Davidson MH, Ballantyne CM, Jacobson TA, et al. Clinical utility of inflammatory markers and advanced lipoprotein testing: advice from an expert panel of lipid specialists. *J Clin Lipidol.* 2011;5:338-367.
2. Nordestgaard BG, Chapman MJ, Ray K, et al. Lipoprotein(a) as a cardiovascular risk factor: current status. *Eur Heart J.* 2010;31:2844-2853.

57 Obesity

Are Metabolically Healthy Overweight and Obesity Benign Conditions?: A Systematic Review and Meta-Analysis

Kramer CK, Zinman B, Retnakaran R (Mount Sinai Hosp, Toronto, Ontario, Canada; Univ of Toronto, Ontario, Canada)

Ann Intern Med 159:758-769, 2013

Background.—Recent interest has focused on a unique subgroup of overweight and obese individuals who have normal metabolic features despite increased adiposity. Normal-weight individuals with adverse metabolic status have also been described. However, it remains unclear whether metabolic phenotype modifies the morbidity and mortality associated with higher body mass index (BMI).

Purpose.—To determine the effect of metabolic status on all-cause mortality and cardiovascular events in normal-weight, overweight, and obese persons.

Data Sources.—Studies were identified from electronic databases.

Study Selection.—Included studies evaluated all-cause mortality or cardiovascular events (or both) and clinical characteristics of 6 patient groups defined by BMI category (normal weight/overweight/obesity) and metabolic status (healthy/unhealthy), as defined by the presence or absence of components of the metabolic syndrome by Adult Treatment Panel III or International Diabetes Federation criteria.

Data Extraction.—Two independent reviewers extracted the data. Metabolically healthy people of normal weight made up the reference group.

Data Synthesis.—Eight studies ($n = 61\,386$; 3988 events) evaluated participants for all-cause mortality and/or cardiovascular events. Metabolically healthy obese individuals (relative risk [RR], 1.24; 95% CI, 1.02 to 1.55) had increased risk for events compared with metabolically healthy normal-weight individuals when only studies with 10 or more years of follow-up were considered. All metabolically unhealthy groups had a similarly elevated risk: normal weight (RR, 3.14; CI, 2.36 to 3.93), overweight (RR, 2.70; CI, 2.08 to 3.30), and obese (RR, 2.65; CI, 2.18 to 3.12).

Limitation.—Duration of exposure to the metabolic-BMI phenotypes was not described in the studies and could partially affect the estimates.

Conclusion.—Compared with metabolically healthy normal-weight individuals, obese persons are at increased risk for adverse long-term

outcomes even in the absence of metabolic abnormalities, suggesting that there is no healthy pattern of increased weight.

▶ It is well recognized that individuals in the same body mass index (BMI) category can have substantial heterogeneity of metabolic features, including glucose tolerance, lipid profiles, blood pressure, and waist circumference. Up to 30% of obese individuals are considered "metabolically healthy" and some have suggested that this subgroup of healthy obese patients are protected against metabolic and cardiovascular comorbidities and may not need treatment.[1] In this systematic review and meta-analysis, the authors identified 12 prospective or cross-sectional studies that evaluated all-cause mortality or cardiovascular events and clinical characteristics of 6 patient groups defined by BMI category (normal weight/overweight/obesity) and metabolic status (healthy/unhealthy) as defined by the presence or absence of components of the metabolic syndrome by Adult Treatment Panel III or International Diabetes Federation criteria. The most important finding was that the metabolically healthy obese group had 24% increased mortality rate and cardiovascular risk compared with the metabolically healthy normal-weight subjects when studies with 10 or more years of follow-up were considered. The metabolically healthy overweight group, however, had similar risk to the healthy, normal-weight individuals. All metabolically unhealthy groups regardless of BMI category had a 2- to 3-fold increased cardiovascular risk. When they compared persons with the same metabolic status (healthy or unhealthy), those with higher BMI had increased levels of systolic blood pressure, diastolic blood pressure, waist circumference, and Homeostasis Model Assessment of Insulin Resistance. A similar inverse association was observed for high-density lipoprotein cholesterol.

This meta-analysis has limitations. The studies did not account for other factors possibly associated with mortality, such as smoking or physical activity, and they did not have data on weight gain, age, or ethnicity of subjects. Higher BMI has been reported to provide lower relative mortality risk in elderly persons than in young and middle-aged populations; thus, results of this meta-analysis may not be generalizable to older people. Similarly, people of certain ethnic backgrounds are at higher risk of metabolic syndrome despite being normal weight.

It should be noted that complications of obesity are not limited to metabolic syndrome. Obese people are at risk for other medical conditions such as sleep apnea, osteoarthritis, gallbladder disease, infertility, and certain types of cancer.[2] Obese people may experience social stigma, discrimination, and overall reduced quality of life.[3] Even though preventing cardiovascular disease and death is very important, it should not be the only reason obese people should be encouraged to lose weight.

L. Khaodhiar, MD

References

1. Blüher M. The distinction of metabolically 'healthy' from 'unhealthy' obese individuals. *Curr Opin Lipidol.* 2010;21:38-43.

2. Bray GA. Risks of obesity. *Endocrinol Metab Clin North Am.* 2003;32:787-804.
3. Puhl RM, Heuer CA. Weight bias: a review and update. *Obesity (Silver Spring).* 2009;17:941-964.

Review of the key results from the Swedish Obese Subjects (SOS) trial – a prospective controlled intervention study of bariatric surgery

Sjöström L (The Univ of Gothenburg, Sweden)

J Intern Med 273:219-234, 2013

Obesity is a risk factor for diabetes, cardiovascular disease events, cancer and overall mortality. Weight loss may protect against these conditions, but robust evidence for this has been lacking. The Swedish Obese Subjects (SOS) study is the first long-term, prospective, controlled trial to provide information on the effects of bariatric surgery on the incidence of these objective endpoints. The SOS study involved 2010 obese subjects who underwent bariatric surgery [gastric bypass (13%), banding (19%) and vertical banded gastroplasty (68%)] and 2037 contemporaneously matched obese control subjects receiving usual care. The age of participants was 37–60 years and body mass index (BMI) was ≥34 kg m^{-2} in men and ≥38 kg m^{-2} in women. Here, we review the key SOS study results published between 2004 and 2012. Follow-up periods varied from 10 to 20 years in different reports. The mean changes in body weight after 2, 10, 15 and 20 years were 23%, −17%, −16% and −18% in the surgery group and 0%, 1%, −1% and −1% in the control group respectively. Compared with usual care, bariatric surgery was associated with a long-term reduction in overall mortality (primary endpoint) [adjusted hazard ratio (HR) = 0.71, 95% confidence interval (CI) 0.54– 0.92; $P = 0.01$] and decreased incidences of diabetes (adjusted HR = 0.17; $P < 0.001$), myocardial infarction (adjusted HR = 0.71; $P = 0.02$), stroke (adjusted HR = 0.66; $P = 0.008$) and cancer (women: adjusted HR = 0.58; $P = 0.0008$; men: n.s.]. The diabetes remission rate was increased severalfold at 2 years [adjusted odds ratio (OR) = 8.42; $P < 0.001$] and 10 years (adjusted OR = 3.45; $P < 0.001$). Whereas high insulin and/or high glucose at baseline predicted favourable treatment effects, high baseline BMI did not, indicating that current selection criteria for bariatric surgery need to be revised.

▶ Overweight and obesity are associated with increased morbidity and mortality. Several short-term studies have demonstrated beneficial effects of moderate weight loss, defined as 5% to 10% weight loss, on many cardiovascular risk factors. The review and meta-analysis of prospective cohort studies showed that intentional weight loss achieved by diet and lifestyle changes had a neutral effect on all-cause mortality.[1] The Look AHEAD (Action for HEAlth in Diabetes) trial, a large randomized controlled study, was stopped early on the basis of futility after 9.6 years when the investigators found no effect of an intensive lifestyle intervention on cardiovascular events in overweight or obese adults with type 2 diabetes.[2] In contrast, the results of retrospective cohort studies in obese subjects have shown that long-term mortality is markedly reduced after gastric bypass surgery in patients both with and without diabetes.[3,4] The Swedish Obese Subjects (SOS) trial is a prospective, nonrandomized controlled intervention study of bariatric surgery. The study involved more than 2000 obese patients who had surgery, compared with more than 2000 obese patients who received usual care. Majority of the patients underwent vertical banded gastroplasty (68%), whereas the remainder underwent either gastric banding (19%) or gastric bypass (13%).

The author has reviewed the results of SOS study published between 2004 to 2012 when the follow-up periods varied from 10 to 20 years. The mean weight losses were 23%, 17%, 16%, and 18% at 2, 10, 15, and 20 years after surgery. Compared with usual care, patients who underwent bariatric surgery had an almost 30% reduction in overall mortality and significantly decreased risks of diabetes, myocardial infarction, stroke, and cancer. The most common cause of death in this cohort was cancer, and fatal myocardial infarction was the second.

Patients with diabetes and/or insulin resistance seem to have multiple benefits from weight loss surgery. Data from the SOS study showed that 72% of patients who had type 2 diabetes at baseline went into remission after 2 years, although about half of these patients had relapsed after 10 years. More importantly, the reduction in cardiovascular death after bariatric surgery was intensified in patients who had higher fasting serum insulin levels. The incidence of myocardial infarction also decreased after surgery in patients with diabetes. In subjects without diabetes, the risk of development of type 2 diabetes diminished by 96%, 84%, and 78% after 2, 10, and 15 years, respectively. The reduction in diabetes risk was more pronounced in people with impaired fasting glucose at baseline than people with normal fasting glucose. These numbers are striking considering the risk reduction reported in several intensive lifestyle intervention studies has been on the order of 40% to 60% over 2 to 6 years.[5,6] Serum insulin was a main predictor for the treatment effect after surgery with regard to mortality, cardiovascular events, and incidence of diabetes, whereas body mass index (BMI) did not predict the effect of surgery on any of these end points. The author has suggested current guidelines for bariatric surgery should be modified, giving more importance to metabolic parameters than the BMI value. Similarly, a recent study of the UK General Practice Research Database reported that factors such as type 2 diabetes status and age may be better predictors of 10-year mortality and eligibility for bariatric surgery in obese patients.[7] They concluded that type 2 diabetes mellitus is the most important mortality predictor and suggested prioritizing it over BMI or other comorbidities.

L. Khaodhiar, MD

References

1. Harrington M, Gibson S, Cottrell RC. A review and meta-analysis of the effect of weight loss on all-cause mortality risk. *Nutr Res Rev.* 2009;22:93-108.
2. Look AHEAD Research Group, Wing RR, Bolin P, Brancati FL, et al. Cardiovascular effects of intensive lifestyle intervention in type 2 diabetes. *N Engl J Med.* 2013;369:145-154.

3. Macdonald KG Jr, Long SD, Swanson MS, et al. The gastric bypass operation reduces the progression and mortality of non-insulin-dependent diabetes mellitus. *J Gastrointest Surg.* 1997;1:213-220.
4. Adams TD, Gress RE, Smith SC, et al. Long-term mortality after gastric bypass surgery. *N Engl J Med.* 2007;357:753-761.
5. Knowler WC, Barrett-Connor E, Fowler SE, et al. Diabetes Prevention Program Research Group. Reduction in the incidence of type 2 diabetes with lifestyle intervention or metformin. *N Engl J Med.* 2002;346:393-403.
6. Yamaoka K, Tango T. Efficacy of lifestyle education to prevent type 2 diabetes: a meta-analysis of randomized controlled trials. *Diabetes Care.* 2005;28:2780-2786.
7. Padwal RS, Klarenbach SW, Wang X, et al. A simple prediction rule for all-cause mortality in a cohort eligible for bariatric surgery. *JAMA Surg.* 2013;148:1109-1115.

58 Thyroid

Embryonic exposure to excess thyroid hormone causes thyrotrope cell death

Tonyushkina KN, Shen M-C, Ortiz-Toro T, et al (Baystate Med Ctr, Springfield, MA; Univ of Massachusetts, Amherst)

J Clin Invest 124:321-327, 2014

Central congenital hypothyroidism (CCH) is more prevalent in children born to women with hyperthyroidism during pregnancy, suggesting a role for thyroid hormone (TH) in the development of central thyroid regulation. Using the zebrafish embryo as a model for thyroid axis development, we have characterized the ontogeny of negative feedback regulation of thyrotrope function and examined the effect of excess TH on thyrotrope development. We found that thyroid-stimulating hormone β subunit (*tshb*) and type 2 deiodinase (*dio2*) are coexpressed in zebrafish thyrotropes by 48 hours after fertilization and that TH-driven negative feedback regulation of *tshb* transcription appears in the thyroid axis by 96 hours after fertilization. Negative feedback regulation correlated with increased systemic TH levels from the developing thyroid follicles. We used a transgenic zebrafish that expresses GFP under the control of the *tshb* promoter to follow thyrotrope fates in vivo. Time-lapse imaging revealed that early exposure to elevated TH leads to thyrotrope cell death. Thyrotrope numbers slowly recovered following the removal of excess TH. These data demonstrate that transient TH exposure profoundly impacts the thyrotrope population during a critical period of pituitary development and may have long-term implications for the functional reserve of thyroid-stimulating hormone (TSH) production and the TSH set point later in life (Figs 2-4).

▶ Thyroid hormone (TH) is essential for normal development of the brain, liver, heart, intestine, blood, and bone, both before and after birth. In the present study, the authors report the impact of excess TH on early thyrotrope development and define the onset of negative regulation of TSH transcription by TH in thyrotropes. To image thyrotropes in live embryos, the authors generated a zebrafish transgenic line in which the GFP was inserted into the genome under *tshb* promoter regulation. Unexpectedly, the authors found that elevated TH levels trigger thyrotrope cell death before, but not after, the onset of negative feedback regulation of *tshb* expression. As shown in Fig 2, embryonic exposure to elevated T4 reduces the number of cells expressing *tshb* and *dio2*. Figs 3 and 4 show that early embryonic exposure to high T4 levels leads to thyrotrope cell

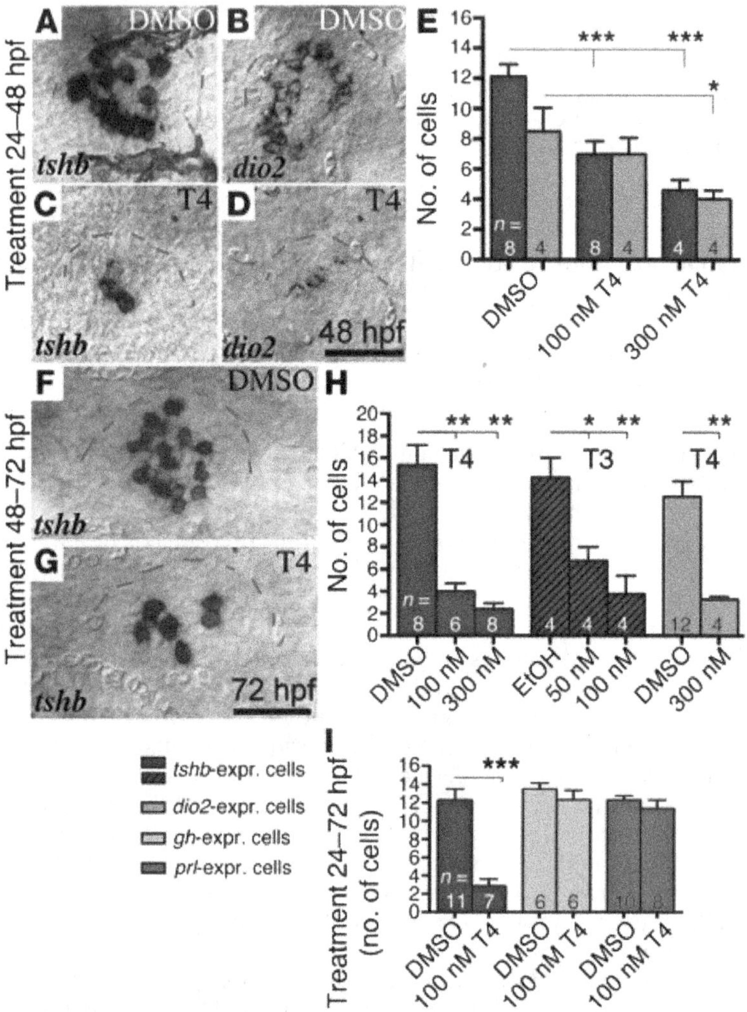

FIGURE 2.—Embryonic exposure to elevated T4 reduces the number of cells expressing *tshb* and *dio2*. (**A–D**) *tshb*- and *dio2*-expressing thyrotropes by 48 hpf following exposure to 300 nM T4 or DMSO (carrier) starting at 24 hpf, as visualized by ISH. (**E**) Graph showing decreases in *tshb*- (blue) and *dio2*-labeled (green) cells. (**F** and **G**) *tshb*-expressing thyrotropes by 72 hpf following a 24-hour exposure to 300 nM T4 or DMSO. (**H**) Graph showing decreases in *tshb*- (blue) and *dio2*-labeled (green) cells after a 24-hour exposure to T4 and T3. (**I**) Graph showing a decrease in *tshb*-labeled (blue) cells and no changes in *gh*- and *prl*-labeled cells after a 48-hour exposure to 100 nM T4 or DMSO (carrier) started 24 hpf. $^{*}P < 0.05$; $^{**}P < 0.01$; $^{***}P < 0.001$. (**A–D**, **F**, and **G**) Ventral views of the left anterior head; red dashed lines outline the left half of the pituitary placode. Scale bars: 25 μm. For Interpretation of the references to color in this figure legend, the reader is referred to web version of this article. (Reprinted from Tonyushkina KN, Shen M-C, Ortiz-Toro T, et al. Embryonic exposure to excess thyroid hormone causes thyrotrope cell death. *J Clin Invest.* 2014;124:321-327, © 2014, American Society of Clinical Investigation.)

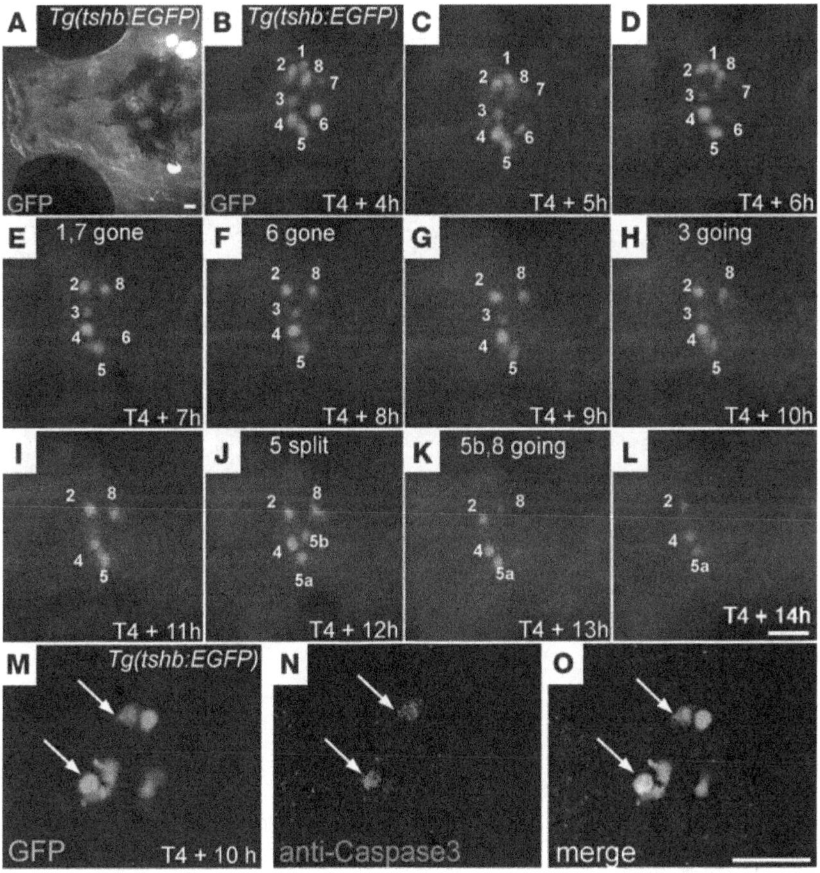

FIGURE 3.—Early embryonic exposure to high T4 levels leads to thyrotrope cell death. (**A**) Ventral view of the zebrafish head in a 6-dpf *Tg(tshb:EGFP)* embryo showing GFP-labeled thyrotropes in the pituitary. (B–L) Single frames from a time-lapse movie (see Supplemental Video 1) of GFP-expressing thyrotropes (numbered) in a *Tg(tshb:EGFP)* embryo 4–14 hours after the application of 300 nM T4 48 hpf. (**B**) Eight GFP-expressing thyrotropes were present 4 hours after application of T4. (**D** and **E**) GFP-expressing thyrotropes began to disappear 6–7 hours after T4 application. (**L**) Only 3 cells remained 14 hours after application of T4. (**M–O**) Example of anti–activated caspase 3 labeling of 2 GFP-expressing thyrotropes (arrows) in a *Tg(tshb:EGFP)* embryo 10 hours after the application of 300 nM T4. Single focal plane images show GFP (**M**), caspase 3 (**N**), and merged channels (**O**). All panels show ventral views of the left anterior forebrain between the eyes. Scale bars: 25 µm. (Reprinted from Tonyushkina KN, Shen M-C, Ortiz-Toro T, et al. Embryonic exposure to excess thyroid hormone causes thyrotrope cell death. *J Clin Invest*. 2014;124:321-327, © 2014, American Society of Clinical Investigation.)

death. This study identifies an important developmental window of TH action and uncovers thyrotrope cell death as a potential mechanism underlying central congenital hypothyroidism and altered set points in mammalian neonates exposed to high levels of maternal TH during embryogenesis, as occurs in poorly controlled Graves' disease in humans.

M. Schott, MD, PhD

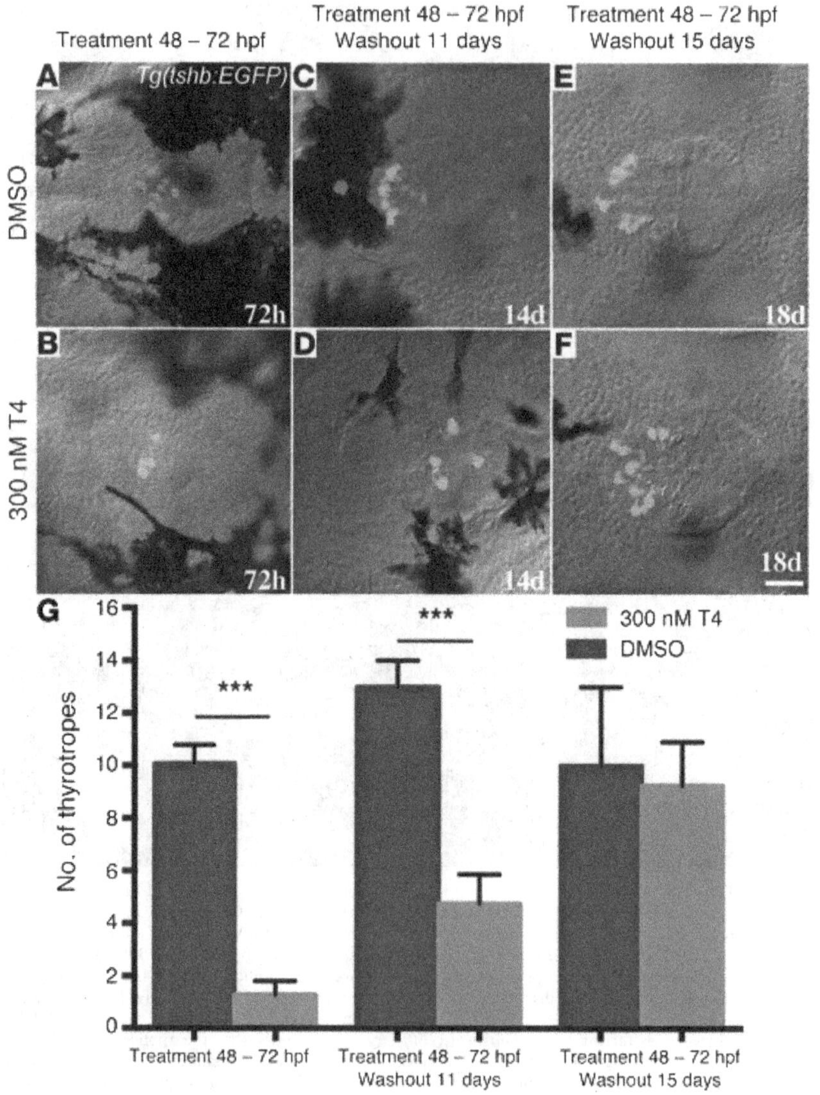

FIGURE 4.—Lasting effects of T4 exposure on thyrotrope numbers. (**A**) Approximately 10 thyrotropes were present in the pituitary by 72 hpf in DMSO-treated control embryos, as visualized by GFP fluorescence in the *Tg(tshb:EGFP)* line. (**B**) Example of decreased thyrotrope numbers by 72 hpf immediately following a 24-hour exposure to 300 nM T4. (**C**) Approximately 13 thyrotropes were present by 14 dpf in DMSO-treated control embryos. (**D**) Example of a 14-dpf larva with 4 thyrotropes that was treated with 300 nM T4 from 48 to 72 hpf, followed by an 11-day washout period. (E) Approximately 10 thyrotropes were present in the pituitary by 18 dpf in DMSO-treated control embryos. (F) Example of a larva with normal thyrotrope numbers that was treated with 300 nM T4 from 48 to 72 hpf, followed by a 15-day washout period. (G) Graph showing thyrotrope numbers, with a minimum of 20 embryos scored for each treatment. $^{***}P < 0.001$. (**A–F**) Ventral views of pituitary in the left anterior forebrain. Scale bar: 25 μm. (Reprinted from Tonyushkina KN, Shen M-C, Ortiz-Toro T, et al. Embryonic exposure to excess thyroid hormone causes thyrotrope cell death. *J Clin Invest.* 2014;124:321-327, © 2014, American Society of Clinical Investigation.)

Does *BRAF* V600E Mutation Predict Aggressive Features in Papillary Thyroid Cancer? Results From Four Endocrine Surgery Centers

Li C, Aragon Han P, Lee KC, et al (The Johns Hopkins Univ School of Medicine, Baltimore, MD; et al)

J Clin Endocrinol Metab 98:3702-3712, 2013

Background.—Existing evidence is controversial regarding the association between *BRAF* mutation status and aggressive features of papillary thyroid cancer (PTC). Specifically, no study has incorporated multiple surgical practices performing routine central lymph node dissection (CLND) and thus has patients who are truly evaluable for the presence or absence of central lymph node metastases (CLNMs).

Methods.—Consecutive patients who underwent total thyroidectomy and routine CLND at 4 tertiary endocrine surgery centers were retrospectively reviewed. Descriptive and bivariable analyses examined demographic, patient, and tumor-related factors. Multivariable analyses examined the odds of CLNM associated with positive *BRAF* status.

Results.—In patients with classical variant PTC, bivariate analysis found no significant associations between *BRAF* mutation and aggressive clinicopathologic features; multivariate analysis demonstrated that *BRAF* status was not an independent predictor of CLNM. When all patients with PTC were analyzed, including those with aggressive or follicular subtypes, bivariate analysis showed *BRAF* mutation to be associated with LNM, advanced American Joint Committee on Cancer (AJCC) stage, and histologic subtype. Multivariable analyses showed *BRAF*, age, size, and extrathyroidal extension to be associated with CLNM.

Conclusion.—Although *BRAF* mutation was found to be an independent predictor of central LNM in the overall cohort of patients with PTC, this relationship lost significance when only classical variant PTC was included in the analysis. The usefulness of *BRAF* in predicting the presence of LNM remains questionable. Prospective studies are needed before *BRAF* mutation can be considered a reliable factor to guide the treatment of patients with PTC, specifically whether to perform prophylactic CLND (Table 14).

▶ A high proportion of papillary thyroid carcinomas (PTC) are characterized by somatic aberrations in the *BRAF* kinase gene. The most frequent mutation is caused by an amino acid change (T1799A/p.V600E) and associated with gain of function. This study aims to address the important controversy regarding the prognostic value of *BRAF* mutation status, with particular emphasis on lymph node metastases, by incorporating patients from 4 tertiary endocrine surgery centers whose surgeons perform routine central lymph node dissection for all patients with PTC. The authors investigated 315 patients with classical variant PTC (CVPTC). In the subgroup of patients with CVPTC only, the bivariate analysis found no significant associations between *BRAF* mutation and aggressive clinicopathologic features, including the presence of lymph node metastases (LNM). Multivariable analysis in our CVPTC subgroup found that only

TABLE 14.—Multivariate Analysis of Predictors Available Preoperatively of Central LNM in All Patients With PTC

Preoperative Features	Odds Ratio	95% Confidence Interval	*P*
BRAF mutation	2.20	1.34–3.61	.002[a]
Gender (female)	1.47	0.87–2.48	.150
Age (≥45 y)	0.43	0.28–0.67	<.001[b]
Tumor size (>2 cm)	1.82	1.16–2.85	.010[a]

[a]Denotes significant positive association.
[b]Denotes significant negative association.
Reprinted from Li C, Aragon Han P, Lee KC, et al. Does BRAF V600E Mutation Predict Aggressive Features in Papillary Thyroid Cancer? Results From Four Endocrine Surgery Centers. J Clin Endocrinol Metab. 2013;98:3702-3712.

increased tumor size and extrathyroidal extension (ETE) were independent predictors of central LNM (Table 14). When similar analyses were applied to patients with follicular variant PTC, significant bivariate associations between *BRAF* mutation and older age as well as advanced American Joint Committee on Cancer stage were seen. *BRAF* mutation and ETE were also found to be independent predictors of central LNM in this subgroup.

As stated by the authors, the results of this study emphasize that the existing evidence behind the use of *BRAF* V600E mutation as a prognostic indicator, specifically to guide whether to perform a central lymph node dissection in patients with PTC, is insufficient. Although *BRAF* mutation was found to be an independent predictor of central LNM in the overall cohort of patients with PTC, this relationship lost significance when follicular and aggressive variants were excluded from the analysis, and only patients with CVPTC, the most common subtype, were examined. Based on these results, the usefulness of *BRAF* mutation in the management algorithm of patients of PTC remains questionable. Prospective, multi-institutional studies should be carried out before *BRAF* mutation can be considered a reliable factor to guide the treatment of patients with PTC.

M. Schott, MD, PhD

Effect of inadequate iodine status in UK pregnant women on cognitive outcomes in their children: results from the Avon Longitudinal Study of Parents and Children (ALSPAC)

Bath SC, Steer CD, Golding J, et al (Univ of Surrey, Guildford, UK; Univ of Bristol, UK)
Lancet 382:331-337, 2013

Background.—As a component of thyroid hormones, iodine is essential for fetal brain development. Although the UK has long been considered iodine replete, increasing evidence suggests that it might now be mildly iodine deficient. We assessed whether mild iodine deficiency during early pregnancy was associated with an adverse effect on child cognitive development.

Methods.—We analysed mother-child pairs from the Avon Longitudinal Study of Parents and Children (ALSPAC) cohort by measuring urinary iodine concentration (and creatinine to correct for urine volume) in stored samples from 1040 first-trimester pregnant women. We selected women on the basis of a singleton pregnancy and availability of both a urine sample from the first trimester (defined as ≤13 weeks' gestation; median 10 weeks [IQR 9–12]) and a measure of intelligence quotient (IQ) in the offspring at age 8 years. Women's results for iodine-to-creatinine ratio were dichotomised to less than 150 μg/g or 150 μg/g or more on the basis of WHO criteria for iodine deficiency or sufficiency in pregnancy. We assessed the association between maternal iodine status and child IQ at age 8 years and reading ability at age 9 years. We included 21 socioeconomic, parental, and child factors as confounders.

Findings.—The group was classified as having mild-to-moderate iodine deficiency on the basis of a median urinary iodine concentration of 91·1 μg/L (IQR 53·8–143; iodine-to-creatinine ratio 110 μg/g, IQR 74–170). After adjustment for confounders, children of women with an iodine-to-creatinine ratio of less than 150 μg/g were more likely to have scores in the lowest quartile for verbal IQ (odds ratio 1·58, 95% CI 1·09–2·30; $P = 0{\cdot}02$), reading accuracy (1·69, 1·15–2·49; $P = 0{\cdot}007$), and reading comprehension (1·54, 1·06–2·23; $P = 0{\cdot}02$) than were those of mothers with ratios of 150 μg/g or more. When the less than 150 μg/g group was subdivided, scores worsened ongoing from 150 μg/g or more, to 50–150 μg/g, to less than 50 μg/g.

Interpretation.—Our results show the importance of adequate iodine status during early gestation and emphasise the risk that iodine deficiency can pose to the developing infant, even in a country classified as only mildly iodine deficient. Iodine deficiency in pregnant women in the UK should be treated as an important public health issue that needs attention (Fig 1).

▶ The World Health Organization considers iodine deficiency to be the single most important preventable cause of brain damage worldwide. Although iodine deficiency is often thought to be a problem of developing countries, industrialized countries are not immune. Indeed, concern is emerging that iodine deficiency might be widespread in industrialized countries. The aim of this study was to investigate whether women with low iodine status in early pregnancy would have children with poorer cognitive outcomes than would those with higher status. A previous Avon Longitudinal Study of Parents and Children (ALSPAC) found a positive association between maternal seafood consumption and child intelligence quotient (IQ), which the authors suggest could at least partly have been driven by the high iodine content of seafood.[1]

As shown in Fig 1 there was a significant difference in the verbal IQ, the total IQ, and reading comprehension in children of iodine-deficient mothers compared with children of mothers with normal iodine intake.

As discussed by the authors, this study has several limitations. First, because it is observational, residual confounding by factors that the authors either have

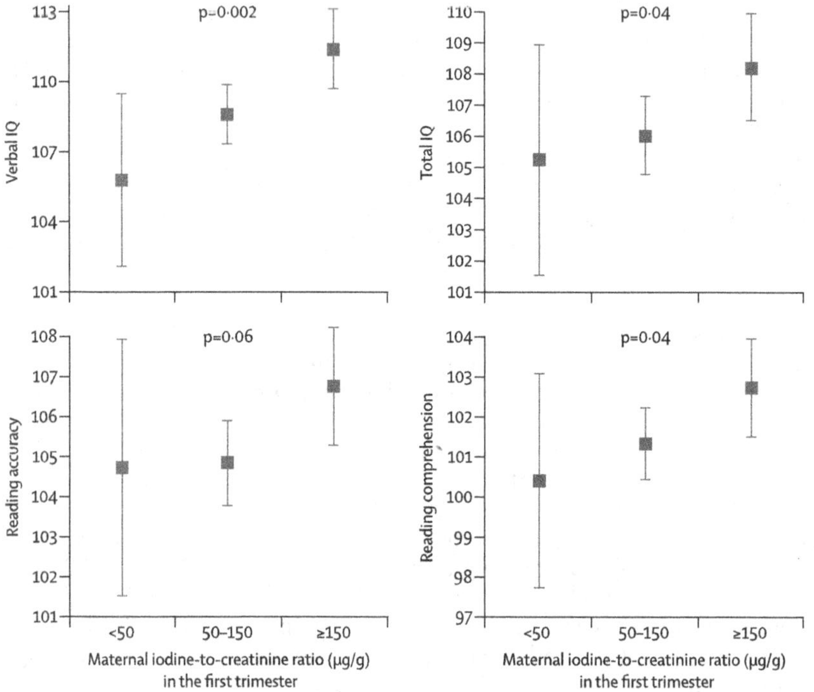

FIGURE 1.—Means (95% CIs) for child cognitive outcomes according to maternal iodine status in the first trimester Values are adjusted for the effect of confounders (model three). Child verbal and total IQ were assessed at age 8 years and reading accuracy and comprehension at age 9 years. IQ = intelligence quotient. (Reprinted from Bath SC, Steer CD, Golding J, et al. Effect of inadequate iodine status in UK pregnant women on cognitive outcomes in their children: results from the Avon Longitudinal Study of Parents and Children (ALSPAC). *Lancet.* 2013;382:331-337, Copyright 2013, with permission from Elsevier.)

not measured or not considered is a possibility; however, adjustment for up to 21 variables mostly made little difference to overall effect sizes. The authors did not control for potential iodine deficiency in the child, but this deficiency is likely to be less of an issue than in pregnancy because the iodine requirement in childhood is substantially lower and more likely to be met by children's high consumption of milk. Second, use of one spot-urine sample has limitations for measurement of iodine status in an individual. However, these limitations were minimized by correcting for urinary volume with use of iodine-to-creatinine ratio and by broad grouping of women into 2 categories of iodine status, effectively giving 2 populations and reducing the effect of any misclassification of status. Third, measurement of iodine status at one time point in pregnancy might not represent dietary iodine intake during the entire pregnancy and does not give specific information about maternal thyroid function, of which the authors have no measure.

Because of the observational nature of this study, these findings need to be replicated by others. Evidence from a randomized placebo-controlled trial of the effect of iodine supplementation in pregnancy on child cognition is needed from regions of mild-to-moderate iodine deficiency because existing evidence from trials in such regions is weak.

M. Schott, MD

Reference

1. Hibbeln JR, Davis JM, Steer C, et al. Maternal seafood consumption in pregnancy and neurodevelopmental outcomes in childhood (ALSPAC study): an observational cohort study. *Lancet*. 2007;369:578-585.

Five-Year Follow-Up for Women With Subclinical Hypothyroidism in Pregnancy

Shields BM, Knight BA, Hill AV, et al (Univ of Exeter, UK)

J Clin Endocrinol Metab 98:E1941-E1945, 2013

Context.—Increasing numbers of women are being treated with L-thyroxine in pregnancy for mild thyroid dysfunction because of its association with impaired neuropsychological development in their offspring and other adverse obstetric outcomes. However, there are limited data to indicate whether treatment should be continued outside of pregnancy.

Objectives.—We aimed to determine whether subclinical hypothyroidism and maternal hypothyroxinemia resolve postdelivery.

Design, Setting, and Participants.—A total of 523 pregnant healthy women with no known thyroid disorders were recruited during routine antenatal care and provided blood samples at 28 weeks of pregnancy and at a mean of 4.9 years postpregnancy.

Main Outcome Measures.—TSH, free T_4, free T_3, and thyroid peroxidase antibody levels were measured in serum taken in pregnancy and at follow-up.

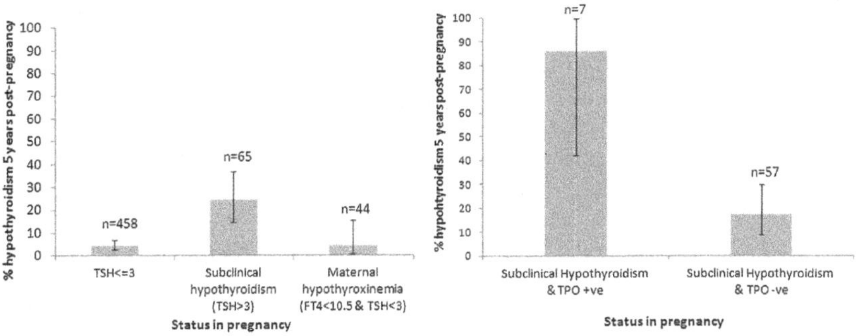

FIGURE 1.—Prevalence of hypothyroidism 5 years postpregnancy. Bar charts show the prevalence of hypothyroidism 5 years postpregnancy in (A) women with TSH ≤3 mIU/L, subclinical hypothyroidism (TSH >3 mIU/L), or maternal hypothyroxinemia in pregnancy (FT4 <10.5 pmol/L and TSH ≤3 mIU/L) ($P < .0001$ (by χ^2 test) for comparison between those with TSH ≤3 mIU/L and TSH >3 mIU/L) and (B) women with subclinical hypothyroidism in pregnancy with (+ve) and without (-ve) TPO-Abs ($P < .001$). Error bars represent 95% confidence intervals. One TPO-Ab result for a patient with subclinical hypothyroidism was unavailable. (Reprinted from Shields BM, Knight BA, Hill AV, et al. Five-Year follow-Up for women with subclinical hypothyroidism in pregnancy. *J Clin Endocrinol Metab*. 2013;98:E1941-E1945, Copyright 2013, with permission from the Author[s] and The Endocrine Society.)

Results.—Subclinical hypothyroidism in pregnancy (TSH >3 mIU/L) was present in 65 of 523 (12.4%) women. Of these, 49 (75.4%) women had normal thyroid function postpregnancy; 16 of 65 (24.6%) had persistent high TSH (TSH >4.5 mIU/L postpregnancy) with 3 women receiving L-thyroxine treatment. A total of 44 of 523 (8.4%) women had isolated maternal hypothyroxinemia in pregnancy (free T_4 <10th centile and TSH ≤3 mIU/L). Only 2 of 44 (4.5%) had TSH >4.5 mIU/L outside pregnancy. Of the women with subclinical hypothyroidism in pregnancy with antibody measurements available, those with thyroid peroxidase antibodies in pregnancy were more likely to have persistently elevated TSH or be receiving L-thyroxine replacement after pregnancy (6 of 7 [86%] vs 10 of 57 [18%], $P < .001$).

Conclusions.—The majority of cases of subclinical hypothyroidism in pregnancy are transient, so treatment with L-thyroxine in these patients should be reviewed because it may not be warranted after pregnancy (Fig 1).

▶ Increasing numbers of clinicians and hospitals are testing thyroid function in pregnancy to detect and treat mild thyroid dysfunction. The use of trimester-specific reference ranges in routine clinical practice results in milder forms of thyroid dysfunction (subclinical hypothyroidism and isolated maternal hypothyroxinemia) being diagnosed in as many as 15% of pregnant women.[1,2] The aim of the study by Shields and coworkers was to investigate the natural history of mild thyroid hormone deficiency during pregnancy and after delivery. The authors performed the first systematic follow-up study of subclinical hypothyroidism in pregnancy. They found that the majority (75%) of women identified as having subclinical hypothyroidism in pregnancy had normal thyroid-stimulating hormone (TSH) levels after pregnancy, and only 2 of 44 (4.4%) women with maternal hypothyroxinemia had high TSH levels outside pregnancy (Fig 1). The biggest risk factor for raised TSH levels after pregnancy was the presence of thyroid peroxidase antibodies. A TSH level > 5 mIU/L in pregnancy was also a risk factor, but a history of cesarean delivery was not (Table 2 in the original article). This study has a number of limitations. First, the authors only measured thyroid function at a single time point during and after pregnancy. However, this is not likely to have a significant impact on the conclusions of this study because it has been demonstrated that variations in an individual's thyroid function over a short duration tends to be narrow both in and outside pregnancy. Irrespective of the limitations, these results highlight the need for reassessment of the thyroid status of pregnant women after pregnancy.

M. Schott, MD, PhD

References

1. Blatt AJ, Nakamoto JM, Kaufman HW. National status of testing for hypothyroidism during pregnancy and postpartum. *J Clin Endocrinol Metab*. 2012;97:777-784.
2. Altomare M, La Vignera S, Asero P, et al. High prevalence of thyroid dysfunction in pregnant women. *J Endocrinol Invest*. 2013;36:407-411.

Analysis of 754 Cases of Antithyroid Drug-Induced Agranulocytosis Over 30 Years in Japan

Nakamura H, Miyauchi A, Miyawaki N, et al (Kuma Hosp, Chuo-ku, Japan; Nihonbashi-Muromachi 2-Chome, Chuo-ku, Tokyo, Japan)
J Clin Endocrinol Metab 98:4776-4783, 2013

Background.—Agranulocytosis is a rare but serious complication of antithyroid drug (ATD) therapy. Characteristics of agranulocytosis have been reported in only a small number of patients.

Method.—We studied 754 cases of ATD-induced agranulocytosis reported over 30 years. The age distribution and sex ratio were compared with those in 12 503 untreated Graves' patients at Kuma Hospital. The annual number of new Graves' patients in Japan was estimated from the Japan Medical Data Center Data Mart-Pharmacovigilance health insurance receipt database.

Results.—Agranulocytosis developed within 90 days after starting ATD therapy in most patients (84.5%). The methimazole dose given at onset was 25.2 ± 12.8 mg/d (mean ± SD). The mean age was 43.4 ± 15.2 years, and the male to female ratio was 1:6.3. When compared with patients at Kuma Hospital, patients with agranulocytosis were older ($P < .001$) and more females ($P < .0001$). Of 211 patients with more than 1 granulocyte measurement before onset, 131 (62%) showed normal counts (>1000/μL) within 2 weeks before onset, demonstrating real sudden onset of agranulocytosis. In contrast, some of the 20 patients with more than 4 measurements showed gradual decreases in granulocyte counts. Analysis of physician reports for 30 fatal cases revealed that some deaths might have been prevented. The number of new Graves' patients treated with ATD was estimated at about 35 000 per year, and the incidence rate of agranulocytosis was 0.1% to 0.15% in Japan.

Conclusion.—This is the largest study of agranulocytosis. Agranulocytosis tends to occur abruptly within 3 months after initiation of ATD therapy, although it develops gradually in some patients. Providing every patient with sufficient information on agranulocytosis is critical.

▶ Antithyroid drug (ATD) therapy is associated with several adverse reactions. Among them, agranulocytosis is the most serious life-threatening event. It can occur abruptly, and prediction and prevention are very difficult. Agranulocytosis is a rare event, occurring in 0.1% to 0.5% of Graves' patients. The authors of this study studied 754 reports of ATD-induced agranulocytosis. In accordance with the frequency of hyperthyroidism, there is a clear peak of ATD-induced agranulocytosis in the third up to the fifth decade (Fig 1 in the original article). The mean onset of agranulocytosis is between the 20th and about the 40th day after initiation of ATD therapy (Fig 2 in the original article). Importantly, only a few patients died from agranulocytosis during the follow-up since 1986 (Fig 3 in the original article). As stated by the authors, limitations of this study are that data are completely dependent on physician reports, and necessary data are missing in a considerable number of reports. The distinction between agranulocytosis and pancytopenia was not necessarily rigorous, and, in some cases, it was unclear whether symptoms or even death were caused by agranulocytosis. Despite these limitations, the authors believe that this study, the largest to date in patients with agranulocytosis, provides important and thought-provoking information.

M. Schott, MD, PhD

Article Index

Chapter 9: Systemic Sclerosis

Chapter 10: Vasculitis

Chapter 11: Bacterial Infections

Chapter 12: Human Immunodeficiency Virus

Chapter 13: Vaccines

Chapter 18: Gynecologic Cancers

Chapter 19: Breast Cancer

Chapter 20: Prostate Cancer

Chapter 26: Acute Kidney Injury

Chapter 27: Clinical Nephrology

Chapter 28: Chronic Kidney Disease

Chapter 29: Dialysis and Transplantation

Chapter 30: Diabetes

Chapter 31: Asthma, Allergy, and Cystic Fibrosis

Chapter 36: Pleural, Interstitial Ling, and Pulmonary Vascular Disease

Chapter 37: Sleep Disorders

Chapter 38: Critical Care Medicine

Chapter 39: Chronic Coronary Artery Disease

Chapter 40: Risk Factors

Chapter 41: Arrhythmias

Chapter 42: Acute Coronary Syndromes

Chapter 43: Coronary Intervention Procedures

Chapter 44: Cardiomyopathy

Chapter 45: Valvular Heart Disease

Chapter 46: Esophagus

Chapter 47: Stomach

Chapter 48: Small Bowel

Chapter 49: Colon

Chapter 50: Liver

Chapter 51: Calcium and Bone Metabolism

Chapter 52: Adrenal Cortex

Chapter 53: Reproductive Endocrinology

Chapter 54: Pediatric Endocrinology

Chapter 55: Neuroendocrinology

Chapter 56: Lipoproteins and Atherosclerosis

Chapter 57: Obesity

Chapter 58: Thyroid

Author Index

E

F

G

H

I

J

K

L

X

Y

Z